The Essential Guide
to Nonprescription Drugs

The Essential Guide to Nonprescription Drugs

DAVID R. ZIMMERMAN

1817

HARPER & ROW, PUBLISHERS, New York

Cambridge, Philadelphia, San Francisco, London

Mexico City, São Paulo, Sydney

FIRST EDITION

Designer: C. Linda Dingler

Library of Congress Cataloging in Publication Data

Zimmerman, David R.
  The essential guide to nonprescription drugs.

  Includes index.
  1. Drugs, Nonprescription. I. Title.
RM671.A1Z55 1983   615′.1   82–48139
ISBN 0–06–014915–9
ISBN 0–06–091023–2 (pbk.)

           83 84 85 86 10 9 8 7 6 5 4 3 2 1
           83 84 85 86 10 9 8 7 6 5 4 3 2 1

For my Tobias

Contents

Contents   xi

Acknowledgments

This guide derives from a federally sponsored, decade-long review of nonprescription drugs. My principal source are the many reports—unadopted, adopted, tentative final, final, and supplements—that in final form have been or will be published in the *Federal Register*, the official record of government actions.

I am especially indebted to some two hundred medical and scientific advisers who participated in the review process (Panel members are listed on pages xxv to xxxi); the administrators who organized meetings; analysts who surveyed results; editors and writers who prepared the various reports; and any number of federal employees who skillfully shaped and guided the review.

Particularly I want to thank Gerald M. Rachanow, Deputy Director of the Division of OTC Drug Evaluation, and his assistant, Mrs. Mary White; Edward R. Nida (FDA Public Affairs); Wayne L. Pines, Associate Commissioner for Public Affairs; Marc Stern, Chief of the News Branch of the National Institutes of Health (NIH) in Bethesda; and Irwin Rosenberg, M.D., who early on consented to read and comment on the unit "Vitamins and Minerals."

In condensing the mountains of material generated by the nonprescription drug review, it was necessary to work with material in varying stages of development over a period of several years. To ensure that this whole guide reflects current status of medical knowledge—and also as a check of my "translation"—the completed text of this guide was read and checked for factual accuracy by information specialists, physicians, and scientists at the National Institutes of Health in Bethesda, Maryland, an agency of the United States Public Health Service. It is important to note, however, that these experts were not asked to read—and did not read—the product ratings that conclude each unit. These ratings represent my own opinion of individual brand-name products based on the current findings of the independent OTC Review Panels and the FDA about active ingredients and combinations of active ingredients which are in these products.

Finally, for their help and support, I want to thank my friend Ted Klein; my agent, Connie Clausen, and her associate, Nancy Trichter; and my colleague and friend, Fay Webern. This venture has enjoyed continuing support from John Heuston, for which I am grateful. The monumental task of typing, retyping and proofing five thousand pages of manuscript and tables has been graciously managed and skillfully executed by Alice Warwick and her associates at Heuston Typing.

Words cannot express my thanks to my family—Veva, J.B., Toby— for their patience with me, and with this endeavor. Years have gone by! Finally, special thanks are due to Dr. Emily Sisley, whose assistance, advice and help has contributed immeasurably to this final work.

DAVID R. ZIMMERMAN
January 1983

A NOTE FROM THE EDITOR

Putting together a complex reference is never simple. For all their hard work, help and support thanks are due to Mary Chadwick and Pat Slesarchik for their superb handling of production; to production editors Kathleen Hyde and Coral Tysliava, who more than ably put all the pieces together; to Bill Reynolds, Bernie Borok, and Martha Schwartz, superior copyeditors and proofreaders; to Georgia Wiedmann, who expertly typed the entire manuscript on a word processor; to Jean Palmer, who efficiently inserted all changes and corrected the discs; to assistant editor Helen Moore; to Lois Merman; to indexer Sydney Cohen; to designer C. Linda Dingler; to Dave Davis, Manager of the Graphic Systems and Programming at ComCom; and to Jim Fox for his advice, good humor, and patience through some very trying times.

Carol Cohen, Editor
Harper & Row
January 1983

Unit Sources

Acne Medications: PR, *FR* 12430–77, 1982.
Antacids: PR, *FR* 8714–24, 1973; TFM, *FR* 31260–9, 1973; FM, *FR* 19862–83, 1974; WU, *FR* 39427–8, 1978; Addenda, *FR* 24328–44, 1975; *FR* 54731–3, 1979; 21 *CFR* 331.
Antacids for Controlling Phosphate Levels (Box): PR, *FR* 81154–8, 1980.
Antibiotics for Skin Infections: PR, *FR* 17642–81, 1977; TFM, *FR* 29986–30000, 1982.
Anti-Gas Agents: *See* Antacids; 21 *CFR* 332.
Antimicrobial Bar Soaps: PR, *FR* 33102–41, 1974; TFM, *FR* 1210–49, 1978.
Antiperspirants: PR, *FR* 46694–732, 1978.
Antiseptics: PR, *FR* 33102–41, 1974; TFM, *FR* 1210–49, 1978; PR, *FR* 436–42, 1982; PR, *FR* 22324–33, 1982.
Aphrodisiacs: UDR, June 1979.
Asthma Drugs: PR, *FR* 38312–424, 1976.
Bleaches for Skin Blemishes: PR, *FR* 51546–55, 1978.
Boil Ointments: PR, *FR* 28306–9, 1982.
Camphor: Special Warning: PR, FDA Preamble, Statement, etc., *FR* 63869–79, 1980.
Cold, Cough, and Allergy Drugs: PR, *FR* 38312–424, 1976; TFM, *FR* 30002–10, 1982.
Cold Sore Balms: UDR, August 1980; PR, *FR* 502–10, 1982.
Contraceptives: PR, *FR* 82014–49, 1980.
Corn and Callus Removers: PR, *FR* 522–30, 1982.
Cradle Cap Removers: UDR, November 1980.
Dandruff & Seborrheic Scale Shampoos: UDR, November 1980.
Daytime Sedatives: PR, *FR* 57292–329, 1975; FM, *FR* 36378–80, 1979; 21 *CFR* 310.519.
Deodorants for Ostomies and Incontinence: PR, *FR* 512–20, 1982.
Diaper Rash Medications: UDR, November 1980.
Diarrhea Remedies: PR, *FR* 12902–44, 1975.
Digestive Aids: PR, *FR* 454–87, 1982.
Douches and Other Vaginal Applications: UDR, November 1978.
Ear-Care Aids: PR, *FR* 63556–66, 1977; TFM, *FR* 30012–21, 1982.
Eye Drops and Ointments: PR, *FR* 30002–50, 1980.
Eyes: Artificial Tears: *Ibid.*
Eyewash: *Ibid.*
First Aid Preparations for Skin Wounds: PR, *FR* 33102–41, 1974; TFM, *FR* 1210–49, 1978; PR, *FR* 17642–81, 1977; TFM, *FR* 29986–30000, 1982.
Gum Treatments: PR, *FR* 63270–90, 1979; PR, *FR* 22712–59, 1982.
Hair Growth Stimulants and Baldness Preventives, PR, *FR* 73955–60, 1980.
Hangover and Overindulgence Remedies: UDR, May 1981.
Hemorrhoid Medication and Other Anorectal Applications: PR, *FR* 35576–677, 1980.
Hormone Skin Creams and Oils: PR, *FR* 430–9, 1982.
Ingrown-Toenail Relievers: PR, *FR* 69128–33, 1980.
Insect Bite and Sting Treatments: UDR, May 1980; PR, *FR* 424–7, 1982.
Itch and Pain Remedies Applied to the Skin: PR, *FR* 69768–866, 1979.
Jock Itch, Athlete's Foot, and Ringworm Cures: PR, *FR* 12480–566, 1982.
Kidney and Bladder Drugs: Preliminary Report: Status of Ingredients in the OTC Drug Review, FDA, November 13, 1980.
Laxatives: PR, *FR* 12902–44, 1975.
Lice Poisons: PR, *FR* 28312–21, 1982.
Liniments and Poultices for Aches and Pains: PR, *FR* 69768–866, 1979.
Menstrual Distress Preparations: UDR, July 1981.
Motion-Sickness Medicines: PR, *FR* 12902–44, 1975; TFM, *FR* 41064–73, 1979.
Mouthwash for Oral Hygiene: PR, *FR* 22760–930, 1982.

Nail-Biting and Thumb-Sucking Deterrents: PR, *FR* 69122–8, 1980.

Pain, Fever, and Anti-Inflammatory Drugs Taken Internally: PR, *FR* 35346–494, 1977.

Pancreatic Enzyme Supplements: PR, *FR* 75666–70, 1979.

Phenol: Special Warning: PR, *FR* 33102–41, 1974; TFM, *FR* 1210–49, 1978.

Poisoning Antidotes: PR, *FR* 12902–44, 1975; TFM, *FR* 39544–6, 1978; PR (Acute Toxic Ingestion), *FR* 444–51, 1982.

Poison-Ivy Preventives and Palliatives: PR, *FR* 444–51, 1982.

Premature Ejaculation Retardants: UDR, February 1980.

Psoriasis Lotions: UDR, November 1980.

Reducing Aids: PR, *FR* 8466–84, 1982.

Appetite Stimulants (Box): Status of Ingredients in the OTC Drug Review, FDA, November 13, 1980.

Salt Supplements and Substitutes: Preliminary Report: *Ibid.*

Sleep Aids: PR, *FR* 57292–329, 1975; TFM, *FR* 25544–602, 1978.

Smelling Salts: Preliminary Report: Status of Ingredients in the OTC Drug Review, FDA, November 13, 1980.

Smoking Deterrents: PR, *FR* 490–500, 1982.

Sore Throat and Mouth Medicines: PR, *FR* 22760–930, 1982.

Stimulants: PR, *FR* 57292–329, 1975; TFM, *FR* 25544–602, 1978.

Stomach Acidifiers: PR, *FR* 60316–20, 1979.

Styptic Pencils and Other Astringents: UDR, November 1980.

Sunscreens: PR, *FR* 38206–69, 1978.

Sweet Spirits of Nitre: Special Warning: PR, *FR* 11846–9, 1980; FM, *FR* 43400–1, 1980; 21 *CFR* 310.525.

Teething Easers: PR, *FR* 22712–59, 1982.

Toothache Relievers: PR, *FR* 22712–59, 1982.

Unguents and Powders for the Skin: PR, *FR* 34628–48, 1978.

Vitamins and Minerals: PR, *FR* 16126–201, 1979.

Wart Paints: PR, FR 65609–18, 1980.

Worm-Killers for Pinworms: PR, *FR* 59540–8, 1980.

"Yeast" Killers for Feminine Itching: UDR, November 1978; PR, *FR* 12480–566, 1982.

Introduction

More than 200,000 nonprescription drug products are offered for sale in the United States. Yet, large as this number is, the really striking fact is that, until the federally sponsored review of nonprescription drugs began—a review described below—information to evaluate these drugs was not available. Now, almost all of the active ingredients in these drugs have been assessed by panels organized by the FDA. Here in this complete and authoritative Guide to nonprescription drugs you can find the information about the active ingredients in over-the-counter drugs.

"Are they appropriate for the symptom or condition I am suffering?"

"Are they effective?"

"Are they safe?"

"Are they safe for my children?"

"How much should I take—and how often?"

"How long should I treat myself with a nonprescription product before consulting a doctor?"

A nonprescription drug, also called an over-the-counter (OTC) drug, is a drug product that you can buy without a prescription and use when *you* think it is useful or necessary. It differs from a prescription (Rx) drug, which is selected by a doctor and then used under his or her supervision.

Nonprescription drugs differ from prescription medicines in another important regard: a prescription drug may effectively relieve symptoms or it may cure the underlying disease. Most nonprescription drugs are *not* curative. Rather, they relieve symptoms—such as pain, inflammation, itching. They essentially provide *comfort* so that people can continue their daily routine while time and the body's natural healing powers provide the cure.

Surveys show that almost everyone uses nonprescription drugs. Retail sales are projected to reach $8 billion a year by 1984—up from the $4 billion to $5 billion range set at the start of the decade. In 1974, Dr. Alexander M. Schmidt, then the commissioner of the Food and Drug Administration (FDA), declared: "An underlying premise . . . of the sales of drugs over-the-counter, rather than on prescription, is that the consumer is capable of making an intelligent choice of a drug product if he possesses adequate information about the products offered for treatment of specific conditions or symptoms."

The problem was that in the past there was no source that the consumer could refer to for this information. In 1962 Congress mandated a review of over-the-counter drugs. Now the review is about halfway finished and most of the Panels convened by the FDA to evaluate the active ingredients in the over-the-counter drugs have published their reports. *The Essential Guide to Nonprescription Drugs* provides information from these reports—published and unpublished—and from follow-up FDA documents which can help the consumer make intelligent choices about over-the-counter drugs. The Guide describes many different symptoms and conditions as well as the groups of nonprescription drugs that are sold to relieve them. It offers help on differentiating self-treatable conditions from those that require a doctor's attention, and indicates which drugs are safe and effective—and which are not—for treating each condition. The guide translates review-process judgments (described below) into three categories: *approved, disapproved,* and *conditionally approved.*

Information about these drugs are summarized in charts that cover single active ingredients and combinations of active ingredients. This Guide includes information from the Panel reports such as warnings and information about side effects, time limits beyond which one should seek professional care if a condition still remains, and a series of product ratings based on information in these Panel reports—ratings prepared by the author, not the FDA or the Advisory Panels.

Most units in this Guide include a Claims section. Here recommended labeling claims drafted by the Advisory Panels are given. These approved and allowed statements contain the best objective estimate that is available concerning the benefit that can—or cannot—be expected from self-treatment with safe and effective drugs. Included also is a sampling of disapproved, conditionally approved and misleading claims for over-the-counter drugs.

THE REVIEW PROCESS: NONPRESCRIPTION DRUGS ON THE LINE

The review upon which this Guide is based has been in progress for more than a decade. It is mandated by Congress in amendments to the Federal Food, Drug, and Cosmetic Act passed in 1962 and conducted by the Food and Drug Administration (FDA)—an agency of the United States Public Health Service. Each medically active ingredient in every nonprescription drug legitimately marketed in the United States is being assessed. These evaluations were initially made by some 200 medical and scientific independent experts who served on 17 Advisory Review Panels convened by the FDA.

Massive amounts of data were collected for this project. The cost is estimated by the FDA at 12 million dollars for the first ten years (January 1972 through December 1981). This cost is being borne by taxpayers, who, as health-product consumers, are the review's beneficiaries.

Until recently there was limited control over the safety and effectiveness of nonprescription drugs. The FDA lacked legal authority to require that they be effective. It did have the authority to remove a product from the market if it could show that the product was unsafe. The goal for this review, set by Congress, is to require that nonprescription drug products be proved safe, effective and be correctly labeled as a condition of entering or remaining on the market.

Since the FDA already held responsibility for regulating prescription drugs and their labeling, it was decided that the agency should exercise similar control over nonprescription medications. In short, the FDA would use the Advisory Panels' recommendations as the basis for writing new regulations that will control both the medicinal contents and label information of all nonprescription drugs. When the review is complete, all nonprescription drug products that one buys over-the-counter in stores will be safe, effective, and correctly labeled on the basis of currently accepted medical knowledge. Unsafe or ineffective drugs will be banned and inaccurate labels will be forbidden by law.

The hundreds of thousands of nonprescription drug products contain *far fewer* active ingredients. For example, among roughly 50,000 pain relievers, there are only about a dozen active ingredients. Three of them—aspirin, acetaminophen, and phenacetin—accounted for the bulk of all sales. (So despite great advertising ballyhoo about "special" or "unique" formulas, most internal pain-relieving drugs contain one or more of only a very few ingredients. And they're there in more or less comparable amounts.) In fact, in *all* nonprescription products marketed in the United States, the experts had by late 1980 identified only 750 active ingredients. Some are used for two or more purposes. For example, camphor is sold to relieve itching and also to kill germs. By one recent rough count, these 750 active ingredients are sold for some 1400 specific medicinal uses.

At the start, in 1972, the FDA divided all nonprescription drug products into 17 classes. Rather than assessing the more than 200,000 products—an impossible task—the FDA decided that the drug products' active ingredients should be assessed. Then the FDA appointed 17 Panels of outside experts—that is, people not affiliated with the FDA or with drug companies—to make these assessments.

Great care was taken in selecting the panelists: most are distinguished academic medical specialists, including deans of medical or pharmacology schools, department heads, and other medical educators. Panels also included private practitioners—doctors and dentists who see many patients in their private offices. These professionals are familiar with commonplace complaints of patients that are rarely referred to hospital-based specialists. These are the kinds of medical/dental problems for which self-treatment with nonprescription drugs may be especially appropriate.

Each Panel further included a pharmacist (the man or woman who fills prescriptions at the drugstore and often advises health consumers on the choice and use of nonprescription drugs) and either a pharmacologist (an expert on drugs) or a toxicologist (a specialist in drugs' adverse effects). Every Panel had at least one expert on the design and interpretation of scientific studies.

Consumers and the drug industry were both represented on all the Panels by nonvoting members. The Consumer Federation of America nominated consumer representatives. The Proprietary Association (the trade organization of OTC drug manufacturers) and other manufacturers' groups nominated the industry representatives.

The Panels were assisted in their work by special consultants hired by the FDA and by FDA staff workers. These people provided information from the agency's files and from exhaustive searches into the medical, drug, and chemical literature available at federal research libraries. Staff work was done by FDA officials and employees.

Considerable information came from interested parties. For example, drug manufacturers and their Washington lawyers and lobbyists presented evidence to the Panels in support of various active ingredients—and, thus, the products that contain them. Doctors and consumer advocates also contributed information and points of view. The FDA states that everyone who asked to present data or suggestions to a Panel was able to do so.

Methods

The Panels started with several thousand nonprescription products submitted by manufacturers. They considered labels and lists of ingredients as well as studies submitted by the drug makers to demonstrate safety and effectiveness. But, independent scientific or medical reports and reviews culled from the literature were the Panels' principal sources of data. (For many ingredients this record was found wanting, and new tests were called for.) Less heed was paid to manufacturers' sales records and complaint files, though this information received some consideration. And testimonials not backed by scientific data were discounted.

The drug data available to the reviewers varied in quantity and in quality. For aspirin—the most widely used and carefully studied active ingredient—there were hundreds of scientific reports to study. For some traditional remedies—like herbs and grasses—little or no credible information was to be had.

In their deliberations, the panelists decided which ingredients are *active* (providing medicinal benefit) and which are *inactive*. (The latter may be present as fillers, preservatives, flavors, colors, or for other nontherapeutic purposes.) The reviewers met many times before drafting evaluations of each active ingredient; inactive ingredients were not assessed. The evaluators were required to place each active ingredient into one of three categories:

1. The ingredient is safe and effective for the purpose for which it is being sold; it is not misbranded.
2. The ingredient is not safe and not effective for the purpose for which it is being sold; it is misbranded.
3. The available information is not sufficient to permit final classification at this time. This amounts to a form of "conditional approval" that allows manufacturers a grace period to prove scientifically that the ingredient really is safe and effective. If they fail to do so, the FDA will declare the ingredient unsafe and ineffective; steps will be taken to remove it from the market.

According to one official tally made in 1982, one-third of the 1400 specific uses (or indications) for active ingredients in nonprescription drugs were considered safe and effective; another third, conditionally safe and effective; a final third, unsafe and/or ineffective.

The reviewers' evaluations go well beyond individual active ingredients: combinations of two or more active ingredients were also graded. Generally speaking, however, Panel members and the FDA believe that products containing a single active ingredient are preferable to those that contain two or more, where one active ingredient is sufficient for a particular symptom and unnecessary medication can be avoided.

The Panels also scrutinized the labels on the thousands of drug products submitted by manufacturers for review. Many claims were rejected as false, misleading, unclear, unjustified—or because they were not based on scientifically sound data. Reviewers were further asked to determine doses—how much of the drug should be taken, how often, and for how long—for each active ingredient classified as safe and effective.

Phases of Review

As the Panels complete their review, the evaluators' recommendations for each active ingredient are published as "Panel reports" in the *Federal Register*. Each active ingredient is described and there is a summary of the evidence upon which each Panel decision was based.

Then a review period follows. Manufacturers, scientists, doctors, and consumers are invited to write to the FDA to agree or disagree with any of the Panel's recommendations—and the FDA must respond. The record is also open for new information from manufacturers or other sources.

When this review period ends, the FDA assesses for itself the Panel recommendations and the new information it has received. It then issues the Panel's principal findings as modified or revised by the FDA in a "tentative final monograph," which is also published in the *Federal Register*.

The tentative final monograph includes a draft set of rules—framed according to the scientific record—that the FDA proposes for controlling the contents and labeling for each active ingredient in each class of drugs. The FDA states its view as to whether each ingredient is safe and effective, not safe and not effective, or requires still further study. At this stage manufacturers have a fairly clear picture of the FDA's judgment of the active ingredients in their products. If need be, they can conduct more tests—using methods suggested by the original Panel and by the FDA—to try to prove that an ingredient is safe and effective. Or they can drop the ingredient from their product and put an approved ingredient in instead.

The review process then allows for another round of comment and review after the publication of the tentative final monograph in the *Federal Register*. The gist of the FDA's findings—with any changes based on new evidence—is then published in the *Federal Register* along with a final draft of the regulations. This publication is called the "final monograph." Within 6 months of publication of final monographs, manufacturers must remove drugs containing disapproved active ingredients from the market or face FDA seizures of products or other legal actions. The conditionally approved ingredients also must be established as safe and effective by this time or they, too, must be removed from the market. The final regulations—which at this time have the force of law—are added to the *Code of Federal Regulations*.

Results and Comments

When the review process reaches completion, consumers can have the same confidence in nonprescription drugs that they now can have about prescription drugs (which are regulated in essentially the same way). The question is: When will this happen?

At the outset, FDA officials now wryly concede, the feeling in the agency was that the entire review might be completed in two or three years. That was in 1972. Today, more than 10 years later, the Panel phase of the project is just ending: a final Panel held its last meeting in October 1981. And it may be two or three more years before all Panel reports can be edited and be published in the *Federal Register*.

In an accounting in July, 1982, ten and a half years after the review began, the FDA said that it had received panel reports or the equivalent on 78 categories of drugs, and had published the reports for 63 of them. But only 8 were issued as final monographs. Only one major group, antacids—an early starter and an early finisher—had reached this stage. At the present rate, another decade may go by before the OTC Review is complete. It may well be 1990, or later, before Congress's 1962 mandate is fulfilled. This Guide is based on the latest reports available and the reader will find, at the bottom of each page where a new unit begins, the nature of the reports on which the particular unit is based.

Why the process is taking so long could be the subject for another book. Briefly, the wheels of government turn very slowly—particularly when hundreds of commercial interests have major stakes in the outcome. The sheer volume of information and paperwork, not to mention the number of decisions that must be reached and approved, is awesome, and resources and time required were grossly underestimated.

Although the FDA has taken some steps to speed up the process, it must be recognized that only recently has the present administration pushed for its early completion. On the other hand, nonprescription drug manufacturers (through their trade organization, the Proprietary Association)—who might be thought to oppose regulatory efforts—are actually supporting the drug-review process. They believe they stand to gain from legitimization of what once were dubbed "patent medicines."

What This Review Means to Consumers

One result of this review has been the change in status of some drugs. Consumers can now buy some drugs without prescription that were available previously by prescription only. The Panels proposed roughly 3 dozen of these switches in status. The most dramatic of these changes is the one that allows weak concentrations of the corticosteroids, hydrocortisone and hydrocortisone acetate, to be sold over-the-counter. Within a year of this change hydrocortisone became the best-selling nonprescription anti-itch medication.

Another result of the review for consumers is the change in the range of nonprescription products available to consumers. The leaf, bark, and root extracts that were the principal ingredients of nineteenth-century patent medicines usually do not meet evaluators' scientific standards, so they are being disapproved. Ginseng, the traditional Oriental remedy, fails in this way, as do rhubarb, dandelion, and golden seal. The medicinal value of turpentine, eucalyptus, and other aromatic plant substances is also being strongly questioned.

Too, some ingredients that have long been doctors' favorites are being found to be dangerous or ineffective when sold and used for self-treatment. These drugs include phenol (carbolic acid) and mercury.

However, not all old drugs are being discarded. Aspirin, derived originally from birchbark, is approved as a pain reliever. Sulfur, a remedy used since ancient times, continues to be approved as safe and effective for treating acne and dandruff.

It is still too soon for final judgments on the over-the-counter drug review. But despite delays, it continues to receive high marks from consumers and consumer activists on the one hand, and from the drug industry and its representatives on the other. The publisher of the *Physicians' Desk Reference for Nonprescription Drugs*—an industry-supported drug guide for doctors—stated the matter clearly a few years ago: "The FDA's OTC Review is unprecedented—for this or any other industry—in its scope, its thoroughness and its openness. It is probably the most extensive scrutiny of an industry's products ever conducted."

Even though the review is not complete, consumers should know that if a drug is extremely hazardous, the FDA can hasten the removal process. For example, the antihistamine drug methapyrilene was taken off the market within months after it was found to cause cancers in test animals, and sweet spirits of nitre was banned when it was found to have killed several children.

Consumers should also be aware of the fact that when the review process is finally completed, all nonprescription drug labels will have to conform to the new standards. But TV, radio, and print advertising for these same products probably will not—because advertising is regulated by a different agency, the Federal Trade Commission (FTC). For a while there was sentiment inside the FTC that all ad claims should conform to the FDA-approved labeling. But blanket application of FDA-sanctioned label language to FTC-regulated ads was ruled out in 1981. So it remains unclear how closely the FTC will require manufacturers to adhere to FDA standards in their promotional campaigns. Fortunately, consumers can make these judgments for themselves by using this Guide.

Categories for Active Ingredients in Nonprescription Drugs

The FDA-sponsored OTC Review places the ingredients evaluated into three categories: I, II, and III. The Review defines as category I those ingredients which are "generally recognized as safe and effective" for the use indicated; category II, those ingredients which are "not generally recognized as safe and effective or [are] misbranded"; category III, those ingredients for which "the available data are insufficient to classify [them] as category I or category II."

The organization of the units in this Guide is centered around these classifications. Category I ingredients are given under the heading *approved*, and are listed or described in the discussions in the units and the charts following the units as "safe and effective." Category II ingredients are given under the heading *disapproved* and are listed or described in the discussions in the units and in the charts as "not safe," "not effective," "not safe and/or not effective" (when it was not clear from the reports on which basis the ingredient was not approved), "disapproved," or "summarily dismissed." Category III ingredients are found in this Guide under the heading *conditionally approved* and are listed or described in the discussions and tables as "not proved safe," "not proved effective," "not proved safe or effective," "not proved safe and/or not proved effective" (when it is not clear from the reports on which basis conditional approval was granted). In each case the description of safety or effectiveness given for the ingredient is based on the characterizations of the ingredient at the stage in the review process indicated by the report given in the footnote at the beginning of each unit.

Ratings of Brand Name and Generic Products

Ratings of over-the-counter drug products appear at the end of most units. These ratings represent the author's opinion of these products, based on a comparison of the ingredients in the products to the OTC Review categorization of their ingredients.

In the Ratings Tables a drug product is rated **A** if the ingredient or ingredients and dosages per unit have been approved by the Panel or the FDA as safe and effective for the purpose listed. They are rated **B** if an ingredient or ingredients or dosages have been conditionally approved by the Panel or the FDA for the purpose listed. They are rated **C** if in the process of the OTC Review an ingredient or ingredients have been found to be not safe, not effective, or both for the purpose listed, or if the dosage has been found not safe, not effective, or both. Readers should note that in some cases an ingredient was summarily disapproved because no information was submitted to the Panel about it, and none could be found.

Some products which contain pain- and fever-relieving active ingredients are rated **C** because the amount of active ingredient contained in them is greater or less than the standard dose recommended by the Panel on internal pain-relieving drugs. This panel says that nonstandard tablets, capsules, or other dosage units that exceed the recommended standard amounts may be unsafe, and those which contain less than the standard may be ineffective.

Under the *Comment* in the tables at least one reason is cited for each **B** or **C** rating. The ratings for combination products are based on the rules formulated by the panels and the FDA as summarized in the Combination Tables that appear in most units.

These ratings are the author's opinion and do not come directly from the OTC Drug Review since the review did not pass on specific brand name products. The ratings also have not been submitted to the NIH vetters who did review the rest of the book.

It would be impossible to rate all of the hundreds of thousands of nonprescription drug products available. A selection of approximately 1500 products was made by the author from information provided by Facts and Comparisons, Inc., of St. Louis, Missouri, a loose-leaf information service for pharmacologists and pharmacists, from other reference sources, and from drug products on drugstore shelves.

In a few instances, chemical names used in the OTC Review are used in the Ratings Tables rather than the alternative name found on the product label. In most cases, the reader will find the alternate names for these ingredients in the text under the names used in the OTC Review.

The FDA-sponsored OTC Review is a one-time effort, intended to fulfill the Congressional mandate that all currently marketed nonprescription drugs be shown to be safe and effective or taken off the market. New information—good and bad—is continually becoming available, however, on available drugs. How the FDA plans to transform the OTC Drug Review into an ongoing regulatory process has not been announced.

This Guide includes all unadopted Panel Reports, all adopted Panel Reports and Tentative Final Monographs published in the *Federal Register* through August 1, 1982, and all Final Monographs or the equivalent published in the *Federal Register* through September 7, 1982. The Ratings Tables reflect updates through September 1982.

Advisory Review Panels and Their Members

The Advisory Review Panel on OTC Anatacid Drugs included:

Franz J. Ingelfinger, M.D., Chairman, *Editor of the New England Journal of Medicine*, Boston, MA; Howard C. Ansel, Ph.D., *Professor of Pharmacy and Head of School of Pharmacy, University of Georgia*, Athens, GA; Morton I. Grossman, M.D., *Internist, Veterans Administration Center*, Los Angeles, CA; Stewart C. Harvey, Ph.D., *Associate Professor of Pharmacology, University of Utah College of Medicine*, Salt Lake City, UT; Edward W. Moore, M.D., *Professor of Medicine, Medical College of Virginia*, Richmond, VA; John F. Morrissey, M.D., *Professor of Medicine, University of Wisconsin School of Medicine*, Madison, WI; Howard M. Spiro, M.D., *Professor of Medicine, Yale University School of Medicine*, New Haven, CT.

The Advisory Review Panel on OTC Antimicrobial Drug Products for Repeated Daily Human Use (Antimicrobial I Panel) included:

Harvey Blank, M.D., Chairman, *Professor of Dermatology, University of Miami School of Medicine*, Miami, FL; Frank B. Engley, Jr., Ph.D., *Professor and Chairman, Department of Microbiology, University of Missouri School of Medicine*, Columbia, MO; William L. Epstein, M.D., *Chairman of the Department of Dermatology, University of California San Francisco Medical Center*, San Francisco, CA; Wallace L. Guess,

Ph.D., *Dean, School of Pharmacy, University of Mississippi,* University, MS; Florence K. Kinoshita, Ph.D., 1810 Frontage Road, Northbrook, IL; Mary Marples, M.D., D.T., M. & H., 1 Van Bruch Close, Old Woodstock, Oxfordshire, England; Paul D. Stolley, M.D., *Johns Hopkins School of Hygiene and Public Health,* Baltimore, MD.

The Advisory Review Panel on OTC Antimicrobial Drug Products (Antimicrobial II Panel) included:

Wallace L. Guess, Ph.D., Chairman, *Dean, School of Pharmacy, University of Mississippi,* University, MS; W. Kenneth Blaylock, M.D., *Assistant Dean for Graduate Medical Education, Medical College of Virginia,* Richmond, VA; Ruth E. Brown, R. Pharm., *Director of Pharmacy, Retired, Group Health,* Seattle, WA; Frank B. Engley, Jr., Ph.D., *Professor and Chairman, Department of Microbiology, University of Missouri School of Medicine,* Columbia, MO; Zenona W. Mally, M.D., *Dermatologist,* Washington, DC; James E. Rasmussen, M.D., *Department of Pediatrics, Buffalo Children's Hospital,* Buffalo, NY; William F. Schorr, M.D., *Director, Dermatologic Residency Training Program, Marshfield Clinic,* Marshfield, WI; E. Dorinda Loeffel Shelley, M.D., *Assistant Professor of Dermatology, University of Illinois Medical Center,* Chicago, IL; Paul D. Stolley, M.D., M.P.H., *Johns Hopkins School of Hygiene and Public Health,* Baltimore, MD; Anne N. Tucker, Ph.D., *Department of Pharmacology, Medical College of Virginia,* Richmond, VA; George B. Youngstrom, M.D., *Dermatologist and Allergist,* Everett, WA.

The Advisory Review Panel on OTC Antiperspirant Drug Products included:

E. William Rosenberg, M.D., Chairman, *Professor and Chairman, Department of Dermatology, University of Tennessee College of Medicine,* Memphis, TN; J. Wesley Clayton, Ph.D., *Director, Toxicology Program, The University of Arizona,* Tucson, AZ; Charles Evans, M.D., Ph.D., *Professor, Department of Microbiology, University of Washington,* Seattle, WA; Zenona Mally, M.D., 1835 I Street, N.W., Washington, DC; Jane Rosenzweig, M.D., *Clinical Instructor, The Permanent Medical Group,* 2200 O'Farrell Street, San Francisco, CA; Robert Scheuplein, Ph.D., *Principal Associate in Biophysics, Department of Dermatology, Massachusetts General Hospital,* Boston, MA; Eli Shefter, Ph.D., *Associate Professor of Pharmaceutics, School of Pharmacy, State University of New York at Buffalo,* Buffalo, NY.

The Advisory Review Panel on OTC Cold, Cough, Allergy, Bronchodilator, and Antiasthmatic Products included:

Francis C. Lowell, M.D., Chairman, *Chief, Allergy Unit, Massachusetts General Hospital*, Boston, MA; Hylan A. Bickerman, M.D., *Associate Clinical Professor of Medicine, College of Physicians and Surgeons, Columbia University*, New York, NY; Halla Brown, M.D., *Chief, Allergy Unit, George Washington University Hospital*, Washington, DC; Robert K. Chalmers, Ph.D., *Associate Dean for Professional Education Program, School of Pharmacy and Pharmacal Science, Purdue University*, Lafayette, IN; Mary Jo Reilly, M.S., *Assistant Executive Director, American Society of Hospital Pharmacists*, Washington, DC; James R. Tureman, M.D., *Professor of Pharmacology, Department of Pharmacology, College of Medicine, Howard University*, Washington, DC; Colin R. Woolf, M.D., *Director, Tri-Hospital Respiratory Service, Toronto General Hospital*, Toronto, Ontario, Canada.

The Advisory Review panel on OTC Contraceptives and other Vaginal Drug Products included:

Elizabeth B. Connell, M.D., Chairman, *Associate Director for Biomedical Sciences, The Rockefeller Foundation*, New York, NY; Evelyn M. Benson, R.Ph., *Pharmacist, Mission Pharmacy*, Seattle, WA; Cynthia W. Cooke, M.D., *Obstetrician-Gynecologist*, Bryn Mawr, PA; Myron Gordon, M.D., *Associate Professor of Obstetrics and Gynecology, New York Medical College*, New York, NY; William A. Mac-Coll, M.D., *Pediatric Allergist*, Berkeley, CA; William H. Pearlman, Ph.D., *Professor of Pharmacology, University of North Carolina School of Medicine*, Chapel Hill, NC; Louise B. Tyrer, M.D., *Vice-President for Medical Affairs, Planned Parenthood World Population*, New York, NY.

The Advisory Review Panel on Dentifrice and Dental-Care Drug Products included:

Louis P. Gangarosa, Ph.D., D.D.S., Chairman, *Professor of Oral Biology, Medical College of Georgia*, Augusta, GA; Joseph J. Aleo, Ph.D., *Assistant Dean, Temple University Dental School*, Philadelphia, PA; Arthur N. Bahn, Ph.D., *Department of Microbiology, Southern Illinois University*, Edwardsville, IL; Howard H. Chauncey, D.M.D., Ph.D., *Veterans Administration Outpatient Clinic*, Boston, MA; Valerie Hurst, Ph.D., *Associate Professor of Microbiology, University of California*

School of Dentistry, San Francisco, CA; Joy B. Plein, Ph.D., *Associate Professor of Pharmacy, University of Washington College of Pharmacy,* Seattle, WA; Delos E. Raymond, D.D.S., *Dentist,* Inkster, MI; Roger H. Scholle, D.D.S., M.S., *Assistant Secretary, Council of Dental Therapeutics, American Dental Association,* Chicago, IL; Lawrence E. Van Kirk, Jr., D.D.S., M.P.H., *Department of Restorative Dentistry, University of Detroit School of Dentistry,* Detroit, MI.

The Advisory Review Panel on OTC Hemorrhoidal Drug Products included:

Claude E. Welch, M.D., Chairman, *Senior Consulting Surgeon, Massachusetts General Hospital,* Boston, MA; Leon Banov, Jr., M.D., *Colonic and Rectal Surgeon,* Charleston, SC; Eugene A. Castiglia, M.D., *Gastroenterologist,* Albuquerque, NM; Winston H. Gaskin, R.Ph., *Veterans Administration Hospital,* Syracuse, NY; Jean Dace Golden, M.D., *General and Plastic Surgeon,* East Stroudsburg, PA; Thaddeus S. Grosicki, Ph.D., *Professor of Pharmaceutics, School of Pharmacy, University of Arkansas,* Little Rock, AR; Judith Karen Jones, M.D., Ph.D., *Internist and Clinical Pharmacologist,* San Francisco, CA.

The Advisory Review Panel on OTC Internal Analgesic, Antipyretic, and Antirheumatic Products included:

Henry W. Elliott, M.D., Ph.D., Chairman, *Professor and Chairman, Department of Medical Pharmacology and Therapeutics, Orange County Medical Center,* Orange, CA; J. Weldon Bellville, M.D., Chairman, *Department of Anesthesiology, University of California School of Medicine,* Los Angeles, CA; William H. Barr, Ph.D., *Department of Pharmacy, Medical College of Virginia,* Richmond, VA; Julius M. Coon, M.D., Ph.D., *Professor of Pharmacology, Thomas Jefferson University,* Philadelphia, PA; Ninfa I. Redmond, Ph.D., *Department of Pharmacology, Faculty of Medicine, University of Montreal,* Montreal, Quebec, Canada; Naomi F. Rothfield, M.D., *Chief, Arthritis Section, Professor of Medicine, University of Connecticut School of Medicine,* Farmington, CT; George Sharpe, M.D., 10400 Connecticut Avenue, Kensington, MD.

The Advisory Review Panel on OTC Laxative, Antidiarrheal, Emetic and Antiemetic Drug products included:

Nicholas C. Hightower, Jr., M.D., *Director of Research and Education, Scott and White Memorial Hospital,* Temple, TX; Carol R. Angle,

M.D., *Professor of Pediatrics, University of Nebraska,* Omaha, NE; James C. Cain, M.D., *Gastroenterologist and Internist, Mayo Clinic,* Rochester, MN; Ivan E. Danhof, M.D., Ph.D., *Associate Professor of Physiology, University of Texas Medical School,* Dallas, TX; James W. Freston, M.D., Ph.D., *Chairman, Division of Gastroenterology, University of Utah Medical Center,* Salt Lake City, UT; Albert L. Picchioni, Ph.D., *Head, Department of Pharmacology and Toxicology, University of Arizona,* Tucson, AZ; Sheila West, Pharm. D., *Program Director, Pharmacy Studies, Johns Hopkins Medical Institutions,* Baltimore, MD.

The Advisory Review Panel on OTC Miscellaneous External Drug Products included:

William E. Lotterhos, M.D., Chairman, *Director, Montgomery Family Practice Program,* Montgomery, AL; George C. Cypress, M.D., *Pediatrician,* Private Practice, Newport News, VA; Rose Dagirmanjian, Ph.D., *Professor of Pharmacology, University of Louisville,* Louisville, KY; Vincent J. Derbes, M.D., *Dermatologist,* Private Practice, New Orleans, LA; J. Robert Hewson, M.D., *Department of Family Practice, University of South Carolina School of Medicine,* Columbia, SC; Yelva L. Lynfield, M.D., *Chief, Dermatology Section, Veterans Administration Hospital,* Brooklyn, NY; Harry E. Morton, Sc.D., *Professor Emeritus of Microbiology, University of Pennsylvania School of Medicine,* Philadelphia, PA; Marianne N. O'Donoghue, M.D., *Dermatologist,* Private Practice, River Forest, IL; Chester L. Rossi, R.Ph., D.P.M., *Podiatrist, Torno Medical Clinic,* Pasadena, TX.

The Advisory Review Panel on OTC Miscellaneous Internal Drug Products included:

John W. Norcross, M.D., Chairman, *Internist,* Belmont, MA; James L. Tullis, M.D.; Chairman, *Department of Hematology, New England-Deaconess Hospital,* Boston, MA; William R. Arrowsmith, M.D., *Department of Internal Medicine, Ochsner Clinic,* New Orleans, LA; Elizabeth C. Gablin, N.N., Ed.D., *Professor of Physiological Nursing, University of Washington,* Seattle, WA; Richard D. Harshfield, M.D., *Associate Professor of Pharmacology, University of Illinois,* Rockford, IL; Theodore L. Hyde, M.D., *General Surgeon,* The Dalles, OR; Diana F. Rodriguez-Calvert, Pharm. D., *Pioneer Pharmacy,* Wagoner, OK; Claus A. Rohweder, D.O., *Director of Medical Education, Kirksville College of Osteopathic Medicine,* Kirksville, MO.

The Advisory Review Panel on OTC Ophthalmic Drug Products included:

Philip Ellis, M.D., Chairman, *Chairman of Ophthalmalogy, University of Colorado Medical School,* Denver, CO; Donald E. Cadwallader, Ph.D., *Professor of Pharmacy, University of Georgia School of Medicine,* Athens, GA; Calvin Hanna, Ph.D., *Department of Pharmacology, University of Arkansas Medical Center,* Little Rock, AR; William H. Havener, M.D., *Chairman of Ophthalmology, Ohio State University,* Columbus, OH; James F. Koetting, O.D., *Professor of Optometry, University of Houston College of Optometry,* Houston, TX; Pearl A. Watson, M.D., *Ophthalmologist,* Washington, D.C.

The Advisory Review Panel on OTC Oral-Cavity Drug Products included:

Lawrence Cohen, M.D., Ph.D., D.D.S., Chairman, *Emergency Medicine Specialist,* Wilmette, IL; John Adriani, M.D., *Clinical Professor of Anesthesiology, Charity Hospital,* New Orleans, LA; Arthur N. Bahn, Ph.D., *Microbiologist, Southern Illinois University,* Edwardsville, IL; Roy C. Darlington, Ph.D., Washington, DC, Martin J. Goldberg, D.D.S., *Dentist,* Kensington, MD; Valarie Hurst, Ph.D., *Professor of Microbiology, School of Dentistry, University of California,* San Francisco, CA; Walter E. Loch, M.D., *Associate Professor of Otolaryngology, School of Medicine, Johns Hopkins University,* Baltimore, MD.

The Advisory Review Panel on OTC Sedative, Tranquilizer, and Sleep-Aid Drug Products included:

Karl E. Rickels, M.D., Chairman, *Professor of Psychiatry and Pharmacology, Department of Psychiatry, University of Pennsylvania,* Philadelphia, PA; Carleton K. Erickson, Ph.D., *School of Pharmacy, University of Kansas,* Lawrence, KS; Helen Dun Goiun, R.Ph., M.S., 916 Crystal Square West, 1515 S. Jefferson Davis Highway, Arlington, VA; Ernest L. Hartmann, M.D., *Professor of Psychiatry, Tufts University School of Medicine,* Boston, MA; Sumner M. Kalman, M.D., *School of Medicine, Stanford University,* Stanford, CA; Lester C. Mark, M.D., *Professor of Anesthesiology, College of Physicians and Surgeons, Columbia University,* New York, NY; Frances S. Norris, M.D., *Medical Director, Division of Licensing and Certification, Maryland Department of Health,* Baltimore, MD.

The Advisory Review Panel on OTC Topical Analgesic, Antirheumatic, Otic, Burn, and Sunburn Prevention and Treatment Drug Products included:

Thomas G. Kantor, M.D., Chairman, *Associate Physician, New York University Medical Center,* New York, NY; John Adriani, M.D., *Clinical Professor of Anesthesiology, Charity Hospital,* New Orleans, LA; Col. William A. Akers, M.C., U.S.A., *Commander, Letterman Army Institute of Research,* San Francisco, CA; Maxine E. Bennett, M.D., *Professor of Otolaryngology, University of Wisconsin Hospitals,* Madison, WI; Minerva S. Buerk, M.D., *Dermatologist,* Wynnewood, PA; Walter L. Dickison, Ph.D., *Dean, School of Pharmacy, Southwestern Oklahoma State University,* Weatherford, OK; Jerry M. Shuck, M.D., *Associate Professor of Surgery, University of New Mexico School of Medicine,* Albuquerque, NM.

The Advisory Review Panel on OTC Vitamin, Mineral and Hemantic Drug Products included:

Irwin H. Rosenberg, M.D., Chairman, *Chief, Gastroenterology Section, University of Chicago School of Medicine,* Chicago, IL; Louis V. Avioli, M.D., *Director, Metabolic Clinic, Washington University School of Medicine,* St. Louis, MO; George M. Briggs, Ph.D., *Professor of Nutrition, University of California,* Berkeley, CA; Robert S. Goodhart, M.D., *Executive Secretary, Committee on Medical Education, The New York Academy of Medicine,* New York, NY; Mary Anne Kimble, Pharm. D., *Assistant Clinical Professor of Pharmacy, University of California,* San Francisco, CA; Carroll M. Leevy, M.D., *Director, Division of Hepatic Metabolism, College of Medicine and Dentistry of New Jersey,* Newark, NJ; Mary Susanne Roscoe, M.D., *Emergency Medicine Specialist,* Aurora, IL.

In addition to the Panel members listed here, the Advisory Panels included a number of nonvoting liaisons some of whom represented the interests of consumer organizations and some, the nonprescription drug industry.

OTHER SOURCES OF INFORMATION FOR CONSUMERS

In addition to the *Federal Register,* where the completed reports described above are published, other helpful references for drug consumers include:

Blakiston's New Gould Medical Dictionary, 2nd ed. (New York: McGraw-Hill, 1956); the *AMA Drug Evaluations,* 4th ed. (Chicago: American Medical Association, 1980); the *Handbook of Nonprescription Drugs,* 7th ed. (Washington, DC: American Pharmaceutical Association, 1982); *The United States Pharmacopoeia,* 19th rev. (Rockville, MD: U.S. Pharmacopoeial Convention, 1975); *Physicians' Desk Reference for Nonprescription Drugs,* 3rd ed. (Oradell, NJ: Medical Economics, 1982), as well as the same publisher's *Drug Topics* and *Drug Topics Red Book;* a biweekly called *The Medical Letter* (published in New Rochelle, NY); and the *FDA Consumer* as well as the *FDC Reports* ("The Pink Sheets").

AUTHOR'S NOTE

The information about self-treatment of certain conditions contained in this book is taken from panel and FDA reports. The panels and the FDA based their recommendations on what is generally suitable for the average individual. Before using the information in this book you should take into account your personal medical history and be aware of the basis on which the recommendations have been made and also be aware that some individuals have idiosyncratic reactions to some medications. In addition, any individual should carefully monitor self-treatment of any condition and should keep in mind that OTC drugs are *medicines* and should be used with care according to direction; if any condition for which you are treating yourself persists, professional care should be sought.

Finally, an individual who has a chronic condition or who is taking medication under a doctor's direction for any reason should always seek medical advice before engaging in any course of self-treatment.

The author has chosen the brand name products for each unit for evaluation in as random a manner as the author could devise and with an effort to select products from a variety of manufacturers.

The author has no interest in any company which manufactures, distributes, or sells over-the-counter drugs.

How to Use This Guide

Since this book answers many questions about over-the-counter drugs, there are several ways it can be used. The column on the left gives some of the reasons why you have turned to this Guide for answers and the column on the right tells you how to use the guide to find those answers.

You have a certain symptom or ailment. You want to know more about it, and more about the active ingredients in drugs that are used to treat it. (Active ingredients are what make a drug work —or not work.)

Check the Contents (pp. vii–xii). The unit titles listed under the heading OVER-THE-COUNTER DRUGS tell you what groups of drugs are included in this Guide. The drugs are arranged either by what they're *for* (example: Acne Medications) or what they *do* (example: Reducing Aids).

You're not sure which products will help your particular problem.

Check the Unit Finder list following this section. There you'll find the drugs grouped by the problem for which you may be seeking relief.

You know what's wrong and you have a product you think may help. How can you be sure?

Check the product label to see what the active ingredient is. Examples: the active ingredient in Datril is acetaminophen; in Pepto-Bismol it is bismuth subsalicylate. Then turn to the index to find where you can read about the ingredient.

Check the Safety and Effectiveness chart at the back of each unit about that ingredient.

You've checked the Guide and find that you have a condition which is self-treatable with non-prescription drugs. You're on your way to the drugstore. What product to buy?

Check the Safety and Effectiveness chart at the back of the unit. In most cases only a handful of ingredients are safe and effective. Jot them down—you needn't carry the guide to the drugstore!

You think you know what product you want, because you've seen an ad on television or you once used it. Is it all it's cracked up to be?

Check the Product Ratings that conclude each unit.

Check the Claims section near the beginning of each unit. Forget about products with false or misleading claims.

You think a drug sounds good for one medicinal use. Will it work for others?

Check the index and turn to the appropriate unit—note text descriptions as well as Safety and Effectiveness charts and the Product Ratings. For example, aspirin rates **A** for pain relief when taken internally, **B** when applied to itches, **C** as a sleep aid.

You need to upgrade your medicine chest.

Use this Guide to evaluate every nonprescription drug you have on hand.

You want to know more about nonprescription drugs in general. Can they really help? How do they work? Isn't it always better to go to a doctor?

The main text of this Guide explains in everyday language many symptoms and ailments. It tells how nonprescription drugs can be effective, when a doctor should be consulted, and when and why experts say that self-medication is often appropriate.

UNIT FINDERS

The unit titles in this Guide are arranged alphabetically. If you are looking for help with a toothache, simply turn to the unit "Toothache Relievers" in the Ts. However, you may also want to know what other over-the-counter remedies are available for teeth problems. In the following list of unit finders, the unit titles are arranged under general problems or conditions for which you may be seeking help, specific kinds of products or drugs, or a common subject matter. So, for teeth, look under "Teeth and Mouth." Once you find the unit title that interests you, just turn to that unit. For a complete list of unit titles, see the Contents pages.

Baby-Care Products

Camphor: Special Warning
Cradle-Cap Removers
Diaper-Rash Medications
Nail-Biting and Thumb-Sucking Deterrents
Phenol: Special Warning
Sweet Spirits of Nitre: Special Warning
Teething Easers
Unguents and Powders for the Skin

Body-Odor Control

Antiperspirants
Deodorants for Ostomies and Incontinence
Soaps, Antimicrobial

Eye- and Ear-Care Products

Ear-Care Aids
Eye Drops and Ointments
Eyes: Artificial Tears
Eyes: Corneal Edema
Eyewash

Gastrointestinal Drugs

Antacids
Anti-Gas Agents
Diarrhea Remedies
Digestive Aids
Hangover and Overindulgence Remedies
Laxatives
Motion-Sickness Medicines

Teeth and Mouth

Cold, Cough, and Allergy Drugs
Cold-Sore Balms
Gum Treatments
Mouthwash for Oral Hygiene
Sore-Throat and Mouth Medicines
Teething Easers
Toothache Relievers
Toothpastes, Rinses, and Gels for Cavity Prevention

Women's Products

Contraceptives
Douches and Other Vaginal Applications
Menstrual-Distress Preparations
"Yeast" Killers for Feminine Itching

The FDA commissioner recommends that before buying or using a nonprescription medication, a consumer:

1. Look for broken seals, open or damaged boxes, or other signs of tampering.
2. Check to see if the product has loose, torn, or missing wrapping, or is discolored or has an unusual odor.
3. Take to the pharmacist or store manager any product for which the wrapping or the drug itself seems suspect in any way.

The Essential Guide
to Nonprescription Drugs

Acne Medications

"There is no single disease which causes more emotional injury, more maladjustment between parents and children, more general insecurity and feelings of inferiority, and greater sums of emotional suffering than does acne."

—MARION B. SULZBERGER, M.D.

The principal sufferers of acne are teen-agers, for whom this report on nonprescription acne medications is especially written. Older persons with deep, pitting acne that will not go away know by now most of the simple facts about this disease. They should be under a dermatologist's care—as should any younger person who is or thinks he or she is suffering from severe acne. Women in their twenties and thirties who develop patches of tiny but unsightly acne papules on their chins and foreheads can probably blame the cosmetics they use. If a change from oil-base to water-base products and avoidance of face creams does not bring relief after 6 or 8 weeks, these women, too, should probably see a dermatologist.

There are few teen-agers who have not been bothered—indeed, mortified—by the sudden emergence of a pimple or other blemish before an important social event. The Panel has important news for teens about acne. Unfortunately not all of it is good news.

Bad news: Acne cannot be cured.

Good news: It can be effectively treated in most individuals.

Bad news: Treatment can be long and costly because many effective medications work slowly and are available only by prescription—so their use must be monitored by a doctor.

Good news: Simple self-care steps and one or two nonprescription drugs can be used to clear up or markedly improve many cases of acne.

Bad news: No method is effective against all acne cases. Each young person needs individualized treatment, which may consist of nonpre-

ACNE MEDICATIONS is based on the report "Topical Acne Drug Products for OTC Human Use" by the FDA's Advisory Review Panel on OTC Antimicrobial Drug Products (Antimicrobial II Panel).

1

scription drugs, prescription drugs, other measures, or a combination of all available remedies.

Good news: Many of the old myths about what causes acne have no basis in fact—so they no longer need be a reason for concern to adolescents.

Bad news: Many of the drugs that are heavily promoted for self-treatment of acne are worthless. Some are even dangerous and should be crossed off the list by teen-agers who are trying to decide which products to buy. The following discussions will help in assessing available products.

CLAIMS

Accurate

for "the treatment of acne"

"anti-acne formula"

"dries and clears acne blemishes [or pimples]"

"reduces blackheads"

"clears up most blackheads"

"helps remove acne pimples"

"unplugs pores to help clear acne"

"penetrates follicles [or pores] to eliminate most blackheads and acne pimples"

"helps keep skin clear of new acne lesions"

"helps prevent new blackheads or acne pimples"

"helps prevent new acne pimples"

Unproved

"antibacterial" (germ-killing activity not yet proved)

"kills acne bacteria and helps clear acne pimples"

"penetrates follicles [or pores] to kill bacteria associated with acne"

"reduces the bacterial products associated with the irritation of acne"

False or Misleading

modifiers such as "prompt" or "fast"

"clears up more pimples faster"

"works fast against surface pimples"

"clinically proven for prompt effective relief of acne"

"makes externally caused skin flareups look better while they're getting better"

"helps involute inflamed pustules"

"fights acne pimples"

"kills facial germs"

"strips away oils and waxy buildup that can lead to pimples and blackheads"

"helps pull loosened oils from pores"

"helps prevent the reinfection of pimples"

"Aids in removing greasy oils from your skin. This can prevent the pores from becoming clogged again."

"hypoallergenic"

"an effective antimicrobial against a wide variety of both gram negative and gram positive bacteria and fungi"

"special medicated skin cleanser"

"helps heal and clear acne by molecular action"

"produces a soft, light peeling of the skin"

"contains time-proved ingredients"

WARNING   These preparations are for external use only and should be kept out of children's reach. Other topical acne medications should not be used at the same time.

MYTHS AND FACTS ABOUT ACNE

A lot has been learned about acne in recent years. It is time to squelch many myths about the disorder and also to summarize (particularly for teen-agers) some research findings the Panel cites:

- Chocolate and "junk foods" do not cause acne or make it worse, and for the most part other foods don't either. New theories about diet and skin blemishes pop up all the time and then, after a few years, are shot down by scientific studies. Unless there is some food that you, individually, find routinely causes your face to break out, you should stop worrying about your choice in foods. On the other hand, one recent study suggests that overeating and undereating—in terms of *quantity*—may both cause acne in males, though it seems not to in females.
- Neither too little sex nor too much is responsible for acne. Neither does it matter what kind of sex you are getting—or not getting.
- Soap and water will cure acne, adults tell adolescents. But the Panel sides with kids who say "No, it won't!" Simply leaving acne alone is no better. Treatment with drugs, which may have to continue for many months, will probably be needed.
- Three out of four teen-agers have some acne, and in one in every four the condition is moderate to severe.

- Facial acne is as common in teen-age girls as it is' in boys. It starts earlier in girls, but is less severe.
- Half of the teen-agers who have acne say they are bothered by it, and more than half treat their faces in one way or another. But only 1 in 10 has consulted a doctor.
- Moderate to severe acne is more common in white adolescents than in blacks. But mild acne—that is, blackheads and whiteheads but no inflammation—is more common in blacks.
- The more "nervous" an adolescent is, the more likely it is that acne will occur. Moments of high stress—when you want things under control—tend to be just those moments when, infuriatingly, a blemish appears.

WHY ACNE DEVELOPS

The increased production of sex hormones in adolescence is the principal stimulus for acne. Androgens (male sex hormones), particularly testosterone, are to blame.

The androgens circulate through the body in the bloodstream, in both males and females, and act upon tiny glands in the pores (or hair follicles) of the skin. These are called the *sebaceous glands,* and their principal function is to secrete the oily substance called *sebum.* Sebum naturally softens and lubricates the skin. When the sebaceous glands are stimulated by testosterone, they produce more sebum—which is discharged through a tiny duct into the hair follicle, and then moves outward to the skin's surface. Sebaceous glands are most numerous on the face, shoulders, and upper back—areas where most acne develops. People with acne tend to have larger sebaceous glands than persons whose skin remains clear. It's also been shown that the more sebum one secretes, the more severe the acne is.

If sebum simply flowed on outward to the skin, where it could be wiped away, it would pose no problems. But there are complicating factors. A "plug" can form in the pore. It consists of sebum and dead skin cells, and may also contain bacteria, hair fragments, and other debris. As more material accumulates, these plugs swell.

In this initial, hard-to-see stage, this plug is called a whitehead. If some of the accumulated material pushes outward and becomes visible where the hair follicle opens onto the skin surface, the plug is called a blackhead. The black color appears to come from a skin pigment called melanin.

Blackheads and whiteheads are bad enough, but there may be

worse to come. Enter here several species of microorganisms, the best known of which is a germ called *Propionibacterium acnes*, or *P. acnes* for short. It lives on the skin, and seems to dote upon sebum, which it eats. In the process of dining, it releases enzymes that break sebum down into greasy substances called free fatty acids.

These acids are extremely irritating. When whiteheads or blackheads that contain these acids leak into—or burst out into—surrounding tissues, they provoke an inflammatory reaction. The tissue reddens and red-colored blemishes (papules) appear. Affected areas may feel painful, irritated, or itchy. Swelling occurs. Rubbing, pushing, or scratching only increases the inflammation.

Because *P. acnes* bacteria are infectious organisms, the body mobilizes its defense forces—including white blood cells—to fight it. Many white blood cells die in combat; their remains are pus. This explains why many a red papule takes on a greenish-white head before it finally breaks open and drains, or recedes gradually back into the body. These pus-filled blemishes are called pustules, or, more simply, pimples.

In some cases the inflammation fails to subside. Then irregular red blemishes called nodules develop on the face and form scars. Cosmetic surgery may be required to remove or reduce them.

This, in brief, is how Panel members and other experts believe acne starts and progresses. But many questions remain unanswered, and theories may change as new information becomes available.

TREATMENTS FOR ACNE

Early treatment may reduce the severity of the disease, but, reviewers caution, there is no evidence that any treatment program built around scrubs or soaps and other nonprescription products—or anything else—can wholly prevent acne.

Left alone, most blemishes will vanish within 2 to 4 weeks. A drug that shortens this recovery time is, according to the experts, effective in treating acne. A drug that reduces the number of new eruptions between week 4 and 8 is *protectively* beneficial as well. Evaluators say that drugs which are effective in treating acne will also prevent new eruptions.

Effective acne treatment slows down the cellular turnover rate and the accumulation of cellular debris in the hair follicle, slows down the production of sebum, and kills or inhibits *P. acnes* and other microorganisms in the pores, stifling the inflammatory activity of the enzymes they produce.

There are several methods now used in efforts to treat acne:

Applying these nonprescription drugs to the skin:

abrasives (e.g., soaps, granules, polyester fiber sponges)
benzoyl peroxide 2.5 to 10 percent lotions and creams
salicylic acid 0.5 to 5 percent
sulfur-resorcinol combinations
Vleminckx' solution (sulfurated lime solution)

Applying these prescription drugs to the skin:

antibiotics (clindamycin, erythromycin, tetracycline)
benzyl peroxide 2.5 to 10 percent gels and lotions
tretinoin (vitamin A acid) 0.05 to 0.1 percent

Taking these prescription drugs internally:

antibiotics (tetracycline, erythromycin, minocycline)
corticosteroids
estrogens
13-*cis* retinoic acid, sold as Accutane (Roche), for severe cystic acne

Using these skin treatments:

acne surgery (comedone extraction and lancing of pimples)
dermabrasion (skin peeling)
fibrin injections to build up concave scars
freezing (cryotherapy with carbon dioxide in the form of dry ice
   or slush, or with liquid nitrogen)
steroid injections into acne nodules and cysts

Only nonprescription treatments are assessed here. If such a product doesn't work satisfactorily, or if you feel you might do better with more intensive therapy, then the person to see is your pediatrician or adolescent-medicine specialist, your family doctor, or, preferably, a dermatologist. The key thing to remember is that many of the methods discussed here do work—but only if you adhere religiously to the treatment plan that you—or you and your doctor—have decided to try, and give the program enough time (weeks or even months).

First Aid for Pimples

A few methods are available to provide fast clearance of one or two large, juicy pimples, or large blackheads or whiteheads. The bad stuff can often be forced out by using a tool called a comedone extractor. It can be bought at a drugstore.

Dermatologists are of two minds about this pimple-squeezing tool. Some warn that it is dangerous, because the infected material may be forced back into the bloodstream and carried to other parts of the body. They particularly warn against squeezing pimples that erupt in the triangular area between the top of the nose and the corners of the mouth, because underlying blood vessels drain directly into the brain.

Not all dermatologists take this dire view, however. At least one nationally known skin doctor says it is safe to carefully drain these lesions using a comedone extractor. The middle course—if a really important social event looms—is to schedule an emergency visit with a dermatologist and let him "squeeze" the pimple for you. The other alternative is temporarily covering up the blemish with makeup available for this purpose.

ABRASIVE SCRUBS

A wide variety of antiacne soaps, pastes, and cleansers contain mildly abrasive substances like aluminum oxide or polyethylene granules. These abrasives are very popular, perhaps because they provide something one can *do* about acne—scrub out clogged pores.

The studies that have been conducted on these ingredients are inconclusive. One researcher found in a 10-year study of 1000 patients that aluminum oxide fused to soap paste was the most effective of several abrasives. But he failed to keep accurate blemish counts between those who used this abrasive system and those who didn't. He said that scrubbing with an abrasive replaces one's urge to pick and squeeze the pimples—which could be an advantage.

Two other highly regarded acne specialists carefully tested five abrasive preparations in patients with moderate to conspicuous whiteheads and blackheads. None of the abrasives provided a clinically significant benefit. The abrasives all reduced the number of papules and pustules in the first weeks of treatment, but some test subjects ended up with *more* of these blemishes after eight weeks than they had when they started. Because acne sufferers' skin is sensitive to physical injury, the researchers warned against use of abrasives.

The Panel's view is that abrasives like aluminum oxide and polyethylene "do not have an effect on acne lesions," so they are categorized as "inactive ingredients."

Will Zinc Supplements Help?

One currently popular self-treatment for acne is zinc tablets, which can be obtained from drug-or health-food stores. Zinc is an essential trace element; the body needs about 15 mg per day, and most people get at least this amount in their diets.

A person who each day takes 3 tablets of 220-mg zinc sulfate to treat acne is getting 150 mg of elemental zinc—or 10 times the daily requirement. This may lead to unpleasant side effects, including nausea, vomiting, stomach cramps, and diarrhea. The Panel says effervescent zinc heptahydrate (citrate) salt, mixed in water, may cause fewer of these problems than zinc sulfate monohydrate tablets or capsules.

While a dietary deficiency of zinc has been shown to cause acne, Panel members doubt that large numbers of teen-age Americans are zinc-deficient, and there is no good explanation of how zinc supplements relieve this condition—if in fact they do.

A number of scientifically controlled, double-blind studies have been conducted on oral zinc therapy. Some show significant improvement that is not duplicated either by dummy medication or by other acne treatments. Other results are equivocal. Until more conclusive evidence emerges, the Panel says it cannot recommend oral zinc as a treatment for acne.

Assessing Products

Two problems bedevil efforts to assess anti-acne active ingredients and products. One is that the vehicle (base) in which the active ingredient(s) is formulated influences effectiveness. The Panel did not offer any suggestions on which bases to choose. Also difficult—for scientists trying to rate acne medications as well as for sufferers who use them—is the method of evaluating test results.

Some scientists—and some sufferers—count the blemishes before and after treatment. Others break down the blemishes into types before counting. Still others grade the severity of each blemish, while an alternative method is to venture an overall estimate. As yet there is no universally accepted way to measure acne's severity or assess treatment benefits.

Combination Products

For the most part, the fewer active ingredients in a drug product, the safer it is. Based on this philosophy, the Panel views combination products unfavorably and, generally speaking, would require that each be proved more effective—yet not more toxic—than the single active ingredients used alone.

Panel members found few well-run clinical studies which demonstrate a clear advantage to combination preparations. So they approved as safe and effective only one combination, and one close variant of it:

The combination of sulfur 8 percent + resorcinol 2 percent and the equivalent combination of sulfur 8 percent + resorcinol monoacetate 3 percent   Although the origins and mechanisms of these combinations remain unclear, the resorcinol seems to enhance sulfur's ability to clear up acne (*see* SULFUR, under APPROVED ACTIVE INGREDIENTS, below). Resorcinol by itself is not effective. Several studies show that sulfur + resorcinol is as effective as sulfur alone, and one shows that the combination is more effective than pure sulfur against some acne lesions. Thus the Panel evaluates these combinations as safe and effective, but warns that they should be applied "to affected areas only." It adds: "Do not use on broken skin or apply to large areas of the body."

The combination of sulfur 5 percent + aluminum chlorohydrex 10 percent   Though judged safe, this combination has not been proved to be wholly effective. It helps clear up papules and pimples but is not convincingly effective against whiteheads when they develop.

The combination of benzoyl peroxide 7.5 percent + sulfur 5 percent   This combination is certainly effective. But the sulfur appears to significantly increase the risk of developing an allergic sensitivity to the benzoyl peroxide. For this reason the Panel wants this combination to remain a prescription drug to be used only under medical supervision.

The combination of calcium polysulfide + calcium thiosulfate   This combination is called sulfurated lime solution, or Vleminckx' solution. It is a weak skin-peeling agent. Despite a century's use for a variety of skin conditions, there is still no convincing evidence that the mixture effectively combats acne.

Several other combinations are rejected more summarily (*see* SAFETY AND EFFECTIVENESS: COMBINATION PRODUCTS chart at the end of this unit).

PREPARATIONS FOR ACNE

Approved Active Ingredients

Benzoyl peroxide   This compound has been used in a variety of medicines since the 1920s. It appears to act in two ways that are possibly related. The drug mildly irritates the blemished outer layer of skin and causes it to peel away. It then kills underlying microorganisms—particularly *P. acnes*—perhaps by overwhelming their environment with oxygen, which they cannot tolerate.

The safety of benzoyl peroxide has been carefully studied in many tests on lab animals and humans. When the drug is applied to the skin, little of it is absorbed; most of that is excreted. It does not appear to pose a risk of cancer, birth defects, or genetic damage.

Benzoyl peroxide causes allergic reactions in a very small percentage of users. Persons with very light, sensitive, or dry skin may be easily irritated by benzoyl peroxide. Black persons are less likely to have this reaction, but they may be disturbed by the ashy gray cast it gives to their skin.

The higher the concentration of benzoyl peroxide that is used in an acne preparation, the greater the irritation. The Panel suggests that consumers find and use the lowest dose that effectively controls their symptoms.

However, despite the drug's reputation for causing irritation, evaluators judge benzoyl peroxide as safe.

Many studies have been conducted to determine whether benzoyl peroxide is effective. After evaluating test results, the Panel concluded that the chemical decreases counts of all types of acne blemish—including blackheads, whiteheads, papules, and pimples—in a much greater percentage of users than do dummy medications. In one study, for example, benzoyl peroxide was tested in patients with moderate to severe acne. The number of facial blemishes dropped from an average of 10.5 to 6.6 per person in the group that used a 5.5 percent benzoyl peroxide preparation 1 or more times daily. By comparison, in a control group who treated themselves with the dummy, nonmedication preparation, blemish counts *rose*, from 10.4 to 11.1 per person. In another study, two-thirds of persons using the active ingredient improved while only one-third of the control individuals did.

A few studies indicate that a weaker 2.5 percent concentration of benzoyl peroxide, which is relatively nonirritating to the skin, is almost as effective as a more potent 10 percent concentration. So concentrations of 2.5 to 10 percent are safe and effective for self-treating acne.

WARNING Persons with very sensitive skin or a known allergy to benzoyl peroxide should not use this medication. If uncomfortable irritation or excessive dryness and/or peeling occurs, reduce the frequency of use or the amount of dosage. If excessive itching, redness, burning, or swelling occurs, discontinue use. If these symptoms persist, consult a doctor promptly. Keep away from the eyes, lips, and other mucous membranes. Some preparations may bleach hair or dyed fabrics.

Resorcinol and resorcinol monoacetate in combination with sulfur There are doubts about the safety and strong doubts about the effectiveness of resorcinol and resorcinol monoacetate. They are not—and the Panel believes they should not be—used in single-ingredient products (*see* page 16).

Resorcinol and resorcinol monoacetate are, however, widely used in combination antiacne medications, particularly with sulfur, in formulations legitimized as much by a long history of use as by scientific evidence. They may enhance sulfur's efficacy. So the Panel grants a safe and effective label to resorcinol 2 percent and resorcinol monoacetate 3 percent when they are used in combination with sulfur 8 percent.

Sulfur For thousands of years people have used this pungent yellow element as medicine. Yet its safety and effectiveness in controlling acne are less well studied than the safety and effectiveness of benzoyl peroxide, which has been marketed only for several decades. How sulfur acts in helping to clear acne remains unclear. It is believed that sulfur causes the outer layer of dead and dying skin to peel away, and that it kills microorganisms like *P. acnes*.

The Panel judges sulfur to be safe—largely on the basis of its years of use and acceptance by dermatologists, as well as the scarcity of reports of severe side effects.

Evaluators say that as yet too few controlled tests have been conducted. Nevertheless, the handful of studies that are available show that sulfur—usually in combination with one or more other ingredients—is superior to placebo drugs. In one study, 3 percent sulfur twice daily cut blemish counts by half or more in 12 weeks in one-third of those treated. The reduction was only one-tenth in the patients treated with a dummy mixture. Conclusion: sulfur is a safe and effective acne treatment at concentrations of 3 to 10 percent.

WARNING Keep away from the eyes. If excessive skin irritation develops, or increases, discontinue use and consult a doctor or pharmacist.

Conditionally Approved Active Ingredients

Povidone-iodine This is iodine in a slow-release medication applied to the skin. The Panel assessed it as safe for treating acne although another Panel has raised questions about its safety (*see* IODOPHORS, page 335).

In one small study, povidone-iodine 7.5 percent was compared with its inactive base for a treatment period of several months. Among 10 subjects who applied povidone-iodine, 9 were improved or much improved. In the control group, who applied the base only, only 3 of 7 participants were better. In the other tests submitted for review, participants either received a second medicine besides povidone-iodine —which confounded the results—or the test had some other serious flaw in its structure. So the Panel says that while 7.5 percent povidone-iodine is safe—and *may* be of value—its effectiveness needs to be proved.

Resorcinol and resorcinol monoacetate in combination with salicylic acid   There are doubts about the safety and the effectiveness of these phenollike compounds. They are not—and the Panel believes they should not be—used in single-ingredient products (*see* page 16).

Resorcinol and resorcinol monoacetate are, however, widely used in combination antiacne medications, with salicylic acid in formulations sanctioned more by long usage than by scientific evidence. So, pending proof of effectiveness, resorcinol and resorcinol monoacetate are granted conditional approval when combined with salicylic acid.

Salicylic acid   A skin-peeling agent chemically related to aspirin, salicylic acid was assessed as safe for treating certain fungus conditions. The absorption rate is low, so even widespread use of current salicylic-acid preparations is unlikely to cause serious harm to acne sufferers.

Salicylic acid has been used to treat acne and other skin disorders for more than a century. But the way it works has never been precisely explained. Worse, no definitive study has ever been conducted on its effectiveness as a single active ingredient (rather than as part of a combination). The current belief is that the acid peels away overlying skin so that other ingredients formulated with it can reach and act on bacteria and sebum in the pores.

In one of the better studies, 2 percent salicylic-acid lotion was compared with a nonmedicated bar soap. The 109 subjects all had mild acne. After 2 weeks' treatment, the salicylic-acid lotion proved to be far superior in reducing blackheads, but there was no significant difference between the two groups in terms of papule counts, frequency of new blemishes, or overall improvement. The researchers decided that 14 days was too short a time to measure improvement, so they ran a second, 3-month test on 177 acne sufferers. Three-quarters of the participants treated with the salicylic-acid lotion had good to excellent results, compared with only 10 percent in those who used the soap. The treatment group had fewer blackheads and pimples, and their faces were significantly less oily.

This study, and several others in which supplemental treatments were used in addition to salicylic acid, led evaluators to believe that salicylic acid may be an effective ingredient. But it was decided that definitive testing needs to be done to confirm this. Verdict: safe but not proved effective.

Disapproved Active Ingredients

Many acne products contain ingredients that won't work or are unsafe. Teen-agers and other acne sufferers can save themselves a lot of aggravation by simply shunning products that contain these substances.

Alkyl isoquinolonium bromide This germ-killing agent is used in food processing as well as in drugs. But the Panel found the available safety data to be inadequate, although it chose not to make a conclusive ruling on this issue. Nor was any evidence submitted (and the Panel could find none) to show that alkyl isoquinolonium bromide relieves acne. Verdict: not proved safe and not effective.

Aluminum compounds: alcloxa, aluminum chlorohydrex, aluminum hydroxide, and magnesium aluminum silicate These aluminum compounds have been assessed by several Panels concerned with a variety of medicinal purposes. Basing its judgment on the earlier analyses, the present Panel lists the compounds as safe.

Alcloxa has been used for half a century to treat many different skin disorders. But no data was furnished to the Panel to show the drug's effectiveness. Aluminum chlorohydrex inhibits perspiration, and allegedly dries up sebum. But no test has demonstrated that it is effective, as a single ingredient, in clearing up acne. Nor was any evidence available on aluminum hydroxide's role, if any, in *curbing* acne. Magnesium aluminum silicate is thought to absorb oil from the skin—but no acceptable studies have been conducted to show that it clears up acne blemishes. For all of these aluminum compounds the Panel's verdict is: safe but not effective.

Benzocaine As topical anesthetics go, this one is very safe; but with its use lies some risk of allergic reactions and other side effects. Since the Panel could think of no good reason for including a short-acting anesthetic in an acne preparation, it decided that benzocaine is not safe. As to effectiveness, the concentrations of benzocaine in products marketed for acne are too low to be effective. Furthermore, neither manufacturers nor researchers provided any evidence that benzocaine really works in combatting acne. Verdict: unsafe and ineffective.

Benzoic acid   This compound is widely used as an antifungal skin medication. No side effects have been reported, so the Panel judges it safe. But no investigations demonstrated its value, if any, in clearing up acne. The Panel concludes that benzoic acid is safe but not effective.

Boron compounds: boric acid and sodium borate   While high levels of these compounds may irritate damaged skin, the Panel calculates that the low doses (up to 5 percent boric acid or sodium borate) formulated into acne products cannot cause serious skin damage or internal poisoning.

The handful of studies that are cited in an effort to prove that borates are helpful in acne were too poorly constructed to merit the evaluators' approval. They think that sodium borate might work against superficial pimples but not acne lesions. Conclusion: safe but not effective.

Calcium polysulfide   This compound of sulfur has been used for a century in treating acne. It is one of the ingredients of Vleminckx' solution, or sulfurated lime solution. The Panel says that its principal breakdown product is elemental sulfur. And since that is safe, calcium polysulfide is considered safe. However, absolutely no evidence is available to support calcium polysulfide's effectiveness against acne, so the Panel judges it safe but not effective.

Calcium thiosulfate   This chemical is formulated into sulfurated lime solution, or Vleminckx' solution. Since, when moistened, its principal breakdown product is sulfur, which is safe in low doses, the Panel judges calcium thiosulfate to be safe. But no controlled clinical trial has demonstrated that calcium thiosulfate is effective acne medicine. Conclusion: safe but not effective.

Camphor   This ingredient—discussed in many sections of this book—is considered safe for application to the skin in concentrations of up to 2.5 percent. However, lacking any test results to prove, or even suggest, that the drug effectively relieves acne, the Panel decided to rank it safe but not effective.

Chlorhydroxyquinoline   No safety information is available on this compound, so the Panel rates it as not safe. Nor has it been well studied as a single active ingredient for the treatment of acne. So the decision is: not safe or effective.

Chloroxylenol   The Panel assessed this ingredient as an antifungal drug and found it safe—a judgment repeated in its use on acne. Chloroxylenol's effectiveness against acne has not been studied. So the ingredient is ranked safe but not effective.

Coal tar   There is an unresolved question of whether this substance promotes or causes skin cancer, for which reason the Panel labels it unsafe. The fragmentary medical record on the relation of this drug to acne is that coal tar is more likely to *cause* the disorder than to cure or relieve it. Conclusion: not safe and not effective.

Dibenzothiophene   Little safety information is available on this compound, but it is known that some of its chemical derivatives are highly toxic and can cause cancer. The Panel therefore judges it unsafe for treating acne.

While the drug appears to be effective against acne, careful scientific study is needed to confirm this. And especially because of the serious reservations that it has about dibenzothiophene's safety, the Panel says: not proved effective and not safe.

Estrone   This is an estrogen, a female hormone. Studies to show that it effectively combats acne do not meet the Panel's standards. At the same time, a bias against nonprescription use of any hormonal products shows through in the Panel's report.

The rationale for using female hormones is that they counteract the male hormones (androgens) that stimulate the skin's sebaceous glands to produce sebum. To have an anti-androgen effect, evaluators say, the estrone must be absorbed through the skin and then act on the androgen-producing internal organs. The dosage required to achieve this result is so large, however, that the Panel claims there is a risk of blood clots and other side effects.

The estrone cream evaluated contains only a very small amount of estrone (3.333 International Units per ounce). Nevertheless, favorable —although inconclusive—studies have been published on its use against acne. Results suggest that estrone acts locally on the sebaceous glands in the skin (as manufacturers claim) and does not have to act internally on androgen-producing organs. However, the value of these studies is questionable because the cream product that was tested also contained a second active ingredient, salicylic acid. But some experts believe that, contrary to the Panel's analysis, it is not inconceivable that low doses of estrogen in acne creams may be helpful.

In other tests, higher dosages of estrogens were found to be more effective in relieving acne in men than in women. These studies, too, are inconclusive because other treatments were administered at the same time.

The Panel's conclusion is that estrone is neither safe nor effective for use as an active ingredient in nonprescription acne medication.

Magnesium sulfate   Better known as epsom salts, this compound is widely used to treat skin inflammations. No adverse effects have been reported, and the evaluators judge it safe for treating acne. Magnesium sulfate is thought to act by "drawing inflammation to the surface of the skin by osmotic pressure." The Panel doubts this, and says there are no studies to show that the drug is of any benefit against acne. It lists magnesium sulfate as safe but not effective.

Phenolates: phenol and phenolate sodium   The Panel is not convinced that phenolates are safe, even in the low concentrations of under 1.5 percent that the FDA has decided are not hazardous. The reviewers believe there is a lack of reliable data about absorption of phenolates into small areas of skin and too little information about their effects on wound healing and on the risk of causing allergic rashes or other unanticipated reactions. No proof is available to show that phenolates effectively clear acne from the skin. So the Panel's verdict is that these substances have not been proved safe and definitely are not effective.

Phenyl salicylate   The toxicologic information available on this compound is far too sparse to support a conclusion about its safety. No data could be found—anywhere—to justify its use against acne. In short, phenyl salicylate is not proved safe and it is ineffective.

Pyrilamine maleate   This is an antihistamine. No toxic reactions have been reported from its use on the skin, so it is listed as safe. But no clinical trials show it is effective in relieving acne. The Panel says it makes no sense to use an anti-itch medication like pyrilamine maleate to treat this disorder. Conclusion: safe but not effective.

Resorcinol and resorcinol monoacetate   For the treatment of acne, these drugs are long-standing items in the old medicine chest. They almost always are combined with one or more other ingredients (one of which is usually sulfur), so it's difficult to separate their particular contribution to a preparation.

Despite the drug's wide usage without untoward side effects, evaluators have strong reservations about resorcinol. It is a phenollike compound and, like phenol, acts as a poison on the central nervous system when large amounts are absorbed through the skin. Some of the better animal studies undertaken to prove resorcinol's safety are deficient. So while the Panel cautiously approves low concentrations of resorcinol 2 percent and resorcinol monoacetate 3 percent as safe, it warns they should not be used over large surfaces of the body.

As to its effectiveness, no study has examined the therapeutic value of resorcinol as a single ingredient in treating acne patients. Results of testing sulfur in combination with resorcinol are not wholly convincing. The Panel therefore concludes that resorcinol and resorcinol monoacetate are ineffective as single ingredients. (It grants them its approval as safe and effective when combined with sulfur and conditional approval when used in combination with salicylic acid.)

Sodium thiosulfate　This compound, which is used to treat mange in dogs, is nonirritating to the skin. The Panel says it is safe. Its effectiveness in peeling the skin over the acne blemish and in killing bacteria has not been demonstrated. None of the studies reported meets the Panel's criteria for effectiveness: all involve the use of combination products, rather than single ingredients, and none provides comparison between the sodium thiosulfate and the inactive base in which it is formulated. In sum: this drug is safe but it is not effective.

Tetracaine hydrochloride　A topical anesthetic, tetracaine hydrochloride may cause allergic reactions. The risks of using it on large body surfaces over prolonged periods of time have not been adequately assessed. Further, no studies have been conducted to show that tetracaine hydrochloride actually combats acne. In fact, the Panel believes that it makes no sense to use an anesthetic for this purpose. Conclusion: unsafe and ineffective.

Thymol　This ingredient is of questionable safety because its absorption through wound surfaces has not been well studied. Neither has its irritancy. The very low concentrations of thymol used in some acne preparations probably are too weak to kill microorganisms (as they are purported to do). While a few studies of thymol suggest that it has some value against acne, it has never been tested against a look-alike dummy preparation that lacks only the thymol. Wanting such evidence, the Panel lists thymol as not safe and as not effective.

Vitamin E　This vitamin is found in high concentrations in wheat germ, sunflower seeds, soybean oil, and other plant products. The Panel's view is that applying vitamin E to the face poses some risk of creating an allergic reaction—particularly when the vitamin is used with a skin-peeling agent. No study has ever been reported that demonstrates the effectiveness of vitamin E as a single active ingredient. The Panel could think of no reason to support its use against acne, and lists it as not proved safe and ineffective.

Zinc compounds: zinc oxide, zinc stearate, and zinc sulfide　These zinc compounds have long been used in baby powders. While little toxicity information is available on zinc as a drug applied to the skin, the Panel notes that no ill effects have been reported following its use.

Zinc oxide is used as a protectant, astringent, or antiseptic. But the Panel says neither it nor the other zinc compounds have ever been scientifically studied as an acne treatment. Lacking adequate test data, it calls the zinc compounds ineffective, although safe.

Inactive Ingredients

Many impressive-sounding chemicals are formulated into acne products, but in reality they play no active role in clearing one's skin. They are used, among other reasons, to provide bulk, as preservatives, or to lend the product cosmetic appeal. Some of these inactive ingredients are:

alcohol
allantoin
aluminum oxide
bentonite
benzalkonium chloride
benzethonium chloride
calcium phosphate
carbomer 940
carboxyvinyl polymer
cetyl alcohol
cholesterol
citric acid
colloidal alumina
cosmetic colors
dioctyl sodium sulfosuccinate
edetate disodium
glycerin
glycerol monostearate
glyceryl monostearate
hexachlorophene
hydrocarbon hydrotropes

isopropyl alcohol
isopropyl palmitate
laureth-4 (polyoxyethylene lauryl ether)
menthol
methylbenzethonium chloride
methylparaben (methyl parasept)
methyl salicylate
polyethylene
polyethylene glycol monostearate
polyethylene glycol 1000 monostearate
propylene glycol
propylparaben (propyl parasept)
purified water
soapless cleansers
sodium hydroxide
sodium lauryl sulfate
stearic acid
sulfated surfactants
sulfonated alkyl benzenes
wetting agents

Safety and Effectiveness: Active Ingredients
in Over-the-Counter Acne Medications

Active Ingredient	Panel's Assessment
alkyl isoquinolinium bromide	not proved safe and not effective
aluminum compounds: alcloxa, aluminum chlorohydrex, aluminum hydroxide, and magnesium aluminum silicate	safe but not effective
benzocaine	not safe or effective
benzoic acid	safe but not effective
benzoyl peroxide	safe and effective
boron compounds: boric acid and sodium borate	safe but not effective
calcium polysulfide	safe but not effective
calcium thiosulfate	safe but not effective
camphor	safe but not effective
chlorhydroxyquinoline	not safe or effective
chloroxylenol	safe but not effective
coal tar	not safe or effective
dibenzothiophene	not safe
estrone	not safe or effective
magnesium sulfate	safe but not effective
phenolates: phenol and phenolate sodium	not proved safe and not effective
phenyl salicylate	not proved safe and not effective
povidone-iodine	safe but not proved effective
pyrilamine maleate	safe but not effective
resorcinol 2 percent and resorcinol monoacetate 3 percent in combination with sulfur 8 percent	safe and effective
resorcinol and resorcinol monoacetate as single ingredients	safe but not effective
resorcinol and resorcinol monoacetate in combination with salicylic acid	safe but not proved effective
salicylic acid	safe but not proved effective
sodium thiosulfate	safe but not effective
sulfur	safe and effective
tetracaine hydrochloride	not safe or effective
thymol	not safe or effective
vitamin E	not proved safe and not effective
zinc compounds: zinc oxide, zinc stearate, and zinc sulfide	safe but not effective

Safety and Effectiveness: Over-the-Counter Combination Products Used to Treat Acne

Safe and Effective

sulfur 8% + resorcinol 2%
sulfur 8% + resorcinol monoacetate 3%

Conditionally Safe and Effective

calcium polysulfide + calcium thiosulfate
  (Vleminckx' solution, or sulfurated lime solution)
sulfur 5% + aluminum chlorohydrex 10%
sulfur + resorcinol + alcloxa
sulfur + resorcinol + thymol + zinc oxide
sulfur + salicylic acid
salicylic acid + resorcinol
salicylic acid + resorcinol + alcloxa
salicylic acid + resorcinol + sodium thiosulfate
benzoic acid + boric acid + zinc oxide-zinc
  stearate

Not Safe and/or Not Effective

benzoyl peroxide 7.5% + sulfur 5%*

*This combination *is* approved as a prescription drug.

Acne Medications: Product Ratings

Single-Ingredient Products

Product and Distributor	Dosage of Active Ingredients	Rating[1]	Comment
benzoyl peroxide			
Benoxyl 5 (Stiefel)	**lotion:** 5%	A	
benzoyl peroxide (generic)		A	
Dry and Clear (Whitehall)		A	
Persadox (Owen)		A	
Zeroxin (Syosset Labs)		A	
Benoxyl 10 (Stiefel)	**lotion:** 10%	A	
benzoyl peroxide (generic)		A	
Oxy 10 (Norcliff Thayer)		A	
Topex (Vicks Toiletry Products)		A	
Zeroxin (Syosset Labs)		A	

Acne Medications: Product Ratings *(continued)*

Single-Ingredient Products

Product and Distributor	Dosage of Active Ingredients	Rating[1]	Comment
Clearasil BP Acne Treatment (Vicks Toiletry Products)	cream: 10%	A	
Persadox HP (Owen)		A	
Persadox (Owen)	cream: 5%	A	
salicyclic acid preparation			
Saligel Acne Gel (Stiefel)	gel: 5%	B	not proved effective
sulfur preparations			
Acne Aid (Stiefel)	lotion: 10%	A	
Noxzema 12-Hour Acne Medicine (Noxell)		A	
Fostex CM (Westwood)	cream: 2%	C	not enough sulfur
Postacne (Dermik)	lotion: 2%	C	not enough sulfur
Xerac (Person & Covey)	gel: 4% (microcrystalline)	A	

Combination Products

Product and Distributor	Dosage of Active Ingredients	Rating[1]	Comment
Acno (Baker-Cummins)	lotion: 3% sulfur + 2% salicylic acid	B	not proved effective
Acnomel (Menley & James)	cream: 8% sulfur + 2% resorcinol	A	
Acnotex (C & M Pharm.)	lotion: 8% sulfur + 2.25% salicylic acid	B	not proved effective
Akne Drying (Alto)	lotion: 6% sulfur + 2% salicylic acid + 10% urea with zinc oxide	C	urea not assessed by Panel
Clearasil (Vicks Toiletry Products)	stick: 8% sulfur + 1% resorcinol	C	too little resorcinol
Fostril (Westwood)	lotion: 2% sulfur + zinc oxide	C	less-than-effective dose of sulfur
Klaron (Dermik)	lotion: 5% colloidal sulfur + 2% salicylic acid	B	neither salicylic acid nor this combination proved effective

Acne Medications: Product Ratings *(continued)*

Product and Distributor	Dosage of Active Ingredients	Rating[1]	Comment
Komed Mild (Barnes-Hind)	**lotion:** 2% sodium thiosulfate + 1% salicylic acid	C	sodium thiosulfate not effective
Loroxide (Dermik)	**lotion:** 5.5% benzoyl peroxide + 0.25% chlorhydroxyquinoline	C	chlorhydroxyquinoline not safe or effective
Lotalba (Durel)	**ointment:** (Lotio alba + glycerine + mineral gums)	C	contains no effective anti-acne drugs, according to Panel assessments
Microsyn (Syntex)	**lotion:** 8% sodium thiosulfate + 2% salicylic acid + 2% resorcinol	C	sodium thiosulfate not effective
R.A. (Medco Labs)	**lotion:** 3% resorcinol + 6% calamine	C	too much resorcinol; calamine not effective
Vlem-Dome (Miles Pharm.)	**packets:** calcium polysulfide + calcium thiosulfate (Vleminckx' solution)	B	not proved effective
Vlemasque (Dermik)	**solution:** calcium polysulfide + calcium thiosulfate (Vleminckx' solution)	B	not proved effective

Medicated Bar Soaps

Product and Distributor	Dosage of Active Ingredients	Rating[1]	Comment
Acnaveen Cleansing Bar (Berlex)	**soap:** 2% sulfur + 2% salicylic acid + 50% colloidal oatmeal	C	colloidal oatmeal not submitted for Panel's assessment; too little sulfur
Buf Acne Cleansing Bar (Riker)	**soap:** 1% sulfur + 1% salicylic acid	C	less-than-effective concentration of sulfur
Clearasil Antibacterial Soap (Vicks Toiletry Products)	**soap:** 0.75% triclosan	C	not proved safe or effective, according to Antimicrobial I Panel
Fostex Cake (Westwood)	**soap:** 2% sulfur + 2% salicylic acid	C	not enough sulfur; combination is not proved effective

Acne Medications: Product Ratings *(continued)*

Product and Distributor	Dosage of Active Ingredients	Rating[1]	Comment
Fostex 10% Benzoyl Peroxide Cleansing Bar (Westwood)	**soap:** 10% benzoyl peroxide	A	
Salicylic Acid and Sulfur (Stiefel)	**soap:** 10% precipitated sulfur + 3% salicylic acid	B	neither salicylic acid nor this combination proved effective
SAStid (Stiefel)		B	
Sulfur Soap (Stiefel)	**soap:** 10% precipitated sulfur	A	

Liquid Cleansers

Product and Distributor	Dosage of Active Ingredients	Rating[1]	Comment
Acne-Dome Cleanser (Miles)	**liquid:** 2% colloidal sulfur + 2% salicylic acid	C	ineffectively low concentration of sulfur
Exzit Cleanser (Miles)		C	
Acno (Baker-Cummins)	**lotion:** 3% sulfur + 2% salicylic acid	B	salicylic acid not proved effective; combination not proved effective
Dry and Clear Medicated Acne Cleanser (Whitehall)	**liquid:** 0.5% salicylic acid + 0.5% benzoic acid	C	benzoic acid not effective
Drytex Lotion (C & M Pharm.)	**lotion:** 10% salicylic acid	B	salicylic acid not proved effective
Fomac Foam (Dermik)	**foam:** 2% salicylic acid	B	salicylic acid not proved effective
d-Seb Gel Skin Cleanser (Berlex)	2% chloroxylenol	C	ingredient not effective
Seba-Nil Liquid Cleanser (Owen)	**liquid:** no active anti-acne ingredients	C	not safe or effective as a drug, since contains no medicinal ingredients
Tyrosum Liquid (Summers)		C	not safe or effective as a drug, since contains no medicinal ingredients
Therapads (Parke-Davis)	**medicated pads:** 1.5% salicylic acid	B	salicylic acid not proved effective

1. Author's interpretation of Panel criteria. Based on contents, not claims.

Alcohol

See ANTISEPTICS

Allergy Drugs

See COLD, COUGH, AND ALLERGY DRUGS

Antacids

Millions of people use over-the-counter antacids—liquids, gels, tablets, capsules, chewing gums, and powders—to relieve symptoms of upper gastrointestinal distress. An antacid neutralizes hydrochloric acid.

When a person smells, tastes, chews, or swallows food—or sometimes even thinks about it—hydrochloric acid is produced. This is a potent gastric acid that is secreted by glands in the lining of the stomach to aid in the digestion of food. Why the same amount of acid secretions plagues some people but not others remains unclear.

The only symptoms that can be safely and effectively self-diagnosed and self-treated with nonprescription antacids are those that are caused by excess stomach acid. These symptoms have been described as a burning distress that is felt in the upper abdomen, behind the chest, and as high up as the throat.

CLAIMS

Accurate

   for relief of any of the following:
   "heartburn"

ANTACIDS is based on the report of the FDA's Advisory Review Panel on OTC Antacid Drugs, the FDA's Tentative Final Order for Antacid Products, the FDA's Final Order for Antacid and Antiflatulent Products Generally Recognized as Safe and Effective and Not Misbranded, and official addenda of the OTC drug review process. The section entitled "Antacids for Controlling Phosphate Levels" is based on the report "Hypophosphatemia and Hyperphosphatemia Drug Products" by the FDA's Advisory Review Panel on OTC Miscellaneous Internal Drug Products.

"sour stomach"

"acid indigestion"

"upset stomach" that occurs in association with any of the previous symptoms

False or Misleading

for the relief of any of the following:

"gas"

"upper abdominal pressure"

"full feeling"

"nausea"

"excessive eructations [belching]"

"sour breath"

"nervous and emotional disturbances"

"excessive smoking"

"food intolerance"

"consumption of alcoholic beverages"

"nervous-tension headaches"

"cold symptoms"

"morning sickness of pregnancy"

HOW THEY WORK

Antacids do *not* act by forming a protective, physical "coating" to keep acid away from the stomach wall. They work by means of the old saying "Opposites attract." That is, the antacid's negatively charged particles (negative ions) link with the positively charged hydrogen particles in the molecules of hydrochloric acid. Neutralization results.

In terms of acidity and its opposite, alkalinity, the chemical scale —called pH—ranges from 0 to 14. A pH of 7 is neutral. A substance that has a pH lower than 7 is acid. The lower the pH, the greater the acidity. The higher the pH above 7, the greater the alkalinity.

The stomach's normal pH is acidic to begin with. But in persons with gastric acidity, the pH may be somewhat below normal. There is also an increase in the *amount* of acid in the stomach.

Antacids raise the pH in the direction of pH 7, but they do not— and need not—completely neutralize the acids. An antacid that raises the stomach contents from pH 1.5 to pH 3.5 has produced a hundredfold reduction in the concentration of acid. In other words, 99 percent of the acid has been neutralized. This in turn inhibits pepsin, another potent component of the digestive juice. Pepsin's potentially irritating effect on the stomach lining has been largely stopped when the stomach contents reach a pH of 3.5.

POTENCY AND PALATABILITY

The Panel stipulated that one dose of an antacid product must be able to neutralize the amount of gastric juice that is present in a normal stomach at rest between meals: about 1 to 2 ounces. This must be measured in a lab test in which a comparable amount of pure hydrochloric acid must be raised to pH 3.5 within 10 minutes. The tight time requirement was set because antacids must act rapidly to be of value. When taken between meals, most of a standard dose has passed out of the stomach in 15 minutes.

The neutralizing capacity of the added substance (the antacid) is expressed in milliequivalents (meq) of hydrochloric acid. Every antacid product must have a total neutralizing capacity of at least 5 meq of hydrochloric acid per dosage unit. This is roughly enough to raise the pH in an essentially empty stomach to 3.5 The more potent a product is, the more acid it will neutralize. A product that neutralizes 7.5 meq acid per dose is half again as potent as one that neutralizes 5 meq; one that neutralizes 10 meq is twice as potent.

As of 1981, the FDA required that all manufacturers test their antacids and that potency information be included on product information intended for doctors. But manufacturers are *not* allowed to list the neutralizing capacity on labels of products sold over-the-counter to consumers. The reason? Publicizing this information might lead users to place undue reliance on an antacid's potency when there are other important considerations in choosing a product—for example, constipating effect, sodium content, and suitability for use over a certain length of time. (These subjects are discussed throughout this unit.)

Nevertheless, consumers may wish to know this information since the more potent the antacid, the less one has to take—and, by and large, the cheaper an effective dose is. The *acid-neutralizing capacity,* or *ANC,* for a number of antacid products is listed below.

The ANCs reveal great disparity in potency between antacid products. The widely respected *Medical Letter on Drugs and Therapeutics* (vol. 24, June 25, 1982, page 61) points out that there is a sevenfold difference in ANC between Amphojel (Wyeth), which is a weak antacid (ANC 6.5) and Delcid (Merrell-National), which is a strong one (ANC 42).

These differences become highly dramatic if one considers the antacid dose required to neutralize the acid present between meals in the stomach of a person with highly acidic digestive juices. The dose that will usually relieve pain in a person with a gastric ulcer must provide an ANC of roughly 152. If one uses Delcid, less than 4 teaspoonsful of antacid would be required. With Amphojel, by contrast, 23 teaspoonsful of the product would be required. Similarly, it would take 15 or 16 Tums (Norcliff Thayer) tablets, ANC 10, or 9 Camalox Tablets (Rorer), ANC 18, to achieve this result.

In using antacids to treat ulcers there clearly is a major advantage in selecting a more potent antacid—one with a high ANC. This advantage is enhanced by the fact that, by and large, the more potent the antacid, the *less* expensive an effective dose will be. One analysis shows, for example, that an effective dose of Delcid costs less than a quarter as much as an effective dose of Amphojel.

These potency differences also present a challenge to individuals who use antacids to self-treat heartburn, sour stomach, and other less-serious symptoms that appear to be related to acid. The *Medical Letter* points out that most manufacturers recommend doses of 1 to 2 teaspoonsful of liquid antacid, which would provide very different acid-neutralizing capacity, depending on the product. At these doses, which are approved by the FDA, the weaker antacids may deliver precious little neutralizing capacity. This suggests that relatively insignificant neutralization will suffice to quell these symptoms or, alternatively, as the Panel maintains, that acid and its neutralization may not be the whole story in the appearance or the relief of these symptoms.

Potency is not the only factor to consider in selecting an antacid. Palatability may be even more important. Antacids taste bad to many people, who thus may tend to take too little rather than too much of a product. The way to circumvent this problem is to choose the product that you, as an individual, find most palatable.

Acid-Neutralizing Capacity of Liquid Antacids

Product	Acid-Neutralizing Capacity in Meq Acid/Tsp Antacid	Standard Dose (To Neutralize 152 Meq Acid)
AlternaGEL (Stuart)	12	12 tsps
Aludrox (Wyeth)	14	11 tsps
Amphojel (Wyeth)	6.5	25 tsps
A-M-T (Wyeth)	11	14 tsps
Camalox (Rorer)	18	8 tsps
Delcid (Merrell-National)	42	4 tsps

Acid-Neutralizing Capacity of Liquid Antacids (continued)

Product	Acid-Neutralizing Capacity in Meq Acid/Tsp Antacid	Standard Dose (To Neutralize 152 Meq Acid)
Di-Gel (Plough)	12.5	12 tsps
Gelusil (Warner-Chilcott)	11.5	13 tsps
Gelusil II (Warner-Chilcott)	23.5	6 tsps
Kolantyl (Merrell-National)	10.5	14 tsps
Maalox (Rorer)	13.5	11 tsps
Maalox Plus (Rorer)	13.5	11 tsps
Maalox Therapeutic Concentrate	28.5	5 tsps
Mylanta (Stuart)	12.5	12 tsps
Mylanta II (Stuart)	25.5	6 tsps
Riopan (Ayerst)	11	14 tsps
Riopan Plus (Ayerst)	11	14 tsps
Simeco (Wyeth)	22	7 tsps
Titralac (Riker)	19	8 tsps

Acid-Neutralizing Capacity of Antacids in Tablets

Product	Acid Neutralizing Capacity in Meq Acid/Tablet	Number of Tablets (To Neutralize 152 Meq Acid)
Alka-Seltzer Effervescent (Miles)	10.6	15
Aludrox Tablets (Wyeth)	11.5	14
Amphogel Tablets (Wyeth)	9	17
Camalox Tablets (Rorer)	18	9
Gelusil Tablets (Parke-Davis)	11	14
Gelusil II Tablets (Parke-Davis)	21	8
Mylanta II Tablets (Stuart)	23	7
Riopan Tablets (Ayerst)	13.5	12
Tums (Norcliff Thayer)	10	16

SAFETY AND EFFECTIVENESS

There is great variability in the dosage needs for antacids—acid secretion varies widely from person to person and it also varies in the same person from time to time. Antacids are relatively nontoxic, and have a low potential for abuse. For these reasons the Panel decided not to set a maximum daily dosage limit based on effectiveness. Some ingredients, however, are potentially more toxic than others, and dosage limits were set in terms of safety. Sodium, for example, promotes water retention and high blood pressure—particularly in older persons and people whose kidneys may be failing. Sodium content of antacids now must appear on product labels.

An officially required label warning cautions users not to exceed the maximum daily dose and not to use the product for more than 2 weeks unless under a doctor's direction.

ANTACIDS AND PEPTIC ULCERS

Evaluators did not try to relate gastric-acid symptoms to underlying causes or disease states. They did note, however, that the over-the-counter antacid products used for the self-treatment of acid indigestion also are prescribed—often in much higher dosages—to treat peptic ulcers. Peptic ulcers are serious, often painful, erosions into the wall of the stomach or upper small intestine (duodenum). These disorders are believed to be caused, in part at least, by excessive gastric acid.

A clinical study published in 1977 demonstrated that extremely large dosages—up to 7 1-ounce doses of antacid products containing aluminum hydroxide or a combination of aluminum hydroxide and magnesium hydroxide each day—will heal most duodenal ulcers within 7 weeks' time. This therapy was found equal in effectiveness to the use of a potent prescription drug (Tagamet).

However, these investigators concurred with the Panel's earlier conclusion that ulcers should not be self-treated. Persons with diagnosed or presumed ulcer disease—or any other acid-related gastrointestinal disorders—should be under the care and supervision of a physician, even if the medication they are taking is a nonprescription antacid.

ANTACIDS FOR CONTROLLING PHOSPHATE LEVELS

Two aluminum-containing antacids are used—and are effective—in regulating levels of phosphates. Phosphates are compounds normally present in the body. There are, however, several illnesses that cause abnormally low or abnormally high levels of phosphate in the blood and other body tissues.

Two nonprescription antacid products carry labels that say the preparations can correct these defects. One raises and one lowers phosphate levels. Recent research findings strongly indicate that the aluminum in these drugs can cause serious brain degeneration (encephalopathy). What is worse, according to the FDA's Panel reviewers, this risk is especially great in some of those patients who need the most help in regulating phosphate levels. For example, individuals with impaired kidney functioning are unable to adequately filter aluminum out of the bloodstream.

The phosphate disturbances for which these antacids are used cannot be self-diagnosed or self-treated. Evaluators recommend that nonprescription product labels not be allowed to list these uses. They maintain that antacid products should be used for phosphate regulation only under a doctor's supervision.

Specific Conditions

Hypophosphatemia When there is *too little* phosphate in the bloodstream and other body tissues, one refers to hypophosphatemia. This condition tends to occur in persons who have severe kidney disease or who have received kidney transplants. Their parathyroid glands secrete too much parathyroid hormone; this in turn depletes the body's phosphate levels. Phosphate is needed to balance calcium levels, and when too little is available to the body, the calcium builds up to dangerously high levels in the bones, blood vessels, and in some organs.

Depleted phosphate levels can be successfully restored by treating patients with phosphate in the form of aluminum phosphate gel; this is a standard antacid. In one study of kidney-transplant patients cited by reviewers, the gel corrected the problem in 8 out of 9 patients.

The risk of brain damage from using this drug without a doctor's advice is much too great—especially in those patients whose aluminum-clearing organs, the kidneys, are not working well. The Panel recommends that aluminum phosphate gel be made a prescription drug for supplementing phosphate levels. They also note that the only aluminum-phosphate-gel product for which a phosphate-supplementing claim has been made is Phosphaljel (Wyeth). If the FDA concurs in the Panel's proposal, this claim will no longer be allowed.

Hyperphosphatemia Excessively *high* levels of phosphate (hyperphosphatemia) are found in the bloodstream and in other body tissues of persons suffering from phosphate kidney stones, renal osteodystrophy (a serious disease that causes bone deterioration), inadequate output of parathyroid hormone, and other medical conditions—all of which require a doctor's diagnosis and management. Hyperphosphatemia can be corrected by taking aluminum carbonate, a standard antacid preparation. The drug is judged safe for prescription use, although it may cause temporary constipation and might produce symptoms of weakness, dizziness, and loss of appetite if used to excess. But aluminum carbonate is not safe for over-the-counter use in treating conditions requiring medical care—labels should not carry phosphate-lowering indications. Apparently the only aluminum carbonate antacid labeled this way is Basaljel (Wyeth), sold in capsules, tablets, and liquid suspensions.

COMBINATION PRODUCTS

The 4 principal neutralizing ingredients in antacids are sodium bicarbonate, calcium carbonate, aluminum compounds, and magnesium compounds. Almost all antacid products contain at least one of the four; most contain at least two. The ingredients and the products into which they are formulated vary considerably in potency. Sodium bicarbonate and calcium carbonate are more potent than the magnesium compounds, which in turn tend to be more potent than the aluminum ones.

Some combination products treat acid indigestion and closely related symptoms. Others are intended to simultaneously treat gastric acidity and other problems, such as headache.

Antacids Combined with Other Antacids

The FDA permits up to four antacid active ingredients to be combined, provided that each contributes at least 25 percent of the product's acid-neutralizing capacity. (A number of inactive ingredients are used in formulating the products, but they were outside the reviewers' purview.)

A modest amount of a laxative that has been categorized as safe and effective can be added to an antacid product to correct its constipating effect. But no laxative effect can be claimed for such a product, nor can a substance like mineral oil be used since too few people experience acid indigestion and constipation simultaneously.

Antacids Combined with Other Active Ingredients

Approved combinations A drug that safely and effectively relieves symptoms of intestinal gas (flatulence) can be combined with an antacid. This antacid-antiflatulent combination is to be used—and must be labeled—only for the relief of gas that is experienced with heartburn, sour stomach, or acid indigestion. One drug, simethicone, is approved as a safe and effective over-the-counter drug for treating gas pains, and so it may be combined with antacids.

The FDA also permits the combination of antacid ingredients with safe and effective pain-killing ingredients (analgesics). These combinations are approved only when acid indigestion and headache occur together, and they must be sold in a form that can be taken as a liquid.

Disapproved combinations   It is not safe or effective to combine antacids with drugs of the class called anticholinergics. These drugs are used in nonprescription products as drying agents for runny nose or watery eyes. The dosages of antacids and anticholinergics must be individually determined.

The same ban applies to the combination of an antacid with a sedative or relaxant; with drugs to prevent nausea and vomiting; and with antipeptic agents. Combining an antacid with an antipeptic or with bile or bile salts could contribute to a user's developing ulcers.

ANTACID INGREDIENTS

Approved Active Ingredients

Most traditional antacid ingredients have been approved for over-the-counter use in the FDA's review process. They are judged to be effective on the basis of reports in the scientific literature and on tests which show that each tablet, capsule, or other dosage unit has the capacity to neutralize the acid present between meals in an essentially empty stomach.

Compared with other groups of drugs, like pain-killers, antacids are considered very safe. Nevertheless, they may pose a threat to some persons—particularly if taken in large amounts for extended periods of time.

Aluminum compounds   Compounds that contain aluminum tend to be very safe as antacid ingredients because very little aluminum is absorbed from the gastrointestinal tract into the body. So no dosage limits have been established—except for aluminum phosphate (8 grams per day), because phosphate intake should be limited.

The complications that do occur when taking aluminum-containing antacids usually are the result of their obstructive effect in the intestines. These products tend to be viscous, and since they are relatively weak as antacids, large doses may be required—which could induce intestinal blockage. Simple constipation, however, is the more common occurrence.

Some manufacturers counteract the constipating tendency of aluminum antacid ingredients by combining them with magnesium ingredients or other substances that have the opposite (laxative) effect.

Aluminum interferes with the absorption of some prescription drugs, most notably the antibiotic tetracycline. It should not be taken by patients for whom tetracycline has been prescribed by a doctor.

Even though the FDA concurred with the Panel in approving aluminum-containing compounds as safe and effective, more recent studies indicate that they could be risky for individuals with kidney problems, and persons on kidney dialysis, in whom they can cause a severe neurologic disturbance called dialysis dementia. Of wider concern is recent evidence which suggests that heavy use of aluminum-containing antacids may adversely affect the metabolism of the minerals phosphorus, calcium and fluoride in the body, and cause or intensify bone abnormalities. Evidence also suggests that aluminum may cause or contribute to development of a common form of early senility called *Alzheimer's disease.* These concerns prompted the Associated Pharmacologists & Toxicologists to petition the FDA in 1982 asking the Agency to restudy the safety of aluminum-containing antacids.

Bicarbonate compounds   The bicarbonate compounds used as antacids include sodium bicarbonate (ordinary baking soda) and potassium bicarbonate. Both are potent neutralizers of stomach acid. So are sodium carbonate and potassium carbonate, which are used in effervescent preparations that are drunk as bubbling liquids.

The principal drawback of bicarbonates is that they are readily absorbed into the body. There they can measurably increase the alkalinity of blood plasma and other body tissues. They probably cannot raise the pH of plasma beyond a range that is normal, but the effects of their prolonged use are largely unknown. Bicarbonates could be particularly risky for persons with impaired kidney function. When carbonate is taken as sodium bicarbonate, the sodium is absorbed from the intestine into the body. For people with defective kidneys who have trouble ridding their bodies of sodium, the buildup can be a hazard.

Sodium bicarbonate—which is widely used as a food product, tooth cleanser, and mouthwash, as well as an antacid—has an extremely low potential for causing injury by overdose. But the suggested upper dosage limit is 10 grams per day for persons up to age 60; 5 grams per day for persons over 60.

Bismuth compounds   The bismuth-containing compounds marketed as antacids are considered safe in the amounts commonly used. The oral dose for adults is 1 gram, and the usual daily dosage is 4 grams —so 4 doses can be taken each day.

Calcium compounds   The 2 approved ingredients—calcium carbonate and calcium phosphate—are fast-acting neutralizers of gastric acid. They also are quite potent. Very small doses are as effective as far larger amounts of other antacid ingredients.

However, safety considerations suggest limiting one's intake of calcium. It can cause constipation. It also is readily absorbed from the gut into the body and may form calcium kidney stones or trigger other toxic consequences. For these reasons, the Panel recommended that no more than 8 grams of calcium carbonate be taken daily. The limit for calcium phosphate is 13.1 grams (about half an ounce).

Consumers should also be aware of a somewhat puzzling dual action. While calcium-containing antacid ingredients relieve acidity, they can also stimulate the secretion of stomach acids—which is the opposite effect of that sought. Some experts say, therefore, that calcium-containing compounds should not be used as antacids. But the information thus far available does not warrant such a restriction. So these active ingredients are fully approved as safe and effective for self-treatment.

Citrates   Neither the Panel nor the FDA has much to say about citrate-containing antacid ingredients like citric acid, except that they are safe and effective. The recommended maximum daily dosage is 8 grams, a bit less than a third of an ounce.

Glycine (aminoacetic acid)   This amino acid is practically nontoxic. It is judged safe without dosage restriction for nonprescription use as an antacid when taken for up to 2 weeks. Research studies indicate that amino acids like glycine are quite effective in initially neutralizing sour stomach contents, but they are less effective in providing further neutralization after a pH of 2.5 has been achieved.

Magnesium compounds   The magnesium antacid substances for the most part are less potent than calcium or sodium carbonates. When they neutralize hydrochloric acid, the compound magnesium chloride is formed. Some of it is absorbed into the body, but then it is rapidly and safely excreted by the kidneys except for those people whose kidney function is impaired. For them, lowered blood pressure, nausea, vomiting, respiratory distress, and even coma may result from these magnesium compounds.

Magnesium is an essential nutrient that is contained in food. About one-third of dietary magnesium is absorbed. Even less of the magnesium in antacids is absorbed. This unabsorbed magnesium has the effect of pulling water into the intestine, causing diarrhea. To counteract this effect, materials that have the opposite (constipating) effect—particularly calcium or aluminum—are often mixed with magnesium in antacid products.

Panel reviewers believe magnesium-containing antacids are, in commonly used dosages, unlikely to cause other side effects. No restriction has been placed on daily intake, and they may be used for up to 2 weeks. However, products that contain relatively large amounts of magnesium should not be used by persons with kidney problems except under medical supervision.

Milk solids, dried Milk solids are used as antacid active ingredients. They are safe for this purpose in the amounts usually taken in antacid products, so that no dosage limit has been set on their use.

Phosphate compounds The amounts of phosphates usually taken orally for antacid purposes are relatively low and safe. Products formulated with mono- or dibasic calcium phosphate as the phosphate source usually contain 200 mg per tablet; the customary dosage is up to 8 tablets per day. Products that contain aluminum phosphate are formulated with up to 2 grams per tablet, with a recommended dosage of up to 4 tablets daily. When the phospate source is tricalcium phosphate, each tablet contains 1 to 4 grams, and the package directions suggest up to 6 tablets daily. All these dosages are safe, provided the product is not used longer than 2 weeks without the individual's seeing a doctor.

An aluminum phosphate gel long has been marketed over the counter as an antacid and currently is assessed as safe and effective by the FDA. But data submitted to the FDA and evaluted by the Miscellaneous Internal Drug Products Panel indicates that this gel fails to meet the acid-neutralizing test and so "is not acceptable" as an antacid.

Potassium compounds Several antacids contain potassium, usually in the form of sodium potassium tartrate or potassium citrate. While the buildup of potassium in the body can be dangerous to health, this is a rare problem that tends to occur only in people with inadequate kidney function. There is no evidence that normal persons risk potassium toxicity (hyperkalemia) when they use the popular antacids that contain this ingredient. No maximum daily intake level has been set, but products that contain relatively large amounts of potassium must carry the warning that persons with kidney disease should take them only under the advice and care of a physician.

Silicates Antacid active ingredients that carry silicates—including magnesium aluminosilicates and magnesium trisilicate—appear relatively safe. While there are reports of patients' developing kidney stones, there is insufficient evidence to conclude that a maximum daily dosage needs to be set.

Magnesium trisilicate, however, may interfere with the absorption of some other drugs. Persons who are taking other medications should consult their doctor.

Sodium compounds   The problem with sodium, which principally concerns older persons, is that it triggers and exacerbates high blood pressure. This risk is increased when a person has poor kidney function and cannot quickly excrete sodium from the body. Thus, limits have been set on the amount that should be taken each day in nonprescription antacid products, including sodium bicarbonate (baking soda), sodium carbonate, and sodium potassium carbonate. If one were taking pure sodium bicarbonate powder—baking soda—this limit would be 2 to 2½ teaspoonsful for persons over age 60, and 4½-teaspoonsful for younger persons.

Tartrate compounds   Although tartrates—which include tartaric acid and its salts—are found in baking powder and a variety of other foods, and seem safe, the effect of their repeated day-to-day medicinal use in antacids has not been adquately studied. In high doses, they conceivably could cause kidney problems.

It still is not clear whether tartrate is absorbed into the body; tartrate metabolism is poorly defined. Balancing both this lack of knowledge and possible risk against traditional usage, evaluators set a maximum daily dose limit of 15 grams—just over half an ounce—even though tartrate and its equivalents are assessed as safe and effective.

Conditionally Approved Active Ingredient

Alginic acid   Ten years after the start of the review process, the status of one active ingredient of antacid products—alginic acid—remained to be determined.

Alginic acid is not an antacid. Rather, according to a manufacturer's petition, it is a substance that reacts with sodium bicarbonate (with which it is formulated) to form a floating foam that rises to the top of the stomach. It thus may be partially effective in relieving heartburn, or inflammation of the esophagus—provided the person is standing, sitting, or reclining with his head and trunk in a relatively upright position. The FDA does not believe manufacturers have adequately demonstrated that alginic acid contributes to the effectiveness of antacid products that contain it. But the agency extended its deadline to give them added time for presentation of acceptable data.

Disapproved Active Ingredients

Several ingredients that formerly were used in antacid products have been banned by the FDA as ineffective as antacids. They are:

attapulgite, activated
carboxymethylcellulose
charcoal, activated
gastric mucin
kaolin
methylcellulose
pectin

Safety and Effectiveness: Active Ingredients
in Over-the-Counter Antacids

Neutralizing Agent	Panel and FDA† Assessment
alginic acid	safe but not proved effective
aluminum compounds	
aluminum carbonate	safe and effective
aluminum hydroxide	safe and effective
aluminum hydroxide-hexitol, stabilized polymer	safe and effective
aluminum hydroxide-magnesium carbonate, co-dried gel	safe and effective
aluminum hydroxide-magnesium trisilicate, co-dried gel	safe and effective
aluminum hydroxide sucrose powder, hydrated	safe and effective
aluminum phosphate*	safe and effective
dihydroxyaluminum aminoacetate	safe and effective
dihydroxyaluminum aminoacetic	safe and effective
dihydroxyaluminum sodium carbonate	safe and effective
attapulgite, activated	not effective
bismuth compounds	safe and effective
bismuth aluminate	safe and effective
bismuth carbonate	safe and effective
bismuth subcarbonate	safe and effective
bismuth subgallate	safe and effective
bismuth subnitrate	safe and effective
calcium compounds	
calcium carbonate	safe and effective
calcium phosphate	safe and effective
carboxymethylcellulose	not effective
charcoal, activated	not effective
citrate compounds	
citric acid	safe and effective
citric salts	safe and effective
gastric mucin	not effective
glycine (aminoacetic acid)	safe and effective
kaolin	not effective

Safety and Effectiveness: Active Ingredients in Over-the-Counter Antacids *(continued)*

Neutralizing Agent	*Panel and FDA† Assessment*
magnesium compounds	safe and effective
hydrate magnesium aluminate,	
activated sulfate	safe and effective
magaldrate	safe and effective
magnesium aluminosilicate	safe and effective
magnesium carbonate	safe and effective
magnesium glycinate	safe and effective
magnesium hydroxide	safe and effective
magnesium oxide	safe and effective
magnesium trisilicate	safe and effective
methylcellulose	not effective
milk solids, dried	safe and effective
pectin	not effective
phosphate compounds	
aluminum phosphate	safe and effective
mono- or dibasic calcium salt	safe and effective
tricalcium phosphate	safe and effective
potassium compounds	
potassium bicarbonate	safe and effective
potassium carbonate	safe and effective
sodium potassium tartrate	safe and effective
silicates	
magnesium aluminosilicate	safe and effective
magnesium trisilicate	safe and effective
sodium compounds	
sodium bicarbonate	safe and effective
sodium carbonate	safe and effective
sodium potassium tartrate	safe and effective
tartrate compounds	
sodium potassium tartrate	safe and effective
tartaric acid	safe and effective
tartrate	safe and effective

†Judgments reaffirmed or modified by the FDA, or originated by it.
*Recent data indicate that a widely marketed aluminum phosphate gel may not be an acceptably strong antacid.

Safety and Effectiveness: Active Ingredients in Over-the-Counter Phosphate-Regulating Drugs

Active Ingredient	*Action*	*Panel's Assessment*
aluminum carbonate	depletes phosphates	not safe
aluminum phosphate gel	supplements phosphates	not safe

Antacids: Product Ratings[1]

Single-Ingredient Products

Product and Distributor	Dosage of Active Ingredients	Rating[2]	Comment
aluminum carbonate gel, basic			
Basaljel (Wyeth)	**capsules and swallow tablets:** dried basic aluminum carbonate gel equivalent to 608 mg dried aluminum hydroxide gel or 500 mg aluminum hydroxide	A	
aluminum hydroxide gel			
Alternagel (Stuart)	**liquid:** 600 mg per teaspoonful	A	
Alu-Cap (Riker)	**capsules:** 475 mg	A	
Aluminum Hydroxide Gel (Schein)	**tablets, chewable:** 487 mg, 450 mg	A	
aluminum hydroxide gel, USP (generic)	**suspension**	A	
Amphojel (Wyeth)	**tablets:** 300 mg, 600 mg	A	
	suspension: 320 mg per teaspoonful		
aluminum phosphate gel			
Phosphaljel (Wyeth)	**suspension:** 233 mg per teaspoonful	A[3]	
calcium carbonate			
Alka-2 (Miles Labs.)	**tablets, chewable:** 500 mg	A	
Chooz (Plough)		A	
Tums (Norcliff Thayer)		A	
Amitone (Norcliff Thayer)	**tablets, chewable:** 350 mg	A	
calcium carbonate (generic)	**tablets:** 650 mg	A	
Mallamint (Mallard)	**tablets, chewable:** 420 mg	A	

Antacids: Product Ratings[1] (continued)

Single-Ingredient Products

Product and Distributor	Dosage of Active Ingredients	Rating[2]	Comment
dihydroxyaluminum aminoacetate			
Robalate (Robins)	**tablets, chewable:** 500 mg	A	
dihydroxyaluminum sodium carbonate			
Rolaids (Warner-Lambert)	**tablets, chewable:** 334 mg	A	
magaldrate (hydroxymagnesium aluminate)			
Riopan (Ayerst)	**swallow tablets:** 480 mg	A	
	tablets, chewable: 480 mg	A	
	suspension: 480 mg per teaspoonful	A	
magnesium carbonate			
magnesium carbonate (generic)	**powder**	A	
magnesium hydroxide (magnesia)			
milk of magnesia (generic)	**tablets:** 325 mg	A	
	liquid	A	
Milk of Magnesia (CMC)	**tablets:** 650 mg	A	
Phillips' Milk of Magnesia (Glenbrook)	**tablets:** 311 mg	A	
	suspension: approx. 360 mg per teaspoonful	A	
magnesium oxide			
Mag Ox 400 (Blaine)	**tablets:** 400 mg	A	
Maox (Kenneth Manne)	**tablets:** 420 mg	A	
Par-Mag (Parmed)	**capsules:** 140 mg	A	

magnesium trisilicate
magnesium trisilicate (generic)   tablets: 488 mg   A

sodium bicarbonate (contains 27% sodium)
Arm and Hammer Baking Soda (Church and Dwight)   powder: bicarbonate of soda, USP   A
Soda Mint (Schein)   tablets: 487.5 mg   A
sodium bicarbonate (generic)   tablets: 325 mg, 650 mg   A

Combination Products

Product and Distributor	aluminum hydroxide	magnesium hydroxide	calcium carbonate	magnesium trisilicate	Other Content[1]	Rating[2]
capsules and tablets						
Alkets Tablets (Upjohn)			780 mg		130 mg magnesium carbonate + 65 mg magnesium oxide	A
Alma-Mag #4 Tablets (Rugby)	260 mg			488 mg		A
Aludrox Tablets (Wyeth)	233 mg	83 mg				A
Bisodol Tablets (Whitehall)		178 mg	194 mg			A
Calcilac Tablets (Schein)			420 mg		180 mg glycine	A
Di-Gel Tablets (Plough)		85 mg			282 mg (aluminum hydroxide + magnesium carbonate) + 25 mg simethicone	A
Estomul-M Tablets (Riker)					500 mg (aluminum hydroxide + magnesium carbonate) + 45 mg magnesium oxide	A
Gaviscon Tablets (Marion)	80 mg			20 mg	200 mg alginic acid + sodium bicarbonate	B[1]

Antacids: Product Ratings[1] (continued)

Product and Distributor	aluminum hydroxide	magnesium hydroxide	calcium carbonate	magnesium trisilicate	Other Content	Rating[2]
capsules and tablets						
Gelusil Tablets (Parke-Davis)	200 mg	200 mg			25 mg simethicone	A
Gustalac Tablets (Geriatric)			300 mg		200 mg defatted skim-milk powder	A
Kolantyl Tablets (Merrell-Dow)	300 mg	170 mg				A
Kolantyl Wafers (Merrell-Dow)	180 mg	200 mg			185 mg magnesium oxide	A
Maalox No. 1 Tablets (Rorer)	200 mg	200 mg				A
Maalox No. 2 Tablets (Rorer)	400 mg	400 mg				A
Maalox Plus Tablets (Rorer)	200 mg	200 mg			25 mg simethicone	A
Mylanta Tablets (Stuart)	200 mg	200 mg			20 mg simethicone	A
Mylanta-II Tablets (Stuart)	400 mg	400 mg			30 mg simethicone	A
Neosorb Plus Tablets (Lemmon)	300 mg	150 mg			tartrazine	A
PAMA # 2 Tablets (No. American)			420 mg		180 mg glycine	A
Riopan Plus Chew Tablets (Ayerst)					480 mg magaldrate + 20 mg simethicone	A
Spastosed Tablets (No. American)			226 mg		162 mg magnesium carbonate	A
Trimagel Tablets (Columbia Med.)	250 mg			500 mg		A
Titralac Tablets (Riker)			420 mg		180 mg glycine	A

Product and Distributor	Dosage of Active Ingredients	Rating[2]	Comment
Liquids and Suspensions: contents given mg per teaspoonful (5 ml)			
Almacone II Liquid (Rugby)	400 / 400	A	30 mg simethicone
Aludrox Suspension (Wyeth)	307 / 103	A	
Alumid Plus Suspension (Vangard)	200 / 200	A	20 mg simethicone
Camalox Suspension (Rorer)	225 / 200 / 250	A	
Delcid Suspension (Merrell-National)	600 / 665	A	
Di-Gel Liquid (Plough)	282 / 87	A	25 mg simethicone
Maalox Suspension (Rorer)	225 / 200	A	
Maalox Plus Suspension (Rorer)	225 / 200	A	25 mg simethicone
Maalox Therapeutic Concentrate (Rorer)	600 / 300	A	
Mylanta Liquid (Stuart)	200 / 200	A	20 mg simethicone
Riopan Plus Suspension (Ayerst)		A	480 mg magaldrate + 20 mg simethicone
Rolox Suspension (Purepac)	200 / 200	A	
Simeco Suspension (Wyeth)	365 / 300	A	30 mg simethicone
Titralac Liquid (Riker)	1000	A	300 mg glycine
Tralmag Suspension (O'Neal)	150 / 150	A	200 mg dihydroxyaluminum aminoacetate
WinGel Liquid (Winthrop)	180 / 160	A	
powders and effervescent tablets			
Alka-Seltzer without Aspirin (Miles Labs.)	effervescent tablets: 958 mg sodium bicarbonate + 832 mg citric acid + 312 mg potassium bicarbonate	A	

Antacids: Product Ratings[1] (continued)

Product and Distributor	Dosage of Active Ingredients	Rating[2]	Comment
Bisodol (Whitehall)	**powder and effervescent tablets** **powder:** 644 mg sodium bicarbonate + 475 mg magnesium carbonate per 5 g	A	
Bromo Seltzer (Warner-Lambert)	**effervescent granules:** 325 mg acetaminophen + 2.781 g sodium bicarbonate + 2.224 g citric acid per dosage measure	A	
Citrocarbonate (Upjohn)	**effervescent salt:** 1.82 g sodium citrate + 0.78 g sodium bicarbonate per 3.9 g dose	A	

Antacids Used to Manipulate Phosphate Levels

Product and Distributor	Dosage of Active Ingredients	Rating[2]	Comment
aluminum carbonate gel, basic Basaljel (Wyeth)	**capsules and swallow tablets:** dried basic aluminum carbonate gel equivalent to 608 mg dried aluminum hydroxide gel or 500 mg aluminum hydroxide	C	not safe for self-treatment to lower phosphate levels in body
aluminum phosphate gel Phosphaljel (Wyeth)	**suspension:** 233 mg per teaspoonful	C	not safe for self-treatment to raise phosphate levels in body

1. All currently-marketed antacid products are required to meet final standards of the Over the Counter Drug Review, except that one ingredient, alginic acid, which may be formulated as sodium alginate, still has not been proved to be effective—so products containing it are rated "B."
2. Author's interpretation of Panel/FDA criteria. Based on contents, not claims.
3. Does not meet FDA acid-neutralizing standard, according to OTC Miscellaneous Internal Drug Panel.

Antibiotics for Skin Infections

Pus-filled bumps surrounded by reddened, warmish skin can be surprisingly painful—and ugly. No one is wholly spared these skin infections. They are unpleasant enough that one wants to be rid of them at the earliest possible moment.

NATURAL HEALING NEEDS LITTLE HELP

Fortunately, most minor skin infections heal by themselves, within a week; the major and unresolved question is whether (and to what extent) self-treatment with potent germ-killing drugs may be helpful in treatment or prevention.

Infections are caused by bacteria and other types of microorganisms. In the last half-century scientists have developed potent drugs, called antibiotics, that kill bacteria or control their growth. They are of life-saving value in curing major infections, and most antibiotics are available only by prescription. But a few older ones are now sold over-the-counter—usually in ointment form—as self-medication for small skin infections.

Millions of people buy and use these ointments, which typically combine two or more antibiotic agents. Yet surprisingly, the Panel found little evidence to demonstrate that these products are necessary or effective. The FDA, assessing these findings, decided that they are "inappropriate" for self-treatment of skin infections, since the average person has no means of determining what kind of bacteria is causing a particular infection, and so cannot select the right antibiotic to treat it. Treatment of an infection usually involves oral or injected antibiotics, the FDA added, rather than topically applied drugs.

The FDA does approve first-aid use of these antibiotics on fresh skin wounds in an attempt to *prevent* infections. This preventive usage is assessed in the unit FIRST-AID PREPARATIONS FOR SKIN WOUNDS.

If the FDA sticks by its position that antibiotics are inappropriate —as well, apparently, as ineffective—for treating skin infections, it eventually will forbid manufacturers to make treatment claims on these products' labels.

ANTIBIOTICS FOR SKIN INFECTIONS is based on the report "Topical Antibiotic Products" by the FDA's Advisory Review Panel on OTC Antimicrobial Drug Products (Antimicrobial II Panel), and the FDA's Tentative Final Order on these drugs.

CLAIMS

False or Misleading
"treats infection"
"decreases bacteria"
"helps reduce the number of bacteria in the treated area"
"aid," "speed," "augment," or "hasten" healing

TYPES OF INFECTION

Skin infections, collectively, are called pyoderma, which means "pus in the skin." The infected area usually is red and warm, and painful or tender. There are two types of these infections: primary, which arise in apparently normal or uninjured skin, and secondary, which develop when bacteria take hold where the protective upper layers of the skin have been broached by a cut, scrape, or burn; by poison ivy or a similar allergic eruption, or insect bites; or by chronic skin problems like diaper rash, eczema, or the ulcers that sometimes plague older persons who suffer from poor circulation. Some skin infections are of added medical concern because they may provide a breeding ground for bacteria that can travel through the bloodstream and seriously damage the kidneys and other internal organs.

Primary Infections

Several primary skin infections are often self-treated with nonprescription antibiotic preparations.

Impetigo   This is a common, very contagious, skin infection that afflicts many children. Blisters emerge on the skin and break open to form thick, yellowish-red crusts. The cause is usually either *Staphylococcus aureus* ("staph") or Group A beta-hemolytic streptococcus ("strep").

Ecthymas   Ecthymas are deeper, spreading, pus-filled sores that can arise on the legs in insect bite sites. They may leave lasting scars in their wake. Strep is the usual cause.

Folliculitis   A small, tight, red, pus-filled blister can arise from a hair follicle. Staph is often the cause. If left alone, these infections open, dry up, and go away—but if scratched, they fester and spread.

Boils   A boil—referred to in medicine as a furuncle—is a skin-follicle infection that swells into a large, deep, red, and often very painful pus-filled bump. Staph is the most probable bacteria. Boils should not be self-treated with nonprescription drugs (*see* BOIL OINT-MENTS).

Acute paronychia   A staph infection can occur around or under a fingernail or toenail. It causes a red, tender, pus-filled swelling.

CAUSES, EFFECTS, TREATMENT OF SKIN INFECTIONS

Primary infections tend to erupt unexpectedly. Little can be suggested to prevent them other than paying basic respect to cleanliness and good skin care. Consequently these infections must be treated after they appear. A secondary infection, however, sometimes can be prevented by applying antibiotics or other antimicrobial drugs to cut, bruised, burned, or otherwise wounded skin.

Primary infections in the skin for the most part are caused by gram-positive bacteria. This designation is based on their penchant for absorbing a dye (called Gram's stain) that colors them purple, making them clearly visible under a microscope. Secondary infections very often are caused by gram-negative bacteria, which show up with a faint pink color. Gram-negative organisms tend to be more dangerous than gram-positive ones. They also tend to be susceptible to different antibiotics.

The best medicine for a small, isolated skin infection may well be to keep it clean and leave it alone. Hot soaks may help relieve the discomfort and cause the pus to "point" and drain.

Should you lance a small infection with the point of a clean needle to speed drainage? Many people do. Doctors say it is better to let a health professional do it for you.

If an infection continues to worsen, spreads, deepens, becomes more painful, or induces a fever, then there is no question what to do: see a doctor.

Safe, effective prescription drugs are available for treating common infections. It is a mistake to dally and risk the infection's spread when this treatment easily can be had from a doctor.

ANTIBIOTIC INGREDIENTS

Approved Active Ingredients

None

Conditionally Approved Active Ingredients

None

Disapproved Active Ingredients

The following antibiotics—each of which is described more fully as an "Approved" or "Conditionally Approved" ingredient in FIRST-AID PREPARATIONS FOR SKIN WOUNDS—are evaluated by the FDA as inappropriate and apparently ineffective for the self-treatment of self-diagnosed skin infections:

> bacitracin
> gramicidin
> neomycin
> polymyxin
> tetracyclines
> > chlortetracycline hydrochloride
> > oxytetracycline hydrochloride
> > tetracycline hydrochloride

Combination Products

Topical antibiotics are often sold in products that contain two or three antibiotic active ingredients. Since all individual ingredients are disapproved, it follows that all combinations are also disapproved. The disapproved combinations include the following:

> bacitracin + neomycin
> bacitracin + polymyxin + neomycin
> bacitracin + polymyxin
> neomycin + gramicidin
> polymyxin + gramicidin
> tetracycline + bacitracin
> tetracycline + polymyxin
> tetracycline + gramicidin

All combinations of antibiotics with other active ingredients are similarly disapproved. The Panel notes that it is particularly unwise to combine an antibiotic with a pain-reliever, since pain is a signal that an infection is growing worse—so that one should seek medical care.

Safety and Effectiveness: Antibiotics in Over-the-Counter Medications For Treating Skin Infections

Antibiotic Ingredient	FDA's Assessment
bacitracin	not safe and/or not effective
gramicidin	not safe and/or not effective
neomycin	not safe and/or not effective
polymyxin alone	not safe and/or not effective
polymyxin + bacitracin or a tetracycline*	not safe and/or not effective
tetracycline*	not safe and/or not effective

*chlortetracycline hydrochloride, oxytetracycline hydrochloride, or tetracycline hydrochloride

Antibiotics for Treating Skin Infections: Product Ratings[1]

Single-Ingredient Products

Product and Distributor	Dosage of Active Ingredients	Rating[2]	Comment
bacitracin			
bacitracin (generic)	ointment: 500 units per g	C	not safe and/or not effective
Baciguent (Upjohn)		C	not safe and/or not effective
chlortetracycline hydrochloride			
Aureomycin (Lederle)	ointment: 3%	C	not safe and/or not effective
neomycin sulfate			
neomycin (generic)	ointment: 5 mg per g (0.5%)	C	not safe and/or not effective
Myciguent (Upjohn)		C	not safe and/or not effective
tetracycline hydrochloride			
Achromycin (Lederle)	ointment: 3%	C	not safe and/or not effective

Antibiotics for Treating Skin Infections: Product Ratings[1] *(continued)*

Combination Products

Product and Distributor	Dosage of Active Ingredients	Rating[2]	Comment
Bacimycin (Merrell-National)	**ointment:** 500 units zinc bacitracin + 3.5 mg neomycin base (as sulfate) per g	C	not safe and/or not effective
Baximin (Columbia Med.)	**ointment:** 5000 units polymyxin B sulfate + 3.5 mg neomycin base (as sulfate) + 400 units bacitracin per g	C	not safe and/or not effective
Hysoquen (Tutag)		C	not safe and/or not effective
Neo-Polycin (Dow)		C	not safe and/or not effective
Neosporin (Burroughs-Wellcome)		C	not safe and/or not effective
Epimycin "A" (Delta Drug)	**ointment:** 5000 units polymyxin B sulfate + 3.5 mg neomycin base (as sulfate) + 400 units bacitracin + 10 mg diperodon hydrochloride per g	C	not safe and/or not effective
Spectrocin (Squibb)	**ointment:** 2.5 mg neomycin base (as sulfate) + 0.25 mg gramicidin per g	C	not safe and/or not effective
Terramycin with Polymyxin B Sulfate (Pfipharmecs)	**ointment:** 30 mg oxytetracycline (as hydrochloride) + 10,000 units polymyxin B sulfate per g	C	not safe and/or not effective
Tri-Salve (Rexall)	**ointment:** 5000 units polymyxin B sulfate + 3.5 mg neomycin base (as sulfate) + 500 units zinc bacitracin per g + 3% benzocaine	C	not safe and/or not effective

1. For use of these products in preventing skin infection, *see* FIRST AID PREPARATIONS, p. 330.
2. Author's interpretation of FDA criteria. Based on contents, not claims.

Antidotes for Poison
See POISONING ANTIDOTES

Anti-Gas Agents

A drug that expels gas from the stomach and intestines is often called an antiflatulent, since *flatus* is the technical—and "polite"—word for gastrointestinal-tract gas.

One active ingredient, simethicone, is approved as safe and effective for this purpose. It works by lowering the surface tension of small gas bubbles in the stomach and intestines. This causes the bubbles to combine into larger ones that are more easily expelled.

CLAIMS

Accurate
"antiflatulent"
"relieves the symptoms of gas"

False or Misleading
references to "bloating," "belching," and "colic"

SIMETHICONE

Simethicone has been marketed for a number of years, often in combination with antacid ingredients. Evaluators who assessed it accepted it as safe but raised questions about its effectiveness. They believed it reasonably certain that the surface action causes small gas bubbles to coalesce, forming larger ones—but they had reservations about whether this action is truly beneficial. The Panel wondered if the sensations of which patients complain really result from accumulations of gas.

ANTI-GAS AGENTS is based on the report of the FDA's Advisory Review Panel on OTC Antacid Drugs, the FDA's Tentative Final Order for Antacid Products, the FDA's Final Order for Antacid and Antiflatulent Products Generally Recognized as Safe and Effective and Not Misbranded, and official addenda of the OTC drug review process.

These doubts were allayed by two studies in which neither patients nor doctors knew whether the preparation being used contained simethicone or was a similar-tasting dummy substance. Participants in one study were primed with gas-inducing meals. "In both studies," the FDA reported, "the patients showed a statistically significant preference for simethicone." This decision notwithstanding, the Panel on Miscellaneous Internal Drug Products, which took a later look at simethicone, remained unconvinced that the drug relieves digestive distress due to gas. So the FDA now plans to rethink the whole question of simethicone's effectiveness.

Simethicone can be combined with safe and effective antacids, provided the product is labeled both for the relief of "gas" and concurrent symptoms of sour stomach, heartburn, or acid indigestion, and accompanying upset stomach. The maximum daily dosage recommended in over-the-counter preparations is 500 mg. (Higher dosages can be prescribed by doctors.)

Safety and Effectiveness: Active Ingredients in Over-the-Counter Anti-Gas Agents

Ingredient	Panel and FDA Assessment
simethicone	safe and effective

Anti-Gas Agents: Product Ratings

Product and Distributor	Dosage of Active Ingredient	Rating[1]
simethicone		
Mylicon (Stuart)	**tablets, chewable:** 40 mg	**A**
Mylicon-80 (Stuart)	**tablets, chewable:** 80 mg	**A**
Silain (Robins)	**tablets:** 50 mg	**A**

1. Author's interpretation of Panel/FDA criteria. Based on contents, not claims.

Anti-Inflammatory Drugs

See PAIN, FEVER, AND ANTI-INFLAMMATORY DRUGS TAKEN
INTERNALLY

Antimicrobial Bar Soaps

See SOAPS, ANTIMICROBIAL

Antiperspirants

Body odor is not new. Neither are attempts to subdue it. Early Egyptian, Greek, and Roman literature records efforts to control it through bathing, grooming, and perfuming practices. The French of the seventeenth century, who rarely bathed, raised to an art the use of perfumed oils and waters to disguise the smell of their unclean bodies.

The link between sweat and odor began to be more clearly understood when the sweat glands were discovered in the nineteenth century. The first product marketed specifically for underarm odor was Mum, introduced in 1888. This preparation used zinc oxide in a cream base. Everdry in 1902 and Hush in 1908 were the first to use aluminum chloride solutions. In 1914, Odo-Ro-No was the first product to be launched with national magazine advertising that claimed it would remedy excessive perspiration and keep dresses "clean and dainty." Five years later, Odo-Ro-No advertising again led the way. It was the first to assert that perspiration and body odor—or "B.O." as it later came to be called—are socially shocking and offensive.

In the first 50 years, antiperspirants were used mainly by women, who came to consider them almost as essential as soap. In recent decades, more and more men have begun to use antiperspirants—one reason sales have increased anywhere from 4 to 25 percent every year

ANTIPERSPIRANTS is based on the preliminary and final reports of the FDA Advisory Review Panel on OTC Antiperspirant Drug Products, and on the FDA final regulation on aerosol drug and cosmetic products containing zirconium.

since 1945. Such products now generate more than four-fifths of a billion dollars in sales in the United States each year. Sales are spurred on by highly competitive advertising that creates a strong sense of need for these products in the consumer's mind.

Underarm preparations perform two functions: they reduce the amount of perspiration secreted under the arms and they mask or control odor—although the same ingredients in the products can, and do, perform both these functions. Evaluators were faced with a peculiar problem in judging these two functions. Because they affect body secretions, antiperspirants are defined as drugs under the Federal Drug and Cosmetic Act. Products that mask or control odor are defined as cosmetics. The latter are not considered in the over-the-counter review process and they—and the claims made for them—are much less stringently regulated than drugs are. So consumers have been denied a rigorous scientific evaluation of the deodorant effect of these products. This is unfortunate because many people believe their anti-odor function is the most important.

CLAIMS

Accurate
"helps reduce underarm wetness"
"helps reduce underarm dampness"
"helps reduce underarm perspiration"

False or Misleading
"completely guards your family"
"helps stop wetness"
"really helps keep you dry"
"stops," "halts," or "ends" underarm perspiration
"dry formula"
"dry"
"extra-strength"

Unproved
references to "problem" or "especially troublesome" sweat
references to "longer-lasting" or "24-hour" protection or to "emotional" sweating

(It should be noted that two panelists—in a minority statement—said that to list approved and disapproved words in this way is unduly restrictive and unworkable. "These phrases," they said, "are historically and correctly part of American competitive marketing.")

PERSPIRATION

Sources

Human perspiration is produced by two kinds of sweat glands, the apocrine and the eccrine.

Apocrine glands These structures lie close to the hair follicles and are found all over the body's surface at birth. Most of them gradually disappear. In adults, the remaining glands are concentrated in the armpit (axilla) as well as in areas around the anus and around breast nipples.

These glands are inactive during childhood. They develop and begin to function during puberty—apparently due to sex-hormone stimulation—and they tend to atrophy or "wither" in old age. Their exact function remains unknown.

Sweat secretion from the apocrine glands is scant and slow. After an apocrine gland produces its single small droplet of sweat, a long period follows before the same gland is ready to secrete another droplet. Droplets dry into gluelike granules that stick to the skin and under-arm hairs. They are normally odorless.

Eccrine glands Most of the body's sweat is produced by the eccrine glands. These glands appear in abundance on all body surfaces except the lips and parts of the sexual organs. Since babies have much smaller skin surfaces than adults, their eccrine glands are much more closely spaced—which may be why they seem to sweat more freely.

Eccrine sweat is copious and consists mostly of water. But it also contains small amounts of salt, potassium, urea, lactate, and glucose. In extreme heat and with high water intake, human subjects have been reported to secrete up to 3 gallons of sweat in 24 hours, most of it through the eccrine glands.

The eccrine glands have a clear physiological role: they regulate body heat. (The popular notion that people need to sweat to "purify" their bodies is mistaken.) Evaporation of eccrine sweat from the skin rapidly cools the body. Persons who are unable to sweat cannot tolerate ambient temperatures much above 80°F; neither can they very well endure the heat generated by vigorous physical exercise.

The eccrine glands function in response to nerve impulses. They can be stimulated by external heat or fever, eating spicy foods, and by emotional stress. Sweating induced by emotional reactions is particularly noticeable in the armpits and on the palms of the hands and soles of the feet.

Excessive sweating—technically called hyperhidrosis—principally involves the eccrine glands. The condition is most common from early adolescence to the mid-twenties. Most heavy sweating follows overheating, or fear and embarrassment or other emotional responses. However, it may also accompany conditions such as shock, diabetes, hyperthyroidism, and nausea or overconsumption of alcohol.

It takes several minutes or longer for physical heat to produce perspiration, but heated emotions can generate an almost instantaneous sweat response.

Armpit Odor

Because the armpits are normally warm and moist, they create a hospitable environment for bacteria. Convincing scientific evidence exists to show that armpit odor arises from bacteria that grow in secretions of the apocrine glands. One research group collected fresh apocrine sweat from unwashed armpits and showed that it was odorless. When kept for 6 hours at room temperature, the bacteria present were able to grow and the sweat acquired that characteristically rank "armpit" odor. When sweat from the same source was refrigerated, no odor developed.

Apocrine sweat collected from armpits that had been shaved and disinfected with alcohol developed no odor at room temperature. In other tests, armpits treated with an antibacterial cleanser remained odor-free for 18 hours longer than untreated armpits.

The copious moisture provided by the eccrine glands facilitates the growth of the bacteria and contributes to the dispersal of odor. The hair tuft under the arm acts as a kind of wick from which mixed eccrine and bacterially decomposed apocrine sweat evaporates into one's personal environment.

Few attempts have been made to discover exactly which bacteria cause underarm odor and how many of them need to be present for the odor to be detectable—even though, The Panel pointedly commented, "the American public spends hundreds of millions of dollars annually to combat these bacteria."

What purpose these odors may serve in human beings is only beginning to be investigated. The currently favored view is that apocrine-gland secretions function as chemical signals—pheromones—

that activate specific behavioral responses in other members of the same species. If one believes antiperspirant and deodorant advertisements, one is repelled by underarm odor—particularly when it emanates from a member of the opposite sex. But it is possible that at an unconscious (or perhaps even at a conscious) level these odors are sexual attractants.

How Antiperspirants Work

These products reduce underarm wetness. This effort additionally retards bacterial growth. Decreased wetness and fewer bacteria probably account for the fact that antiperspirants prevent or decrease armpit odor for meaningful periods of time when they are applied once or twice daily on a fairly regular basis. While they reduce underarm wetness—so that it's more difficult for bacteria to grow—their effectiveness against odor depends on their ability to kill bacteria. The evidence for direct antibacterial action is fragmentary.

The manner in which aluminum compounds—the principal components of antiperspirants—act on sweat glands is unknown. One theory maintains that they penetrate some distance into the sweat duct. There they bind with the outer layer of the duct wall in such a way as to block the passage of water. Pressure then builds up in the duct. This action, through a biofeedback mechanism, stops further sweat secretion. A competing theory suggests that the sweat duct is made more permeable to water. In this way—like a leaky hose—more moisture is dispersed into the surrounding skin rather than emerging from it in large droplets. A third view holds that aluminum chloride and comparable chemicals block transmission of the nerve impulses that turn on the sweat glands. Finally, one industry representative claimed that his product acts like glue to block up the sweat duct—a concept that was received skeptically by reviewers.

Whatever the mechanism, antiperspirants act only on the eccrine glands. They have no effect on the apocrine glands, whose bacterially altered secretions are the principal source of underarm odor. In fact, no known nonprescription product can halt or control apocrine sweat, and antiperspirants were not specifically evaluated on their ability to quell underarm odor because this is technically a cosmetic action, not a drug action. But evaluators were satisfied by industry "sniff tests" and other evidence that aluminum and zirconium salts—the ingredients in antiperspirants that reduce underarm moisture—also reduce underarm odor.

REDUCING UNDERARM MOISTURE

Antiperspirant Effectiveness

Antiperspirant effectiveness is often tested by applying the product to one armpit, and the base alone—that is, the cream, liquid, or spray in which the active ingredient is usually formulated—to the other. A dozen or more persons may participate in each test. Cotton pads are placed in each armpit, and the subjects either go about their daily routines or are put into a hot, humid room. Some testers challenge subjects with mental puzzles or try to upset them to enhance sweating. After a set time the pads are collected and weighed. If the pads in the treated armpit weigh less than the others, the ingredient is judged to have antiperspirant activity. The greater the difference in weight between the two pads, the more effective the ingredient. Most antiperspirants reduce wetness by 20 to 40 percent.

Reviewers considered this a low overall level of effectiveness, but when tests showed that a reduction of less than 20 percent cannot be detected, they chose that as a standard. An effective product must provide at least a 20 percent reduction in underarm perspiration in at least half of its users who apply it once a day.

The effectiveness of antiperspirants depends upon regular use. They do not usually become effective immediately; some take hours, others require even more time and repeated applications. To achieve maximum levels of effectiveness, they must be used at least once daily.

Forms of Antiperspirants

Test results submitted for review showed that, as a class, aerosol products are the *least* effective and lotions the *most* effective. A few antiperspirant products are marketed to reduce sweat on body surfaces other than the armpits—particularly the feet and hands. The decrease was not shown to be enough to be noticed by the user, and the Panel regarded these products as no more than conditionally effective. The ranges in average sweat reduction in tests with various types of underarm products are shown below.

aerosols	20 to 33 percent
liquids	15 to 54 percent
sticks	35 to 40 percent

creams   35 to 47 percent
roll-ons   14 to 70 percent
lotions   38 to 62 percent

Even with the information that a particular ingredient or product reduces sweat by 20 percent or more in the majority of users, consumers have to try out different products themselves. People vary greatly in their responses to antiperspirants—even one person's responses may change at different times. To make matters more confusing, unnoted changes in manufacturers' formulation—even in an inactive ingredient —can significantly change a product's effectiveness. So the Panel suggests that consumers would do well to try out several products and change brands from time to time if they are not fully satisfied.

Are Aerosols Safe?

In the early 1960s, the introduction of active ingredients that contain the metal zirconium in combination with aluminum coincided with the introduction of aerosol sprays. The two together—zirconium in aerosol dispensers—soon became the cause of considerable alarm.

Aerosols, while convenient, have the disadvantage of producing airborne particles that are likely to be inhaled. These particles enter the lungs, where they tend to remain. In animal tests, one exposure to aluminum chlorohydrate spray left aluminum particles in the lungs for two months or longer. Regular users thus almost certainly accumulate these particles and this accumulation may require months or years to be cleared even after use is discontinued.

Risk depends to some extent on what kind of antiperspirant particles lodge in the lungs. Products made with zirconium may be far more dangerous than those that contain only aluminum salts as their active ingredient. One company recalled a new zirconium-containing antiperspirant after 4 months because it received 249 consumer complaints that the product caused coughing, choking, shortness of breath, and other forms of respiratory distress.

Aerosolized zirconium products were banned by the FDA on the Panel's recommendation. The fate of spray products containing aluminum remains undecided. While short-term tests in animals show no danger, evaluators doubted that the results can be applied to long-term use of these products by humans. It proposed an inhalation toxicity test to determine long-term risk and granted aluminum-containing aerosols only conditional approval.

In one of these tests, conducted by Becton-Dickinson, a medical products manufacturer, continued exposure to extraordinarily high doses of aerosolized aluminum chlorohydrate caused tumors in some test rats. But lower exposure levels, equivalent to 100 times the amount humans might inhale, did not.

The FDA, dissatisfied with these findings, originally asked that another two-year cancer study be conducted on rats. It then changed its mind and said it probably would rule the sprays safe without further testing. "The existing safety data provide a broad toxicological profile that can be used to establish general recognition of safety of aerosolized aluminum antiperspirants," the FDA declared.

This easing of safety test requirements cheered manufacturers. But it could be cause for consumers' concern. As the "Pink Sheet"—the Washington newsletter that serves drug company executives—noted in its May 17, 1982 issue:

"The . . . decision may indicate that the agency is beginning to move away from the more rigid Rx-style technical requirements for establishing OTC ingredient safety and efficacy."

It is these stiff requirements that, for the first time, had provided consumers with assurance that no stone would be left unturned to confirm the safety and effectiveness of nonprescription products.

COMBINATION PRODUCTS

Many antiperspirants contain substances with jawbreaking names like *aluminum zirconium trichlorohydrate* that seem to be combinations of two or more active ingredients. These are, however, considered single ingredients. No product submitted for review contained more than one active ingredient for the reduction of perspiration.

The only currently marketed combination containing antiperspirants and other types of drugs that were submitted for review are combinations of antifungal active ingredients + an antiperspirant for the prevention and treatment of athlete's foot. The Panel and the FDA agree that, in principle, this could be a safe and effective combination. But data are sparse, and the Panel did not approve any specific antiperspirant ingredient as safe and effective for this purpose. Rather, it granted them only conditional approval. Of the few such products currently marketed, the FDA adds, none appears to contain a safe and effective approved antifungal ingredient—so that these combinations, for now, are at best only conditionally approved.

ANTIPERSPIRANTS REVIEWED

The standard name of the ingredient may differ from the name used on a label, so consumers may want to consult the Antiperspirant Ingredient Names chart.

Antiperspirant Ingredient Names

Standard Names	*Alternate Names*
aluminum chlorohydrate	aluminum chlorhydrate
	aluminum chlorhydrate compound
	aluminum chlorhydroxide
	aluminum chlorhydroxide complex
	aluminum chlorohydroxide
	aluminum hydroxychloride
aluminum chlorohydrex PG[1]	aluminum chlorhydroxide—propylene glycol complex
aluminum dichlorohydrate	aluminum chlorhydroxide, aluminum chloride
	aluminum chlorhydrol, aluminum chloride
	aluminum hydroxychloride, aluminum chloride
aluminum sesquichlorohydrate	aluminum chlorhydroxide, aluminum chloride
	aluminum chlorhydrate, aluminum chloride
	aluminum chlorhydrol, aluminum chloride
aluminum sulfate, buffered	aluminum sulfate, sodium aluminum lactate
aluminum zirconium tetrachlorohydrex Gly[2]	aluminum chlorhydrate zirconium oxychloride aluminum glycinate
	aluminum-zirconyl hydroxychloride complex
aluminum zirconium trichlorohydrate	aluminum chlorhydrate, zirconium chlorhydrate
	aluminum chlorhydrate, zirconium chlorohydrate
	aluminum-zirconium chlorohydrate complex
aluminum zirconium trichlorohydrex Gly	zirconium chlorhydrate-aluminum chlorhydrate-glycine complex
	zirconium-aluminum-glycine complex
aluminum zirconium pentachlorohydrex Gly	zirconium chlorhydrate-aluminum chlorohydrate-glycine complex
sodium aluminum chlorohydroxy lactate	sodium aluminum chlorhydroxy lactate

[1]PG=polyethylene glycol complex.
[2]Gly=glycine complex.

Approved Active Ingredients

Many active ingredients are approved as safe and effective for reducing underarm wetness—provided they are used in nonaerosol products. All are aluminum compounds or aluminum and zirconium compounds.

Aluminum chloride   Antiperspirant products containing aluminum chloride are potent inhibitors of underarm moisture. But they tend to be more irritating to the skin and more damaging to clothing than aluminum chlorohydrate products.

In one comparative test, under everyday conditions, a 13.3 percent aluminum chloride preparation was compared with a 22 percent aluminum chlorohydrate preparation. The latter was more effective an hour after application. But after 12 hours, the aluminum chloride had reduced sweat production by half—compared with only a one-third reduction by the aluminum chlorohydrate. After 3½ days and several applications, the aluminum chloride still provided a 49 percent reduction in sweat compared with a barely effective 22 percent reduction with aluminum chlorohydrate.

The Panel concluded from this and other tests that 15 percent or less aqueous solutions of aluminum chloride show more reduction in perspiration when compared with other antiperspirant compounds, but there is a significantly greater potential for producing skin irritation. Consumers need to be warned of this on labels.

Aluminum chlorohydrates   Many aluminum chlorohydrate ingredients are approved as safe and effective when formulated in liquids, creams, and other products that are applied directly to the skin. Although these forms vary chemically, their effect on the skin is much the same. So they are discussed as one group here.

The safety of the aluminum chlorohydrates has been demonstrated by skin tests in animals and humans, as well as by marketing experience. Manufacturers receive about 6 complaints of adverse reactions for every million product units sold—a very low complaint rate for skin products. A concentration of over of 25 percent of aluminum chlorohydrate in the base can be dangerous.

The effectiveness of aluminum chlorohydrate has been established by hot-room tests. Some tests were conducted under emotionally stressful conditions that enhance sweating, ones designed to produce tension, fear, frustration, and embarrassment. Sweat reductions were in the range of 26 to 46 percent. Tests also showed that different formulations of the same ingredient can produce significantly different levels of sweat inhibition. In some instances formulations that contained a relatively high percentage of an aluminum chlorohydrate were less effective than those of lower concentration.

Aluminum sulfate, buffered   Used by itself, aluminum sulfate is highly irritating. But the addition of sodium aluminum lactate acts as a buffer. A product that contains 8 percent each of these aluminum ingredients has been widely used for years. Test results with buffered aluminum sulfate show that this ingredient produces neither irritation nor allergic responses. In one allergy test of 204 subjects, reactions to the buffered aluminum sulfate were milder and less numerous than the reactions to a widely marketed mild soap.

Hot-room tests showed that buffered aluminum preparations are effective, reducing underarm wetness by 25 to 31 percent.

However, because various inactive ingredients can change a preparation's effectiveness, evaluators recommended that the final formulation of buffered aluminum sulfate products be tested further.

Aluminum zirconium chlorohydrates   These compounds have been banned from spray products in the United States. However, they are safe and effective antiperspirant ingredients when applied directly to the underarm skin. Bumps and other irritant reactions occur in a small number of people, but these minor problems are easily recognized and disappear when use of the product is discontinued.

Conditionally Approved Active Ingredients

Aluminum chlorohydrates, aerosolized, and aluminum chloride, aerosolized   The aerosol forms of the aluminum compounds listed below have been rated only conditionally acceptable pending tests that might conclusively demonstrate their safety and effectiveness. The Panel suggested various periods of time for manufacturers to provide data, failing which these ingredients would be banned when used in aerosol products.

Aluminum sulfate (cake alum) and potassium aluminum sulfate   Also granted only conditional approval—pending further test data—are two other active ingredients. Aluminum sulfate can be highly irritating when used in an antiperspirant. Potassium aluminum sulfate, often used in styptic pencils (to stop bleeding from small cuts such as razor nicks), is quite acidic.

Sodium aluminum chlorohydroxy lactate   This compound, used in antiperspirant sticks, has the advantage in that it does not react with soaps. Although it may irritate the eyes, it appears not to react with or injure the skin, and the Panel judges it safe when used in nonaerosol products. In hot-room tests, however, it was not very effective in reducing perspiration. Verdict: safe but not proved effective.

Disapproved Active Ingredients

Several types of antiperspirant active ingredients were disapproved by the Panel as being unsafe or ineffective or both. Some of them already have been removed from the market by the FDA.

Aluminum bromohydrate   This substance has never been marketed in the United States as an antiperspirant—meaning, legally, that it is a *new drug*. Preliminary findings indicate that it is safe and effective when applied to the skin to control underarm moisture, but it cannot be approved until well-controlled scientific studies provide proof of positive results.

Aluminum chloride, alcoholic solutions   A 20 percent aluminum chloride solution in alcohol is used by doctors to treat severe cases of excess sweating. This solution—available only on prescription—is applied at bedtime and the armpits are then wrapped in an impermeable plastic cover.

Physicians who use this method claim it provides total control of armpit wetness. These results suggest that this potent aluminum chloride formulation is very effective. But the available data do not show that the method or the material can be safely used for self-treatment, so the ingredient is not approved for nonprescription products.

Aluminum zirconium chlorohydrates, aerosolized   While these compounds are safe and effective when applied directly to the skin in liquid, cream, or roll-on bases, they are disapproved for use in spray products. The FDA banned them from the United States market in September 1977.

Safety and Effectiveness: Active Ingredients in Over-the-Counter Antiperspirants

Active Ingredient	Panel's Assessment	
	In Nonaerosol Dosage Form	In Aerosol Dosage Form
aluminum bromohydrate	not proved safe or effective	not proved safe or effective
aluminum chlorohydrates (dosage: up to 25% in the base)		
aluminum chlorohydrex PEG[1]	safe and effective	effective but not proved safe
aluminum chlorohydrex PG[2]	safe and effective	effective but not proved safe
aluminum dichlorohydrate	safe and effective	effective but not proved safe
aluminum dichlorohydrex PEG	safe and effective	effective but not proved safe
aluminum dichlorohydrex PG	safe and effective	effective but not proved safe
aluminum sesquichlorohydrex PEG	safe and effective	effective but not proved safe
aluminum sesquichlorohydrex PG	safe and effective	effective but not proved safe
aluminum chloride (dosage: 15% or less in aqueous solution)	safe and effective	effective but not proved safe
aluminum chloride, alcoholic solution	not safe	not safe
aluminum sulfate	not proved safe or effective	not proved safe or effective
aluminum sulfate, buffered	safe and effective	effective but not proved safe

Safety and Effectiveness: Active Ingredients in Over-the-Counter Antiperspirants *(continued)*

	Panel's Assessment	
Active Ingredient	*In Nonaerosol Dosage Form*	*In Aerosol Dosage Form*
aluminum zirconium chlorohydrates		
aluminum zirconium octachlorohydrate	safe and effective	not safe
aluminum zirconium octachlorohydrex Gly[3]	safe and effective	not safe
aluminum zirconium pentachlorohydrate	safe and effective	not safe
aluminum zirconium pentachlorohydrex Gly	safe and effective	not safe
aluminum zirconium tetrachlorohydrate	safe and effective	not safe
aluminum zirconium tetrachlorohydrex Gly	safe and effective	not safe
aluminum zirconium trichlorohydrate	safe and effective	not safe
aluminum zirconium trichlorohydrex Gly	safe and effective	not safe
potassium aluminum sulfate	not proved safe or effective	not proved safe or effective
sodium aluminum chlorohydroxy lactate	safe but not proved effective	

[1]PEG = polyethylene glycol complex
[2]PG = propylene glycol complex
[3]Gly = glycine complex

Antiperspirants: Product Ratings[1]

Product and Distributor	Dosage of Active Ingredients	Rating[2]	Comment
aluminum chlorohydrates			
Arrid Extra Dry Antiperspirant, Deodorant Spray (Carter)	**aerosol spray:** aluminum chlorohydrate	**B**	sprays not proved safe
Arrid Extra Dry Cream (Carter)	**cream:** aluminum chlorohydrate + aluminum chloride	**A**	
Ban Super Solid (Bristol-Myers)	**stick:** aluminum chlorohydrate	**A**	
Brut 33 Anti-Perspirant Spray (Faberge)	**aerosol spray:** aluminum chlorohydrate	**B**	sprays not proved safe
dial Long-Lasting Anti-Perspirant Deodorant (Armour-Dial)	**aerosol spray:** aluminum chlorohydrate	**B**	sprays not proved safe
5-day Anti-Perspirant/ Deodorant Pads (J. B. Williams)	**medicated pads:** 25% aluminum chlorohydrate	**A**	
Mitchum Cream anti-perspirant (Mitchum)	**cream:** aluminum chlorohydrate + aluminum chloride	**A**	
Mum (Bristol-Myers)	**cream:** aluminum chlorohydrate	**A**	
Right Guard (Gillette)	**powder in spray:** aluminum chlorohydrate	**B**	sprays not proved safe
Secret Antiperspirant (Procter & Gamble)	**aerosol spray:** aluminum chlorohydrate	**B**	sprays not proved safe
aluminum zirconium chlorohydrates			
Arrid Extra Dry (Carter)	**stick:** aluminum-zirconyl hydroxychloride complex	**A**	
Right Guard Roll-On Antiperspirant (Gillette)	**roll-on:** aluminum-zirconyl hydroxychloride complex	**A**	
Secret (Procter & Gamble)	**cream:** zirconium-aluminum-glycine-hydroxychloride complex	**A**	

1. Evaluated as antiperspirants, not as deodorants.
2. Author's interpretation of Panel criteria. Based on contents, not claims.

Antiseptics

An antiseptic is a drug that kills germs and other microorganisms on the skin or other body surfaces, or retards their growth and spread. People use antiseptics mainly to prevent bacterial, viral, and fungal infections —and because of the sense of cleanliness they confer.

Antiseptics are formulated as swab-on liquids, sprays, powders, moist paper-wipes, as well as other ways. They are commonly used to wipe babies' bottoms and to remove germs after contact with human or animal wastes and other disagreeable and presumably germ-laden substances. Their most important use may be in first aid—to cleanse and de-germ the skin around splinters, cuts, scratches and other superficial wounds (*see* FIRST-AID PREPARATIONS FOR SKIN WOUNDS).

Antiseptic products are specifically defined by the FDA as nonirritating antimicrobial-containing preparations that prevent overt skin infection.

There is a distinction between antiseptics and disinfectants. They may contain identical chemicals, though an antiseptic is intended to cleanse and de-germ the skin and other body surfaces. A disinfectant is used to clean and de-germ inanimate objects—from surgical instruments to toilet seats and hospital floors.

Because of these distinctions, the FDA would disallow the claim that antiseptic products will "disinfect" or "sanitize" the skin. And since no antiseptic can kill *all* germs on the skin, the FDA also disapproves of claims that these drugs can "sterilize" or "ensure bacterially clean" skin. Accurate statements for nonalcoholic preparations include: "prevents skin infection," for "de-germing," "reduces the risk of infection and cross-infection," and "first-aid product."

The FDA plans to require that every product sold over-the-counter as a skin antiseptic contain an active antimicrobial, an ingredient that will kill or inhibit microorganisms. Eventually these antimicrobials will have to be shown safe and effective in order for such products to remain on the market. As of late 1982, however, only two of them—ethyl alcohol and isopropyl alcohol—have met this test.

ANTISEPTICS is based on the report of the FDA's Advisory Review Panel on OTC Antimicrobial Drug Products for Repeated Daily Human Use (Antimicrobial I Panel); the FDA's initial "Temporary Final Monograph on OTC Antimicrobial Products," and two reports by the FDA's Advisory Review Panel on OTC Miscellaneous External Drug Products: "Alcohol Drug Products for Topical Antimicrobial OTC Use" and "Mercury-Containing Drug Products for Topical Antimicrobial OTC Human Use."

ALCOHOLS

Some of the most impressive antiseptics are alcohols. They kill bacteria on contact, within seconds. They are, however, less effective against viruses and even less effective against funguses.

Besides killing "germs," alcohols are solvents and astringents. They loosen, dissolve, and remove grease and oil, protein-type matter, and other dirt and debris from the skin. And they evaporate quickly. The mild burning sensation felt when alcohol is rubbed on the skin offers a relaxing counterirritant effect for persons suffering from aches and pains.

Alcohols are colorless and do not stain clothing or the skin. This means that skin-color changes—and particularly the inflammatory redness that may signal a developing infection—are not masked by alcohol as they are when Mercurochrome or other dark-staining antiseptics are used. Finally, plain alcohol is likely to be far less expensive than other, less effective antiseptic products.

On the deficit side, alcohols may irritate underlying tissues. They therefore should not be used on deep or wide wounds, or on puncture wounds, and should not be used to irrigate deeply embedded splinters before an attempt is made to remove them. These deep wounds require medical care. Mucosal tissue is more sensitive to alcohol than regular skin, and so should not be treated with strong alcohols. Because it is irritating, alcohol should not be used for treating burns.

CLAIMS

Accurate

for "first-aid use to decrease germs in minor cuts and scrapes"

"to decrease germs on the skin prior to removing a splinter or other foreign objects and prior to an injection"

False or Misleading

Use "as a local antiseptic in such conditions as simple sunburn, hand iron burns, mouth burns caused by hot foods, kitchen burns caused by hot pots, etc."

WARNING   Alcohol is for external use only. It should be kept out of children's reach. If it is swallowed, professional help should be sought from a doctor, emergency room, or poison-control center.

MERCURIALS

The heavy liquid metal mercury and its salts have been used medicinally for thousands of years. But unlike alcohols, the mercurials' use as drugs—and particularly as skin antiseptics—is now fast waning.

A major difficulty with mercury is that it is readily absorbed through broken or unbroken skin, as well as from the gastrointestinal tract when swallowed, and from the respiratory tract when inhaled as mercury vapor. Mercury is highly toxic. Once absorbed it can cause major damage—even death. Small amounts applied to minor skin wounds probably do not pose a serious or lethal hazard. But they can produce an itchy contact dermatitis and may provoke an allergic reaction.

However, the principal complaint against mercury as an antiseptic is not its lack of safety but its lack of effectiveness. Although Mercurochrome, Merthiolate (also called thimerosal), and related compounds were the standard applications for minor cuts and scratches a generation ago, they have since fallen into disuse. The reason is that experiments conducted in the 1940s show that mercurials do stop bacteria from growing but they often fail to kill them. The organisms revive and multiply anew once the mercury compound is removed, diluted, or neutralized.

The most striking discovery in this regard was that human serum —the clear liquid portion of the blood—inactivates mercurial antiseptics. When Merthiolate is suspended in human serum, it requires 14,000 times more of the antiseptic to inactivate a test dose of infectious bacteria (*Salmonella typhosa*) than is needed when the antiseptic is suspended in salt water. Since mercurials used on the skin are likely to come into contact with serum, pus, and other body fluids, their effect on the bacteria they are supposed to kill may be voided.

For these reasons, the Panel declared that all topical mercurials are ineffective as antiseptics; some are dangerous as well. Given that they are worthless, all medical claims for them are misleading and examples of misbranding. If the Panel's view prevails, all mercurial antiseptics will be removed from the nonprescription drug-marketplace in the United States within the current decade.

ASSESSING DRUGS AND CLAIMS

Alcohol and mercurial antiseptics were assessed by the FDA's Advisory Panel on Miscellaneous External Drugs. This Panel also was asked to evaluate hydrogen peroxide 3 percent and gentian violet 1 to 2 percent, but it appears not to have done so. The other antiseptics described in this unit were evaluated by the Antimicrobial I Panel, which also assessed them as active ingredients in antimicrobial bar soaps and first-aid preparations. In many cases, readers can refer to other units for more detailed descriptions of each ingredient, and discussion here will be limited to the evaluators' ranking of safety and effectiveness as antiseptics.

COMBINATION PRODUCTS

Antimicrobial active ingredients may be combined with external pain-relievers and with other active and inactive ingredients—including perfumes and other aromatics that may have a "clean" smell even if they kill no germs. The Panel approves combinations in which safe and effective antimicrobials are combined with other safe and effective active ingredients in a way that will serve a real need in a significant number of people. But these combinations must not interfere with the effectiveness or safety of any of the individual active ingredients.

Combinations that contain conditionally approved or disapproved individual ingredients merit the same rating. Since ethyl alcohol and isopropyl alcohol are the only two safe and effective antiseptics, it follows that they are the only ones that can be included in combination products that could hope to win the FDA's full approval.

ANTISEPTIC PREPARATIONS

Approved Active Ingredients

Ethyl alcohol (60 to 95 percent by volume)   This is the oldest and best-known alcohol. It is the alcohol in liquor and wine, and has been used for centuries for its nutritional, intoxicant, and medicinal properties. When sold in drugstores for medicinal use it contains additives that make it unpalatable. Ethyl alcohol may also be called absolute alcohol, alcohol, denatured alcohol, or ethanol.

The long and universal use of ethyl alcohol in beverages attests to its relative lack of toxicity when taken in small quantities. As to external applications, it is not safe to use ethyl alcohol on large, open wounds—both because it is irritating and because it kills white blood cells. However, evaluators say it is safe to use for small wounds; allergic reactions and other side effects are extremely rare.

Ethyl alcohol starts killing bacteria within seconds. Dipping one's hands into it for 1 minute kills more bacteria than scrubbing them in water for 6 minutes. Ethyl alcohol also will kill or inactivate many common viruses, including flu virus and some herpes viruses. It is less effective against funguses, so it is not used to treat conditions like athlete's foot.

Daily or routine use of alcohol as an antiseptic is unwise. It kills the normal bacteria on skin surfaces so effectively that it may make the skin susceptible to the growth of other, disease-causing, bacteria.

Ethyl alcohol works best in the presence of water. So the Panel stipulates that these preparations contain at least 5 percent water by volume. The safe and effective concentrations of ethyl alcohol are 60 to 95 percent by volume.

Isopropyl alcohol (50 to 91.3 percent by volume) Obtained principally from petroleum, isopropyl alcohol (also called isopropanol) is unfit to drink. It is more toxic than ethyl alcohol if accidentally swallowed, and the vapors are poisonous enough that it should be used for alcohol rubs only in a well-ventilated room. But there is little if any risk in using isopropyl alcohol as an antiseptic, so the Panel lists it as safe.

When swabbed on the skin, isopropyl alcohol begins killing *Staphylococcus aureus*, *Escherichia coli*, and other bacteria within seconds. It works more slowly and less effectively against viruses, and does even more poorly against funguses (for which other antiseptics are needed).

This alcohol, too, works better in the presence of water—which should be present in no less than approximately 9 percent. At a concentration of 50 to 91.3 percent, isopropyl alcohol is assessed as both safe and effective.

Conditionally Approved Active Ingredients

Benzalkonium chloride Not proved safe or effective as an antiseptic for use on the skin.

Benzethonium chloride Similar to benzalkonium chloride; not proved safe or effective as an antiseptic for use on the skin.

Chloroxylenol (PCMX) Not proved safe or effective as an antiseptic for use on the skin.

Hexylresorcinol Not proved safe or effective as an antiseptic for use on the skin.

Iodine complexed with phosphate ester of alkylaryloxy po-

lyethylene glycol   Not proved safe or effective as an antiseptic for use on the skin.

Methylbenzethonium chloride   Not proved safe or effective as an antiseptic for use on the skin. It is similar to benzalkonium chloride.

Nonylphenoxypoly (ethylenoxy) ethanoliodine   Not proved safe or effective as an antiseptic for use on the skin.

Phenol (0.5 to 1.5 percent in aqueous or alcoholic solution) Not proved effective as an antiseptic for use on the skin.

Poloxamer-iodine   Not proved safe or effective as an antiseptic for use on the skin.

Povidone-iodine   Not proved safe or effective as an antiseptic for use on the skin.

Tincture of iodine   Not proved safe for use on the skin.

Triclosan   Not proved safe or effective as an antiseptic for use on the skin.

Undecoylium chloride–iodine complex   Not proved safe or effective as an antiseptic for use on the skin.

The above ingredients are used in a variety of products. To locate where these ingredients are discussed elsewhere in this book, consult the index.

Disapproved Active Ingredients

Benzyl alcohol   This alcohol is not harmful to the skin. But it has only weak antiseptic properties, so the Panel rules that it is safe but not effective.

Calomel   When identified by its alternate name, mercurous chloride, this drug is more readily recognizable as a mercurial compound. It is practically insoluble in water, and therefore not very toxic when applied to the skin. So it may be safe. But like all mercurials, it is not effective.

Chlorobutanol   Although this alcohol is quite toxic, the evaluators say that in concentrations under 5 percent it will not injure the skin. But it acts too slowly against bacteria to be considered an effective antiseptic. Verdict: safe but not effective.

Cloflucarban   Not safe or effective for use on the skin.

Ethyl alcohol (under 60 percent)   Low concentrations of this alcohol do not kill bacteria with the certainty and speed that the Panel requires of a safe and effective antiseptic. Conclusion: ineffective.

Fluorosalan   Not safe for use on the skin.

Hexachlorophene   Not safe for use on the skin.

Isopropyl alcohol (under 50 percent)   In these low concentrations, this alcohol fails to destroy bacteria with the sureness or rapidity that the evaluators demand of a safe and effective antiseptic. Verdict: ineffective.

Isopropyl alcohol with ethylene oxide   The Panel could find no data on the safety or the effectiveness of this alcoholic solution. So it is classified—without comment—as not safe and not effective.

Merbromin   See MERCUROCHROME, below.

Mercuric chloride   This compound, also called bichloride of mercury, is highly poisonous to human cells—yet quite nontoxic to microorganisms. The Panel's decision is: not safe and not effective.

Mercuric salicylate and mercuric sulfide   Evaluators could not find any data about these mercurial compounds. So they summarily disapproved them.

Mercurochrome   Another mercurial, also called merbromin, this substance dyes the skin dark red. But it does little else—least of all kill germs with dispatch. One investigator, a half-century ago, discovered that such antiseptic power as Mercurochrome may have might actually come from the alcohol, or acetone, in which it is formulated. While no harm comes of painting the skin with Mercurochrome, no help does either, according to the Panel. So Mercurochrome is listed as safe but ineffective.

Mercury, elemental   As with several mercury compounds noted above, the reviewers could find no data on elemental mercury's use as an antiseptic. So they summarily disapproved it.

Mercury, ammoniated   This is a toxic form of mercury that has been used to treat psoriasis, ringworm, and other skin conditions. The incidence of mercury poisoning is high. Therefore, the Panel concludes that ammoniated mercury is not safe, and, like other mercurials it is not effective as an antiseptic.

Mercury chloride   The reviewers found no data on this compound's use as an antiseptic, so they summarily disapproved it.

Merthiolate   This compound, which is also known as thimerosal, is a mercurial antiseptic. It was once widely used for first aid. Since that time, it has been found to be very damaging to human skin cells. It also is highly allergenic: in one survey, 1 out of every 6 military recruits was found to be allergic to the drug. Apart from the question of safety, Merthiolate has also been found to slow bacterial growth, but not kill the bacteria. So the Panel calls the drug neither safe nor effective.

Nitromersol   Here, too, the reviewers could find no information about the use of this drug. Their reaction: summary disapproval.

Orthochloromercuriphenol Yet another mercury compound about which no meaningful data are available, this preparation was summarily disapproved.

Orthohydroxyphenylmercuric chloride This mercurial is used in burn preparations, and the Panel assesses it as safe in the low concentration of 0.05 percent in which it is currently marketed over-the-counter. But this compound is not effective because it only inhibits and does not kill bacteria.

Para-chloromercuriphenol Like other mercury compounds, this substance is summarily disapproved.

Phenylmercuric nitrate While this compound has been found to be less toxic to human skin cells than some other commonly used mercurial antiseptics, there is no evidence that it effectively combats microorganisms in the low concentrations in which it is formulated into nonprescription products. The Panel's judgment therefore is that it is safe but not effective.

Thimerosal See MERTHIOLATE, above.

Tribromsalan This ingredient is judged not safe for use as an antiseptic.

Triclocarban Because of lack of data concerning triclocarban's safety and effectiveness as an antiseptic, the Panel summarily disapproved it.

Vitromersol One more mercury compound about which evaluators could find no data, vitromersol was summarily disapproved.

Zyloxin This is a mercurial. No data on its value as an antiseptic was found, and it was summarily dismissed.

Some of these ingredients are used in a variety of products. To locate where these ingredients are discussed, consult the index.

Safety and Effectiveness: Active Ingredients in Over-the-Counter Antiseptics

Active Ingredient	FDA* and/or Panel's Assessment
benzalkonium chloride	not proved safe or effective
benzethonium chloride	not proved safe or effective
benzyl alcohol	safe but not effective
calomel	not proved safe and not effective
chloroxylenol (PCMX)	not proved safe or effective
chlorobutanol	safe but not effective
cloflucarban	not safe or effective
ethyl alcohol (60 to 95%)	safe and effective
ethyl alcohol (under 60%)	safe but not effective

**Safety and Effectiveness: Active Ingredients
in Over-the-Counter Antiseptics** *(continued)*

Active Ingredient	*FDA* and/or Panel's Assessment*
fluorosalan	not safe
gentian violet (1–2%)	evaluation pending
hexachlorophene	not safe
hexylresorcinol	not proved safe or effective
iodine, *see* TINCTURE OF IODINE, below	
iodine complexed with phosphate ester of alkylaryloxy polyethylene glycol	not proved safe or effective
isopropyl alcohol (50 to 91.3%)	safe and effective
isopropyl alcohol (under 50%)	not effective
isopropyl alcohol with ethylene oxide	summarily disapproved
merbromin, *see* MERCUROCHROME	
mercuric chloride	not safe or effective
mercuric salicylate	summarily disapproved
mercuric sulfide	summarily disapproved
Mercurochrome	safe but not effective
mercury	summarily disapproved
mercury, ammoniated	not safe or effective
mercury chloride	summarily disapproved
Merthiolate	not safe or effective
methylbenzethonium chloride	not proved safe or effective
nitromersol	summarily disapproved
nonylphenoxypoly (ethyleneoxy) ethanoliodine	not proved safe or effective
orthochloromercuriphenol	summarily disapproved
orthohydroxyphenylmercuric chloride	safe but not effective
para-chloromercuriphenol	summarily disapproved
phenol (0.5 to 1.5% in aqueous or alcoholic solution)	not proved effective
phenol (greater than 1.5% in aqueous or alcoholic solution)	not safe
phenylmercuric nitrate	safe but not effective
poloxamer-iodine	not proved safe or effective
povidone-iodine	not proved safe or effective
thimerosal, *see* MERTHIOLATE	
tincture of iodine	not proved safe
tribromsalan	not safe
triclocarban	summarily disapproved
triclosan	not proved safe or effective
undecoylium chloride-iodine	not proved safe or effective
vitromersol	summarily disapproved
zyloxin	summarily disapproved

*Judgments reaffirmed or modified by the FDA, or originated by it.

Antiseptics: Product Ratings

Single-Ingredient Products

Product and Distributor	Dosage of Active Ingredients	Rating[1]	Comment
benzalkonium chloride			
Bactine (Miles Labs.)	aerosol: 0.13%	B	not proved safe or effective
	squeeze bottle: 0.13%		
Mercurochrome II (Becton Dickinson)	solution: 0.13%	B	not proved safe or effective
Zephiran (Winthrop)	tincture spray: 1:750	B	not proved safe or effective
ethyl alcohol (60% to 95%)			
Alcare (Vestal)	foam: 62%	A	
ethyl alcohol (generic)	liquid: 60% to 95%	A	
Ethyl Alcohol (Blue Cross)	liquid: 70%	A	
Ethyl Rubbing Alcohol (Whiteworth)	liquid: 70%	A	
hexylresorcinol			
S. T. 37 (Beecham Products)	solution: 0.1%	B	not proved safe or effective
iodine			
iodine tincture (generic)	2% + 2.4% sodium iodide (in 50% alcohol)	B	not proved safe
iodine topical solution (generic)	2% + 2.4% sodium iodide (in purified water)	B	not proved safe
Sepp Antiseptic (Marion)	applicators: 2%	B	not proved safe
isopropyl alcohol (50% to 91.3%)			
isopropyl alcohol (generic)	liquid: 50% to 91.3%	A	
Isopropyl Alcohol (Bowman)	liquid: 70%	A	
Isopropyl Alcohol (Lilly)	liquid: 91%	A	
Isopropyl Alcohol (Purepac)	liquid: 70% and 91%	A	
merbromin (*see* mercurochrome)			

Antiseptics: Product Ratings *(continued)*

Single-Ingredient Products

Product and Distributor	Dosage of Active Ingredients	Rating[1]	Comment
Mercurochrome (25% mercury + 20% bromine)			
Mercurochrome (Becton Dickinson)	**liquid:** 2%	**C**	not effective
thimerosal			
Mersol (Century Pharm.)	**tincture:** 1:1,000	**C**	not safe or effective
Merthiolate (Lilly)	**tincture:** 1:1,000 **aeropump:** 1:1,000	**C**	not safe or effective
thimerosal (generic)	**tincture:** 1:1,000	**C**	not safe or effective
phenylmercuric nitrate (63% mercury)			
Phe-Mer-Nite (Beecham Labs.)	**tincture:** 1:3,000	**C**	not effective
povidone-iodine (liberates approximately 10% free iodine)			
Betadine (Purdue-Frederick)	**aerosol antiseptic gauze pads skin cleanser skin-cleanser foam**	**B**	not proved safe or effective
Operand (Redi Products)	**aerosol solution, swab sticks**	**B**	not proved safe or effective
Pharmadine (Sherwood)	**solution spray**	**B**	not proved safe or effective
Polydine (Century)	**solution**	**B**	not proved safe or effective

Combination Products

Product and Distributor	Dosage of Active Ingredients	Rating[1]	Comment
Mercresin (Upjohn)	**tinted tincture:** 0.1% secondary amyltricresols + 0.1% mercufenol chloride	**C**	neither ingredient submitted to or assessed by Panel as antiseptic; other mercury-phenol entities assessed by Panel as not safe or effective

Antiseptics: Product Ratings (continued)

Combination Products

Product and Distributor	Dosage of Active Ingredients	Rating[1]	Comment
Oil-O-Sol (Health Care Industries)	**liquid:** 6.8% camphor + 0.1% hexylresorcinol	C	camphor 6.8% not safe or effective
Sanicide Germicidal Skin Cleanser (Tutag)	**liquid:** cetyldimethylbenzyl ammonium chloride	C	this compound not submitted to Panel, which doubts effectiveness of all similar compounds in this class when used as antiseptics

1. Author's interpretation of Panel/FDA criteria. Based on contents, not claims.

Aphrodisiacs

Love potions, or aphrodisiacs, are at least as old as the Bible. They live on in folklore and once in a while they appear commercially—in bottles with labels that may describe them, more prosaically, as "tonics."

Since no manufacturer submitted an aphrodisiac or sexual tonic for review, the Panel (with the FDA's help) drew up its own list from medical and folkloric literature. Then it evaluated these drugs.

The findings will be a splash of cold water for dreamful lovers. Some prescription preparations do influence sexual desire and performance. But the dried plants and insects and other substances long believed to be erotic stimulants all are either ineffective or unsafe (or both). What is more, they are inappropriate therapy for persons who have sexual problems and who may be most tempted to use such products.

APHRODISIACS is based on the unadopted draft report "OTC Aphrodisiac Drug Products" by the FDA's Advisory Review Panel on OTC Miscellaneous Internal Drug Products.

WHAT DO LOVE POTIONS DO?

An aphrodisiac is defined by the Panel as a drug that is claimed to arouse or increase sexual desire or improve sexual performance. (Wanting and doing are, of course, two very different functions.)

Aphrodisiacs are likely to be sought by persons troubled by frigidity, impotence, or some other sexual problem. These conditions, however, are not amenable to self-treatment. Panel reviewers say the better recourse is psychotherapy—which very often can provide significant help.

Sex hormones, available by prescription but not over-the-counter, can affect sexual behavior. Women who are given the male sex hormone testosterone as a treatment for breast cancer, for example, often experience a stepped-up sex drive. (But they may also grow hair on their face or show other signs of masculinization.) In men who have an actual deficiency of testosterone, hormonal supplements can be effective. But men with normal testosterone levels show little if any changes in feelings or behavior when these supplements are administered. Estrogen, the female sex hormone, does not increase a woman's sexual desire (libido). And it is experienced as a powerful turn-off by men, who sometimes are given the substance as a treatment for prostatic cancers.

Thus both male and female sex hormones can have powerful effects —negative and positive—on libido. But the Panel warns that they are not safe to use except under a physician's supervision.

Few individuals who believe in or sell drugs that are supposed to be aphrodisiacs seem willing to put them to the test of science. After a thorough search, evaluators could find only two studies that assessed applicable ingredients. Both studies, described below, were poorly constructed, so that findings are inconclusive. Thus, no specific ingredient is listed as safe and effective, or even conditionally so. Also, because the reviewers believe that people who suffer from sexual problems are best helped by seeking professional advice, *all* claims for aphrodisiacs are disapproved.

CLAIMS

False or Misleading

"acts as an aphrodisiac"

"arouses or increases sexual desire and improves sexual performance"

"helps restore sexual vigor, potency, and performance"
"improves performance, staying power, and sexual potency"
"builds virility and sexual potency"
"creates an uncontrollable desire for immediate sexual gratification"
"expands nature's gift of love"

SEX STIMULANTS

Approved Active Ingredients

None

Conditionally Approved Active Ingredients

None

Disapproved Active Ingredients

Cantharides preparations: cantharides, Spanish fly, and cantharidin   These are dried, ground-up preparations, made from insects of the genus *Cantharides*. Cantharidin is the pharmacologically active ingredient in these drugs, which are popularly called Spanish fly. When swallowed, such a preparation causes extreme irritation of the genito-urinary tract. This may bring blood to the clitoris, or to the penis, causing an erection. But the Panel says it has found no evidence that this effect is accompanied either by increased sexual desire or by improved sexual performance.

These irritants have been reported to cause serious damage to the genito-urinary tract. The severe gastroenteritis that may occur as a result of taking these substances has even resulted in death. So the evaluation is obvious: not safe and not effective.

Don qual   Finding no mention of this substance in any medical or scientific index in the last 20 years, reviewers judged it not safe or effective as an over-the-counter aphrodisiac.

Estrogens   While estrogens (female sex hormones) are prescribed for various medical reasons, they do not enhance women's sexuality and they decidedly decrease responses when given to men. So, in addition to being ineffective they are also unsafe as aphrodisiacs.

Ginseng   The root of this plant is highly acclaimed in Eastern folklore as an aphrodisiac. It contains substances called panaxosides that have a weak masculinizing effect. But the Panel could find no medical or scientific reports to show that ginseng enhances men's libido or sexual performance; conclusion: not effective.

Golden seal This plant was classified as ineffective because reviewers could find no information on its use as an aphrodisiac.

Gotu kola An Asian plant, gotu kola contains tritarpenes, substances that have mildly masculinizing properties like the panaxosides in ginseng. However, no data could be found to support the notion that these chemicals arouse desire or improve sexual performance. So gotu kola was judged ineffective.

Korean ginseng *See* GINSENG, above.

Licorice This extract from *Glycyrrhiza*, a type of sweet-root plant that is used in candies, contains tritarpenes. There is no evidence of aphrodisiac qualities; conclusion: ineffective.

Methyltestosterone This is a potent masculinizing hormone. As a prescription drug, it can be of value in some instances where a man's lack of desire stems from inadequate levels of natural testosterone. However, because both diagnosis and treatment require medical expertise, reviewers list methyltestosterone as unsafe for availability over-the-counter.

Nux vomica The seeds of the Indian tree *Strychnos nux-vomica* are used as a sexual tonic, often in combination with other substances. The bitter-tasting active ingredient is the poison strychnine, which has been claimed, on the basis of users' testimonials, to act as a sexual stimulant. But no scientific studies support this belief, and the Panel's judgment is that nux vomica is ineffective as well as unsafe.

Pega palo This is one of the few aphrodisiacs that have been tested, with findings reported in a medical publication, in this case the *Journal of the National Medical Association* (Vol. 52, pp. 25–28, 1960). An alcoholic extract of pega palo plant (*Rhynchosia pyramidalis*) was used to treat 50 men with sexual impotence related to partial or complete loss of sexual desire and erections. The researchers claimed the pega palo enhanced sexual desire in 41 of the men and restored 16 of them to normal sexual activity during the period of the test. Dummy medication was used for comparative purposes, but the doctors knew to whom they were dispensing the active drug and to whom the dummy tonic. This situation may have biased the reporting of results. Further, the outcome of treatment with the dummy drug was not given. So Panel reviewers concluded that the study did not meet criteria for properly controlled scientific investigation, and that pega palo cannot be considered effective.

Sarsaparilla This root extract from *Smilax* plants contains, among other chemicals, tritarpenes. These substances have not been shown to act as an aphrodisiac, so sarsaparilla is judged ineffective.

Strychnine See NUX VOMICA, above.

Yohimbine A plant alkaloid derived from the bark of the tree *Coryanthe yohimbe*, yohimbine has been used for centuries as an aphrodisiac. But there is no acceptable medical evidence that it bolsters either desire or performance.

One report has been published in the medical literature. In this study, 41 impotent men were treated with a combination of yohimbine hydrochloride, nux vomica, and methyltestosterone. The investigators claimed "excellent" or "good" responses in 31 of the men, compared with only a single "good" response in a group of 41 men given dummy medication. The Panel believes the study to be quite inadequate. One objection was that the authors do not define what they mean by "good" or "excellent" results. Also, the extremely poor response among the men taking dummy drugs makes the findings questionable because in most medical studies about 25 percent of "controls" experience the sought-after relief—an effect called the placebo response. A final problem was separating the contribution, if any, of the yohimbine from that produced by the methyltestosterone (a potent male hormone). In sum, reviewers rejected the report and judged yohimbine ineffective as an aphrodisiac.

Safety and Effectiveness: Aphrodisiacs Sold Over-the-Counter

Active Ingredient	Panel's Assessment
cantharides preparations: cantharides, Spanish fly, and cantharidin	not safe or effective
don qual	not safe or effective
estrogens	not safe or effective
ginseng	not effective
golden seal	not effective
gotu kola	not effective
Korean ginseng, *see* GINSENG	
licorice	not effective
methyltestosterone	not safe
nux vomica	not safe or effective
pega palo	not effective
sarsaparilla	not effective

**Safety and Effectiveness: Aphrodisiacs Sold
Over-the-Counter** *(continued)*

Active Ingredient	*Panel's Assessment*
Spanish fly, *see* CANTHARIDES PREPARATIONS	
strychnine, *see* NUX VOMICA	
yohimbine	not effective

Aphrodisiacs: Product Ratings

All products marketed over-the-counter as aphrodisiacs are not safe and/or not effective, as stipulated by the Panel, and therefore are rated "C."

Asthma Drugs

Panting? The Greeks had a word for it: *asthma*. Yet the principal signs and symptoms of the disorder that Hippocrates himself called asthma —difficulty in breathing, wheezing, coughing and a frightening sense of constriction that may make the victim feel like he or she is choking— can occur in other disorders. So, no one should attempt to self-diagnose asthma and no one should use asthma drugs unless the medical diagnosis has been clearly established.

Bronchial asthma involves spasmodic contractions of the bronchial tubes. This obstructs the free passage of air in and out of the lungs— which results in the symptoms described above. As difficulty in breathing increases, the victim may look pale or even blue. At first the cough is dry; later, thick phlegm may be produced. During an attack, the asthma sufferer often feels a sense of impending doom.

Asthma usually (but not always) starts in childhood. Pollens, dust, and other allergy-producing substances have been implicated as causes.

ASTHMA DRUGS is based on the report of the FDA's Advisory Review Panel on OTC Cold, Cough, Allergy, Bronchodilator, and Anti-Asthmatic Products and on related documents in the OTC Drug Review process.

However, both hereditary factors (e.g., a family history of hay fever and the like) and an individual's emotional or psychological state are thought to play important roles.

BRONCHIAL MUSCLE RELAXERS (BRONCHODILATORS)

In asthma, the muscle spasms that cause the narrowing of air passages often abate of their own accord. When the airway is reopened, normal breathing is restored. Drugs that relax these muscles are called bronchodilators. They are administered as tablets, liquids, sprays, or inhalants. Several are quite effective and work quickly.

Because of their potency and the potential for severe side effects, these drugs should be used only in dosages approved by a doctor. Bronchodilators can make the heart race and seem to pound noisily in the chest. They can also elevate blood pressure to dangerous levels. Nervousness, sleeplessness, nausea, and vomiting are other possible side effects. So bronchodilators must be used carefully and treated with extraordinary respect. They must be kept away from small children, who can be seriously hurt by swallowing or inhaling the drugs.

If these products do not provide good, rapid relief—within 20 minutes to an hour at most—the Panel urges asthmatics to call a doctor or go (or be taken) to a hospital emergency room. This is imperative because drugs that are providing only slight relief may be masking a severe and worsening attack that could prove fatal if not treated medically.

Two principal groups of drugs are used as nonprescription bronchodilators. The *sympathomimetics* stimulate the production of an enzyme that relaxes smooth muscle in the bronchial tubes, thus dilating the air passages. The *theophyllines* inhibit a different enzyme that keeps smooth muscle from relaxing. They work well together.

CLAIMS

Accurate
for "temporary relief of bronchial asthma"
for "temporary relief of wheezing attacks and distress of bronchial asthma"

Unproved
"for temporary relief of cough caused by the 'common cold' or 'bronchitis'"

False or Misleading
"relieves gasping for breath"
"free breathing restored"
"breathes a sigh of relief"

WARNING Bronchodilators should be purchased over-the-counter only for medically diagnosed asthma. If relief is not obtained rapidly—within 20 to 60 minutes at most—a doctor should be called or the individual should be taken to a hospital emergency room. (Over-the-counter drugs may mask a worsening attack that could prove fatal.)

Persons who have heart disease, high blood pressure, thyroid, or diabetic conditions or prostatic-gland enlargements should use bronchodilators only under medical supervision.

Combination Products

Theoretically these 2 groups of drugs should be efficient and convenient when combined in a single tablet. However, the Panel says that different persons metabolize theophylline at vastly different rates, so the dosage must be adjusted for each user. This means in turn that it may be difficult to combine the correct doses of a sympathomimetic and a theophylline in one product and yet meet the needs of each individual patient.

The theophyllines are available over-the-counter only in combination products. The Panel proposed that they be marketed as single-entity drugs but the FDA blocked that proposal. The agency cited recent data which it says call into question both the safety and the effectiveness of those compounds when they are used without direct medical supervision.

Nevertheless, combinations of an oral sympathomimetic and an oral theophylline were judged safe and effective for asthmatics. Reviewers also approved combinations of a safe and effective expectorant with these bronchial muscle relaxers, provided the product is labeled for "cough associated with asthma" only.

Combinations that include two sympathomimetics with a theophylline or two theophyllines with a sympathomimetic were disapproved. Evaluators also disapproved combinations of bronchial muscle relaxers with pain and fever relievers. This disapproval was made on the grounds that an asthmatic suffering a cold should probably treat the two illnesses individually.

Other combinations rejected were bronchodilators with a drying agent (anticholinergic) or with an antihistamine. The latter substances dry and thicken the bronchial secretions, possibly making an asthmatic attack more severe.

Finally, formulating a bronchodilator with a cough suppressor—as opposed to an *expectorant*—was judged dangerous because asthmatics *need* to cough to clear bronchial secretions.

ASTHMA DRUGS

Approved airway-widening drugs include ephedrines, epinephrines, and methoxyphenamine hydrochloride (all of which are classified as sympathomimetic agents), and several forms of theophylline. The sympathomimetics—agents that mimic effects of certain impulses of the sympathetic nervous system—can be taken orally or in nasal sprays.

The principal side effects of sympathomimetic drugs are seen in the cardiovascular and the central nervous systems. Sympathomimetics can cause heartbeat irregularities, high blood pressure, dizziness, tremor, nervousness, and insomnia. They can also elevate blood sugar, and, in older men, can slow or obstruct the passage of urine. Clearly those individuals with heart ailments, elevated blood pressure, thyroid or diabetic conditions, or enlarged prostates should excercise caution in use of these medications.

Theophyllines can produce nausea and vomiting. In extreme cases this can result in dehydration and shock.

Approved Active Ingredients

Ephedrine preparations Ephedrine, ephedrine hydrochloride, ephedrine sulfate, and racephedrine hydrochloride are taken orally. They ease breathing rather slowly—not until about 15 to 25 minutes after they are taken. Relief may last 2 to 3 hours. Studies show that these preparations significantly diminish airway constrictions and improve airflow to the lungs. One study showed 10 to 25 percent improvement.

Ephedrine's side effects—on the heartbeat, nervous system, and urinary flow—discourage abuse of these preparations. Persons taking prescription drugs that are monoamine oxidase (MAO) inhibitors—potent drugs used principally as antidepressants—can experience a dangerous rise in blood pressure when they take ephedrine, and so should not use it.

Although the Panel considered ephedrine safe and effective, it also cautioned that its usefulness is limited to the milder forms of asthma.

Epinephrine preparations   Epinephrine, a hormone secreted by the adrenal gland, is popularly known as adrenaline. It stimulates the heart and other organ systems. The familiar increase in heart rate one experiences when faced with physical danger or emotional stress comes from the increase of epinephrine, released into the bloodstream. Epinephrine, epinephrine bitartrate, and epinephrine hydrochloride tend to be safer, faster-acting, and more effective than ephedrine preparations in treating asthma, but results are of much shorter duration. In clinical use and in scientifically controlled trials, epinephrine provided significant relief within 15 minutes. There were measurable improvements in bronchial air flow. These drugs are self-administered as inhalants because they are largely destroyed by stomach acid when swallowed.

A few years ago there was considerable concern about epinephrine's safety because it is chemically related to isoproterenol, a more potent bronchodilator that caused a number of deaths in England. Severe side effects, however, do not appear to occur with epinephrine. This may be because epinephrine is inhaled in more dilute solutions so that only a small amount of the drug is absorbed into the bloodstream. Also, by contracting the blood vessels that pass through the lungs, epinephrine may limit its own distribution through the bloodstream to other parts of the body.

This safe and effective drug can be overused or abused by children and adolescents for the "high" it produces, so intake should be monitored by an adult. Epinephrine should not be taken by persons using prescription drugs that are MAO inhibitors.

Dosage Recommendations for
Safe and Effective OTC Bronchodilators

Active Ingredient	Dosage (Maximum Daily Dosage)	
	Adults	Children
ephedrine preparations (ephedrine, ephedrine hydrochloride, ephedrine sulfate, racephedrine hydrochloride)	12.5 to 25 mg not oftener than every 4 hours (150 mg)	consult doctor

Dosage Recommendations for
Safe and Effective OTC Bronchodilators *(continued)*

Active Ingredient	Dosage (Maximum Daily Dosage)	
	Adults	Children
epinephrine preparations (epinephrine, epinephrine bitartrate, epinephrine hydrochloride [racemic] inhalants)	1 to 3 inhalations of 1% aqueous solution of l-epinephrine or equivalent not oftener than once every 3 hours	over age 4, same as adults; under age 4, consult doctor
methoxyphenamine hydrochloride	100 mg every 4 to 6 hours (600 mg)	consult doctor
theophylline preparations (aminophylline, theophylline anhydrous, theophylline calcium salicylate, theophylline sodium glycinate)	100 to 200 mg anhydrous theophylline equivalent every 6 hours (800 mg)	consult doctor

Methoxyphenamine hydrochloride   Although less potent than ephedrine, so that larger doses are required, methoxyphenamine hydrochloride has fewer and less severe side effects (such as dry mouth and loss of appetite). It may be a good choice for persons who cannot tolerate ephedrine.

The drug is assessed as safe and effective for adults (*not* for children). But persons who have heart disease, high blood pressure, or thyroid or diabetic disorders should not take methoxyphenamine; neither should men with enlarged prostates or people who are using a prescription drug that is an MAO inhibitor.

Theophylline preparations   These potent bronchial muscle relaxants are chemically similar to caffeine. They are judged safe and effective as nonprescription drugs for asthmatics, with research findings showing a definite correlation between ease of breathing and blood levels of theophylline.

The several preparations available are not equally potent. The Panel chose anhydrous theophylline as the standard against which the other preparations are compared. The equivalent of 100 mg of anhydrous theophylline is as follows:

aminophylline anhydrous	116 mg
theophylline calcium salicylate	208 mg
theophylline sodium glycinate	200 mg

The principal side effects of theophylline—loss of appetite, nausea, and vomiting—are unlikely to occur (or to be severe) in asthmatics who take the low doses recommended for nonprescription preparations. However, *overdose*—especially in children—may lead to very serious consequences including convulsions or even death.

The most appropriate dosage should be determined by a doctor because the amount of theophylline needed varies widely from one individual to the next. One carefully conducted study showed the effective dosage to range from 300 mg to as high as 3200 mg per 24 hours. Fortunately, each person's effective dose remains fairly constant, so when a doctor determines an individual's appropriate level, the asthmatic can be reasonably sure of using the correct quantity in over-the-counter products.

At this stage, in the early 1980s, experts within and outside the FDA are divided on the question of whether or not theophylline should be removed from all over-the-counter products. They are in agreement, however, that better medications than fixed-dosage nonprescription combination tablets are available, on prescription, for treating asthmatic emergencies.

Theophylline preparations sold over-the-counter for asthma all are combination products, as required by the FDA. They typically contain 100 to 130 mg of theophylline combined with 24 mg of an ephedrine. Small amounts of the sedative phenobarbital may be formulated into theophylline preparations to counteract the caffeine-like stimulating effect of the theophyllines. The phenobarbital is categorized as safe but not proved effective.

Conditionally Approved Active Ingredient

Euphorbia piluifera   This drug has been marketed for a long time as an asthma and a cold remedy, and it has been popular with users. It does not fall into either class of bronchial muscle relaxants described above. Euphorbia piluifera increases bronchial secretions. In large doses, it can cause vomiting and diarrhea—but its long history of apparently problem-free use persuaded the Panel to list piluifera as safe. But in the absence of well-controlled tests, reviewers believe that effectiveness remains to be proved.

Disapproved Active Ingredients

Two types of products that have been used as bronchial muscle relaxers are disapproved by reviewers. The Panel decided that one is unsafe and the other is ineffective.

Belladonna alkaloids, inhaled   A mixture of dried leaves from the plants *Atropa belladonna* and *Datura stramonia* is marketed as a nonprescription anti-asthmatic drug. The substance is smoked in a cigarette or pipe, or burned and inhaled as incense. This mixture is of unproved value, and it has a great potential for abuse because it is highly psychoactive. It can be quite dangerous: deaths have been reported to follow use of the drug. The Panel judges it unsafe for nonprescription use and recommends that it be banned.

Pseudoephedrine preparations   Two studies have shown that pseudoephedrine—which may be prepared as pseudoephedrine hydrochloride or pseudoephedrine sulfate—is marginally effective, at best, as a bronchodilator. It is far less effective than ephedrine. The Panel judges these preparations safe but not effective.

Safety and Effectiveness: Bronchodilators
Sold Over-the-Counter for Asthma

Active Ingredient	FDA and Panel's Assessment
aminophylline	safe and effective*
belladonna alkaloids, inhaled	not safe
ephedrine	safe and effective
ephedrine hydrochloride	safe and effective
ephedrine sulfate	safe and effective
epinephrine	safe and effective
epinephrine bitartrate	safe and effective
epinephrine hydrochloride (racemic)	safe and effective
euphorbia pilulifera	safe but not proved effective
methoxyphenamine hydrochloride	safe and effective
pseudoephedrine hydrochloride	safe but not effective
pseudoephedrine sulfate	safe but not effective
racephedrine hydrochloride	safe and effective
theophylline, anhydrous	safe and effective*
theophylline calcium salicylate	safe and effective*
theophylline sodium glycinate	safe and effective*

*Approved for purchase without prescription in combination products only.

Asthma Drugs: Product Ratings

Single-Ingredient Products

Product and Distributor	Dosage of Active Ingredients	Rating[1]	Comment
ephedrine sulfate			
ephedrine sulfate (generic)	**capsules:** 25 mg	A	
ephedrine sulfate (generic)	**syrup USP:** 20 mg per teaspoonful	A	
Ephedrine Sulfate (Lilly)	**syrup:** 11 mg per teaspoonful	A	
epinephrine			
Adrenalin Chloride (Parke-Davis)	**solution for nebulization:** 1:100	A	
AsthmaNefrin (Norcliff Thayer)	**solution for nebulization:** racepinephrine (as hydrochloride) equivalent to 2.25% epinephrine base	A	
Vaponefrin (Fisons)		A	
AsthmaHaler (Norcliff Thayer)	**aerosol:** 0.3 mg epinephrine bitartrate equivalent to 0.16 mg epinephrine base per inhalation	A	
Bronitin Mist (Whitehall)		A	
Primatene Mist Suspension (Whitehall)		A	
Bronkaid Mist (Winthrop)	**aerosol:** 0.16 mg epinephrine per spray	A	
pseudoephedrine hydrochloride			
First Sign (J. B. Williams)	**tablets:** 30 mg	C	not effective
pseudoephedrine hydrochloride (generic)	**tablets:** 30 mg	C	not effective
Sudafed (Burroughs-Wellcome)	**liquid:** 30 mg per teaspoonful	C	not effective
Pseudoephedrine sulfate			
Afrinol Repetabs (Schering)	**tablets (repeat action):** 120 mg	C	not effective

Asthma Drugs: Product Ratings *(continued)*

Combination Products

Product and Distributor	Dosage of Active Ingredient	Rating[1]	Comment
capsules and tablets			
Amodrine Tablets (Searle)	**tablets:** 100 mg aminophylline + 25 mg racephedrine hydrochloride + 8 mg phenobarbital	B	phenobarbital not proved effective
Bronkaid Tablets (Winthrop)	**tablets:** 100 mg theophylline + 24 mg ephedrine sulfate + 100 mg guaifenesin	B	expectorant guaifenesin not proved effective
Bronkotabs Tablets (Breon)	**tablets:** 100 mg theophylline + 24 mg ephedrine sulfate + 100 mg guaifenesin + 8 mg phenobarbital	B	expectorant guaifenesin not proved effective
Brontin Tablets (Whitehall)	**tablets:** 120 mg theophylline + 24 mg ephedrine hydrochloride + 100 mg guaifenesin + 16.6 mg pyrilamine maleate	C	antihistamine pyrilamine maleate may thicken bronchial secretions
Lardet Tablets (Halsom)	**tablets:** 130 mg theophylline + 24 mg ephedrine hydrochloride + 8 mg phenobarbital	B	phenobarbital not proved effective
Phedral C.T. Tablets (North American)		B	
Primatene "P" Formula Tablets (Whitehall)		B	
T.E.P. Tablets (Geneva Generics)		B	
Theofenal Tablets (Spencer-Mead)		B	
liquids			
Bronkolixir Elixir (Breon)	**liquid:** 45 mg theophylline + 36 mg ephedrine sulfate + 150 mg guaifenesin + 12 mg phenobarbital per 3 teaspoonsful	B	expectorant guaifenesin not proved effective
Tedral Suspension (Warner-Lambert)	**liquid:** 65 mg theophylline + 12 mg ephedrine hydrochloride + 4 mg phenobarbital per teaspoonful	B	phenobarbital not proved effective

Asthma Drugs: Product Ratings *(continued)*

Combination Products

Product and Distributor	Dosage of Active Ingredient	Rating[1]	Comment
	liquids		
Theofed Pediatric Suspension (Three P Products)		**B**	
Theoral Pediatric Suspension (Vangard)		**B**	

1. Author's interpretation of Panel criteria. Based on contents, not claims.

Athlete's Foot

See JOCK ITCH, ATHLETE'S FOOT, AND RINGWORM CURES

Baldness Preventives

See HAIR-GROWTH STIMULANTS AND BALDNESS PREVENTIVES

Birth-Control Aids

See CONTRACEPTIVES

Bleaches for Skin Blemishes

An Industrial Mishap

Where: a leather tannery. When: 1939. Who: Black working men and women. Problem: White, depigmented spots began appearing on the

BLEACHES FOR SKIN BLEMISHES is based on the report "Skin Bleaching Products" by the FDA's Advisory Review Panel on OTC Miscellaneous External Drug Products.

hands of the workers. Explanation: The cause of the problem was traced to a variant form of the chemical hydroquinone—a constituent of protective rubber work gloves the workers wore. Hydroquinone is the chemical now formulated into over-the-counter preparations used for bleaching small darkened patches of skin. These defects can be freckles, age spots, or facial pigmentation that sometimes results from pregnancy or the use of oral contraceptives. Hydroquinone is the only chemical used in these preparations, and it is safe and effective at low concentrations.

CLAIMS

Accurate

"lightens dark pigment in the skin"

for "the gradual fading of age spots, liver spots, freckles and melasma" (the mask of pregnancy, a condition of the skin that may also result from the use of oral contraceptives)

False or Misleading

"helps skin look fairer, clearer, and younger"

promises of relief from "skin discolorations," "hand spots," "blotches," or "blotchy skin"

references to "fast-acting" or "quick" (bleaching takes weeks or even months)

WARNING Products must be kept away from the eyes. Bleaches should not be used on children under 12 (there are no reports in scientific journals on hydroquinone therapy in this age group). If the skin becomes irritated, discontinue use or see a doctor. If no improvement is seen after 2 months, stop the treatment. Sun exposure should be avoided indefinitely by using a sunscreen agent, a sunblocking agent, or protective clothing to cover bleached skin.

WHY DARK SPOTS ARISE

The normal hues of human skin are due to the dark pigment melanin, produced by skin cells. (Black people simply have more melanin than white people do.)

Freckles appear naturally on many light-skinned young persons, particularly if they spend much time in the sun. Of greater concern to many persons are the larger "age spots" or "liver spots" that develop in middle age on sun-exposed body surfaces. They affect both men and women. The candid—albeit unpleasant—technical name for these spots is *senile lentigines*: freckles of old age.

Hormonal imbalances caused by pregnancy or by the so-called "false pregnancy" created by oral contraceptives can create widespread facial hyperpigmentation. Also, a number of diseases may unevenly darken the skin. Endocrine disorders like Addison's disease and hyperthyroidism cause changes in skin color, as will liver conditions and rheumatoid arthritis. Certain drugs used to treat serious illness—cancer, mental illness, and malaria—may discolor the skin, too. Rubbing the skin, overexposure to the sun, industrial chemicals, and a host of other environmental factors also may darken small skin areas.

The Panel says that "there is valid reason for some people to use skin bleaches" because of the emotional and social problems that can compound the cosmetic disfiguration.

SKIN-BLEACHING AGENTS

Approved Active Ingredient

Hydroquinone   Hydroquinone is the only active ingredient evaluated safe and effective as a skin bleach. It is an industrial chemical, a dihydroxybenzene. Chemicals in this group have a variety of uses. For example, they inhibit oxidation and are therefore mixed into fats to keep them from becoming rancid. Hydroquinone is a principal ingredient of photographic developer.

Although concentrations of 5 percent hydroquinone may seriously and permanently damage human skin when used for prolonged periods of time, the 1.5 to 2 percent concentrations allowed in bleach creams have not been reported to cause damage. A mild, temporary inflammation may initially arise on the treatment site, but this may foretell success for the treatment.

Tests in animals and in humans show that this ingredient can be ingested in fairly high amounts without risk.

The question of *how* hydroquinone fades skin spots has been studied by a number of scientists, but the answer remains unclear. Apparently the compound inhibits or injures melanin-producing skin cells or the melanin granules within them.

Consumers should know that hydroquinone bleach creams produce only a partial change—they lighten dark spots by about 50 percent at best. This means that they are more effective on relatively light spots than they are on relatively dark ones, for which some remaining over-pigmentation can be anticipated even after treatment—which, in itself, takes 3 weeks to 3 months of daily (or nightly) application.

The results of skin-bleaching with hydroquinone are likely not to last. Depigmented areas will darken again when exposed to the sun, which is why users are cautioned to cover up in the sun or apply a sunscreen. (The one type of skin-bleach combination product approved is a mixture of hydroquinone and a sunscreen.)

Conditionally Approved Active Ingredients

None

Disapproved Active Ingredient

Ammoniated mercury This compound was assessed as unsafe and ineffective. (It is the ingredient used in over-the-counter skin-bleaching products before hydroquinone was.) This white, powdery material is also known as ammoniated mercuric chloride.

Mercury passes through the intact skin—particularly when applied in an ointment base—and continued use could cause mercury poisoning. Thus it is extremely dangerous to use it as a skin bleach. Further, evaluators could find no evidence that ammoniated mercury is actually effective for this intended purpose. Verdict: not safe, not effective.

Safety and Effectiveness: Active Ingredients in Over-the-Counter Skin Bleaches

Active Ingredient	Panel's Assessment
ammoniated mercury	not safe or effective
hydroquinone	safe and effective

Bleaches for Skin Blemishes: Product Ratings

Single-Ingredient Products

Product and Distributor	Dosage of Active Ingredient	Rating[1]	Comment
hydroquinone			
Eldoquin (Elder)	cream: 2%	A	
	lotion: 2%	A	
Eldoquin Forte (Elder)	ointment: 4%	C	not safe because too strong

Bleaches for Skin Blemishes: Product Ratings *(continued)*

Single-Ingredient Products

Product and Distributor	Dosage of Active Ingredient	Rating[1]	Comment
Porcelana (Jeffrey Martin)	**cream:** 2%	**A**	
Quinnone (Dermohr)	**cream:** 4%	**C**	not safe because too strong

Combination Products

Product and Distributor	Dosage of Active Ingredients	Rating[1]	Comment
hydroquinone + sunscreen or sunblock			
Eldopaque (Elder)	**ointment:** 2% + opaque base	**A**	
Porcelana with Sunscreen (Jeffrey Martin)	**cream:** 2% + 2.5% octyl dimethyl PABA (also called palimate O)	**A**	

1. Author's interpretation of Panel criteria. Based on contents, not claims.

Boil Ointments

A red, angry-looking, pus-filled eruption on the skin is apt to be a boil (furuncle). These abscesses are usually caused by bacteria, of which *Staphylococcus aureus* is the most common culprit—and they seem to bedevil some individuals much more often than others.

Several nonprescription drug products are sold for the treatment of boils. They sometimes are called drawing ointments, probably because they are intended to help draw the pus together in a raised, pointed bump that will open and drain of its own accord, or can easily be opened with a sterile needle or blade. The Panel reviewing these preparations came to the conclusion that it is unwise to self-treat a boil

BOIL OINTMENTS is based on the report "Boil Ointment Drug Products for OTC Human Use," by the FDA's Advisory Review Panel on OTC Miscellaneous External Drug Products.

with over-the-counter drugs. Therefore it ruled that all ingredients in nonprescription products claimed to provide boil care are not safe and not effective. If the Panel's view prevails, boil products will be banned from interstate commerce by the FDA at the last stage of the over-the-counter review process.

BOIL CARE

The Panel believes that boils should always be diagnosed by a doctor since they may be caused by bacteria other than *Staphylococcus aureus*; more important, bacteria from a badly treated (or untreated) boil can enter the bloodstream, causing blood poisoning. Boils can also seed serious secondary infections in vital internal organs, including the brain. Boils on the face are particularly dangerous, since underlying blood vessels also serve the brain. Another reason why the Panel discourages self-medication is that antimicrobial drugs are often required to stop the infection and cure the boil. And since different strains of *staphylococci* respond to different drugs, only a lab test can indicate with certainty which drug is best for any particular boil. In short, since self-treatment may delay effective professional treatment, allowing the infection to spread, the reviewers caution against it.

Very small boils sometimes recede without any specific treatment. Soaking a boil in hot water or covering it periodically with hot cloths will sometimes bring it to a point and cause it to drain spontaneously. But the boil will heal faster if a doctor opens and drains it; he or she may then decide to treat it with prescription drugs.

OVER-THE-COUNTER MEDICATIONS FOR BOILS

Approved Active Ingredients

None

Conditionally Approved Active Ingredients

None

Disapproved Active Ingredients

The Panel, with the FDA's help, developed a list of about 2 dozen ingredients in nonprescription boil medications. All are disapproved as unsafe and ineffective, as noted in the chart that follows.

**Safety and Effectiveness: Active Ingredients
in Over-the-Counter Boil Ointments**

Active Ingredient	Panel's Assessment
aminoacridine hydrochloride	not safe and/or effective
benzocaine	not safe and/or effective
bismuth subnitrate	not safe and/or effective
camphor	not safe and/or effective
cholesterol	not safe and/or effective
hexachlorophene	not safe and/or effective
ichthammol	not safe and/or effective
isobutyl para-aminobenzoate	not safe and/or effective
lanolin	not safe and/or effective
magnesium sulfate	not safe and/or effective
menthol	not safe and/or effective
mercurous chloride	not safe and/or effective
methyl salicylate	not safe and/or effective
oil of cade (juniper tar)	not safe and/or effective
oil of sassafras	not safe and/or effective
oxyquinoline sulfate	not safe and/or effective
petrolatum	not safe and/or effective
phenol	not safe and/or effective
pine tar	not safe and/or effective
rosin	not safe and/or effective
rosin cerate	not safe and/or effective
thymol	not safe and/or effective
zinc oxide	not safe and/or effective

Boil Ointments: Product Ratings

All products marketed over-the-counter as boil ointments are not safe and/or not effective, as stipulated by the Panel, and therefore are rated "C."

Callus Removers

See CORN AND CALLUS REMOVERS

Camphor: Special Warning

Over-the-counter drugs that contain high concentrations of camphor are dangerous. Furthermore, they are of little or no medicinal value.

These Panel conclusions are outlined below, in terms of three levels of risk:

- Products containing more than 11 percent camphor are *extremely dangerous*. The FDA, acting on the Panel's recommendation, already has asked manufacturers to recall these products. The agency has also taken steps to ban marketing some such preparations under penalty of law. This ban was formally announced in 1982.
- Products containing 2.5 to 11 percent camphor are *unsafe* and appear to have no appreciable therapeutic value. The Panel believes that these products should also be banned and the FDA is evaluating this recommendation as part of the over-the-counter drug-review process. If the agency agrees with the Panel, eventually, it will ban these products.
- Products containing 2.5 percent or less camphor are *safe*—even if of doubtful effectiveness—if each container holds no more than 360 mg of camphor. This is an amount that probably would not be lethal if eaten by a child (*see* SAFE CAMPHOR PREPARATIONS, below). Even so, the Panel recommends that these products be marketed in containers with child-resistant lids. The FDA is evaluating this recommendation and will mandate these safety steps if it concurs. One manufacturer says the packaging restriction is absurd; the company points out that it would limit camphor products to containers holding no more than about ½ ounce.

EXTREMELY DANGEROUS CAMPHOR PREPARATIONS

The extremely dangerous camphor drugs that the Panel and the FDA want to remove from the over-the-counter market at once contain camphor at concentrations of 11 percent or greater. The FDA has asked manufacturers to recall stock of these preparations, and it

CAMPHOR: SPECIAL WARNING is based on the report "Camphorated Oil and Camphor-Containing Drug Products" by the FDA's Advisory Review Panel on OTC Miscellaneous External Drug Products, on the Panel's "Statement Concerning OTC Drug Products Containing Camphor," on the FDA's Preambles to these documents, and on the FDA's Final Order on Camphorated Oil.

banned further sales of camphorated oil on September 21, 1982. In the same spirit, consumers may wish to check their medicine cabinets and destroy any such products on hand. These highly dangerous substances may be labeled with any of the names that follow—or names like them:

camphor 11% (or above)
camphorated oil
camphor liniment

Note: Camphorated oil is 20% camphor in cottonseed oil. *Camphor liniment* is another name for camphorated oil.

Camphor has been used medicinally for thousands of years, for a variety of purposes. This may be surprising, given the evaluators' declaration—backed by the FDA and other medical authorities—that it "appears to have little, if any, therapeutic benefit." Perhaps camphor's popularity rests on its sensory effects on the body: it has a pungent odor, associated with healing, which may be particularly appreciated by a person who has been cut off from smells by a cold or stuffed-up nose. Camphor creates feelings of both coolness and warmth when applied to the skin. It is irritating enough to cause visible reddening of the skin when it is applied as a liniment or rub. This latter effect appears to be the principal use for the strong preparation called camphor liniment, which is of particular concern to the Panel and the FDA.

Camphor liniment was dropped from the official *National Formulary* of drugs in the United States as long ago as 1970. Yet it has continued to be marketed over-the-counter. The FDA twice asked drug makers to submit their products for evaluation in the over-the-counter drug-review process but no submissions were received. The camphor 20-percent preparations were brought to the reviewers' attention by a pharmacist in Jersey City, New Jersey—Carmine Varano. He wrote to the FDA that a number of persons, most of them children, are poisoned each year by camphor products, particularly camphorated oil. Some die as a result.

The number of poisonings from *all* camphor products appears to be increasing. In one recent year, there were 805 such cases reported to the National Clearinghouse for Poison Control Centers. The following year there were 855.

Many poisonings caused by camphorated oil are accidental. People take it themselves or give it to their children in the mistaken belief that the bottle they have plucked from the medicine cabinet is castor oil, or cod-liver oil, or cough medicine. Young children may find and swallow these drugs. Less commonly, poisonings occur from therapeutic use of camphor liniment or other external products: camphor is readily absorbed through the skin and may be conveyed throughout the body in the bloodstream when it is used as a chest rub or steam inhalant.

The symptoms of camphor poisoning may appear within minutes or they may be delayed several hours if the victim has just eaten food. These symptoms include a feeling of warmth, headache, dizziness, mental confusion, restlessness, delirium, and hallucinations. They may be accompanied by increased muscular excitability, tremors, jerky movements, convulsions, central nervous system depression, and coma. In severe poisoning, respiratory failure or extreme convulsons are usually the cause of death.

If you suspect someone has ingested camphor, smell his or her breath, mouth, and saliva. If you believe camphor may have been taken, phone your doctor, hospital, or the National Poison Center Network at (412) 647–5600.

Banning camphor products containing 11 percent or more camphor will represent little therapeutic loss, assuming the FDA succeeds in this goal. The American Pharmaceutical Association, which represents the nation's pharmacists, testified that not once in camphor's long history—it was officially noted in the first *United States Pharmacopeia*, published in 1820—has the literature shown a single reference concerning the drug's effectiveness.

Conclusion: hazards outweigh by far any medicinal value, and camphorated oil by any name, as well as all other products with greater than 11 percent camphor, are neither safe nor effective.

UNSAFE CAMPHOR PREPARATIONS

A wide variety of single and combination products contain concentrations of camphor between 2.5 percent and 11 percent. They are used as cough suppressors, nasal decongestants, and itch and pain remedies, and are formulated as steam inhalants, as well as liniments and rubs.

The Panel is particularly concerned about a camphor preparation called *camphor spirit*. It consists of 9 to 11 percent camphor in alcohol. Camphor spirit continues to be listed in the two official drug compendia, the *National Formulary* and the *United States Pharmacopeia* (1980 edition). Evaluators are worried that when camphorated oil (20 percent camphor) disappears from the nonprescription market, camphor spirit—which is also hazardous—may replace it.

Many camphor-containing drug products for external use were

submitted for evaluation. Reviewers found little scientific evidence of medicinal value but considerable data to support the viewpoint that camphor products of 2.5 to 11 percent concentration also pose a hazard to health. A past president of the National Clearinghouse for Poison Control Centers recommends that any nonprescription medication containing camphor be limited to 2.5 percent concentration to reduce the risk of accidental poisoning. The American Academy of Pediatrics Committee on Drugs maintains that even relatively small amounts of camphor taken orally have resulted in deaths. This group also emphasized the significance of absorption through the skin or by inhalation, and noted that camphor used by a pregnant woman can cross the placenta and poison a fetus.

The Panel concluded that camphor spirit and all other camphor preparations with between 2.5 and 11 percent concentration are unsafe and ineffective. It has recommended to the FDA that such products be removed from the over-the-counter market. The FDA is assessing this recommendation within the guidelines of the whole over-the-counter drug-review program, and if it concurs, these products will eventually be banned from interstate commerce under penalty of law.

SAFE CAMPHOR PREPARATIONS

Although evaluators are skeptical that camphor has any beneficial value, they referred judgment on products containing concentrations of less than 2.5 percent camphor to Panels considering these types of products.

The present Panel says these preparations would be safe for marketing over-the-counter if each jar or tube contained less than 360 mg of camphor. This is the highest amount that one of the reviewers calculates a 2-year-old, 27-pound child would be reasonably certain to survive if the youngster ate the entire contents of a container. As a further safety measure, the Panel recommends that *all* camphor-containing products have child-resistant lids.

Safety and Effectiveness: Active Ingredients in Over-the-Counter Camphor Products

Active Ingredient	Panel's Assessment*
camphor under 2.5%	safe and *possibly* effective†
camphor 2.5 to 11%	not safe or effective
camphor 11 to 20%	not safe or effective‡
camphor spirits	not safe or effective
camphorated oil (camphorated liniment)	not safe or effective‡

*FDA's Advisory Review Panel on OTC Miscellaneous External Drug Products.
†If properly labeled and packaged.
‡The FDA concurs.

Camphor: Product Ratings—Rated for Safety Only[1]

Product and Distributor	Camphor Dosage	Rating[2]
Caladryl Lotion (Parke-Davis)	2%	A
Campho-Phenique Liquid (Winthrop)	10.8%	C
Camphor Spirit (Humco Lab)	9%	C
Camphor Spirit (McKesson Labs)	9%	C
Deep-Down (J. B. Williams)	0.5%	A
Heet Spray (Whitehall)	3%	C
Panalgesic Rub (Poythress)	2%	A
Rhulicream (Lederle)	0.3%	A

1. Based on *Facts & Comparisons* and industry sources.
2. Author's interpretation of Panel/FDA criteria. Based on contents, not claims.

Cold, Cough, and Allergy Drugs

Americans buy a billion dollars' worth of cold, cough, and allergy drugs over-the-counter annually. Many of the 50,000 products sold for this purpose are complex combinations of several active ingredients—for which a puzzling variety of claims are made, confusing for the pharmacist as well as for the person who is ill. By sorting out the specific symptoms for which people buy and use these products, identifying the group or groups of drugs that could be expected to relieve each type of symptom, and then evaluating the safety and effectiveness of the drugs' active ingredients in each of these groups, the Panel that reviewed these drugs has set criteria by which consumers can choose their medications more intelligently. Shoppers will be in a better position to assess what drug ingredients are actually needed (singly or in combination form), sparing them the risk and cost of those they do not need.

HOW TO FIND THE DRUG THAT RELIEVES SPECIFIC SYMPTOMS

The Symptom Key to Drugs for Colds, Coughs, and Allergies gives the general group of drugs that offers relief for specific symptoms and tells under what unit in this book and under what heading these medications are described.

Symptom Key to Drugs for Colds, Coughs, and Allergies

Symptom	Drug Group	See Page
aches (generalized)	pain-fever relievers	575
bronchospasm	bronchial muscle relaxers	
	(bronchodilators)	125
cough	cough suppressors	113
	expectorants	120
fever	pain-fever relievers	575
nasal congestion	nasal decongestants	133
runny nose	antihistamines	127
	drying agents	126

COLD, COUGH, AND ALLERGY DRUGS is based on the report of the FDA's Advisory Review Panel on OTC Cold, Cough, Allergy, Bronchodilator, and Anti-Asthmatic Products, the FDA's Tentative Final Order on OTC Anticholinergic and Expectorant Drug Products, and official addenda.

**Symptom Key to Drugs for Colds,
Coughs, and Allergies** *(continued)*

Symptom	Drug Group	See Page
sinus congestion	nasal decongestants	133
	pain-fever relievers	575
sneezing and watery, itchy		
eyes caused by allergy	antihistamines	127
sore throat	pain-fever relievers	575
	sore-throat medicines	685

Charts at the end of the unit are set up to help consumers select safe and effective drugs to meet their specific needs of the moment. The prospective purchaser must keep in mind what these drugs can and cannot do. They cannot cure the common cold, or any other condition. But they can—and do—partially relieve some of the principal symptoms associated with colds and minor upper-respiratory infections. They also can relieve symptoms caused by hay fever and other allergies.

CLAIMS

The Panel is concerned that the consumer clearly understand that these remedies can relieve some symptoms but *cannot* cure colds. Claims of special effectiveness are also banned.

False or Misleading
    "cold medicine"
    "cold formula"
    for "relief of colds"
    "specially improved" or "specially formulated"
    "selected ingredients"
    "extra strength" or "stronger than"
    "contains more active ingredients"
    "gets to the roots of" or "fights"
    "multi-action" or "teamed components"

SOME SPECIFIC CONDITIONS

Allergy

An allergic reaction often includes inflamed nasal membranes (rhinitis), runny nose, itchiness in the nose and eyes, coughing, and spitting. More serious responses may include severe shortness of breath and coma, requiring emergency medical care.

Allergy is a form of immune reaction, in which the individual becomes hypersensitive to a particular substance (an allergen) that may be touched, swallowed, or carried by air into the lungs. Common allergens include pollens, mold spores, household dust, animal dander, and industrial emissions. Foods, drugs, and toxic plants like poison ivy are also common allergens. Authorities say that 15 percent of the population is significantly allergic to one or more of these substances.

When allergens touch or enter the body, they trigger the production of a reactive substance (an antibody) that attaches itself to certain types of body cells: mast cells in the blood and basophils in other tissues. The allergens then become "stuck" to these complexes. This reaction prompts the cells to secrete histamine, which acts as an irritant that causes itchiness, tear formation, and other allergic symptoms. As their name implies, antihistamines interrupt the allergic process by blocking histamine's access to the secretory cells. These drugs thus provide direct relief for allergic symptoms—and allergic relief is their principal therapeutic value. The Panel says they are of little or no value when runny nose and watery eyes are the result of a cold.

The best way to relieve allergic complaints is to have an allergist identify the offending substance(s) and then, if possible, avoid it (or them). But when avoidance is impossible, nonprescription antihistamines will often provide substantial relief. If they fail, stronger drugs —including injections of epinephrine and corticosteroids—can be provided by a doctor. It now is possible to tame certain allergies—including those caused by some pollens and by bee stings—with the use of desensitizing injections (preparations that dampen the person's sensitivity to the allergen).

Sore Throat

A sore throat frequently accompanies cough, nasal congestion, and other cold symptoms. It can be treated with aspirin and other pain relievers that are taken internally, and with drugs specifically designed for use in the mouth and throat (see SORE-THROAT AND MOUTH MEDICINES and PAIN, FEVER, AND ANTI-INFLAMMATORY DRUGS TAKEN INTERNALLY).

The Common Cold

Common colds, or, simply, colds, are respiratory infections that are self-limiting—meaning that sooner or later they get better all by themselves. Colds rarely are serious illnesses; but they can be quite annoying and unpleasant.

A cold often starts abruptly with a sore throat, sneezing, and runny nose, followed by nasal congestion. The nasal discharge then may become thick and disagreeable. The eyes begin to water; the voice becomes husky; the nose feels increasingly stuffy. One's senses of smell and taste temporarily vanish, and the cold may spread to the sinuses, producing headache. A wide variety of other aches and pains—to say nothing of fever and lethargy—may follow. This misery can continue for a week or two, with cough and other symptoms coming and going. Discouraging though it may be, the Panel says there is "no generally accepted treatment that can prevent, cure, or shorten the course of the 'common cold.' Treatments which are available only relieve symptoms."

Once over, cold miseries may soon return, because of reinfection by exposure to other people. Many individuals have several colds a year.

Coughing

A cough's main purpose is to clear the airway. It is a protective physiological reflex—part voluntary, part involuntary—that occurs often in healthy people, as well as in sick ones. Infections, chemical irritants, retained body secretions, and the presence of foreign bodies that block one's airway, all can—and do—cause coughing by stimulating the nerve endings in the respiratory tract. (Curiously, tickling the outer ear also sets some people to coughing.)

Drugs that reduce the number and intensity of coughs are called cough suppressors or, technically, antitussives. A few of them are safe and very effective. But because coughing is one of the ways that the body fights illness, it is not always wise to suppress it with drugs. The Panel offers this guidance:

Irritative cough   A *dry* cough, which may be caused by colds or by inhalation of irritating dust or gases, is readily recognizable. It is a hacking kind of cough that produces no sputum or other discharge. Consumers can effectively self-treat these coughs with nonprescription products.

Productive cough   This sputum- or exudate-producing cough (i.e., a *productive* cough) is often associated with asthma and bronchitis. It indicates that phlegm and other secretions are being retained. Suppressing this kind of cough is a bad—even dangerous—idea; the Panel goes so far as to warn against using suppressants but it suggests that an expectorant may be helpful. Evaluators also reiterate this time-honored rule: *any cough that persists more than a week should be investigated by a physician to rule out the possibility of a serious underlying illness.*

Sinus Congestion

The paranasal sinuses—so called because they connect with the nasal cavity—are mucous-membrane-lined air cavities in the bony structure of the skull. When the nose becomes congested, drainage of the sinuses is also impaired. The sinus membranes become inflamed—a condition called *sinusitis*—and may become infected. This situation produces headache, facial pain, and tenderness over the affected sinuses.

Nasal decongestants relieve congested sinuses by opening up the nasal passages so that they can drain. Pain relievers like aspirin will reduce the discomfort. If the symptoms persist, or are accompanied by fever, a doctor should be consulted.

Rhinitis

Rhinitis is nasal inflammation. Marked by a reddening of the nose, it characteristically occurs when one is suffering a cold—but it can occur under some other circumstances.

Allergic rhinitis   This is one of the commonest allergic responses; it tends to recur at the same season each year. The symptoms include sneezy, watery discharge from the nose—which may become thicker if a respiratory infection sets in—and an itchy, stuffed-up feeling. The eyes may itch, redden, and water. Puffy eyelids and headaches are less common consequences. The sinuses may fill with mucus. ·

People who frequently suffer these symptoms usually begin to have some sense of what allergen they are responding to. Their suspicions often can be confirmed by an allergist who uses standard tests.

The most effective drugs for treating allergic rhinitis are antihistamines. Nasal decongestants and anticholinergics may be of some help, too.

Vasomotor rhinitis   This is a nonseasonal problem, unlike many forms of allergic rhinitis. But it tends to recur. The blood vessels of the nasal lining appear to become extremely sensitive and reactive—for reasons that remain unclear. The symptoms are like those of allergic rhinitis, but allergen testing yields no clear-cut categorization. Antihistamines are less effective against vasomotor rhinitis than allergic rhinitis, but nasal decongestants and anticholinergics may offer some relief.

SINGLE VERSUS COMBINATION PRODUCTS

The Panel takes a dim view of the shotgun approach to the treatment of colds and related ailments with combinations of several active ingredients in a single product. This wariness is the more remarkable in that the vast majority of cold, cough, and allergy products contain two or more active ingredients.

When drug firms submitted product data for review, they included information on 152 active ingredients. Yet only 24 of these 152 were formulated as single-ingredient products.

Single-ingredient products are considered preferable by the Panel because they are safer. They allow the consumer to vary the dose of each ingredient individually and they give the consumer an opportunity to select a single drug for a specific symptom. This way people can more easily recognize the drug's action on their bodies and learn to adjust the dosage as necessary—gaining experience in using the drug that can be very useful if such a symptom recurs.

Commenting on the apparent shortage of such single-ingredient medications, the Panel strongly recommends that all components of combination products be made readily available as single ingredients to allow consumers the opportunity to make a more discriminating selection.

However, despite reservations about combining ingredients, the Panel states that, at demonstrably safe and effective doses, combinations "may offer a convenient and rational approach for [relieving] concurrent symptoms." These combinations can include one—but not more than one—safe and effective active ingredient from each of two or three drug groups, as long as the doses are within safe and effective limits. Acceptable and unacceptable combinations are summarized in a table at the end of this unit.

The Panel's concern about combination products extends to the wide and varied list of inactive ingredients—including blood root, licorice, and yerba santa—that they contain. Some of these ingredients may be needed for marketing purposes, the Panel says, but their safety should be evaluated. For a list of inactive ingredients, *see* page 141.

TIMED-RELEASE PRODUCTS

Cold-cough drugs and other medicines taken orally are dissolved in the stomach and intestines. They then are absorbed through the gut wall and into the bloodstream, which carries them to the head, lungs, nose, and other target organs. This action generally occurs within an hour or two. So a drug's peak activity—as defined by its maximal levels in the bloodsteam—typically occurs about 1 or 2 hours after ingestion. A drug may continue to be present and active for several more hours —up to about 6 hours after it is taken.

Many cold-cough remedies are formulated as timed-release products, to spread out and delay absorption of the drug from the gastrointestinal tract. The aim is to provide effective drug action for up to 8 to 12 hours, rather than the 3 to 6 hours obtainable from ordinary medication. Timed-release drugs have the advantage of being easier to take since fewer doses are necessary. They may provide longer-acting relief and also entail fewer and less severe side effects because blood levels of the drugs can be kept fairly constant.

The principal problem has been that it is hard to manufacture uniformly effective timed-release products. The capsules or pills tend to dissolve irregularly, depending in part on the acidity of the user's stomach. They may dissolve too slowly and travel too far down into the gut to be effective. Or they may dissolve too rapidly to be wholly safe.

Nevertheless, with the exception of glyceryl guaiacolate and the theophyllines, all the drugs reviewed were assessed as suitable for timed-release formulation. However, timed-release drugs used for cough-cold-allergy products are granted only *conditional* approval from the standpoint of safety and effectiveness—pending submission of more satisfactory evidence.

Note: The Schering Corporation subsequently obtained approval from the FDA of a repeat-action tablet of chlorpheniramine maleate (Chlor-Trimeton), an antihistamine. Similar approval was granted Menley and James Laboratories for chlorpheniramine maleate sustained-release capsules (Teldrin). Two pseudoephedrine continuous-release allergy relievers were approved, the FDA says: Sudafed S.A. (Abbott) and Sudafed S.A. (Burroughs Wellcome). Finally, one combination of chlorpheniramine maleate and pseudoephedrine sulfate as a repeat-action decongestant tablet was approved by the FDA in 1981 (Chlor-Trimeton Decongestant Tablets, Schering).

DOSAGE

Dosage recommendations for approved active ingredients in cough suppressors, antihistamines, and nasal decongestants are found in the discussions for each of these drug groups below.

Dosages for Children

Children are commonly given cold-cough preparations, yet very little is known about how children react to these drugs or how much they should take. With the help of an *ad hoc* committee of pediatric drug specialists, the Panel established these general guidelines for children:

under age 2   dosage to be determined by a physician
ages 2 to 6   ¼ the adult dose
ages 6 to 12   ½ the adult dosage

Some ingredients should not be taken by children. For example, nonprescription products that contain over 10 percent alcohol by weight should not be given to youngsters under the age of 6—except under a doctor's supervision.

COUGH SUPPRESSORS

As its name implies, a cough suppressor or suppressant (antitussive) suppresses or inhibits the act of coughing. Some of these agents act in the brain to depress the activity of the cough center in the medulla, suppressing the impulse to cough. The narcotic, codeine, and dextromethorphan (a potent nonnarcotic) both act in this way.

A second group of cough suppressors acts on the throat and bronchial passages. They deaden or lessen pain, relax the smooth muscles that are involved in coughing, or thin out sticky phlegm deposits so that fewer coughs are required to expel them.

CLAIMS FOR COUGH SUPPRESSORS

Claims are often made that cough-suppressing ingredients have a "demulcent" or "soothing" effect on irritated throats, which reduces coughing. It has not been proved, however, that soothing the throat reduces coughing. Nor is there a scientific explanation of *how* a drug might act to "soothe" the throat and bronchial passages.

Accurate
"cough suppressant which temporarily reduces the impulse to cough"
"temporarily helps you cough less"
for "the temporary relief of coughs due to minor throat and bronchial irritation as may occur with the common cold or inhaled irritants"
"temporarily quiets coughing by its antitussive action"

Cough suppressors sold over-the-counter are intended—and should be used—to diminish coughs that arise suddenly, due to bronchial irritation. They should not be used for more than one week. Once again, coughs that last longer or are accompanied by high fever, rash, or persistent headache, may signal the presence of serious disease; they should be investigated by a doctor.

Persons with asthma, emphysema, and other diseases characterized by overproduction of bronchial secretions need to cough to keep their airways clear. They should not take cough suppressors except under medical supervision. Similarly, coughs caused by smoking should not be treated with these agents.

Cough suppressors are tested by the straightforward method of comparing the number of coughs that cough sufferers or test subjects emit when they are using the drug compared with when they are using a dummy drug. These tests are more scientifically reliable in blind studies—that is, when the subjects (and preferably the testers, too) do not know when the active drug or the dummy is being used. In these experiments, a number of throat irritants—including ammonia vapor and sprays of peppermint water and citric acid—are used to stimulate coughing so that the efficacy of the drug can be quickly and conveniently assessed.

Approved Active Ingredients

Evaluators decided that two widely marketed types of cough suppressants, codeine preparations and dextromethorphan, are safe and effective for over-the-counter use. It also recommended that a third drug—the antihistamine diphenhydramine hydrochloride, which long had been sold as a prescription cough medicine—be categorized as a safe and effective nonprescription suppressor. But the FDA disagreed, citing the high incidence of drowsiness in those who use diphenhydramine and the paucity of tests showing its effectiveness. After long and costly administrative review and litigation, the FDA agreed late in 1981 to approve over-the-counter sales of Parke-Davis' Benylin, which contains diphenhydramine hydrochloride as an antitussive.

Codeine preparations   Whether in healthy volunteers who are subjected to cough-inducing agents or in patients with chronic coughs, codeine's effectiveness in suppressing coughs has been demonstrated time and again. It is an extremely effective drug. But since most clinical tests have been in adults with chronic coughs, its effectiveness against acute coughs, in colds, or for coughs in children are not nearly so well documented—though it is judged effective.

Codeine may be formulated in nonprescription cough preparations as codeine, codeine alkaloid, codeine phosphate, or codeine sulfate. They are of esssentially equal potency, and all are safe and effective.

One possible side effect is severe constipation. However, the major issue that surrounds codeine's use is its safety. It is a narcotic drug and when large amounts are taken, it can be addictive. But the Panel believes that potential for abuse is negligible and that the drug has a low risk of inducing dependency in the small doses in which—under regulation of the Federal Drug Enforcement Agency—it is formulated in over-the-counter cough remedies. Nonetheless, purchasers now must sign a special register in the drugstore when they buy a codeine cough preparation and in many states they cannot buy any codeine preparations without a prescription.

Because it *suppresses* coughing, codeine should not be taken by people with thick, wet coughs who need to clear their respiratory passages. Neither should it be taken by those with chronic lung disorders or shortness of breath, except under medical supervision.

CLAIMS FOR CODEINE PREPARATIONS

Accurate
"calms the cough control center and relieves coughing"

Recommended Dosage for Over-the-Counter Cough Suppressors

Active Ingredient	Adults	Children 6 to 12	Children 2 to 6
codeine	10 to 20 mg every 4 to 6 hrs (120 mg daily maximum)	5 to 10 mg every 4 to 6 hrs (60 mg daily maximum)	2.5 to 5 mg every 4 to 6 hrs (30 mg daily maximum)
dextromethorphan, dextromethorphan hydrobromide	10 to 20 mg every 4 hrs or 30 mg every 6 to 8 hrs (120 mg daily maximum)	5 to 10 mg every 4 hrs or 15 mg every 6 to 8 hrs (60 mg daily maximum)	2.5 to 5 mg every 4 hrs or 7.5 mg every 6 to 8 hrs (30 mg daily maximum)
diphenhydramine hydrochloride	25 mg every 4 hrs (150 mg daily maximum)	12.5 mg every 4 hrs (75 mg daily maximum)	as recommended by a doctor

Dextromethorphan and dextromethorphan hydrobromide
These variants of morphine lack morphine's pain-killing and addictive traits. But they are highly effective cough suppressants and are used in cough medicines as nonnarcotic alternatives to codeine.

Overdoses of dextromethorphan have produced bizarre behavior and other symptoms, but not physical dependence or death. Because of the drug's low order of toxicity, it was assessed as being possibly the safest nonprescription cough suppressor available.

CLAIMS FOR DEXTROMETHORPHAN

Accurate
"calms cough impulses without narcotics"
"non-narcotic cough suppressant for the temporary control of coughs"

Diphenhydramine hydrochloride   This antihistamine was introduced clinically in the United States as a prescription drug more than three decades ago. The Panel found that it is as effective a cough suppressor as codeine, but the FDA disagreed, saying that there was inadequate evidence to show that it acts directly on the cough center in the brain—as an approved antitussive is required to. The FDA also questioned diphenhydramine hydrochloride's safety, noting that drowsiness is a side effect in 30 percent of those who use this drug. This side effect is particularly dangerous in those who take this drug while driving a car or operating machinery.

On the basis of new studies—supplied predominantly by the drug manufacturer Parke-Davis & Co.—the FDA reversed its view in 1981 and approved the company's Benylin Cough Syrup, in which diphenhydramine hydrochloride is the cough-suppressing active ingredient, as safe and effective.

WARNING FOR DIPHENHYDRAMINE HYDROCHLORIDE   The FDA mandates the important warning: "May cause marked drowsiness . . . Avoid driving a motor vehicle or operating heavy machinery, or drinking alcoholic beverages."

Conditionally Approved Active Ingredients

Most of the cough-suppressing ingredients used in nonprescription drugs are plant extracts. They continue to be used because long experience suggests that they may be helpful. But scientific studies to confirm this belief and demonstrate the safety and effectiveness of these substances have not been done. So only conditional approval was granted.

Beechwood creosote   This is a pungent, smoke-colored distillate of wood tar that has prompted few safety complaints in the many years it has been marketed. But only one contemporary scientific study was submitted to establish its effectiveness—and it was flawed. It is unlikely that lozenges containing 3 or 4 mg of creosote each are effective. Verdict: safe but not proved effective.

Camphor (applied to the skin or inhaled)   Extracts of this irritating plant substance are formulated into salves and ointments that are applied to the skin. The body warms the salve or ointment and the camphor fumes are inhaled from the skin. This substance is also found in steam-inhalant products and lozenges.

Camphor has a paradoxical effect when applied topically: it first produces a menthollike feeling of coolness, then a sense of warmth, particularly when rubbed vigorously onto the skin. It also has a mild numbing effect.

Long experience indicates that topical and inhalant camphorated products are safe in low doses. But camphor is highly toxic when ingested; it should be kept where children cannot reach it (*see* CAMPHOR).

The Panel questions camphor's effectiveness—which has not been convincingly demonstrated. Thus far, there is more evidence to confirm its value as a chest rub than as a lozenge or inhalant. *Note:* The FDA has indicated that it will designate camphor (4.73–5.3 percent) as safe and effective as a cough suppressor when formulated as an ointment to be rubbed on the chest. This will occur at the next stage of the review of these ingredients. The FDA also plans to upgrade—to safe and effective—ointments containing menthol (2.6–2.8 percent) alone, and combinations of camphor, menthol, and eucalyptus oil (1.2–1.3 percent).

Caramiphen edisylate (caramiphen ethanedisulfonate)   This drug acts in the brain to suppress the cough reflex, but it is not a narcotic. It is safe; however, it has a drying effect on the body and should not be used by persons whose conditions (e.g., glaucoma or enlarged prostate gland) it would complicate. No acceptable studies confirm its effectiveness.

Carbetapentane citrate   Besides being a cough suppressant, carbetapentane may relieve bronchial spasms, dry up runny noses, and act —albeit weakly—against pain.

Side effects are rare and for the most part mild—so the Panel says it is safe. Dry mouth is the commonest complaint. Carbetapentane is not a narcotic and it appears not to be habit-forming, but further tests are needed to prove its effectiveness.

Cod-liver oil   This a good natural source of vitamin A and vitamin D, and there is no significant evidence of serious toxicity. But there is virtually no evidence that cod-liver oil can inhibit or suppress coughing.

Elm bark   The bark of the slippery-elm tree, once called "salve bark," traditionally was used by American Indians and early settlers to treat fevers, colds, and coughs. One recipe called for one ounce of powdered bark in a pint of hot water, to be taken at will.

Long use confirms elm bark as safe for use in teas, inhalants, and poultices—but there is no sound evidence that it effectively relieves coughing.

Ethylmorphine hydrochloride   Like codeine, this is a morphine derivative. But it is less potent than codeine as a cough suppressor, and is not widely used. It can be addictive, and may cause severe constipation. However, it is considered safe in doses used in cough medicine, although scientific studies are needed to demonstrate effectiveness.

Eucalyptol and eucalyptus oil (topical or inhaled)   Extracts of the eucalyptus tree are used in ointments, medicated steam inhalants, lozenges, and mouthwashes. Experiments have shown that these extracts do not damage the skin or produce other symptoms, even when taken in higher doses and for periods longer than recommended on product labels. But, the effectiveness of eucalyptus has not been convincingly demonstrated—although a mouthwash containing eucalyptus and other volatile oils reduced cough and nasal cold symptoms in schoolchildren in a long-term, carefully controlled study. Eucalyptus's value is better established for ointments and salves than for other formulations, but all require further evidence of effectiveness. *Note: See* Note under CAMPHOR, above.

Horehound (horehound fluid extract)   Horehound has been used for centuries as a folk medicine in candies, teas, and in other steeped liquids. No adverse effects have been reported, so it is judged safe. But no evidence shows that it effectively suppresses coughing—there is not even an established dosage.

Menthol and peppermint oil   Menthol is the principal constituent of natural peppermint oil. Menthol/peppermint preparations are put into ointments and salves, inhalants, lozenges, and mouthwashes. They are safe in customary dosages—although high doses and accidental overdoses are hazardous. Like camphor, menthol/peppermint produces a first-cool-then-warm feeling when it is applied to the skin and mucosal tissues. Whether inhalation or other exposure to menthol/peppermint—which also has a mild pain-killing effect—really relieves coughing remains to be seen. Test findings were not conclusive.

Noscapine (noscapine hydrochloride)   Although it is an opium derivative, like codeine, noscapine lacks codeine's addictive liability and its constipating side effect. In cough-medicine doses, clinical experience confirms its safety but its effectiveness is less well established.

Thymol   This is a weaker, menthollike compound that can be derived chemically from coal tar. It is formulated into ointments, medicated steam-inhalant products and sprays, and in lozenges and mouthwash. Little scientific data is available on its toxicity in humans, but long clinical use indicates that it is safe in usual dosages—but effectiveness has not been proved.

Turpentine oil (spirits of turpentine) (topical or inhaled)   The volatile oil of turpentine, derived from pine resin, has been widely used in ointments and other combination cold-cough products for many years. The customer complaint rate has been low and no side effects were uncovered by safety tests. It is considered safe for topical and inhalant use, but studies are needed to show it effectively curbs coughing.

Disapproved Active Ingredients

Two cough-suppressant active ingredients were found unsafe for nonprescription use.

Hydrocodone bitartrate (dihydrocodeinone)   This drug is more potent than codeine in relieving coughing and pain. But it also is more addicting than codeine—it is close to morphine in this respect. It is not available over-the-counter, but remains a prescription drug for medically supervised use against severe and persistent coughing disorders.

Turpentine oil (spirits of turpentine) (taken orally)   This distillate of pine-tree resin irritates the throat when taken internally; further, there is no evidence that it effectively prevents coughing. Also, because one-half ounce can fatally poison a child and 5 ounces may be fatal for an adult, turpentine oil is clearly a dangerous substance.

EXPECTORANTS

An expectorant is a drug used to promote or facilitate the removal of secretions from the bronchial airways. Such action should temporarily relieve coughs due to minor throat and bronchial irritations that commonly occur with a cold.

The secretions that expectorants are claimed to act on are the thick respiratory-tract fluids, saliva, and postnasal secretions, which may be referred to as phlegm, mucus, or sputum.

An expectorant may reduce the thickness of bronchial secretions or dilute them so that they are looser and are more easily evacuated. Some expectorants act directly on nerve endings in the bronchial tubes. Others irritate the stomach, triggering a secretory reflex that increases fluid discharges into the stomach and respiratory tract. Still other expectorants stimulate the vomiting center of the brain and other brain areas that are involved in the movement of these thick fluids. When the irritating—sometimes choking—accumulations are gone, the need to cough is diminished.

Expectorants should be useful in relieving irritative, nonproductive coughs, or thick, dry coughs in which little sputum is being expelled. Persons who already are coughing up copious amounts of loose phlegm would be less likely to need these drugs.

Many over-the-counter expectorant drugs have been purchased and used for decades. They have a good safety record and their continued popularity suggests that they are effective. But there is little objective, scientific evidence to confirm this. One reason may be that expectorants are harder to test than cough suppressants, which can be evaluated objectively in cough-counting experiments. With expectorants, the best test method available is to give chronic coughers or persons with acute upper-respiratory infections coded preparations that contain either the active ingredient or a dummy substance. Test subjects then are asked to rate or compare the medications—which clearly makes for more subjective data.

Because of the lack of reliable findings, the Panel did not approve any expectorants as safe and effective. Most were granted conditional approval. The FDA essentially sustained these judgments in 1982, and noted that to the best of its knowledge only one ingredient, guaifenesin, was currently undergoing tests that could qualify it for a "safe and effective" designation within the next few years.

CLAIMS FOR EXPECTORANTS

It is sometimes claimed that expectorants increase the amount of mucus that covers and protects the lining of the throat and bronchial airway. It is claimed, too, that these drugs exert a soothing or demulcent effect on the respiratory passages. The Panel evaluators doubt these claims.

The experts further warn that expectorants should not be taken for persistent or chronic coughs such as occur with smoking, asthma, or emphysema, except with the advice and supervision of a physician. Too, a thick, persistent cough can signal the presence of serious illness; if the coughing continues past a week, medical help should be sought.

If some of these expectorants are shown to be effective, as is claimed, as well as safe, the Panel says the following claims could be made for them.

Accurate

"helps loosen phlegm"

"helps rid the passageways of bothersome mucus"

"helps drainage of the bronchial tubes by thinning the mucus"

"relieves irritated membranes in the respiratory passageways by preventing dryness through increased mucus flow"

Approved Active Ingredients

None

Conditionally Approved Active Ingredients

More than a dozen substances or groups of closely related substances are conditionally approved by the Panel.

Ammonium chloride   In customary dosages, this remedy has been shown by experience to be safe. The most frequent side effects are nausea and vomiting. There are no well-controlled studies documenting ammonium chloride's efficacy as an expectorant. Some tests show no significant change in sputum volume or viscosity following the taking of this drug. Others indicate it makes the sputum more fluid—easier to raise and expel. More definitive studies are needed.

Beechwood creosote   No controlled studies demonstrate effectiveness as an expectorant.

Benzoin preparations   The substances benzoin tincture and compound benzoin tincture, used in medicated steam-inhalant products, are derived from the resin of trees and bushes of the genus *Styrax*. They have a vanillalike odor and an aromatic, slightly acrid taste. Benzoin is often combined with other volatile oils in alcohol. No well-controlled scientific studies are available on its effectiveness as an expectorant.

Camphor   *See* COUGH SUPPRESSORS, above. Its effectiveness as an expectorant is uncertain, since no well-controlled studies could be found in the medical-scientific literature.

Eucalyptol and eucalyptus oil   *See* COUGH SUPPRESSORS, above. There is insufficient evidence concerning effectiveness as an expectorant.

Guaifenesin (glycerol guaiacolate)   This is one of the most widely used cough medications, with few reported adverse reactions. But studies differ on whether in fact it reduces sputum stickiness and improves breathing. And if significant improvement occurs only after 10 days' use, as has been reported, the drug *clearly* is not appropriate where fast action is a requirement. Confirmation of expectorant effectiveness is needed.

Ipecac syrup   Clinical experience indicates that ipecac syrup, in the dosages used in expectorants, is safe, although the Panel could find no scientific study to confirm this. Ipecac is very effective in inducing vomiting in persons who have taken poison. Whether the smaller amounts used in cough medicines can be effective as expectorants remains to be proved. Further, it should not be taken longer than a week because the safety of long-term use remains in question.

Menthol and peppermint oil   *See* COUGH SUPPRESSORS, above. Efficacy as expectorant active ingredients needs to be established.

Pine-tar preparations   These thick, blackish-brown liquids with their characteristic turpentinelike odor and sharp taste have been used for decades. Slightly irritating, these preparations are antiseptic, relieve pain, and seem safe. It is questionable whether they mobilize phlegm. Their inclusion in expectorant products appears a matter of tradition— scientific proof of effectiveness is lacking.
Note: Pine tar may appear on product labels as extract white-pine compound, pine tar, syrup of pine tar, compound white-pine syrup, or, simply, white pine.

Potassium guaiacolsulfonate   Used in expectorant mixtures for many years, this ingredient is considered safe. But there is scant evidence that it is actually effective.

Sodium citrate   In over a half-century, there appears to have been no untoward consequences from the use of sodium citrate as an expectorant. But neither is there acceptable evidence that it is effective. One authoritative pharmacologic text suggests that whatever benefit it does provide is obtained from the fluid (fruit juice or water) with which it must be mixed in order to be palatable.

Terpin hydrate preparations   Whether formulated as terpin hydrate or its elixir, this substance has been used long enough without serious problems to be assessed safe in recommended doses (although it produces nausea and vomiting in some people). The alcohol with which it is formulated may be as strong as that in whiskey, so it is subject to abuse and should not be given to children. The scientific literature shows it is probably harmless—but also of dubious worth as an expectorant.

Tolu preparations   These compounds—which include tolu, tolu balsam, and tolu balsam tincture—are made from an aromatic tree gum with a vanillalike odor; they have been called *Friar's balsam*. There are no documented reports of toxic reactions in humans, but neither are there acceptable studies that show effectiveness as an expectorant in oral or inhalant nonprescription products.

Turpentine oil (spirits of turpentine) (topical or inhaled)   Although safe when applied in salves and ointments, or used to medicate steam for inhalation, these have not been shown, through objective evidence, to be effective as an expectorant.

Disapproved Active Ingredients

Several substances that have been promoted and used as expectorants are clearly unsafe and/or ineffective, according to the Panel. It recommended that these substances be removed from the over-the-counter drug market.

Antimony potassium tartrate   There is no evidence that this compound is effective, and a good deal to suggest that it is hazardous. Compounds of this sort are potent inducers of vomiting; they act both on the brain and on the stomach. Like arsenic, antimony is not excreted; it builds up in the body and causes irritation of the stomach and intestinal walls as well as in the muscles and joints.

Chloroform   Since there is no evidence that chloroform is an expectorant or alleviates coughing, its known toxicity and potential for abuse are both good reasons for banning it as an active ingredient in nonprescription products. This has now been done.

Iodides   Several compounds containing a form of iodide have been used as expectorants, including calcium iodide anhydrous, hydriodic acid syrup, iodized lime, and potassium iodide. While such compounds may be helpful in the medical management of chronic respiratory illnesses, there is no evidence to show that they are effective against acute upper-respiratory infections of the sort that can be self-treated with nonprescription medication. Iodides are highly toxic, and the more one ingests, the more severe the symptoms one can expect. Signs of *iodism*—as iodide toxicity is called—are headache, runny nose, and other cold-like symptoms. So taking an iodide as a cough-medicine ingredient can be dangerously confusing—a kind of "double whammy" that affords little or no therapeutic value.

Ipecac fluid extract   This preparation is 14 times more potent than ipecac syrup (*see* above) and so is *quite* toxic. There is scant evidence that the substance is effective as an expectorant.

Squill and squill extract   In higher concentrations, squill is used as rat poison. It is very toxic, causing nausea and vomiting. Although the low doses used in nonprescription mixtures may be safe, they may also be too low to effect expectorant action. The risks outweigh any possible benefits.

Turpentine oil (spirits of turpentine) (taken orally)   There is no evidence that swallowing turpentine preparations will loosen phlegm. Even more important, turpentine is quite toxic: a half-ounce has been reported to kill a child. Turpentine preparations should not be taken orally as an expectorant—or for any other reason.

BRONCHIAL MUSCLE RELAXANTS (BRONCHODILATORS)

Bronchodilators are drugs that, when spasms occur, relax the smooth muscles lining the bronchial airway. They open the airway and facilitate normal breathing.

Bronchodilators are quite potent and they can be quite dangerous, with side effects ranging all the way to cardiac arrest. The Panel recommends that they be sold over-the-counter for use *only* by people actually diagnosed as suffering from asthma.

These drugs have been included in a number of cold-cough products. But, contrary to claims made for them, the Panel says they:

- do not relieve hay fever
- do not decongest swollen mucosal membranes
- do not relieve bronchitis or the common cold
- do not relieve fear, anxiety, or nervous tension
- do not clear the bronchial passages
- do not contain antiallergen ingredients
- do not ease irritation of bronchial and nasal mucous membranes, or itchy, watery eyes

But despite all these do-*nots*, evaluators could not rule out the possibility that bronchodilators may help relieve some nonasthmatic coughs. They therefore granted *conditional* approval to the claim that these drugs "provide temporary relief of cough caused by the *common cold* or *bronchitis*."

These drugs are discussed elsewhere (*see* ASTHMA) and are evaluated for safety and effectiveness as antiasthmatics in a chart at the end of that unit. None are regarded by the Panel as safe and effective in nonprescription products for use in treating coughs due to the common cold or bronchitis.

DRYING AGENTS (ANTICHOLINERGICS)

Drugs of the class called *anticholinergics* (drying agents) are used to relieve runny nose and rheumy eyes—conditions that commonly accompany colds as well as hay fever and other allergies. They work by blocking the mechanism that allows the glands to emit tears and nasal secretions. The drying agents used to treat runny nose and watery eyes also reduce secretions from the salivary, sweat, and bronchial glands and act, too, on the heart, gastrointestinal tract, and urinary bladder. They can produce dry mouth, reduced sweating, rapid heart rate, and difficulty in urination—as well as restlessness, confusion, and other disconcerting side effects.

When drying agents act on bronchial secretions, they reduce their volume and make them stickier—and thus more difficult to expel from the respiratory passages. This can lead to blockage of the passages. Infections may fester in the impacted phlegm—which can be extremely hazardous for persons with bronchial asthma or chronic lung disorders, who should not use these drugs except under medical supervision.

The anticholinergics are exceptionally potent drugs. Consumers must use them with extreme caution, if they use them at all. None is ranked safe and effective. If an anticholinergic were approved, claims would have to be confined to the following:

"temporary relief of watery nasal discharge and watering of the eyes as may occur in certain allergic conditions and infections of the upper respiratory tract"

"temporary relief from running nose"

The FDA, in accepting the Panel's recommendations, in 1982, noted that no anticholinergic is currently being tested with a view toward proving it safe and effective for use in nonprescription drugs. Most products already have been reformulated to remove these ingredients, and the FDA foresees banning them within the next few years.

Approved Active Ingredients

None

Conditionally Approved Active Ingredients

Two preparations used as drying agents in cold medications are safe when taken in small doses, but their effectiveness needs to be better established.

Atropine sulfate Very small amounts of 0.2 to 0.3 mg atropine sulfate have been used in over-the-counter cold products. While these doses are small enough to be safe, they may be too small to be effective. In one study, a larger dose of 0.6 mg has been shown to marginally reduce nasal discomfort. But there still is little sound evidence to show that even this amount of atropine will effectively relieve cold symptoms.

Belladonna alkaloids These substances are combinations of atropine with smaller amounts of scopolamine, formulated as preparations called *belladonna tincture* and *belladonna extract*. They are common constituents of proprietary cold products. They may provide some symptomatic relief, but, as with atropine sulfate, the small amounts that experience shows to be safe may not be effective.

Disapproved Active Ingredients

Belladonna alkaloids (inhaled) A mixture of *Atropa belladonna* and *Datura stramonia* plant substances is marketed over-the-counter. It is smoked in a cigarette or a pipe mixture, or burned like incense and the smoke inhaled. Like other belladonna formulations, this one is psychoactive—confusion, delirium, and hallucinations may result.

The adverse effects of this powder—including death—have been well described in the medical literature. Against such well-documented risks, there is no scientifically valid evidence that establishes the mixture's effectiveness as a drying agent. Furthermore, its preparation as a smoking material makes it quite susceptible to abuse.

ANTIHISTAMINES

The antihistaminic drugs, developed in France, were first used medically in 1942 and were introduced into the United States a few years later. As a class of medication, they have proved to be extremely safe and extremely useful for several purposes. Close to 50 different antihistamines have been introduced to the prescription and nonprescription markets.

A principal use of antihistamines is to relieve allergic reactions caused by the release of histamine. This irritating body substance attaches itself to secretory cells of the nose, eyes, lungs, and skin—enhancing their fluid-making activity. Antihistamines counteract these distressing effects by blocking histamine receptor sites on these cells.

These drugs also have a mild drying (anticholinergic) effect. For that reason the Panel considers them appropriate in managing allergies. This drying effect is probably what accounts for claims that the drugs are beneficial in relieving cold symptoms.

However, although antihistamines are common ingredients in over-the-counter cold-cough combination products, the Panel says in controlled scientific studies they have never been demonstrated to be effective against cold symptoms. What is more, there is no clear-cut evidence to show that the runny nose and watery eyes that afflict sufferers of the common cold are really caused by the release of histamine, or that the histaminic reaction plays any significant role in colds.

A principal side effect of antihistamines is drowsiness. For this reason they are widely used as sleep aids. According to drug evaluators of the American Medical Association, antihistamines vary in terms of the frequency and severity of the drowsiness they produce. Examples follow:

> *Marked risk of drowsiness*
> diphenhydramine hydrochloride
> doxylamine succinate
> phenyltoloxamine citrate
> *Moderate risk of drowsiness*
> pyrilamine maleate
> thonzylamine hydrochloride
> tripelannamine hydrochloride
> *Low risk of drowsiness*
> brompheniramine maleate
> chlorpheniramine maleate
> pheniramine maleate

Drowsiness from taking antihistamines may be aggravated by drinking alcohol. So users are warned not to drink, as well as to avoid driving a vehicle or operating machinery—precautionary measures stressed by the Panel.

Dry mouth is another fairly frequent side effect of antihistamines.

Fortunately, the more common side effects of these drugs are rarely serious, particularly if the drugs are taken in the dosages recommended for use without prescription.

CLAIMS

Accurate
"alleviates," "decreases," or "for temporary relief of running nose, sneezing, itching of the nose or throat and itchy and watery eyes as may occur in allergic rhinitis [such as hay fever]"

"dries running nose as may occur in allergic rhinitis [such as hay fever]"

Approved Active Ingredients

The Panel approved 10 antihistamines as safe and effective over-the-counter drugs. Two of them, diphenhydramine hydrochloride and promethazine hydrochloride, have been on prescription status and the FDA has declined to reclassify them for nonprescription use as antihistamines. Another such drug, methapyrilene, was abruptly recalled from the over-the-counter drug marketplace in 1979 after animal tests suggested that it might cause cancer in people who use it.

The 7 ingredients that retain the approval of both the Panel and the FDA are discussed below.

Brompheniramine maleate   A half billion dosage units of this antihistamine were sold annually on a prescription basis and very few serious adverse effects were reported. Basing their conclusion on this felicitous clinical experience, as well as on experimental studies in animals, the Panel evaluated brompheniramine maleate as safe and proposed that it be made available in over-the-counter preparations. The FDA agreed.

Studies confirm that brompheniramine acts as an antihistamine in adults suffering from runny noses due to allergy. Some children with persistent runny noses not responsive to other therapies also have been reported to be helped by this drug—although these and other studies of the drug in youngsters did not wholly satisfy the evaluators. The Panel nevertheless rates brompheniramine maleate safe and effective for adults and children over age 2 as a self-treatment drug.

Chlorpheniramine maleate   This antihistamine effectively relieves hay fever and other allergic symptoms. It is safe. In one recent year, 2 billion capsules and other dosage units were sold, and fewer than 2,000 cases of suspected poisoning were reported (none was fatal).

Drowsiness occurs in 10 to 20 percent of users. Chlorpheniramine does not relieve—and in fact may exacerbate—a stopped-up nose.

Recommended Dosage for Over-the-Counter Antihistamines

Active Ingredient	Adults	Children 6 to 12*
brompheniramine maleate	4 mg every 4 to 6 hrs (24 mg daily maximum)	2 mg every 4 to 6 hrs (12 mg daily maximum)
chlorpheniramine maleate	4 mg† every 4 to 6 hrs (24 mg daily maximum)	2 mg every 4 to 6 hrs (12 mg daily maximum)
doxylamine succinate	7.5 mg every 4 to 6 hrs (45 mg daily maximum)	3.75 mg every 4 to 6 hrs (22.5 mg daily maximum)
phenindamine tartrate	25 mg every 4 to 6 hrs (150 mg daily maximum)	12.5 mg every 4 to 6 hrs (75 mg daily maximum)
pheniramine maleate	12.5 to 25 mg every 4 to 6 hrs (150 mg daily maximum)	6.25 to 12.5 mg every 4 to 6 hrs (75 mg daily maximum)
pyrilamine maleate	25 to 50 mg every 6 to 8 hrs (200 mg daily maximum)	12.5 to 25 mg every 6 to 8 hrs (100 mg daily maximum)
thonzylamine hydrochloride	50 to 100 mg every 4 to 6 hrs (600 mg daily maximum)	25 to 50 mg every 4 to 6 hrs (300 mg daily maximum)

*For children 2 to 6, consult doctor.
†8 and 12 mg in sustained-action formulations for use at 8- or 12-hour intervals. Not recommended for children.

Doxylamine succinate   The Panel and the FDA were somewhat at loggerheads over this antihistamine. The Panel said that the *minimum* effective dose against allergic rhinitis is 7.5 mg; in most studies documenting the drug's effectiveness, larger amounts were used. But the FDA believes that 7.5 mg is the *upper* limit for safety in a nonprescription drug because marked drowsiness occurs in up to half of those taking the drug—a higher proportion than in the instance of other effective antihistamines. So, 7.5 mg is the upper limit.

Phenindamine tartrate   This is a fast-acting antihistamine that provides good to excellent relief for two-thirds or more of hay fever victims and other allergy suferers. The reports in the literature over the last 30 years suggest that, compared with some other antihistamines, it may have a wider variety of minor side effects—including dryness of the mouth, overstimulation and nervousness, and, paradoxically, both drowsiness and insomnia.

Pheniramine maleate   This is a widely used and very safe antihistamine. In one recent year in which 291 million dosage units were sold, 358 suspected toxic reactions were reported; half-a-dozen of these people required hospitalization and there were no deaths. This is an "old" drug—it was introduced more than 3 decades ago—and has not been studied as rigorously as some newer ones. But both clinical experience and animal studies indicate that it is effective against hay fever and other allergic symptoms.

Pyrilamine maleate   Relative to several other approved antihistamines, this one produces many side effects—although usually mild ones. These reactions include drowsiness, listlessness, irritability, and loss of appetite. Some users experience nausea and vomiting. On the other hand, even large overdoses appear not to have fatal consequences. About two-thirds of hay fever sufferers who use pyrilamine maleate obtain symptomatic relief.

Thonzylamine hydrochloride   Some studies of this drug, which is more than 30 years old, indicate that it is among the least toxic of its type. In one recent period, during which there were approximately 80 million dosage units sold annually, no suspected poisonings with thonzylamine hydrochloride were reported to the FDA. The other side of the coin is that this drug has been studied less rigorously than some newer antihistamines. Clinical experience over many years suggests, however, that half or more of those who use it will obtain relief of allergic rhinitis.

Conditionally Approved Active Ingredients

Two antihistamines were conditionally approved for want of scientifically sound studies to clearly establish their effectiveness.

Phenyltoloxamine citrate   Data from animal experiments and human trials suggest that this is one of the safest antihistamines currently marketed. The FDA received only one report of an adverse reaction during a recent 5-year period, in which there were sales of between one-third and one-half billion tablets and other dosage units each year. But, despite these huge sales, there is surprisingly little rigorous experimental data to prove the drug's effectiveness or establish the minimum effective dosage level.

Thenyldiamine hydrochloride (taken orally)   This is a safe antihistamine. But there is considerable doubt about its effectiveness in the amounts—2.5 to 7.5 mg—at which it has been included in nonprescription combination products. The effective adult dosage is thought to be from 15 to 30 mg every 4 to 6 hours.

Disapproved Active Ingredients

There are 3 antihistamines that the Panel and/or the FDA contend are unsafe as nonprescription medications.

Diphenhydramine hydrochloride The Panel says this antihistamine is safe and effective against allergic symptoms when used in recommended dosages. It is widely used, but is of no proven benefit, against the common cold.

The major problem with diphenhydramine is that half of those adults who take the maximum approved dose (50 mg) suffer drowsiness as a side effect. More serious side effects, while rare, occasionally do occur. Large overdoses have resulted in psychosis and in deaths. In one recent year in which 187 million dosage units were sold, there were 334 reports of suspected poisoning, including two deaths. This drug has sometimes been abused when formulated as a sedative or sleep aid, but the Panel believes this risk is small in allergy products. The FDA, disagreeing, refuses to approve diphenhydramine hydrochloride for the self-treatment of allergies, although it does allow it to be sold over-the-counter to relieve coughs, and as a sleep aid.

Methapyrilene preparations Methapyrilene fumarate and methapyrilene hydrochloride were used for a quarter-century, with over half a billion dosage units being sold in some years. Commenting on methapyrilene's safety, the Panel cited the drug's "low order of toxicity . . . as compared with other common antihistaminics" assessed in animal studies.

In 1979, however, the National Cancer Institute announced the results of tests at the Oak Ridge National Laboratory: methapyrilene was found to be "a potent cause of liver cancer in rats, and, as such, of potential human hazard." While no cases of cancer in humans have been directly attributed to use of the drug—they would be extremely difficult to document on an individual basis—nonprescription drug makers, prompted by the FDA, removed methapyrilene products from the market within a few months.

Promethazine hydrochloride A few serious side effects have been reported for this drug. However, given that close to 5 billion doses have been prescribed in the past two decades with no reported fatalities, the Panel judged the drug safe. The FDA disagreed, saying that severe central nervous symptoms have been—and continue to be—reported in persons taking promethazine hydrochloride. Psychic changes, convulsions, coma, and death have occurred. So promethazine will be retained as a prescription drug, for use only under a doctor's supervision.

NASAL DECONGESTANTS

A number of drugs—nasal decongestants—will effectively relieve nasal stuffiness and improve breathing in persons suffering acute or chronic rhinitis due to colds, hay fever, and other allergies. They do this not by drying up nasal discharge (which is what antihistamines and anticholinergics may do) but by significantly constricting swollen blood vessels in the mucosal lining of the nose and sinuses. It is the swelling and inflammation of these tissues that are largely to blame for stuffy noses.

The remarkable constrictive effect these drugs can have on blood vessels has one unfortunate result: rebound congestion as the drug wears off. The mucosal blood vessels may swell more than before, so that the nose may feel even more stuffed up than it was. This risk can be reduced by using these drugs no more often than the label advises, and for no more than 3 days at a time. (Oral forms, while less effective, are less likely to produce rebound congestion than nasal sprays.)

Nasal decongestants are formulated for (1) *topical application* as nose drops and sprays, (2) *inhalation* from inhalers or in steam vapors, and (3) *oral ingestion* in liquid or tablets.

When these potent compounds are put directly into the nose—rather than being swallowed—very little drug is absorbed into the bloodstream and carried to the rest of the body. So inhaled decongestants are remarkably free from systemic side effects, unlike orally taken decongestants. The latter preparations, carried throughout the body, can affect major organ systems. Persons with high blood pressure, heart disease, diabetes, or thyroid disease should not take decongestants orally except on a doctor's orders.

There is a different risk for products that are introduced into the nose: the spread of infection via contaminated dispensers. Only one person should use each drug dispenser, in order to prevent the spread of germs.

CLAIMS FOR NASAL DECONGESTANTS

Certain claims can legitimately be made for safe and effective nasal decongestants. Unlike some other cold-cough-allergy drugs, decongestants can be tested objectively: the resistance to airflow through the stuffed-up nasal passage can be measured. In that way, the amount of air flowing through medicated nostrils can easily be compared with the amount passing through nostrils not exposed to the drug.

Accurate

for "the temporary relief of nasal congestion due to the common cold
. . . hay fever or other respiratory allergies"
for "the temporary relief of stuffed-up noses"
"helps clear nasal passages"
"helps decongest sinus openings, sinus passages"

Approved Active Ingredients

Ephedrine preparations (topical)   Ephedrine has been available in the United States for more than half a century. Numerous tests have shown it to be safe and effective when applied as a nasal spray or drops in concentrations of 0.5 to 1 percent. Rebound congestion is unlikely at those low doses if the drug is not used longer than 3 days. Ephedrine acts quickly, reaching its maximal decongestant effect within one hour and losing effectiveness after 4 hours. Approved ephedrine preparations include ephedrine, ephedrine hydrochloride, ephedrine sulfate, and racephedrine hydrochloride.

Recommended Dosage for Over-the-Counter Nasal Decongestants

Active Ingredient	Adults (Drops, Sprays or Inhalations)*	Children 6 to 12*	Children 2 to 6*
Nasal			
ephedrine 0.5%	2 to 3 per nostril every 4 or more hrs	1 to 2 per nostril every 4 or more hrs	consult doctor
naphazoline hydrochloride			
0.05%	1 to 2 per nostril every 6 or more hrs	1 to 2 per nostril every 6 or more hrs	consult doctor
0.025%			
oxymetazoline hydrochloride			
0.05%	2 to 3 per nostril a.m. and p.m.	2 to 3 per nostril a.m. and p.m.	
0.025%			2 to 3 per nostril a.m. and p.m.
phenylephrine hydrochloride			
1%	2 to 3 per nostril every 8 to 10 hrs (daily maximum, 3 doses)		
0.5%	2 to 3 per nostril every 4 or more hrs		
0.25%	2 to 3 per nostril every 4 or more hrs	2 to 3 per nostril every 4 or more hrs	
0.125%			2 to 3 per nostril every 4 or more hrs

Recommended Dosage for Over-the-Counter Nasal Decongestants (continued)

Active Ingredient	Adults (Drops, Sprays or Inhalations)*	Children 6 to 12*	Children 2 to 6*
propylhexedrine 0.4 to 0.5 mg/800 ml air	2 [inhalations] per nostril every 2 or more hrs	2 [inhalations] per nostril every 2 or more hrs	
xylometazoline hydrochloride 0.1%	2 to 3 per nostril every 8 to 10 hrs		
0.05%		2 to 3 per nostril every 8 to 10 hrs	2 to 3 per nostril every 8 to 10 hrs
Oral			
phenylephrine hydrochloride	10 mg every 4 hrs (60 mg daily maximum)	5 mg every 4 hrs (30 mg daily maximum)	2.5 mg every 4 hrs (15 mg daily maximum)
phenylpropanolamine hydrochloride	25 mg every 4 hrs or 50 mg every 8 hrs (150 mg daily maximum)	12.5 mg every 4 hrs or 25 mg every 8 hrs (75 mg daily maximum)	6.25 mg every 4 hrs or 12.5 mg every 8 hrs (37.5 mg daily maximum)
pseudoephedrine	60 mg every 6 hrs (240 mg daily maximum)	30 mg every 6 hrs (120 mg daily maximum)	15 mg every 6 hrs (60 mg daily maximum)

*Nasal application for adults and children 6 to 12 may be by drops or sprays; for children 2 to 6, drops only.

Naphazoline hydrochloride (topical)   This drug has some notable advantages and some notable disadvantages. It is effective and it produces a noticeable decongestant effect within 10 minutes. Relief continues for up to 5 or 6 hours. Tests suggest that most people who use it experience some relief from their symptoms. The disadvantages are that rebound congestion sometimes occurs after even a single treatment and is fairly likely to occur after repeated use. What is more, naphazoline can be habit-forming. If accidentally swallowed, it can cause marked drowsiness. But, despite these problems, naphazoline was evaluated as safe and effective as a nasal decongestant.

Oxymetazoline hydrochloride (topical)   This is a long-acting decongestant. The decongestant effect begins to decline only after 5 or 6 hours. Twice-a-day doses should provide adequate relief without causing rebound congestion. The drug has been shown to be safe and effective in double-blind trials. In one, the nasal airways of 7 out of 14 children treated with the preparation twice daily were completely open for 9 to 12 hours each day. In another study, in 30 children, 3 drops in each nostril 3 times daily provided persistently effective clearance of the nasal passages for 2 weeks.

Phenylephrine hydrochloride (topical or oral)   While potent, this decongestant is both safe and effective. Tests show statistically significant decongestive effect when the drug is administered orally. In one recent study, for example, a 10 mg dose yielded an average reduction of 11 percent in airway resistance at 15 minutes; a 21 percent reduction was shown at 1 and 2 hours. Similar benefit has been reported when the drug is administered in nasal drops and sprays. Oral phenylephrine can raise blood pressure and increase heart rate—but at the low doses taken to clear stuffed-up noses, such effects are unlikely to occur. However, persons taking prescription drugs that contain substances called MAO inhibitors may experience serious cardiovascular effects when they take even the approved oral over-the-counter dose of phenylephrine. The FDA warns, too, that the 1 percent preparations of this drug are especially likely to cause rebound congestion and other side effects.

Phenylpropanolamine preparations (taken orally)   Forms of phenylpropanolamine are among the most frequently used nasal decongestants. Several well-monitored studies have demonstrated their effectiveness. They cause few side effects. Exceptions occur in persons with hypertension (even the recommended amounts of the drug may raise blood pressure slightly) and in persons taking MAO inhibitors (for whom even the normal 25 mg to 50 mg dose can be dangerous). But most users will have no difficulty with phenylpropanolamine; it is evaluated as both safe and effective. Approved forms include phenylpropanolamine bitartrate, phenylpropanolamine hydrochloride, and phenylpropanolamine maleate.

Propylhexedrine (inhaled)   This drug has a wide margin of safety and relative freedom from toxic effects. So it can be used by persons who cannot use ephedrine and similar decongestants.

Pseudoephedrine preparations (taken orally)   The safety and effectiveness of pseudoephedrine hydrochloride and pseudoephedrine sulfate, given orally, has been demonstrated clinically and in scientific studies on cold sufferers. Side effects are minimal; they include drowsiness, headache, and insomnia. In the recommended dosage, pseudoephedrine appears unlikely to cause significant elevations of blood pressure in hypertensive persons. Those taking MAO inhibitors, however, should avoid this drug. (Anyone who is not sure whether his prescribed medication is an MAO inhibitor should check with a doctor.)

Xylometazoline (topical)   This is a potent decongestant that was moved from prescription to nonprescription status after the Panel determined that it is safe and effective for nonprescription use. It is long-acting: a single dosing may provide relief for more than 5 hours. Rebound congestion is less of a problem than with some other nasal decongestants. Tests have shown that xylometazoline produces an objective increase in airflow through the nasal passages and subjective sense of relief from the stuffed-up feeling.

Conditionally Approved Active Ingredients

Many agents are conditionally approved as nasal decongestants pending further testing.

Beechwood creosote topical/oral   As a decongestant, it is believed safe in customary doses, but the Panel decided better studies are needed to establish its effectiveness.

Bornyl acetate (topical)   The safety of bornyl acetate, an aromatic substance, is attested by long clinical use. But there is no well-documented study to show its effectiveness as a nasal decongestant and evaluators could not even determine a suitable dosage for testing purposes.

Camphor (topical or inhaled)   (Described earlier under COUGH SUPPRESSORS, *see* page 118.) Camphor is judged by this Panel to be safe in customary dosages; however, *see* CAMPHOR. Studies on its effectiveness as a decongestant have been in multi-ingredient products, so camphor's contribution, if any, is difficult to determine.

Cedar-leaf oil (topical)   This is a turpentinelike volatile oil that is steam-distilled from the fresh leaves of the cedar tree *Thuja occidentalis*. It is dangerous if eaten, but safe when applied to the chest, neck, and back in the dose used in a widely marketed ointment. Combination products that include cedar-leaf oil significantly reduced congestion, compared with an inert preparation, over a period of several hours. However, the role of cedar-leaf oil needs to be determined by suitably testing it as an individual ingredient. The Panel could not determine a dosage for this substance.

l-Desoxyephedrine (inhaled)   Nose drops and sprays containing this substance cause burning, stinging, sneezing, and runny nose in up to one out of five test subjects. But no serious side effects have been reported, so the Panel considers the drug to be safe. Data on its efficacy are equivocal; results thus far suggest that *l* desoxyephedrine has a relatively brief decongestant effect. *Note:* The FDA indicates that this will be listed as a safe and effective drug in the next stage of the OTC review.

Ephedrine preparations (taken orally)   Ephedrine preparations are safe when taken orally, as they are when inhaled. They can, however, cause tension, nervousness, tremor, and sleeplessness. In high doses they appear to work as nasal decongestants. But no studies have been submitted to show that they are effective for this purpose at the dosage levels recommended for use without prescription.

Eucalyptol and eucalyptus oil (topical or inhaled)   Considered safe, but no well-controlled studies document effectiveness as a nasal decongestant.

Menthol and peppermint oil (topical or inhaled)   Some combination products containing these aromatic substances have been shown to make breathing easier. But menthol's contribution to this therapeutic effect has not been established.

Phenylpropanolamine hydrochloride (topical)   When put into the nose in drops or spray, this substance may sting—but it is safe to use. However, there is no documentation of its effectiveness as a nasal decongestant.

Thenyldiamine hydrochloride (topical)   This antihistamine is included in nonprescription nasal decongestant products although no claims are made for its acting as a nasal decongestant. It is said to block action of the irritant histamine and also to block fluid secretions in the nose. But the antihistaminic activity of the drug, when applied in drops or sprays, has not been tested. It is safe, but it appears to contribute little to the effectiveness of combination nasal decongestants in which it is present.

Thymol (topical or inhaled)   Safe as currently used, but no tests show that it is an effective decongestant.

Turpentine oil (spirits of turpentine) (topical or inhaled)   Ointments, medicated steam preparations, and other dosage forms that contain turpentine preparations are safe, and appear to effectively reduce nasal congestion, but studies fail to demonstrate and quantify the role that turpentine plays in the effectiveness of these products.

Disapproved Active Ingredients

Mustard oil (allyl isothiocyanate) (topical or inhaled)   This volatile oil comes from the seeds of what is called *black mustard*, the same mustard seeds used to prepare a dressing for hot dogs!

Mustard-oil vapors can be quite irritating to the eyes, nose, and throat—and so are not safe. Neither is there acceptable evidence that mustard oil acts as a decongestant.

Turpentine oil (spirits of turpentine) (taken orally)   No evidence confirms effectiveness as a decongestant when taken orally. Worse, it is dangerous as a relatively small amount can poison a child.

MISCELLANEOUS INGREDIENTS

Several ingredients that do not fall under the categories covered above are formulated into combination products used to treat colds, cough, allergy, and asthma. The Panel takes a dim view of their worth.

Approved Miscellaneous Ingredients

None

Conditionally Approved Miscellaneous Ingredients

Ascorbic acid (vitamin C)   Few medical topics have stirred more comment and conversation than the question of whether vitamin C cures the common cold. The Panel says the evidence to show that it does remains inconclusive, so that any *label claim* for this effect is *misbranding*. Vitamin C appears to be essentially safe, even in the extremely high doses that some people take. But until it is proved to be effective, the Panel would grant only conditional approval to vitamin C.

Caffeine   The Panel "presumes" that caffeine is formulated into combination cold-cough remedies to counteract the soporific effects of antihistamines. In the customary low doses, it certainly is safe. But there are no data to show that it is effective.

Phenobarbital   Small amounts of this prescription sleeping medication are formulated into over-the-counter bronchodilator combination products to counteract the caffeinelike stimulation caused by theophylline. They are safe, but evidence is lacking to show that these additives are effective.

Disapproved Miscellaneous Ingredients

None

OTHER INGREDIENTS IN COUGH-COLD-ALLERGY PRODUCTS

The consumer may note that a label lists ingredients not discussed in this unit. Those ingredients listed below are either inactive or may be necessary as pharmaceutical constituents of a product without having any bearing on specific functions evaluated by the Panel (e.g., cough suppression or bronchodilation).

acetic acid
alcohol
alkyl dimethyl
  benzylammonium
  chloride
  (benzalkonium
  chloride)
aluminum hydroxide—
  magnesium
  carbonate (co-dried
  gel)
anethole
anise
banana arome
benzaldehyde
benzalkonium chloride
  (alkyl dimethyl
  benzylammonium
  chloride)
blood root
bryonia tincture
caramel
cedar, natural
cetalkonium chloride
cetylpyridinium
  chloride
cherry flavoring
cherry nut flavoring

chlorobutanol
chloroform (0.4
  percent maximum)
citric acid
citric acid, hydrate
cocillana
dextrose
dipropylene glycol
disodium edetate
drosera tincture
eriodictyon
  fluidextract (yerba
  santa)
glycerin
glycyrrhiza (licorice)
grape flavoring
grindelia
gum arabic
honey
lemon oil
licorice (glycyrrhiza)
lobelia
lobelium
methylcellulose
methylparaben
monocalcium
  phosphate
myristica oil

oleyl alcohol
petrolatum base
phenylmercuric
  acetate
pineapple flavoring
potassium nitrate
propylparaben
rumex
saline phosphate
  buffer solution
sodium bisulfite
sticta pulmonaria
sucrose
sugar
sugar base
syrup base
thimerosol
thonzonium bromide
triethylene glycol
vegetable stearate
wild cherry
  fluidextract
yerba santa
  (eriodictyon
  fluidextract)

Safety and Effectiveness: Active Ingredients in Over-the-Counter Cough Medicines

Active Ingredients	Cough Suppressor	Expectorant	Nasal Decongestant
ammonium chloride			
oral		safe but not proved effective	
antimony potassium tartrate			
oral		not safe or effective	
beechwood creosote			
lozenge	safe but not proved effective	not proved effective	safe but not proved effective
ointment			safe but not proved effective
oral	safe but not proved effective	not proved effective	
benzoin preparations: compound tincture of benzoin and tincture of benzoin			
inhalant		not proved effective	
bornyl acetate			
inhalant			safe but not proved effective
camphor			
inhalant	safe but not proved effective	not proved effective	safe but not proved effective
lozenge	safe but not proved effective	not proved effective	safe but not proved effective
ointment	safe but not proved effective*	not proved effective	safe but not proved effective
caramiphen edisylate (caramiphen ethanedisulfonate)			
oral	safe but not proved effective		
carbetapentane citrate			
oral	safe but not proved effective		
cedar-leaf oil			
ointment			safe but not proved effective
chloroform			
oral		not safe or effective	

codeine preparations: codeine, codeine alkaloid, codeine phosphate, and codeine sulfate			
oral	safe and effective		
cod-liver oil			
oral	safe but not proved effective		
l-desoxyephedrine			
inhalant			safe but not proved effective*
dextromethorphan			
oral	safe and effective		
dextromethorphan hydrobromide			
oral	safe and effective		
diphenhydramine hydrochloride			
oral	safe and effective		
elm bark			
lozenge	safe but not proved effective		
ointment	safe but not proved effective		
oral	safe but not proved effective		
ephedrine preparations: ephedrine, ephedrine hydrochloride, ephedrine sulfate, and racephedrine hydrochloride			
nose drops, sprays			safe and effective
oral			safe but not proved effective
ethylmorphine hydrochloride			
oral	safe but not proved effective		
eucalyptol and eucalyptus oil			
inhalant	safe but not proved effective	not proved effective	safe but not proved effective
lozenge	safe but not proved effective	not proved effective	safe but not proved effective
mouthwash		not proved effective	safe but not proved effective
ointment	safe but not proved effective*	not proved effective	safe but not proved effective

Safety and Effectiveness: Active Ingredients in Over-the-Counter Cough Medicines (continued)

Active Ingredients	Cough Suppressor	Expectorant	Nasal Decongestant
guaifenesin (glycerol guaiacolate)			
oral		not proved effective	
horehound (horehound fluid extract)			
oral	safe but not proved effective		
hydrocodone bitartrate (dihydrocodeinone)			
oral	not safe		
iodides: calcium iodide anhydrous, hydriodic acid syrup, iodized lime, and potassium iodide			
oral		not safe	
ipecac fluid extract			
oral		not safe	
ipecac syrup			
oral		not proved effective	
menthol and peppermint oil			
inhalant	safe but not proved effective	not proved effective	safe but not proved effective
lozenge	safe but not proved effective	not proved effective	safe but not proved effective
mouthwash			safe but not proved effective
ointment	safe but not proved effective*	not proved effective	safe but not proved effective
mustard oil (allyl isothiocyanate)			
inhalant			not safe
ointment			not safe
naphazoline hydrochloride			
nose drops, sprays			safe and effective
noscapine (noscapine hydrochloride)			
oral	safe but not proved effective		

oxymetazoline hydrochloride	
nose drops, sprays	safe and effective
phenylephrine hydrochloride	
nose drops, sprays	safe and effective
oral	safe and effective
phenylpropanolamine preparations: (phenylpropanolamine bitartrate, phenylpropanolamine hydrochloride, and phenylpropanolamine maleate	
nose drops, sprays	safe but not proved effective
oral	safe and effective
pine-tar preparations: extract white-pine compound, pine tar, syrup of pine tar, white pine, and white pine syrup	
oral	not proved effective
potassium guaiacolsulfonate	
oral	not proved effective
propylhexedrine	
inhalant	safe and effective
pseudoephedrine preparations: pseudoephedrine hydrochloride and pseudoephedrine sulfate	
oral	safe and effective
sodium citrate	
oral	not proved effective
squill and squill extract	
oral	not safe or effective
terpin hydrate preparations: terpin hydrate and terpin hydrate elixir	
oral	not proved effective

Safety and Effectiveness: Active Ingredients in Over-the-Counter Cough Medicines (continued)

Active Ingredients	Cough Suppressor	Expectorant	Nasal Decongestant
thenyldiamine hydrochloride			
nose drops, sprays			safe but not proved effective
thymol			
inhalant	safe but not proved effective		safe but not proved effective
lozenge	safe but not proved effective		safe but not proved effective
mouthwash			safe but not proved effective
ointment	safe but not proved effective		safe but not proved effective
tolu preparations: tolu, tolu balsam and			
tolu balsam tincture			
oral		not proved effective	
turpentine oil (spirits of turpentine)			
inhalant	safe but not proved effective	not proved effective	safe but not proved effective
ointment	safe but not proved effective	not proved effective	safe but not proved effective
oral	not safe		not safe
xylometazoline			
nose drops, sprays			safe and effective

*The FDA foresees upgrading to "safe and effective" (*see* Notes with entries in text).

Safety and Effectiveness: Active Ingredients in Over-the-Counter Drying Agents for Colds and Coughs

Active Ingredient	Oral	Inhalant
atropine sulfate	not proved effective	
belladonna alkaloids		
(Atropa belladonna and		
Datura stramonia)	not proved effective	not safe

Safety and Effectiveness: Antihistamines in Over-the-Counter Cold, Cough, and Allergy Medications

Active Ingredient	Panel's Assessment
brompheniramine maleate	safe and effective
chlorpheniramine maleate	safe and effective
diphenhydramine hydrochloride	not safe*
doxylamine succinate	safe and effective
methapyrilene preparations:	
methapyrilene fumarate and	
methapyrilene hydrochloride	not safe*
phenindamine tartrate	safe and effective
pheniramine maleate	safe and effective
phenyltoloxamine citrate	safe but not proved effective
pyrilamine maleate	safe and effective
thenyldiamine hydrochloride	safe but not proved effective
thonzylamine hydrochloride	safe and effective

*FDA assessments.

Safety and Effectiveness: Combination Products Sold Over-the-Counter for Colds and Coughs

Safe and Effective Combinations

Can include 1, but not more than 1, safe and effective active ingredient from each of 2 or 3 drug groups, in safe and effective doses; specifically:
  1 pain-fever reliever + 1 antihistamine
  1 pain-fever reliever + 1 nasal decongestant
  1 pain-fever reliever + 1 antihistamine + 1 nasal decongestant
  1 antihistamine + 1 cough suppressor (label must warn of possible "marked drowsiness")
  1 antihistamine + 1 nasal decongestant
  1 antihistamine + 1 nasal decongestant + 1 cough suppressor
  1 cough suppressor + 1 expectorant (labeled only for "nonproductive coughs")

Safety and Effectiveness: Combination Products
Sold Over-the-Counter for Colds and Coughs *(continued)*

Safe and Effective Combinations

1 cough suppressor + 1 nasal decongestant
1 cough suppressor + local anesthetic or pain-fever reliever (as lozenge only)
1 cough suppressor + 1 expectorant + 1 nasal decongestant (labeled only for "nonproductive coughs")
1 oral bronchodilator + 1 expectorant (labeled only for "cough associated with asthma")
1 sympathomimetic oral bronchodilator + 1 theophylline oral bronchodilator
1 expectorant + 1 nasal decongestant
1 nasal decongestant + 1 local anesthetic or local pain-fever reliever (as lozenge only)
Any of the preceding combinations + safe and effective pain-fever reliever
Any of the preceding combinations + safe and effective local anesthetic (for sore throat)

Conditionally Safe or Conditionally Effective Combinations

1 conditionally approved ingredient or labeling but no disapproved ingredient or labeling less-than-minimally effective dosage in 1 or more ingredients claimed to relieve the same symptom
2 approved ingredients from the same drug group
atropine + a nasal decongestant taken by mouth (safety not established)
an antihistamine + a drying agent (safety not established)
an antihistamine + a nasal decongestant as nose drops or spray (effectiveness not established)
a cough suppressor + a bronchodilator, labeled only for "nonasthmatic cough" (effectiveness not established)
an expectorant + a bronchodilator, labeled only for "nonasthmatic cough" (effectiveness not established)
a cough suppressor + an expectorant, labeled only for "productive cough"
1 cough suppressor + 1 expectorant + 1 nasal decongestant, labeled only for "productive cough"
combinations containing small amounts of a conditionally approved active ingredient intended to counteract side effects of other ingredient(s)—e.g., caffeine or phenobarbital used as a "corrective"
combinations containing an antihistamine for which a conditionally approved sleep-aid claim is made
combinations containing several claimed active ingredients that are mixtures of volatile substances, with overlapping pharmacologic activities for which a minimum effective dose cannot be established for 1 or more ingredient(s)
combinations with 4 or more active ingredients from 4 or more drug groups—e.g., 1 pain-fever reliever + 1 cough suppressor + 1 expectorant + 1 nasal decongestant, or 1 pain-fever reliever + 1 cough suppressor + 1 antihistamine + 1 nasal decongestant

**Safety and Effectiveness: Combination Products
Sold Over-the-Counter for Colds and Coughs** *(continued)*

Conditionally Safe or Conditionally Effective Combinations

combinations containing vitamin C for which no claims of effectiveness against colds
   are made

Not Safe or Not Effective Combinations

a combination with any disapproved ingredient or labeling
a combination of approved ingredients from different groups, each for a different
   symptom, if any ingredient is present at less than the minimum effective dose
a combination containing any active ingredient or carrying labeling not reviewed by the
   Cold-Cough Panel or another panel
3 or more ingredients from the same drug group
a pain-fever reliever + a bronchodilator
a drying agent + an expectorant (ingredients counteract each other)
an antihistamine + an expectorant (ingredients counteract each other)
a bronchodilator + a drying agent (dangerous for asthma sufferers)
a bronchodilator + an antihistamine (dangerous for asthma sufferers)
an oral bronchodilator + a cough suppressor labeled only for "asthmatic cough"
   (dangerous for asthma sufferers)
a cough suppressor approved also as an antihistamine + another antihistamine
   (sedative side effects may be additive)
an antihistamine approved also as a cough suppressor + another cough suppressor
   (the cough-suppressant effect of the 2 drugs may be additive)
combinations containing more than 30 mg of caffeine
combinations containing 2 antihistamines, 1 of which is added and labeled exclusively
   as a sleep aid
combinations containing vitamin C and labeled for prevention or treatment of colds

Cough Suppressors: Product Ratings[1]

Product and Distributor	Dosage of Active Ingredients	Rating[2]	Comment
dextromethorphan hydrobromide			
Congespirin (Bristol-Myers)	**syrup:** 5 mg per teaspoonful	**A**	
Pertussin 8 Hour Cough Formula (Chesebrough-Pond's)	**syrup:** 7.5 mg per teaspoonful	**A**	

Cough Suppressors: Product Ratings[1] *(continued)*

Product and Distributor	Dosage of Active Ingredients	Rating[2]	Comment
Romilar Children's Cough (Block)	**syrup:** 2.5 mg per teaspoonful	A	children's dosage
Symptom I (Parke-Davis)	**liquid:** 10 mg per teaspoonful	A	
diphenhydramine hydrochloride Benylin Cough Syrup (Parke-Davis)	**syrup:** 12.5 mg per teaspoonful	A	
noscapine Tusscapine (Fisons)	**syrup:** 15 mg per teaspoonful	B	not proved effective

1. Also see the cough mixture product ratings table, page 165.
2. Author's interpretation of Panel criteria. Based on contents, not claims.

Expectorants: Product Ratings[1]

Product and Distributor	Dosage of Active Ingredients	Rating[2]	Comment
guaifenesin (formerly glyceryl guaiacolate) Breonesin (Breon)	**capsules:** 200 mg	B	not proved effective
G-200 (Block)		B	not proved effective
Gee-Gee (Bowman)	**tablets:** 200 mg	B	not proved effective
Glytuss (Mayrand)		B	not proved effective
Glycotuss (Vale)	**tablets:** 100 mg	B	not proved effective
Hytuss (Hyrex)		B	not proved effective
guaifenesin (generic)	**syrup:** 100 mg per teaspoonful	B	not proved effective
Anti-Tuss (Century Pharm.)		B	not proved effective
Robitussin (Robins)		B	not proved effective
iodides Hydriodic Acid (Lilly)	**syrup:** 65 to 75 mg hydrogen iodide per teaspoonful	C	not safe

1. Also see the cough mixture product ratings table, page 165.
2. Author's interpretation of Panel criteria. Based on content, not claims.

Antihistamines: Product Ratings

Product and Distributor	Dosage of Active Ingredients	Rating[1]	Comment
brompheniramine maleate			
bromphen (generic)	**elixir:** 2 mg per teaspoonful	A	1 teaspoonful correct for children, 2 for adults
Dimetane (Robins)	**tablets:** 4 mg	A	
	elixir: 2 mg per teaspoonful	A	1 teaspoonful correct for children, 2 for adults
chlorpheniramine maleate			
Chlo-Amine (Hollister-Stier)	**tablets, chewable:** 2 mg	A	children's dosage
Chlor-Niramine (Whiteworth)	**tablets:** 4 mg	A	
Chlor-Trimeton (Schering)		A	
Histrey (Bowman)		A	
Chlor-Mal (Rugby)	**syrup:** 2 mg per teaspoonful	A	
Chlor-Trimeton (Schering)		A	
Chlor-Trimeton Repetabs (Schering)	**tablets, timed-release:** 8 mg	A	
Chlor-Trimeton Repetabs (Schering)	**tablets, timed-release:** 12 mg	A	
Teldrin (Menley & James)	**capsules, timed-release:** 8 mg	A	
diphenhydramine hydrochloride			
Benylin (Parke-Davis)	**syrup:** 12.5 mg per teaspoonful	A	1 teaspoonful is correct dosage for children; 2 is correct for adults
doxylamine succinate			
Decapryn (Merrell-National)	**syrup:** 6.25 mg per teaspoonful	A	
pyrilamine maleate			
pyrilamine maleate (generic)	**tablets:** 25 mg	A	

1. Author's interpretation of Panel criteria. Based on contents, not claims.

Nasal Decongestants: Product Ratings[1]

Single-Ingredient Products

Product and Distributor	Dosage of Active Ingredients	Rating[2]	Comment
ephedrine sulfate			
ephedrine sulfate (generic)	**syrup (USP):** 20 mg per teaspoonful	C	this is double the dosage recommended by Panel for over-the-counter sales and use
Ephedrine Sulfate (Lilly)	**nose drops:** 3%	C	6 times stronger than recommended dosage
	syrup: 11 mg per teaspoonful	B	not proved effective when taken orally
Vatronol (Vicks Health Care)	**nose drops:** 0.5%	A	
epinephrine hydrochloride			
Adrenalin Chloride (Parke-Davis)	**nose drops:** 0.1%	C	not submitted to or approved by Panel as an over-the-counter nasal decongestant
naphazoline hydrochloride			
Privine (Ciba)	**nose drops:** 0.05%	A	
	nasal spray: 0.05%	A	
oxymetazoline hydrochloride			
Afrin (Schering)	**pediatric nose drops:** 0.025%	A	for children
	nose drops: 0.05%	A	
Duration (Plough)	**nasal spray:** 0.05%	A	
	mentholated vapor spray: 0.05%	B	menthol not proved effective
phenylephrine hydrochloride (products listed in order of increasing strength)			
Neo-Synephrine (Winthrop)	**nose drops:** 0.125%	A	dosage for young children
Alconefrin 25 (Webcon)	**nose drops:** 0.25%	A	dosage for older children, adults

Nasal Decongestants: Product Ratings[1] *(continued)*

Single-Ingredient Products

Product and Distributor	Dosage of Active Ingredients	Rating[2]	Comment
doktors (Scherer)	**nose drops:** 0.25%	**A**	
Rhinall (Scherer)	**nasal spray:** 0.25%	**A**	
Super Anahist (Warner-Lambert)	**nasal spray:** 0.25%	**A**	
Alconefrin 50 (Webcon)	**nose drops:** 0.5%	**A**	adult dosage
Allerest Nasal (Pharmacraft)	**nasal spray:** 0.5%	**A**	
Coricidin Nasal Mist (Schering)	**nasal spray:** 0.5%	**A**	
Neo-Synephrine (Winthrop)	**nasal spray** and **nasal jelly** 0.5%	**A**	
Pyracort-D (Lemmon)	**nasal spray** 0.5%	**A**	
Neo-Synephrine (Winthrop)	**nose drops:** 1%	**A**	
phenylpropanolamine hydrochloride			
Propadrine (Merck)	**capsules:** 25 mg, 50 mg	**A**	
	elixir: 20 mg per teaspoonful	**A**	
pseudoephedrine hydrochloride			
First Sign (J. B. Williams)	**tablets:** 30 mg	**A**	
Sudafed (Burroughs-Wellcome)		**A**	
Cenafed Syrup (Century Pharm.)	**liquid:** 30 mg per teaspoonful	**A**	
Novafed (Dow)		**A**	
Symptom-2 (Parke-Davis)		**A**	
pseudoephedrine sulfate			
Afrinol Repetabs (Schering)	**tablets, timed action:** 120 mg	**A**	
xylometazoline hydrochloride (products given in order of increasing strength)			
Neo-Synephrine II Long Acting (Winthrop)	**pediatric nose drops:** 0.05%	**A**	children's dosage

Nasal Decongestants: Product Ratings[1] (continued)

Single-Ingredient Products

Product and Distributor	Dosage of Active Ingredients	Rating[2]	Comment
Chlorohist-LA (Mallard)	**spray:** 0.1%	A	
Dristamead Long Acting (Spencer-Mead)		A	
Sinex Long-Acting (Vicks Health Care)		A	
Sinutab Long-Lasting Sinus (Warner-Lambert)		A	
Neo-Synephrine II Long Acting (Winthrop)	**drops:** 0.1%	A	
Otrivin (Geigy)		A	

Combination Products

Product and Distributor	Dosage of Active Ingredients	Rating[2]	Comment
Benzedrex (Menley & James)	**inhaler:** 250 mg propylhexedrine + menthol + camphor + methyl salicylate + bornyl acetate	C	too many decongestant active ingredients, of which only propylhexedrine is safe and effective The FDA has indicated, however, that at the next stage of the OTC Review it will approve the aromatic ingredients as safe and effective *adjuvants*— which would make this an "A" product.
Efedron Nasal (Hyrex)	**jelly:** 0.6% ephedrine + menthol + cinnamon oil	B	menthol not proved effective
4-Way Nasal (Bristol-Myers)	**nasal spray:** 0.5% phenylephrine hydrochloride + 0.05% naphazoline hydrochloride + 0.2% pyrilamine maleate	B	effectiveness of decongestant + antihistamine not proved

Nasal Decongestants: Product Ratings[1] *(continued)*

Combination Products

Product and Distributor	Dosage of Active Ingredients	Rating[2]	Comment
Neo-Vadrin Nasal Decongestant (Scherer)	**nose drops:** 0.15% phenylephrine hydrochloride + 0.4% phenylpropanolamine hydrochloride	B	2 drugs from same group (decongestants); the second not proved effective
NTZ Nasal (Winthrop)	**nose drops:** 0.5% phenylephrine hydrochloride + 0.1% thenyldiamine hydrochloride	B	combination of decongestant + antihistamine not proved effective; thenyldiamine not proved effective
Sine-Off Once-A-Day (Menley & James)	**nasal spray:** 0.1% xylometazoline hydrochloride + menthol + eucalyptol + camphor + methyl salicylate	C	too many decongestant active ingredients; methyl salicylate not submitted or assessed as decongestant
Sinex (Vicks Health Care)	**spray:** 0.5% phenylephrine hydrochloride + menthol + eucalyptol + camphor + methyl salicylate	C	too many decongestant active ingredients; methyl salicylate not submitted or assessed as decongestant
Vicks Inhaler (Vicks Health Care)	**inhaler:** 50 mg *l*-desoxyephedrine + menthol + camphor + methyl salicylate + bornyl acetate	C	too many decongestant active ingredients, none of which is proved effective
			The FDA, however, has told Vicks that *l*-desoxyephedrine will be approved as safe and effective at the next stage of the OTC Review, and has indicated that the other ingredients are safe and effective as *adjuvants*—which would make this an "A" product.

Nasal Decongestants: Product Ratings[1] (continued)

Combination Products

Product and Distributor	Dosage of Active Ingredients	Rating[2]	Comment
VapoRub (Vicks)	**ointment:** camphor + menthol + turpentine spirits + eucalyptus oil + cedar leaf oil + myristica oil + thymol	C	too many ingredients, none of which is proved effective
VapoSteam (Vicks)	**liquid for vaporizers:** 1.8% poloxyethylene dodecanol + eucalyptus oil + camphor + menthol + tincture of benzoin	C	too many ingredients, none of which is proved effective

1. Also see the cough-mixture products ratings table, page 165.
2. Author's interpretation of Panel criteria. Based on contents, not claims.

Upper Respiratory Drugs: Combination Product Ratings

Decongestant + Pain-Reliever Products

Product and Distributor	Dosage of Active Ingredients	Rating[1]	Comment
Bowman Cold Tablets (Bowman)	tablets: 24 mg phenylpropanolamine hydrochloride + 320 mg acetaminophen + 16 mg caffeine	B	caffeine's value remains unproved
Capex Capsules (Spencer-Mead)	capsules: 18 mg phenylpropanolamine hydrochloride + 325 mg acetaminophen	B	less than the recommended dose of phenylpropanolamine hydrochloride if 1 capsule is taken; more than recommended dose if 2 taken
Deconex Capsules (generic)		B	
Ornex Capsules (Menley & James)		B	
Congesprin Tablets (Bristol-Myers)	tablets: 1.25 mg phenylephrine hydrochloride + 81 mg aspirin	A	correct formulation for young children if 2 taken
Endecon Tablets (Endo)	tablets: 25 mg phenylpropanolamine hydrochloride + 325 mg aspirin	A	
Sine-Aid Tablets (McNeil)		A	
Sinutab-II Tablets (Warner-Lambert)		A	

Antihistamine + Pain-Reliever Products

Product and Distributor	Dosage of Active Ingredients	Rating[1]	Comment
Coricidin Tablets (Schering)	tablets: 2 mg chlorpheniramine maleate + 325 mg aspirin	A	
Rhinate Tablets (Spencer-Mead)		A	

Upper Respiratory Drugs: Combination Product Ratings *(continued)*

Antihistamine + Pain-Reliever Products

Product and Distributor	Dosage of Active Ingredients	Rating[1]	Comment
Coricidin Medilets (Schering)	**tablets:** 1 mg chlorpheniramine maleate + 80 mg aspirin	A	correct formulation for young children
Dasikon Capsules (Beecham Labs.)	**capsules:** 2 mg chlorpheniramine maleate + 195 mg aspirin + 130 mg phenacetin + 0.065 mg atropine sulfate + 32 mg caffeine	C	phenacetin not safe; atropine and caffeine not proved effective
Histadyl and A.S.A. Pulvules (Lilly)	**capsules:** 4 mg chlorpheniramine maleate + 325 mg aspirin	A	
Percogesic Tablets (Endo)	**tablets:** 30 mg phenyltoloxamine citrate + 325 mg aspirin	B	this antihistamine not proved effective
Phenylgesic Tablets (Generix Drug)		B	
Sedadyne Tablets (Spencer-Mead)		B	

Decongestant + Antihistamine

Product and Distributor	Dosage of Active Ingredients	Rating[1]	Comment
	Sustained-Release capsules and tablets		
Allerprop Capsules (Rugby)	**capsules:** 75 mg phenylpropanolamine hydrochloride + 8 mg chlorpheniramine maleate	B	timed-release products not proved safe and effective
Contac Capsules (Menley & James)		B	timed-release products not proved safe and effective

Allerest Timed Release Capsules (Pharmacraft)

capsules: 50 mg phenylpropanolamine hydrochloride + 4 mg chlorpheniramine maleate

B timed-release products not proved safe and effective

Conex D.A. Tablets (O'Neal)

tablets: 50 mg phenylpropanolamine hydrochloride + 50 mg phenyltoloxamine

B timed-release products not proved safe and effective

Chlor-Trimeton Decongestant Repetab Tablets (Schering)

tablets: 120 mg pseudoephedrine sulfate + 8 mg chlorpheniramine maleate

A this drug specifically approved by the FDA

Tablets and Capsules

Aller-Chlor Tablets (Rugby)

tablets: 60 mg pseudoephedrine hydrochloride + 4 mg chlorpheniramine maleate

A

Chlor-Trimeton Decongestant Tablets (Schering)

A

Fedahist Tablets (Dooner)

A

Sudafed Plus Tablets (Burroughs-Wellcome)

Allerest Tablets (Pharmacraft)

tablets: 18.7 mg phenylpropanolamine hydrochloride + 2 mg chlorpheniramine maleate

C 1 tablet delivers less and 2 tablets more than recommended dose of phenylpropanolamine hydrochloride

Spenrest Tablets (Spencer-Mead)

C

Allerstat Capsules (Lemmon)

capsules: 25 mg phenylpropanolamine hydrochloride + 2.5 mg phenylephrine hydrochloride + 12.5 mg pheniramine maleate + 12.5 mg pyrilamine maleate

B less-than-effective dosage of phenylephrine hydrochloride

Upper Respiratory Drugs: Combination Product Ratings (continued)

Decongestant + Antihistamine

Product and Distributor	Dosage of Active Ingredients	Rating[1]	Comment
Tablets and Capsules			
Fedrazil Tablets (Burroughs-Wellcome)	**tablets:** 30 mg pseudoephedrine hydrochloride + 25 mg chlorcyclizine hydrochloride	C	antihistamine chlorcyclizine hydrochloride not submitted to or assessed by Panel
Histatab Plus Tablets (Century Pharm.)	**tablets:** 5 mg phenylephrine hydrochloride + 2 mg chlorpheniramine maleate	A	correct dosage for children 6 to 12
Novahistine Fortis Capsules (Dow)	**capsules:** 10 mg phenylephrine hydrochloride + 2 mg chlorpheniramine maleate	C	2 capsules will deliver less than the recommended 25 mg dose of phenylephrine hydrochloride
Triaminicin Chewable Tablets (Dorsey)	**tablets, chewable:** 6.25 mg phenylpropanolamine hydrochloride + 0.5 mg chlorpheniramine maleate	C	2 tablets deliver correct dose of the decongestant, but less-than-effective amount of antihistamine chlorpheniramine
Liquids: all dosages per teaspoonful			
Alamine Liquid (North American)	18.75 mg phenylpropanolamine hydrochloride + 2 mg chlorpheniramine maleate	C	1 teaspoonful delivers too little, 2 deliver too much phenylpropanolamine
Dehist Elixir (Geneva Generics) Novamor Elixir (H. L. Moore)		C C	
Decohist Syrup (generic)	2.5 mg phenylephrine hydrochloride + 1 mg chlorpheniramine maleate	A	correct proportions for dosages for all age groups
Demazin Syrup (Schering)		A	

Product and Distributor	Ingredients	Rating[1]	Comment
Dimetane Decongestant Elixir (Robins)	5 mg phenylephrine hydrochloride + 2 mg brompheniramine maleate	A	correct proportions for children (1 tsp) or adults (2 tsps)
Hista-Vadrin Syrup (Scherer)	20 mg phenylpropanolamine hydrochloride + 2.5 mg phenylephrine hydrochloride + 2 mg chlorpheniramine maleate	C	no way to get recommended dosages of all 3 ingredients
Noraminic Syrup (North American)	12.5 mg phenylpropanolamine hydrochloride + 2 mg chlorpheniramine maleate	A	1 teaspoonful correct dose for children 6 to 12; 2 teaspoonsful correct for older persons
Ornade 2 Liquid for Children (SKF)		A	
Tri-Mine Syrup (Spencer-Mead)		A	

Decongestant + Antihistamine + Pain-Reliever Products

Product and Distributor	Decongestant	Antihistamine	Analgesic/Other	Rating[1]	Comment
AL-AY Modified Tablets (Bowman)	5 mg phenylephrine hydrochloride	2 mg chlorpheniramine maleate	160 mg acetaminophen + 15 mg caffeine	B	caffeine not proved effective
Alka-Seltzer Plus Tablets (Miles Labs.)	24.08 mg phenylpropanolamine bitartrate	2 mg chlorpheniramine maleate	324 mg aspirin	C	1 tablet gives too little antihistamine; 2 give too much decongestant
Coricidin 'D' Decongestant Tablets (Schering)	12.5 mg phenylpropanolamine hydrochloride	2 mg chlorpheniramine maleate	325 mg aspirin	A	2 tablets give recommended dosage for all 3 ingredients
Coricidin Demilets (Tablets) (Schering)	6.25 mg phenylpropanolamine hydrochloride	1 mg chlorpheniramine maleate	80 mg aspirin	A	for children

Upper Respiratory Drugs: Combination Product Ratings *(continued)*

Decongestant + Antihistamine + Pain-Reliever Products

Product and Distributor	Decongestant	Antihistamine	Analgesic/Other	Rating[1]	Comment
Coricidin Sinus Headache Tablets (Schering)	12.5 mg phenylpropanolamine hydrochloride	2 mg chlorpheniramine maleate	500 mg acetaminophen	C	nonstandard dose of acetaminophen; 2 tablets provide recommended amounts of decongestant, antihistamine, but too much acetaminophen
Colrex Capsules (Rowell)	5 mg phenylephrine hydrochloride	2 mg chlorpheniramine maleate	325 mg acetaminophen	A	correct formulation for children 6–12 (1 tablet) and adults (2 tablets)
Dristamead Tablets (Spencer-Mead) Dristan Tablets (Whitehall)	5 mg phenylephrine hydrochloride	2 mg chlorpheniramine maleate	325 mg aspirin + 16.2 mg caffeine	B	caffeine not proved effective
4-Way Cold Tablets (Bristol-Myers)	12.5 mg phenylpropanolamine hydrochloride	2 mg chlorpheniramine maleate	324 mg aspirin	A	correct formulation for children (1 tablet) or adults (2 tablets)
Hista-Compound No. 5 Tablets (North American)	4 mg phenylephrine hydrochloride	2 mg chlorpheniramine maleate	227.5 mg salicylamide + 162.5 mg phenacetin + 32.5 mg caffeine	C	phenacetin not safe

Product and Distributor	Decongestant	Antihistamine	Drying Agent	Rating[1]	Comment
Histosal Tablets (Ferndale)	20 mg phenylpropanolamine hydrochloride	12.5 mg pyrilamine maleate	324 mg acetaminophen + 30 mg caffeine	C	less-than-recommended dose of phenylpropanolamine hydrochloride and pyrilamine maleate
Sinugesic Tablets (Pharmecon)	25 mg phenylpropanolamine hydrochloride	22 mg phenyltoloxamine citrate	325 mg acetaminophen	B	phenyltoloxamine not proved effective
Sinutab Tablets (Warner-Lambert)				B	
Ursinus Inlay-Tabs (Dorsey)	25 mg phenylpropanolamine hydrochloride	12.5 mg pyrilamine maleate + 12.5 mg pheniramine maleate	382 mg calcium carbaspirin	B	2 approved ingredients from the same group

Decongestant + Antihistamine + Drying Agent

Product and Distributor	Decongestant	Antihistamine	Drying Agent	Rating[1]	Comment
Sustained Release					
Extendac Capsules (Vitarine)	50 mg phenylpropanolamine hydrochloride	1 mg chlorpheniramine maleate + 12.5 mg pheniramine maleate	0.16 mg belladonna alkaloids	B	belladonna not proved effective; 2 approved antihistamines; safety of antihistamine + drying agent unproved
Pronto Capsules (Coastal)				B	

Upper Respiratory Drugs: Combination Product Ratings (continued)

Decongestant + Antihistamine + Drying Agent

Product and Distributor	Decongestant	Antihistamine	Drying Agent	Rating[1]	Comment
		Sustained Release			
Spen-Cold Capsules, Improved (Spencer-Mead)	50 mg phenylpropanolamine hydrochloride	4 mg chlorpheniramine maleate	0.2 mg belladonna alkaloids	B	belladonna not proved effective; antihistamine + drying agent not proved safe

Decongestant + Antihistamine + Other Medications

Product and Distributor	Decongestant	Antihistamine	Other Content	Rating[1]	Comment
Citra Capsules (Boyle)	10 mg phenylephrine hydrochloride	1 mg chlorpheniramine maleate + 6.25 mg pheniramine maleate + 8.33 mg pyrilamine maleate	227 mg salicylamide + 120 mg phenacetin + 50 mg vitamin C + 30 mg caffeine alkaloid	C	3 antihistamines not safe and/or not effective together; phenacetin unsafe
Sinulin Tablets (Carnrick)	37.5 mg phenylpropanolamine hydrochloride	2 mg chlorpheniramine maleate	325 mg acetaminophen + 250 mg salicylamide + 0.75 mg homatropine methylbromide	C	too much of the decongestant; homatropine methylbromide not assessed by Panel as cough-cold or allergy remedy

1. Author's interpretation of Panel criteria. Based on contents, not claims.

Cough Mixture Product Ratings

Cough-Suppressor Combination Products

Product and Distributor	Cough Suppressor	Decongestant	Antihistamine	Other Content	Rating[1]	Comment
Capsules and Tablets						
Alo-Tuss Improved Tablets (North American)	10 mg dextromethorphan hydrobromide	5 mg phenylephrine hydrochloride	2 mg chlorpheniramine maleate	227 mg salicylamide + 100 mg phenacetin + 10 mg caffeine	C	phenacetin not safe
Comtrex Capsules or Tablets (Bristol-Myers)	10 mg dextromethorphan hydrobromide	12.5 mg phenylpropanolamine hydrochloride	1 mg chlorpheniramine maleate	325 mg acetaminophen	C	less-than-effective dose of antihistamine
Contac Severe Cold Formula Capsules (Menley & James)	15 mg dextromethorphan hydrobromide	30 mg pseudoephedrine hydrochloride	3.75 mg doxylamine succinate	500 mg acetaminophen	C	less-than-effective dosage of decongestant, antihistamine; 2 tablets deliver too much of antihistamine, acetaminophen
CoTylenol Cold Formula Capsules or Tablets (McNeil)	15 mg dextromethorphan hydrobromide	30 mg pseudoephedrine hydrochloride	2 mg chlorpheniramine maleate	325 mg acetaminophen	C	1 tablet delivers less-than-effective dose of antihistamine; 2 tablets deliver too much of cough suppressor
DayCare Capsules (Vicks Health Care Div.)	10 mg dextromethorphan hydrobromide	12.5 mg phenylpropanolamine hydrochloride		325 mg acetaminophen	A	1 tablet correct formulation for children 6–12; 2 tablets correct for adults

Cough Mixture Product Ratings *(continued)*

Cough-Suppressor Combination Products

Product and Distributor	Cough Suppressor	Decongestant	Antihistamine	Other Content	Rating[1]	Comment
Rhinex DM Tablets (Lemmon)	10 mg dextromethorphan hydrobromide	5 mg phenylephedrine hydrochloride	2 mg chlorpheniramine maleate		A	1 tablet correct for children 6–12; 2 tablets correct for adults
Tricodene Forte Capsules (Pfeiffer)	10 mg dextromethorphan hydrobromide	12.5 mg phenylpropanolamine hydrochloride	2 mg chlorpheniramine maleate		A	1 tablet correct for children 6–12; 2 tablets correct for adults
Liquids						
Alamine-C Liquid[2] (North American)	10 mg codeine phosphate	18.75 mg phenylpropanolamine hydrochloride	2 mg chlorpheniramine maleate		A	1 tsp correct for children; 2 tsps correct for adults
Co-Histine DH Elixir[2] (Kay Pharm.)					A	
Novahistine DH Liquid[2] (Dow)					A	
Colrex Compound Elixir[2] (Rowell)	8 mg codeine phosphate	5 mg phenylephrine hydrochloride	1 mg chlorpheniramine maleate	120 mg acetaminophen	C	2 teaspoonsful deliver less-than-recommended effective dosage of antihistamine and pain-reliever acetaminophen

Product and Distributor	Expectorant	Decongestant	Antihistamine	Other Content	Rating[1]	Comment
Conar Suspension (Beecham Labs.)	15 mg noscapine				B	noscapine not proved effective
Cosanyl Cough Syrup[2] (Health Care Industries)	10 mg codeine phosphate	30 mg pseudoephedrine hydrochloride			A	1 tsp delivers correct dosage for children 6–12; 2 tsps deliver correct adult dosage
DayCare Liquid (Vicks Health Care Div.)	3.3 mg dextromethorphan hydrobromide	4.17 mg phenylpropanolamine hydrochloride		108 mg acetaminophen	A	suggested 3 tablespoonsful deliver correct dosages
Kolephrin with Codeine[2] Liquid (Pfeiffer)	7.5 mg codeine phosphate	5 mg phenylephrine hydrochloride	10 mg pyrilamine maleate	325 mg sodium salicylate + menthol	B	menthol not proved effective
Phenhist DH Liquid[2] (Rugby)	10 mg codeine phosphate	10 mg phenylephrine hydrochloride	2 mg chlorpheniramine maleate		C	1 tsp delivers too little of antihistamine; 2 tsps deliver too much decongestant
Ryna-C Syrup[2] (Wallace)	10 mg codeine phosphate	30 mg pseudoephedrine hydrochloride	2 mg chlorpheniramine maleate		A	2 tsps provide correct adult dosage
Tricodene Forte Syrup (Pfeiffer)	10 mg dextromethorphan hydrobromide	12.5 mg phenylpropanolamine hydrochloride	2 mg chlorpheniramine maleate		A	2 tsps provide correct adult dosage

Expectorant Combination Products

Capsules and Tablets

Product and Distributor	Expectorant	Decongestant	Antihistamine	Other Content	Rating[1]	Comment
Amocal Tablets (Jenkins)	60 mg ammonium chloride + 30 mg iodized calcium + 4 mg powdered ipecac	2 mg phenylephrine hydrochloride	5 mg pyrilamine maleate		C	3 drugs from same group, one of which, calcium iodide, is not safe.

Cough Mixture Product Ratings (continued)

Expectorant Combination Products

Product and Distributor	Expectorant	Decongestant	Antihistamine	Other Content	Rating[1]	Comment
Broncajen Tablets (Jenkins)	130 mg potassium guaiacolsulfonate + 130 mg ammonium chloride + 8 mg ipecac	2 mg phenylephrine hydrochloride	10 mg pyrilamine maleate		C	3 drugs from same group (none of which is proved effective)
Guaiahist Tablets (Philips Roxane)	100 mg guaifenesin	5 mg phenylephrine hydrochloride			B	guaifenesin not proved effective

Liquids: Contents per teaspoonful (5 ml)

Product and Distributor	Expectorant	Decongestant	Antihistamine	Other Content	Rating[1]	Comment
Atussin Expectorant (Amfre-Grant)	100 mg guaifenesin	5 mg phenylpropanolamine hydrochloride + 5 mg phenylephrine hydrochloride	2 mg chlorpheniramine maleate		B	too little of each decongestant; the expectorant is not proved effective
Chlor-Trimeton Expectorant (Schering)	50 mg guaifenesin + 50 mg sodium citrate + 100 mg ammonium chloride	10 mg phenylephrine hydrochloride	2 mg chlorpheniramine maleate		C	3 is too many ingredients from same group (expectorants)
Fedahist Expectorant (Dooner)	100 mg guaifenesin	30 mg pseudoephedrine hydrochloride	2 mg chlorpheniramine maleate		B	2 tsps would provide approved dosages of all 3 ingredients if guaifenesin were proved effective—which it has not been
Robitussin-PE Syrup (Robins)	100 mg guaifenesin	30 mg pseudoephedrine hydrochloride			B	2 tsps would provide approved dosages of both ingredients if guaifenesin were proved effective—which it has not been

Product and Distributor	Expectorant	Cough Suppressor	Antihistamine	Other Content	Rating[1]	Comment
Tossecol Expectorant (Kenwood)	90 mg ammonium chloride	12.5 mg phenylpropanolamine hydrochloride + 10 mg ephedrine hydrochloride	6.25 mg pheniramine + 6.25 mg pyrilamine maleate		C	antihistamine and expectorant work against each other

Expectorant + Narcotic Cough-Suppressor Products[2]

Product and Distributor	Expectorant	Cough Suppressor	Antihistamine	Other Content	Rating[1]	Comment
Liquids: Contents per teaspoonful (5 ml)						
Calcidrine Syrup (Abbott)	152 mg calcium iodide	8.4 mg codeine			C	calcium iodide not safe
Cheracol Syrup (Upjohn)	100 mg guaifenesin	10 mg codeine phosphate			B	2 tsps would be approved formulation, if guaifenesin were proved effective—which it has not been
Glydeine Liquid (Geneva Generics)					B	
Robitussin A-C Syrup (Robins)					B	
Prunicodeine Liquid (Lilly)	29 mg terpin hydrate + *Pinus strobus*	10 mg codeine		*Prunus virginiana* + sanguinaria	C	2 "other" ingredients not submitted to or assessed by Panel; neither terpin hydrate nor pine preparations are proved effective
terpin hydrate with codeine elixir (generic)	85 mg terpin hydrate	10 mg codeine			B	terpin hydrate not proved effective

Cough Mixture Product Ratings *(continued)*

Expectorant + Narcotic Cough-Suppressor Products[2]

Product and Distributor	Expectorant	Cough Suppressor	Antihistamine	Other Content	Rating[1]	Comment
SKF Terpin Hydrate and Codeine Elixir (SKF)	85 mg terpin hydrate	10 mg codeine			B	

Expectorant + Non-narcotic Cough-suppressor Products

Product and Distributor	Expectorant	Cough Suppressor	Antihistamine	Other Content	Rating[1]	Comment
		Contents per teaspoonful (5 ml)				
Anti-Tuss DM Expectorant (Century Pharm.)	100 mg guaifenesin	15 mg dextromethorphan hydrobromide			B	guaifenesin not proved effective
Dextro-Tuss GG Cough Syrup (Ulmer)					B	
Liquitussin DM Syrup (Three P)					B	
Robitussin-DM Syrup (Robins)					B	
Cheracol D Cough Syrup (Upjohn)	100 mg guaifenesin	10 mg dextromethorphan hydrobromide			B	guaifenesin not proved effective
Glycotuss-dM Tablets (Vale)					B	

Product and Distributor	Expectorant	Cough Suppressor	Antihistamine	Decongestant	Other	Rating[1]	Comment
Novahistine Cough Formula Liquid (Dow)						B	
Ipsatol DM Cough Syrup (Key Pharm.)	22 mg. ammonium chloride	10 mg dextromethorphan hydrobromide				B	ammonium chloride of unproved effectiveness
Robitussin-DM Cough Calmers (Lozenges) (Robins)	50 mg guaifenesin	7.5 mg dextromethorphan hydrobromide				B	guaifenesin not proved effective
Trocal Lozenges (Mallard)		3.5 mg dextromethorphan hydrobromide				B	guaifenesin not proved effective
Vicks Cough Syrup (Vicks Health Care Div.)	25 mg guaifenesin + 200 mg sodium citrate	3.5 mg dextromethorphan hydrobromide				B	2 unproved expectorants

Cough-Suppressor + Expectorant + Other Ingredient Products

Product and Distributor	Expectorant	Cough Suppressor	Antihistamine	Decongestant	Other	Rating[1]	Comment
			Contents per teaspoonful (5 ml)				
C-Tussin (Century)	100 mg guaifenesin	10 mg codeine phosphate		18.75 mg phenyl-propanolamine hydrochloride		B	guaifenesin not proved effective
Midahist Expectorant[2] (Vangard)						B	
Phenhist Expectorant[2] (Rugby)						B	

Cough Mixture Product Ratings *(continued)*

Cough-Suppressor + Expectorant + Other Ingredient Products

Product and Distributor	Expectorant	Cough Suppressor	Antihistamine	Decongestant	Other	Rating[1]	Comment
			Contents per teaspoonful (5 ml)				
Coricidin Cough Syrup (Schering)	100 mg guaifenesin	10 mg dextro-methorphan hydrobromide		12.5 mg phenyl-propanolamine hydrochloride		B	guaifenesin not proved effective
Dimacol Capsules and Liquid (Robins)	100 mg guaifenesin	15 mg dextromethorphan hydrobromide		30 mg pseudoephedrine hydrochloride		C	too little of decongestant in each tablet or tsp; too much dextromethorphan in 2 of them
Effacol Cough Formula (Spencer-Mead)	250 mg sodium citrate	5 mg dextromethorphan hydrobromide	3 mg doxylamine succinate			C	antihistamine and expectorant counteract each other
Endotussin-NN Syrup (Endo)		10 mg dextromethorphan hydrobromide	7.5 mg pyrilamine maleate	40 mg ammonium chloride		C	inadequate amount of pyrilamine maleate; ammonium chloride of unproved value
Formula 44 Cough Mixture (Vicks Health Care Div.)	250 mg sodium citrate	7.5 mg dextromethorphan hydrobromide	3.75 mg doxylamine succinate			C	antihistamine and expectorant counteract each other

Product						Rating	Comment
Lo-Tussin Syrup[2] (Tutag)	100 mg guaifenesin	10 mg codeine phosphate				B	guaifenesin not shown to be effective
Ryna-CX Liquid (Wallace)[2]				30 mg pseudoephedrine hydrochloride			
Midatane DC Expectorant[2] (Vangard)	100 mg guaifenesin	10 mg codeine phosphate	2 mg brompheniramine maleate	5 mg phenylephrine hydrochloride + 5 mg phenyl-propanolamine hydrochloride		C	antihistamine and expectorant counteract each other
N-N Cough Syrup (Vitarine)	65 mg potassium guaiacolsulfonate + 65 mg ammonium chloride	10 mg dextromethorphan hydrobromide	0.5 mg chlorpheniramine maleate			C	too little of antihistamine; antihistamine + expectorant is disapproved combination
Quelidrine Cough Syrup (Abbott)	40 mg ammonium chloride	10 mg dextromethorphan hydrobromide	2 mg chlorpheniramine maleate	5 mg phenylephrine hydrochloride – 5 mg ephedrine hydrochloride		C	antihistamine and expectorant should not be combined
Tussagesic Suspension (Dorsey)	90 mg terpin hydrate	15 mg dextromethorphan hydrobromide	6.25 mg pheniramine maleate + 6.25 mg pyrilamine maleate	12.5 mg phenyl-propanolamine hydrochloride	120 mg acetaminophen	C	less-than-effective dose of acetaminophen; antihistamine should not be combined with expectorant
Viro-Med Tablets (Whitehall)	50 mg guaifenesin	7.5 mg dextromethorphan hydrobromide	1 mg chlorpheniramine maleate	15 mg pseudoephedrine hydrochloride	325 mg aspirin	C	ineffectively low doses of decongestant and antihistamine; antihistamine and expectorant should not be combined

Cough Mixture Product Ratings *(continued)*

Cough Mixtures for Children

Product and Distributor	Expectorant	Cough Suppressor	Decongestant	Other	Rating[1]	Comment
Bayer Cough Syrup for Children (Glenbrook)		7.5 mg dextromethorphan hydrobromide	9 mg phenylpropanolamine hydrochloride		C	less-than-effective dose of decongestant for children 6–12
Contac Jr. Liquid (Menley & James)		5 mg dextromethorphan hydrobromide	9.375 mg phenylpropanolamine hydrochloride	162.5 mg acetaminophen	C	less-than-effective dose of decongestant for children 6–12
Hold (Children's Formula) Lozenges (Beecham Products)		3.75 mg dextromethorphan hydrobromide	6.25 mg phenylpropanolamine hydrochloride		A	1 lozenge is correct for children 2–6; 2 is correct for children 6–12
Kiddi-Koff Syrup[2] (Tutag)	50 mg guaifenesin	5 mg codeine phosphate	15 mg pseudoephedrine hydrochloride		B	guaifenesin not proved effective
Tricodene Pediatric Syrup (Pfeiffer)		10 mg dextromethorphan hydrobromide	12.5 mg phenylpropanolamine hydrochloride		A	½ tsp is right for children 2–6; 1 tsp right for children 6–12

1. Author's interpretation of Panel criteria. Based on contents, not claims.
2. Narcotic products are not available without prescription in some states and if available, may not be displayed on open shelves. Ask your pharmacist.

**Safety and Effectiveness: Miscellaneous Ingredients in
Cold and Cough Combinations**

Ingredient	Panel's Assessment
ascorbic acid (vitamin C) with label claim for curing colds	summarily disapproved*
ascorbic acid (vitamin C) without label claim for curing colds	safe but not proved effective
caffeine	safe but not proved effective
phenobarbital	not proved effective

*Reason: misbranding.

Cold-Sore Balms

A cold sore or fever blister is a painful, itchy, blistering and crusting sore in a corner of the mouth. It comes too often and then goes—too slowly. Such sores are caused by a virus; they tend to recur, and they cannot be wholly prevented. While cold sores cannot be cured, they can be effectively treated to relieve the pain and irritation. Reviewers noted that one self-treatment method that does not use drugs has been reported to curb cold sores at the beginning stage (*see* PREVENTION, below).

HURTFUL HERPES

The virus that causes cold sores is called *herpes simplex* type 1; the sores sometimes are called *herpes labialis* (*labialis* means "lips," which is where they usually occur). The sores particularly seem to favor the corners of the mouth. The *herpes simplex* type 1 virus is spread by mouth-to-mouth and other physical contact.

The *herpes simplex* type 2 virus causes sores on the genitals that are called *herpes genitalis*. This venereal disease is spread mainly by

COLD-SORE BALMS is based on the unadopted draft report "OTC Externally Administered Fever Blister Drug Products" by the FDA's Advisory Review Panel on OTC Miscellaneous External Drug Products and on the report "Orally Administered Drug Products for the Treatment of Fever Blister" by the FDA's Advisory Review Panel on OTC Miscellaneous Internal Drug Products.

sexual contact and has become one of the commonest and most difficult to treat. No cure is known. The discussion in this unit relates solely to *herpes labialis*; persons with *herpes genitalis* should consult a doctor for symptomatic relief.

Most people suffer minor herpes infections early in life, and are immunized by them. Protective substances called *antibodies* combat the infection—but they seem unable to wholly eliminate the virus from the body. The virus remains in a dormant and perhaps incomplete form inside nerve cells near the lips (or at other locations). It rejuvenates and provokes new cold sores when the body's defenses are temporarily under stress or weakened by fever, chilling, sunburn, windburn, menstruation, upset stomach, gastrointestinal distress, emotional pressures, or pure and simple excitement.

The new eruption—called *recurrent herpes*—usually begins with a mild burning or itching; the skin may feel unusually firm because fluid is collecting within the skin. A red bump or *papule* then appears, which enlarges and fills up with clear-colored fluid. Several blisters may coalesce to form a single, large "water blister"—which may then rupture. The fluid it contains is filled with the virus. Care should be taken not to spread it to other parts of one's own body or to somebody else's (as, for example, by kissing).

After several days, the overlying skin layers slough off, scabs form, and the sore finally heals. If healing has not occurred within 7 to 10 days, experts recommend a visit to a doctor—the problem may be something other than a cold sore, for which additional medical care is needed.

COLD SORES AND CANKER SORES

Many people confuse cold sores with canker sores. The two need to be differentiated because they are entirely different diseases. Cold sores can be self-treated with nonprescription medicines (however questionable their effectiveness), while canker sores—which may be called *aphthous stomatitis* or *aphthous ulcers*—need to be examined by a dentist or doctor, who can decide their cause and recommend an appropriate treatment.

The cause of canker sores is unknown. Viruses are among the suspects.

Unlike cold sores, which mainly occur on the outside of the lips, canker sores arise *inside* the mouth—particularly on the inner lining of the lips, the cheeks, or on the tongue, soft palate, or other mucosal surfaces. Canker sores are small, whitish, depressed areas, with red borders. Like cold sores, they can be quite painful.

Canker sores are a recurrent disease. They usually appear for the first time in late childhood or during the teen-age years, though both youngsters and oldsters sometimes are suddenly afflicted with them. They tend to recur when the mucosa has been scratched by a toothbrush bristle or injured in some other way, or as part of an allergic reaction or a hormonal change (such as menstruation). Emotional stress can provoke canker sores. If left untreated, canker sores require 10 to 14 days to heal.

Many topical remedies have been used to treat canker sores. They include dyes, resins such as myrrh, colloidal substances such as aloe, astringents and substances that act on protein (such as alum), and antibacterials (for example, hydrogen peroxide). Both the Miscellaneous Internal Drugs and the Dentifrice and Dental Care Panels believe professional care should be sought for canker sores. Both maintain that these sores cannot safely and effectively be treated with over-the-counter products. (See SORE MOUTH, in SORE-THROAT AND MOUTH MEDICINES).

PREVENTION

A new way of preventing cold sores has been reported in the medical literature. It consists of treating the emerging sore with ice, for periods of 45 to 120 minutes. The treatment will work only if the ice is applied the very same day that the budding new sore first makes itself felt. The ice should be held gently against the sore until the area becomes uncomfortable, then removed briefly before it is applied again. When this treatment is successful—and it often is—the cold sore vanishes by the following morning.

TOPICAL DRUGS FOR COLD SORES

The report on external cold-sore remedies is brief and evaluators did not assess all the active ingredients in preparations used for treatment. The reason is that budgetary constraints in the early 1980s led the FDA to disband the Miscellaneous External Drugs Panel before it could finish its work. So an ingredient-by-ingredient assessment of the compounds found in topical cold-sore remedies will have to be conducted at a later date by the FDA. A list of ingredients in over-the-counter external cold-sore remedies follows:

alcohol
allantoin
   (5-ureido-hydantoin)
ammonia
ammonium carbonate
amyl dimethyl-p-
   aminobenzoate
amyl para-dimethyl-
   aminobenzoate
anhydrous glycerol
aromatic oily solution
beeswax
benzalkonium chloride
benzocaine
BHA

bismuth sodium
   tartrate
calcium silicate
camphor
carbamide peroxide
dyclonine
   hydrochloride
lanolin
lanolin alcohol
menthol
mineral oil
octyldodecanol
paraffin
pectin
peppermint oil

petrolatum, white
phenol
propyl p-benzoate
pyridoxine
   hydrochloride
sorbitan sesquioleate
soya sterol
sesame oil
spermaceti
talcum powder
tannic acid
titanium dioxide
white petrolatum

The Miscellaneous External Drugs Panel believes that ingredients assessed as safe and effective for relieving skin pain or for use as skin protectants are also likely to be safe and effective for treating cold sores. The exceptions are hydrocortisone and hydrocortisone acetate—which the Panel warns should not be used on cold sores because they can spread the virus.

The present Panel was sent one study in which carbamide peroxide 10 percent in anhydrous (water-free) glycerin was compared to the anhydrous glycerin alone. The medicated preparation was reported to reduce pain and reduce healing time. Evaluators also reviewed studies which suggest that drying agents (like alcohols) and astringents may speed cold-sore healing. It's suggested that tannic acid and white petrolatum may prove useful, even though the Topical Analgesic Panel ranked them not safe and not effective.

Conclusions for the time being are summarized in the first of two SAFETY AND EFFECTIVENESS charts at the end of this unit.

INTERNAL DRUGS FOR COLD SORES

CLAIMS

Several drugs taken internally are claimed to relieve cold sores. They were evaluated by the Miscellaneous Internal Drugs Panel, which found some of the claims made for these products misleading or unsupported by scientific data. It specifically disapproves of the claims:

   for "the relief of discomfort of sun blisters"
   "useful for fever blisters of herpetic origin"

"arrests the symptoms associated with cold sores and sun blisters on the lips"

Tentative approval was granted to the following claim, which is still unproved:

"will shorten the duration of fever blisters [cold sores] if taken at the first signs of itching and swelling"

None of the ingredients that are marketed in internal drugs for cold-sore relief was judged safe and effective. If one were to be approved, the Panel would endorse the claim:

for "the relief of the discomfort of fever blisters [cold sores]."

Approved Active Ingredients

None

Conditionally Approved Active Ingredients

The Panel granted tentative approval to three oral-drug ingredients. In the discussion below, two of these substances are considered together.

Lactobacillus acidophilus and Lactobacillus bulgaricus These are bacteria, obtained from milk or from special cultures of yogurt that are dried with milk sugar and then marketed. Some commercial preparations contain *L. acidophilus* alone; at least one contains a mixture of *L. acidophilus* and *L. bulgaricus*. These bacteria are also sold as antidiarrheal drugs, and the present Panel concurs with other reviewers that they are safe in dosages of up to 4 grams daily.

Almost a dozen studies have been conducted on the use of *Lactobacilli* against cold sores; the majority show promising results. But all of the studies failed to meet Panel standards for acceptance.

How *Lactobacilli* might help relieve cold sores has not been explained. One hypothesis is that in some way the bacteria impart a herpes-virus resistance factor to saliva.

While the evaluators held out some hope that the two bacterial preparations *may* effectively treat cold sores, they say that more definitive test results are needed. Until this is accomplished, *L. acidophilus* and *L. bulgaricus*—alone or together—are judged to be safe but not effective against *herpes simplex*, type 1 virus and cold sores.

Lysine (lysine monohydrochloride) An essential amino acid—a constituent of protein—this substance is present in many of the foods we eat. Supplements are given for nutritional and medicinal reasons, and reviewers judge lysine safe in dosages of up to 3 grams a day.

Several clinical studies were reported in which cold-sore patients who were given lysine supplements showed faster healing and had far fewer recurrences. Scientifically controlled studies were then undertaken. Disappointingly, the first such study showed that lysine had no effect on the rate of healing, the appearance of the sores, or the intervals between recurrences. A second study showed that lysine failed to hasten healing once a cold sore appeared. However, significantly fewer participants suffered new cold sores while on the lysine than participants taking the dummy control preparation did. The Panel concludes that lysine may be beneficial in some patients but, pending more conclusive studies, it lists the ingredient as safe but not proved effective as a cold-sore medication.

Disapproved Active Ingredients

The Panel could find no data on the safety or effectiveness of other ingredients in over-the-counter oral preparations for cold-sore relief. It summarily disapproved of them as unsafe and ineffective. They are not discussed here, but they are included in the second of the two SAFETY AND EFFECTIVENESS charts that follow.

Safety and Effectiveness: Active Ingredients in Over-the-Counter Cold-Sore Remedies Applied to the Skin

Active Ingredient	Function	Panels' Assessment*
alcohol (ethyl alcohol 50 to 95%; isopropyl alcohol 60 to 91.3%)	drying agent	safe and effective†
allantoin	protectant	safe and effective
allantoin	wound healer	not proved effective
anhydrous glycerin	protectant	safe and effective
benzocaine	itch-pain reliever	safe and effective
camphor (0.1 to 3%)	itch-pain reliever	safe and effective
carbamide peroxide (in anhydrous glycerin)	pain reliever	appears promising†
lanolin	protectant	safe and effective
menthol (0.1 to 1%)	itch-pain reliever	safe and effective
petrolatum	protectant	safe and effective
petrolatum, white	protectant	safe and effective
phenol (0.5 to 1.5%)	itch-pain reliever	safe and effective
tannic acid	protectant‡	not safe or effective‡

*These judgments pertain to general topical use and may not apply specifically to the treatment of cold sores.
†Judgment by Miscellaneous External Panel. All others by Topical Analgesic Panel.
‡"Appears promising" as a wound healer.

Safety and Effectiveness: Active Ingredients in Over-the-Counter Cold-Sore Remedies Taken Orally

Active Ingredient	Panel's Assessment
acetaminophen	summarily disapproved
caffeine	summarily disapproved
chlorpheniramine maleate	summarily disapproved
Lactobacillus acidophilus	safe but not proved effective
Lactobacillus bulgaricus	safe but not proved effective
lysine (lysine mono-hydrochloride)	safe but not proved effective
phenolphthalein (3,3,-bis *p*-hydroxyphenyl phthalide)	summarily disapproved
phenylephrine hydrochloride	summarily disapproved

Cold-Sore Balms: Product Ratings[1]

Product and Distributor	Dosage of Active Ingredients	Rating[2]	Comment
Taken Internally			
Lactobacilli			
DoFUS (Miller)	**capsules:** at least 100 million viable *Lactobacillus acidophilus* organisms	**B**	not proved effective
Lactinex (H., W. & D.)	**granules** and **tablets:** viable mixed culture of *Lactobacillus acidophilus* + *L. bulgaricus*	**B**	not proved effective
lysine			
Enisyl (Person & Covey)	**tablets:** 334 mg; 500 mg	**B**	not proved effective
L-Lysine (Nature's Bounty)		**B**	not proved effective

1. Since the Panel did not evaluate individual active ingredients in topical cold-sore balms, ratings are given for products taken internally only. The Panel does suggest however that products rated under ITCH AND PAIN REMEDIES APPLIED TO THE SKIN, pages 467–471, and under UNGUENTS AND POWDERS FOR THE SKIN, pages 800–801, may be comparably appropriate for cold sores, except that: hydrocortisone and hydrocortisone acetate-containing products should *not* be used. Tannic acid may be useful and safe, when used in small amounts around the mouth, despite the Topical Analgesic Panel's general disapproval of it.
2. Author's interpretation of Panel criteria. Based on contents, not claims.

Contraceptives

Many women want to buy and use birth-control products freely, without seeing a doctor to get a prescription for oral contraceptives or to be fitted with a diaphragm or an intrauterine device (IUD). This unit focuses on vaginal contraceptives, those contraceptives used by women and bought without prescription.

Rubbers or condoms, contraceptive devices used by men, are also sold over-the-counter. But, since condoms contain no active chemical ingredients, technically they are not drugs and were not evaluated in the review process.

HOW THEY WORK

Vaginal contraceptives work in two ways to prevent pregnancy: they destroy sperm cells and they block the entry of the sperm into the uterus. These contraceptives contain a spermicide (a sperm-killing drug) that quickly kills or immobilizes sperm cells by destroying their ability to break down and use fructose. This sugar, which is present in semen, provides the energy source that sperm require to swim to and impregnate the ovum (egg)—the ultimate act of conception. "Since the activity of sperm depends on the metabolism of fructose," the Panel says, "the blocking of this process effectively destroys [their] capacity . . . to survive." The death of a sperm cell occurs within seconds after it encounters an effective spermicide.

The second line of defense is the cream or other substance with which the spermicide is formulated. This material forms the bulk of the product. It not only holds the spermicide in place during sexual intercourse but it also covers the cervical os, the narrow opening from the vagina into the uterus. It thereby creates a barrier which blocks the path of the sperm through the uterus to the fallopian tubes, where fertilization occurs.

CLAIMS

Accurate
"intended for the prevention of pregnancy"

CONTRACEPTIVES is based on the report on vaginal contraceptives by the FDA's Advisory Review Panel on OTC Contraceptives and Other Vaginal Drug Products.

False or Misleading

"[10-hour] vaginal jelly"
"medically approved" or "medically tested"
"most frequently prescribed by physicians"
"remarkable birth-control invention"
"outstanding sperm effect in tests comparing it to other products"
"instantly lethal to male sperm"

EFFECTIVENESS AND INFLUENCING FACTORS

For women who wish to follow the Panel's guidance, the range of choice is extemely narrow: reviewers approved only two currently marketed compounds, nonoxynol 9 and octoxynol 9, which it says are essentially identical. They are the spermicidal active ingredients in most vaginal contraceptives sold in the United States. These compounds are judged to be safe, as well as effective, because they have been more carefully tested than other spermicides and because major side effects rarely if ever have been reported as the result of their use. (*See* SAFETY AND EFFECTIVENESS chart at the end of this unit; it also lists the alternate chemical names for various substances.)

Vaginal contraceptives that contain nonoxynol 9 or octoxynol 9 may not all be equally effective, however. Products are formulated in different ways—as creams, jellies, aerosol foams, and semisolid vaginal suppositories—and must be inserted into the vagina and used according to different sets of directions. For example, suppositories—recently in vogue—require time to melt, while foams may be used just before intercourse. These differences can affect the comparative effectiveness of the products. The configuration of the vagina influences correct placement of a spermicidal contraceptive—as does a woman's awareness of how much should be used and where it should be placed.

The vagina, 3 to 4 inches long, is not an open, hollow cavity, as is sometimes imagined. Until stretched during sexual activity, the lower third of its length is star-shaped. The middle third is shaped like the letter H. The upper third creates a crescent-shaped space around the cervix, which protrudes into the vagina.

A vaginal-contraceptive product that is not inserted high enough into the vagina or that is spread too thinly over the vaginal walls may not provide an adequate sperm-killing barrier at the critical entrance to the cervix. On the other hand, a suppository inserted high into the back of the vagina immediately before intercourse may not have time to melt and spread to cover the os, the opening in the cervix. Moreover, some women dislike touching their vaginas, which makes it difficult for them to insert a vaginal contraceptive correctly.

Since how these contraceptives are inserted is such an important factor, and among the many variables, it is difficult to declare one more effective than the others. Evaluators say there is "fragmentary evidence" that aerosol foams are better than other preparations because they make correct placement easier. As for suppositories, reviewers expressed concern over the lack of evidence about proper placement, melting time, and the duration of effectiveness of these semisolid products—which have been promoted as being less messy than foams. The Federal Trade Commission, which regulates advertising, has also been concerned about vaginal-suppository contraceptives and the claims made for them. In 1980 the commission told manufacturers that they had to stop saying and suggesting in their ads that the suppositories are as effective as oral contraceptives and IUDs. Instead, they must say suppositories are comparable in effectiveness to vaginal foams, creams, and jellies. Also ads must now state that a waiting period of 10 to 15 minutes is required between the time the suppository is inserted and the time one engages in intercourse.

Another factor influencing the effectiveness of these contraceptives is the care a woman takes in using the product. Studies on product effectiveness made by individual manufacturers are collected and summarized each year in the annual volume *Contraceptive Technology* (Irvington Publishers), edited by Emory University obstetrician Robert A. Hatcher, M.D., and several colleagues. The 1980–81 edition showed that vaginal contraceptives were among the least effective contraceptive methods. Between 20 and 25 of every 100 fertile women who started using vaginal contraceptives became pregnant within a year. (This is a far higher failure rate than was reported in manufacturers' studies, described below, which the Panel used in judging nonoxynol 9 and octoxynol 9 to be effective.) As experts explain it, the lower pregnancy rates can be achieved in well-motivated women who are carefully instructed on the products' use and who are reinforced in their decision to use the products correctly. For example, the high failure rates reported in some field trials using foam are attributed by Hatcher and his colleagues partly to careless use. "The mistakes a foam user can make include using too little, failing to shake the foam container vigorously enough, failing to recognize that the foam bottle is empty, failing to have the foam bottle available, [and] failing to interrupt lovemaking to use the foam. . . ."

Vaginal contraceptives are generally regarded as being *less* effective in preventing pregnancy than oral contraceptives and other medically provided contraceptive methods. But, after an exhaustive search of published and unpublished information, evaluators discovered to their dismay that because there are "no well-controlled studies [of] patients with similar backgrounds who receive their family-planning care at the same time and in the same place," it is not possible at this time to make valid comparisons between the effectiveness of nonprescription products and doctor-prescribed medications or procedures.

UNRESOLVED SAFETY ISSUES

In the sense that few serious adverse effects have been reported from their use, vaginal contraceptives were assessed as apparently being very safe for women and their partners, and for their unborn children. However, reviewers discovered that there were few studies evaluating the safety of spermicidal ingredients. The Panel first studied the literature published between 1950 and 1973—which it found to be wanting. Most published studies were over 10 years old. Worse, none could be found that assessed the effects of the ingredients in vaginal contraceptives directly on an unborn baby carried in the womb, or on future generations through genetic mutation. Neither did the studies evaluate the carcinogenic (cancer-producing) or toxic (poisoning) effects of these ingredients. The effects of medication on an unborn child were dramatically illustrated in the late 1950s, when grossly deformed babies were born to women who had used the sedative thalidomide early in their pregnancies. The thalidomide tragedy led to Senate hearings, conducted in 1962, on the lack of rigorous testing requirements to protect women and their children from defect-causing drugs. These hearings, in turn, led to the federal legislation that mandated the review of over-the-counter drugs.

When the present Panel set out to study serious side effects of nonprescription birth-control products, it quickly discovered that these key safety questions had not been satisfactorily answered. To find more data than the FDA and the contraceptive manufacturers had provided for their use, evaluators conducted their own review of the world literature. Then they asked medical and scientific publications to run notices requesting additional data. Little came in. A medical librarian was hired to continue the search. Companies were asked for additional information. Finally, the reviewers convened two special symposia to explore fundamental issues of female anatomy and reproductive health, and to study proposals for further research into the safety and effectiveness of vaginal contraceptives. The Panel recommended a series of tough new tests. Vaginal contraceptives:

- must act quickly to kill all sperm on contact, or render them incapable of fertilization
- must not be systemically toxic to the woman or irritating either to her vagina or her mate's penis
- must not be harmful to a recently conceived embryo or fetus
- must be free of long-term toxicity to the mother and her offspring

DOUCHING AND CONTRACEPTION

Many women believe douching after sexual intercourse is an effective contraceptive method. *It is not!*

As the American Pharmaceutical Association publication *Handbook of Nonprescription Drugs,* 6th Ed. (1979), explains, douching is not at all reliable because sperm cells from semen enter the uterus too quickly to be washed away by water or other douching solutions. Sperm cells may reach the cervical opening within 30 seconds after ejaculation and enter the cervix and uterus within 90 to 180 seconds. They can be in the fallopian tubes, where conception occurs, within half an hour. "It is highly improbable," the *Handbook* says, "that douching can be initiated quickly or thoroughly enough to remove all traces of semen, and therefore of sperm, from the vagina."

The Panel, concurring in this judgment, wants all douche labels to state quite clearly that the products are *not* intended to prevent pregnancy (*see* DOUCHES AND OTHER VAGINAL APPLICATIONS).

Some women douche after intercourse whether or not they are protected by a contraceptive. This may be a costly mistake for women who use spermicides, for if they douche too soon they may wash the contraceptive material out while living sperm remain in the vagina. Experts recommend waiting at least 6 hours before douching.

SPECIAL NEEDS FOR VAGINAL CONTRACEPTIVES

Some women use vaginal contraceptives on a regular basis. Family-planning experts, manufacturers, and the Panel suggest several specific situations in which these products may be particularly useful:

- when teen-agers who have sex infrequently do not wish to burden their bodies with hormonal oral contraceptives or an IUD

- when older women who have sex infrequently wish to avoid the high risk of heart and artery disease and other complications that they face if they use oral contraceptives (This is of special concern if they also are cigarette smokers)
- for unprotected cycles when a woman is going onto or off the oral contraceptives—or in any cycle when she forgets to take one or two of the pills
- for added protection during highly fertile, midcycle days for couples who usually rely on condoms
- for use with diaphragms if the spermicidal product prescribed with it runs out (The same spermicidal active ingredients are present in *all* vaginal contraceptives)

COMBINATION PRODUCTS

A vaginal contraceptive containing a single active ingredient is safer than one that contains two or more such ingredients, according to the evaluators. No products submitted for review contained two approved spermicidal ingredients. So there are no approved combination vaginal contraceptive products.

One currently marketed combination contains methoxypolyoxy-ethyleneglycol 550 laurate and nonoxynol 9. It was judged safe but not proved effective, since the relative contribution of the two ingredients has not been established. All other combinations were rejected as unsafe or ineffective.

SPERMICIDES

The Panel assessed 7 spermicidal active ingredients—including two mercuric compounds and a combination product that includes two active ingredients, one of which is marketed only in this combined form. Reviewers initially approved three active ingredients as safe and effective, but the FDA turned thumbs down on a new drug, menfegol, because data that show it to be safe and effective were obtained from studies in foreign countries and not in the United States as the drug laws and regulations have required.

Approved Active Ingredients

The two approved surface-acting compounds are closely related chemically.

Nonoxynol 9 This is the active ingredient in the large majority of foams, creams, suppositories, and other over-the-counter vaginal contraceptives. It is the compound upon which the industry is essentially based at this time, and a variety of tests indicate that the substance is safe as well as effective. It has been fed in large doses to rats and dogs, applied to rabbits' sensitive skins and eyes, and inserted in large doses into dogs' vaginas. No significant adverse effects were found. From these findings, as well as clinical experience with human use, reviewers judged it to be safe.

The effectiveness of nonoxynol 9 has been established in a variety of test-tube studies involving precisely measured doses of human semen, and in a variety of more sophisticated experiments in which first the contraceptive and then human semen were introduced into women's vaginas. Afterward samples were collected and assessed to see how many of the sperm cells survived. When an effective dose of nonoxynol 9 is used, most or all sperm cells are immobilized or dead after 20 seconds.

The results have been less spectacular in other human trials. Reviewers summarized the results of 6 clinical experiments covering 425 women who used a nonoxynol cream preparation for a combined total of 4071 months. The pregnancy rate was 2.1 percent per year in women who used the product correctly, and 3.5 percent per year in women who used it incorrectly or irregularly. In other studies involving 1000 women who used nonoxynol 9 foam products for a combined total of 4634 months, the pregnancy rate was as low as 2.2 percent per year with correct use and as high as 5.4 percent when use was incorrect or not regular.

While the pregnancy rates appear low, they also suggest that each group of 100 women who used nonoxynol 9 products correctly throughout their fertile years could anticipate 50 unwanted pregnancies among the group. Women who used the products incorrectly or irregularly could expect as many as 100 pregnancies (among all the 100 women) in this period. Moreover, some reports in the medical literature show considerably higher pregnancy rates than the studies cited by the Panel. However, evaluators concluded that nonoxynol 9 is safe and effective as a vaginal contraceptive. Specific dosages depend on the way that the product is formulated, as do the instructions for use.

Octoxynol 9 This substance is almost identical to nonoxynol 9 (*see* directly above); the Panel says the slight molecular variation between them has no significant effect on the biological or chemical properties of the compound. The failure rates are also quite comparable. Conclusion: octoxynol 9 is safe and effective as a spermicide.

Conditionally Approved Active Ingredients

Two individual spermicides were evaluated as conditionally approved, as was one combination of nonoxynol 9 and a second spermicidal surface-acting substance. In all three cases, it is the spermicide's effectiveness—not its safety—that is in question.

Dodecaethyleneglycol monolaurate This surface-acting substance is less well studied than nonoxynol 9. Evaluators based their decision that it is safe on two studies of rabbits and one of women. In the latter, 50 women used a 5 percent concentration of this active ingredient in a jelly base. They applied it vaginally each night for 10 to 21 days. Neither the women nor the doctors who examined them found any problems in this brief period; so the Panel believes that dodecaethyleneglycol monolaurate is safe.

But data on the effectiveness of this substance were even sparser. One study claiming to show that it blocks the cervical opening for up to 10 hours was conducted on a single human subject. No evidence was submitted showing the drug's sperm-killing ability in test tubes. Nor were there after-intercourse studies on the viability of sperm cells subjected to the substance in either animal or human vaginas. Therefore reviewers decided that, while safe, dodecaethylene's effectiveness remains to be proved.

Laureth 10S Studies in dogs and rabbits showed no significant adverse changes in the animals or in their offspring. In one human study, a 2 percent concentration of laureth 10S in a jelly formulation produced no adverse effects in 10 women who put it into their vaginas daily for 3 weeks.

No evidence was presented on this substance's sperm-killing ability in the test tube or on its effectiveness in after-intercourse tests in animals—let alone in women. The verdict: laureth 10S is safe but its effectiveness is yet to be shown.

The combination of methoxypolyoxyethyleneglycol 550 laurate + nonoxynol 9 While the latter ingredient is both safe and effective (*see* above) no scientific data were submitted on methoxypolyoxyethyleneglycol 550 so that the evaluators could assess its individual safety and efficiency or the contribution it may make to the combination product. The effectiveness of this ingredient and that of the combination product both remain to be established.

Disapproved Active Ingredients

The Panel specifically assessed two sperm-killing compounds as unsafe and the FDA added a third. The condemnation of mercury-containing compounds extends to all other mercury-type substances that might be formulated or labeled for use as vaginal contraceptives.

Menfegol   This surface-acting contraceptive has been successfully marketed outside the United States for more than a decade. Evaluators judged it safe and effective on the basis of fairly extensive tests in mice, rats, rabbits, and dogs, and clinical trials in over 1000 women, although menfegol caused a slight vaginal discharge in some users. The pregnancy rate in various of these human studies ranged from 2.3 to 7.7 pregnancies per 100 woman-years of use. Women and their partners may experience a sensation of warmth from the drug. This is disconcerting to some people, a sexual turn-on to others. Whether menfegol is absorbed through the vaginal wall to enter the bloodstream remains to be determined.

The FDA turned down the Panel's approval of the compound "because menfegol is a new molecular entity, never before marketed as a drug in the U.S." It banned menfegol as unsafe and ineffective until such time as tests conducted under its rules for New Drug Applications demonstrate the safety and effectiveness of this compound for use as a nonprescription spermicide.

Phenylmercuric acetate (PMA)   Weak concentrations of this mercury compound kill sperm, although they are no more effective—and may be less effective—than commonly used concentrations of nonoxynol 9. The major problem with PMA is that mercury is readily absorbed from the vagina into the bloodstream, which carries it throughout a woman's body. It enters her breasts and may contaminate her milk if she is nursing. If, unknown to herself, she is pregnant at the time she uses a PMA vaginal contraceptive product, some of the mercury can pass through the placental barrier into the embryo or fetus—to which it may be quite toxic.

Only a few cases have been reported of very severe prenatal (before-birth) mercury poisoning of children; their mothers had taken the chemical through food or drinking-water. In these tragic cases the babies' nervous systems functioned so poorly that they became grossly crippled idiots.

No documentation is available to show that infants born of mothers who used PMA vaginal contraceptives have been damaged as a result. But evaluators believe that direct proof would be difficult, if not impossible, to obtain. Subtle changes that might show up only years later—for example, in the form of behavioral problems in school—would be particularly difficult to pin to the use of a mercury product. Yet animal studies suggest that such effects might occur.

Although the reviewers advise caution in using animal-study results to predict reactions in humans, they maintain that "the special susceptibility of the fetus and child to chemical pollutants such as mercury and the seriousness of mercury poisoning are generally recognized." So mercury compounds in "vaginal contraceptive preparations are potentially hazardous to the fetus and breast-fed infant."

Thus, the Panel decided that these products are unsafe and should be removed from the market.

Phenylmercuric nitrate   The risks of PMA, described above, extend to phenylmercuric nitrate and *all other mercuric compounds* that might be used in vaginal contraceptive products. The Panel says they are all unsafe.

Inactive Ingredients

The Panel wants to limit inactive ingredients present in vaginal contraceptives to ingredients that either are *essential* for formulating the drug or are for what it terms "product identification"—whatever that means! Reviewers believe the safety of some inactive ingredients is open to question, including the quaternary ammonium compounds benzethonium chloride and methylbenzethonium chloride, which are used as preservatives, and the boron compounds boric acid and sodium borate, which are included for similar reasons.

The following ingredients are inactive, or are required for pharmaceutical purposes in formulating spermicides and other over-the-counter vaginal products:

acacia	hydroxyethylcellulose	propylparaben
alcohol	methylbenzethonium	purified water
benzethonium chloride	chloride	sodium borate
boric acid	methylparaben	starch
butylparaben	methylpolysiloxane	stearic acid
de-ionized water	perfume	tragacanth
glycerin	preservatives	

Safety and Effectiveness: Spermicides
in Over-the-Counter Vaginal Contraceptives

Active Ingredient	Chemical Name*	Panel's Assessment
dodecaethyleneglycol monolaurate	polyethylene glycol 600 monolaurate	safe but not proved effective
laureth 10S		safe but not proved effective
menfegol	p-menthanylphenyl polyoxyethylene (8.8) ether	not safe or effective†
methoxypolyoxyethyleneglycol 550 laurate + nonoxynol 9		safe but not proved effective
nonoxynol 9	nonylphenoxypolyethoxyethanol, nonyl phenoxy polyoxyethylene ethanol, polyoxyethylenenonylphenol	safe and effective
octoxynol 9	p-diisobutylphenenoxypolyethoxyethanol, polyethylene glycol of mono-iso-octyl phenyl ether	safe and effective
phenylmercuric acetate (PMA)		not safe
phenylmercuric nitrate		not safe

*The shortened names are easier and commonly used but package labels may list the longer chemical names, which are included here for consumers' guidance.
†FDA assessment.

Contraceptives: Product Ratings

Product and Distributor	Dosage of Active Ingredients	Rating[1]	Comment
nonoxynol 9			
Conceptrol (Ortho)	vaginal cream: 5%	A	
Dalkon (Robins)	vaginal foam: 8%	A	
Delfen (Ortho)	vaginal foam: 12.5%	A	
Encare (Eaton-Merz)	vaginal suppositories: 2.27%	A	
Emko (Schering)	vaginal foam: 8%	A	
Intercept (Ortho)	vaginal suppositories: 100 mg	A	
Koromex II-A (Holland-Rantos)	vaginal jelly: 2%	A	
Ortho-Gynol (Ortho)	vaginal jelly: 1%	A	for use with vaginal diaphragm
octoxynol 9			
Koromex II (Holland-Rantos)	vaginal jelly: 1%	A	for use with vaginal diaphragm
	vaginal cream: 3%	A	for use with vaginal diaphragm
phenylmercuric borate			
Anvita (A.O. Schmidt)	vaginal suppositories: 1:2000	C	mercurials not safe

1. Author's interpretation of Panel and FDA criteria. Based on contents, not claims.

Corn and Callus Removers

Few pains are as intense as that of a toe-top O-corn—a hard, thick overgrowth of skin encircling a softer center. A bewildering selection of treatment preparations—including adherent films, creams and salves, and medicated pads, disks and plasters—are sold to relieve O-corns and other painful or annoying calluses and corns.

But the choice of which drug to use is easy: the group that studied corn and callus removers came to the conclusion that only salicylic acid is safe and effective. This acid is a keratolytic agent—a drug that eats away the bonds between the cells of the hard, outer portion of skin, causing it to peel.

CLAIMS

Accurate
for "the removal of hard corns and calluses"

False or Misleading
"you are about to make your feet more comfortable"
"you have just purchased one of the finest foot aids available"
"this special liquid preparation helps remove corns quickly"
"walk easy, walk soft"
"makes walking more pleasurable for you"
"absolutely painless"

WARNING   Do not exceed 5 treatments. Do not use if you are a diabetic or have poor blood circulation, because serious complications may result. Do not use on irritated skin or if the area is infected or reddened.

WHAT PRESSURE SORES ARE

Corns and calluses are caused by an overgrowth of the skin's horny outer layer, as a reaction to long-standing friction or pressure. A callus is hard, thickened skin that has no central core. It usually arises on the sole of the foot. Calluses tend to be yellow in color, with normal skin-

CORN AND CALLUS REMOVERS is based on the report "Corn and Callus Remover Drug Products for OTC Human Use" by the FDA's Advisory Review Panel on OTC Miscellaneous External Drug Products.

ridge patterns continuing across their surface. By contrast, corns usually have a definite central area or core, and they are commoner on the toes than on the soles of the feet.

Corns may be hard or soft or, like the O-corn, both hard and soft. They usually arise just over a toe bone, so there is pressure both from above and from below. Hard corns are raised, yellowish-gray sore spots, which are widest on the skin surface and taper inward to a point—like an upside-down volcano that presses (painfully!) on underlying nerve endings. Soft corns are whitish skin thickenings in the toewebs. They tend to stay soft and sore because they are constantly moistened by sweat. Seed corns are tiny ingrowths in callused areas on the soles of the feet: they are rarely painful.

Corns that are red or blue—because they are filled with blood—are called *neurovascular corns*. They do not respond well to self-treatment.

A third major type of pressure sores on the feet are called *bunions*. A bunion is a swelling along the outside rear surface of the big toe. It forces the big toe and other toes out of line; the pressure causes secondary corns. A bunion may well require podiatric or medical care.

TREATMENT

Calluses and corns can often be removed with nonprescription medications. Those that fail to respond can be treated by a podiatrist, a physician, or an orthopedic surgeon who specializes in foot problems.

If you treat a callus or corn with an over-the-counter medication, try at the same time to eliminate the rubbing or pressure that caused it—usually poorly fitting shoes or hosiery. If you don't, the condition is likely to recur. Remember, too, that a callus serves a protective function, so it should not be quickly or abruptly removed, particularly if it is not painful. It may make more sense to correct the underlying problem first. The outgrowth or ingrowth may then slowly recede without further treatment.

Persons who have diabetes or poor circulation should not take care of their own calluses or corns, but rather should let a foot doctor do it. Diabetics are highly vulnerable to infection; professional foot care helps prevent this.

Forms of Treatment

The paucity of active ingredients to relieve corns and calluses is perhaps balanced by the variety of dosage forms in which they are formulated.

- A *collodion* is a solution of nitrocellulose in a solvent, which dries quickly when applied and leaves a thin, cohesive film that contains the active drug in contact with the skin.
- A *foot salve* is an ointment used on the feet.
- A *medicated disk* is a topical medication in a skin-contact adhesive that is backed by a rounded piece of fabric, plastic, or other material. It can be purchased in an appropriate size to cover a corn or callus.
- A *medicated pad* is topical medication in a soft bit of fabric, plastic, or other material that also cushions the callus or corn.
- A *medicated plaster* is a topical drug in a skin-contact adhesive base that is spread on backing of plastic, fabric, or other suitable material.

The Panel says collodions and plaster, disk, and pad dosage forms all are advantageous in treating calluses and corns because they adhere to and keep the medication in contact with the skin. They also hold in moisture, an advantage because salicylic acid works only in the presence of water. (This explains why it is helpful to soak the foot in water for 15 to 30 minutes, then dry it lightly before applying salicylic acid preparations.)

Combination Products

Evaluators could find no products containing two or more active ingredients that it felt could be approved as safe and effective. Conditional approval was granted only to one combination, salicylic acid + zinc chloride. The following combination is rejected as unsafe: Salicylic acid + a local anesthetic is dangerous because the anesthetic can mask the pain that may result from overtreatment with skin-peeling salicylic acid.

SKIN-PEELERS FOR THE FEET

Approved Active Ingredient

Salicylic acid (in collodions, medicated disks, plasters, and pads) This is either the principal active ingredient or the only one in most corn and callus products. It is found in nature in wintergreen leaves and sweet birchbark. Of course, it is also manufactured synthetically—in huge amounts—because it is the parent compound for aspirin and several other pain-relieving drugs. Salicylic acid, however, does not act on corns and calluses as a pain reliever. Rather, it slowly eats away the unwanted skin.

Salicylic Acid for the Treatment of Calluses and Corns

Vehicles (Bases)

recommended	medicated disks, plasters, pads, and collodions
not recommended	ointments and other nonadherent preparations

Approved Dosages

in disks, plasters, and pads	12 to 40%
in collodions	12 to 17.6%

Uses

recommended for	hard corns and calluses
not recommended for	soft corns

Too little salicylic acid is absorbed through the skin from a corn plaster to cause aspirin-poisoning. But it can easily dissolve normal skin as well as the thick skin of a callus and corn, so great care must be taken to apply the drug *only* to overgrown skin areas.

As to safety, in two large studies of foot-clinic patients in the mid-1970s investigators found that salicylic acid products caused few, if any, side effects and none that required a doctor's care. Reviewers accepted these findings and the absence of reported injury as evidence that salicylic acid is safe for nonprescription foot use.

Effectiveness was demonstrated to the Panel's satisfaction in several scientifically controlled tests. In one, 40 percent salicylic acid in medicated disks removed 73 percent of corns after 5 treatments over 11 days. This compares with 4 percent complete removal when the same disk was applied without the active drug. The treatment was less effective against calluses: after 11 days, only 15 percent of calluses were wholly gone. But then, the nonmedicated disks did not remove *any* participant's callus within that time period.

Based on these findings and other studies, evaluators say that salicylic acid is safe and effective for treating hard corns and calluses in concentrations of 12 to 40 percent in medicated pads, plasters, and disks and in concentration of 12 to 17.6 percent in collodion vehicles. If the corn or callus shows no improvement after 14 days, one should see a doctor.

Reviewers claim that they were not given enough data to evaluate salicylic acid's effectiveness against soft corns. They say, too, that they remain unconvinced that salicylic acid in ointment bases is safe and effective, so such preparations are not recommended.

Conditionally Approved Active Ingredients

This category reflects doubts about effectiveness, not safety. The Panel is also unsure about some dosage forms of salicylic acid (*see* below).

Phenoxyacetic acid (phenoxyethanoic acid) This acid is weaker than salicylic acid, and standard tests in laboratory animals and in human volunteers show that it is safe for application to small areas of the body. Two studies, conducted back in 1948, suggest that phenoxyacetic acid is at least as effective as salicylic acid in removing corns and calluses. But these tests used questionable methodology and evaluators feel that new, scientifically sound trials are needed to determine if this substance really works. For now, the verdict is: safe but not proved effective.

Salicylic acid (ointments) The Panel doubts whether foot salves, or ointments, will keep the salicylic acid in close enough contact with the skin, along with water, to remove calluses and corns (*see* the last paragraph under FORMS OF TREATMENT, above). The reviewers believe that the safety and effectiveness of these ointments—and apparently of all other nonadherent dosage forms—remain to be proved.

Zinc chloride This is an irritating, skin-peeling substance. One study, on rabbits' skins, indicates that low doses are not too irritating for human use—a decision seconded by Panel members who cited their own experience with patients.

The chemical is usually formulated with salicylic acid in a combination product. Since the Panel could find no data on the contribution, if any, that zinc chloride makes to the outcome of treatment, the conclusion is: safe but not proved effective.

Disapproved Active Ingredients

Evaluators listed over a dozen chemicals that have been or are being used to treat calluses and corns but for which no safety or effectiveness data could be found. The Panel simply decided to summarily dismiss them.

Inactive Ingredients

A variety of oils, creams, and other soothing ingredients are formulated into corn- and callus-removing products. These balms are treated by the Panel as inactive ingredients. Other therapeutically inactive ingredients act as solvents, vehicles (bases), and preservatives for active drugs. These substances are listed below.

alcohol	chlorophyll	menthol
beeswax	collodion	pyroxylin
benzocaine	cottonseed oil	sodium carbonate
camphor	ether	starch
camphor gum	eucalyptus oil (oil of	thymol
castile soap	eucalyptus)	turpentine
castor oil	lard	

FOOT SALVES: PRELIMINARY NOTES

A variety of salves, creams, lotions, and powders are sold over-the-counter to relieve tired and sore feet and prevent and cure minor foot ailments. Some serve as bases for other, more active drugs. The Panel was planning to write a report on these foot preparations, but it was disbanded before this could be done.

Very preliminary judgments on these ingredients are, however, contained in the reviewers' rough-draft report on these drugs. These tentative judgments follow.

amyl salicylate	not effective
belladonna alkaloids	not effective
benzoic acid	not effective
calcium acetate	not proved safe or effective
camphor gum	not effective
chloroxylenol (PCMX)	not effective
dichlorophenyl trichloroethane	not effective
glyceryl monostearate	not effective
iodized botanical oil	not effective
lard	not effective
magnesium sulfate	not effective
methyl isobutyl ketone	not effective
oil of thyme	not effective
peppermint oil	not effective
pine-needle oil	not effective
potassium iodine	not effective
propylene glycol	not proved effective
salicin	not effective
sassafras oil	not effective
sodium bicarbonate	not effective

sodium chloride	not proved effective
sodium lauryl sulfate	not effective
sodium sesquicarbonate	not effective
sodium sulfate	not effective
tragacanth mucilage	not effective
witch hazel	not effective
zinc sulfate	not effective

Safety and Effectiveness: Active Ingredients in Over-the-Counter Products Sold for Removing Hard Corns and Calluses

Active Ingredient	Panel's Assessment
acetic acid, glacial	summarily disapproved
allantoin	summarily disapproved
ascorbic acid (vitamin C)	summarily disapproved
belladonna, extract	summarily disapproved
chlorobutanol	summarily disapproved
diperodon hydrochloride	summarily disapproved
eucalyptus oil	summarily disapproved
ichthammol	summarily disapproved
iodine	summarily disapproved
methylbenzethonium chloride	summarily disapproved
methyl salicylate	summarily disapproved
panthenol	summarily disapproved
phenoxyacetic acid (phenoxyethanoic acid)	safe but not proved effective
phenyl salicylate	summarily disapproved
salicylic acid (in collodions, medicated disks, pads, and plasters)	safe and effective
salicylic acid (in ointments)	not proved safe or effective
vitamin A	summarily disapproved
zinc chloride	safe but not proved effective

Corn and Callus Removers: Product Ratings

Single-Ingredient Products

Product and Distributor	Dosage of Active Ingredients	Rating[1]	Comment
salicylic acid			
Calicylic Creme (Gordon Labs.)	**cream: 10%**	C	less-than-recommended dosage; creams not recommended

Corn and Callus Removers: Product Ratings *(continued)*

Single-Ingredient Products

Product and Distributor	Dosage of Active Ingredients	Rating[1]	Comment
Mediplast (Beiersdorf)	**plaster:** 40%	A	recommended dosage form
"2" Drop Corn/Callus Remover (Scholl's)	**liquid and pads:** 12.6%	A	recommended dosage form
Wart-Off (Pfipharmecs)	**flexible collodion:** 17%	A	recommended dosage form

Combination Product

Product and Distributor	Dosage of Active Ingredients	Rating[1]	Comment
Freezone Solution (Whitehall)	**flexible collodion:** 13.6% salicylic acid + 2.18% zinc chloride	B	zinc chloride not proved effective

1. Author's interpretation of Panel criteria. Based on contents, not claims.

Cough Drugs

See COLD, COUGH, AND ALLERGY DRUGS

Cradle-Cap Removers

In the first weeks of life, babies often develop a scaly scalp inflammation called *cradle cap*. It may be a residual accumulation of the fatty substance that covers the baby before birth. Or it may be an infantile form of seborrheic dermatitis (*see* FAST SKIN TURNOVER FORMS FLAKES in DANDRUFF AND SEBORRHEIC SCALE SHAMPOOS.) However, it usually goes away within a month and does not return. Occasionally

CRADLE-CAP REMOVERS is based on the unadopted draft report "Dandruff, Seborrheic Dermatitis, Psoriasis Control Drug Products" by the FDA's Advisory Review Panel on OTC Miscellaneous External Drug Products.

it occurs later in infancy and sometimes spreads to other parts of the body.

Cradle cap is not dangerous. But its unsightliness disturbs many new parents. It may thicken because parents are afraid to wash their babies' scalps, even gently, for fear of pressing on the fontanels—the soft spots where the skull has not yet closed. A parent who has this concern should discuss it with a pediatrician, and ask whether to use soap and water or a nonprescription preparation or some other method to remove the cradle cap and prevent its return.

DRUGS FOR CONTROLLING CRADLE CAP

Nonprescription products used to control cradle cap include: (1) an antimicrobial preparation, (2) a skin-peeling (keratolytic) agent, and (3) the unguent petrolatum.

Approved Remedy

The Panel did not list any *active* ingredient as safe and effective for use on infants. But one ingredient, white petrolatum, listed as *inactive*, has been approved as safe and effective by another Panel (the FDA's Advisory Review Panel on OTC Topical Analgesic, Antirheumatic, Otic, Burn and Sunburn Prevention and Treatment Drug Products).

Petrolatum, white This petroleum derivative is widely used on babies to prevent diaper rash and to soften, lubricate, and cover dry skin. It is safe and effective for use as often as necessary. White petrolatum's specific value in dissolving cradle cap and in preventing it from forming again has not been directly assessed by any of the reviewing groups. But in one study white petrolatum was used to prevent cradle cap. Only 6 of 50 babies whose scalps were treated with this protectant developed cradle cap.

Conditionally Approved Remedy

Methylbenzethonium chloride This quaternary ammonium compound, or *quat*, is widely used in first aid; the FDA has approved quats as safe in low concentrations for this use. The Panel finds that this particular ingredient is safe for infants.

Methylbenzethonium chloride (0.07 percent) is included in an infant scalp-care petroleum product said to "soften and separate crusts and scales from the scalp and help prevent and treat local infections." The compound is claimed to inhibit growth of bacteria and other microorganisms.

In one study submitted for review, only 1 in 50 babies treated with this product developed cradle cap—compared with 6 in 50 treated with ordinary white petrolatum and 8 in 50 whose scalps were cleansed with soap and water. In a second study, on babies who already had cradle caps, 29 of 30 were cured or improved by the product containing the methylbenzethonium chloride, compared with 27 of 30 treated with a 1 percent salicylic acid ointment and only 18 of 30 treated with ordinary soap and water. In still another test, a methylbenzethonium chloride product cured twice as many cradle-cap cases as a salicylic acid lotion.

While studies seem to indicate that methylbenzethonium chloride helps prevent or control cradle cap, evaluators concluded that they are not detailed enough to allow a final judgment. Pending better data, the drug is judged to be safe but not proved effective.

Disapproved Remedies

None

Unclassified Remedy

The Panel's draft report did not include an assessment of the following compound used to treat cradle cap.

Salicylic acid   This is a keratolytic or skin-peeling drug that assessors ruled safe and effective for treating dandruff and seborrheic dermatitis in adults. In some comparative tests described by the Panel, salicylic acid appeared to be almost as effective as methylbenzethonium chloride (*see* above) in preventing and relieving cradle cap.

Safety and Effectiveness: Ingredients in Over-the-Counter Cradle Cap Treatments

Ingredient	Panel's Assessment
methylbenzethonium chloride	safe but not proved effective
petrolatum, white	safe and effective*
salicylic acid	not assessed

*Assessed nonspecifically as lubricant, skin-softener, and protectant by Advisory Review Panel on OTC Topical Analgesic, Antirheumatic, Otic, Burn and Sunburn Prevention and Treatment Drug Products.

Cradle-Cap Removers: Product Ratings

Product and Distributor	Dosage	Rating[1]
white petrolatum		
Vaseline (Chesebrough-Pond's)	ointment	**A**

1. Author's interpretation of Panel criteria. Based on contents, not claims.

Dandruff and Seborrheic Scale Shampoos

Dry, white flakes of dandruff falling from one's hair certainly are unsightly. So, too, are the greasier flakes and scales that persistently appear on the scalp, eyebrows, and other hairy areas and body folds of people who suffer from the scalp and skin condition called *seborrheic dermatitis*. Seborrheic dermatitis is a disease. Dandruff is mostly a nuisance.

Neither condition can be wholly cured, but the reviewing Panel says several nonprescription drugs will safely and effectively control both. The list of worthwhile ingredients in the many shampoos, grooming aids, creams, and lotions available is, however, quite short. The list of dubious or worthless ones is quite long. So persons who are pestered by these scalp/skin problems would do well to choose the few among the many that are likely to do the most good.

CLAIMS

Accurate
"relieves the itching and scalp-flaking associated with dandruff"
"relieves the itching, irritation, and skin-flaking associated with seborrheic dermatitis of the scalp and/or body"

False or Misleading
"guaranteed to control dandruff and scalp itch without shampooing"
"proteinized formula time-proven to control dandruff"

DANDRUFF AND SEBORRHEIC SCALE SHAMPOOS is based on the unadopted draft report "Dandruff, Seborrheic Dermatitis, Psoriasis Control Drug Products" by the FDA's Advisory Review Panel on OTC Miscellaneous External Drug Products.

"an exclusive dandruff-control formulation containing a powerful antimicrobial agent".

WARNING   The Panel warns that these products should be kept out of the eyes or rinsed out quickly if they get in, should not be used on children under 2 except as directed by a doctor, and should be kept out of the reach of all children, since some ingredients are poisonous if ingested. If the condition fails to improve or worsens when self-treated, consult the family doctor or a dermatologist.

FAST SKIN TURNOVER FORMS FLAKES

The flakes, or scales, as they are properly called, that characterize dandruff and seborrheic dermatitis principally consist of dead skin shed by the skin's outer layer. This outer layer, called the *epidermis*, and the inner layer, called the *dermis*, are cushioned on an underlying bed of fatty subcutaneous tissue.

Epidermal cells are formed constantly near the border with the dermis. These cells work their way upward and outward as they mature, changing their shapes, their traits, and their functions as they go. The normal life cycle for epidermal cells is 25 to 30 days. As they approach the surface, they harden and die.

The essential defect in both dandruff and seborrheic dermatitis appears to be the same: epidermal skin is being re-created much more rapidly—and so must be shed much more rapidly—than is normal. In dandruff, the turnover rate, about 14 days, is about twice the normal rate. In seborrheic dermatitis it may be even faster. Why these speedups occur is not known—though there are a lot of guesses. The result, though, is clearly visible on victims' heads and shoulders.

The flakes the two conditions produce can be relieved by many of the same drugs. But they can be controlled more effectively when people are aware of which disorder they have. The FLAKE CHARACTERISTICS chart can help one determine that.

Flake Characteristics

Factors	Common Dandruff	Seborrheic Dermatitis
site	scalp only	scalp, face, and body (especially in hairy areas and body folds)
redness (inflammation)	no	yes
appearance of flakes	dry, white to grayish	greasy, yellowish-brown
itching	sometimes	usually
what makes it worse	winter weather	stress and illness

One long-standing explanation for dandruff is that it is caused by a yeastlike fungus, *Pityrosporum ovale*, which resides in the scalp. But virtually everyone has this fungus in his or her hair—and not everyone has dandruff. So experts doubt that the organism causes dandruff.

A long-standing theory put forth to explain seborrheic dermatitis is that excessive sebum (a fatty substance secreted onto the skin's surface by glands) provides a coating of oil that makes it easier for bacteria and yeast to grow. These microorganisms then produce irritating substances that damage the skin and cause it to turn over more quickly, producing scales. Reviewers maintain that it has not been proved that seborrheic dermatitis and seborrhea—the increased production of sebum—always go together. (The names chosen by the Panel to describe these conditions are confusing. Seborrheic dermatitis should mean a skin condition caused by or associated with excess sebum production—in other words, seborrhea. Yet the evaluators claim that seborrheic dermatitis can occur *without* seborrhea—which makes little sense. It is best not to take these terms too literally; the names used for skin conditions are frequently confusing and imprecise.)

Until we have a better understanding of their causes, dandruff and seborrheic dermatitis must be treated symptomatically.

DRUGS USED

Classifications

The drugs used to treat dandruff and seborrheic dermatitis fall into 6 different classes:

- *Cytostatic agents* provide the most direct treatment approach. They slow the growth rate (*-static*) of skin cells (*cyto-*) so that the turnover time for the epidermis is longer. This means that production of dead cells—dandruff and seborrheic scales—is slowed.
- *Keratolytics* cause the flaking outer layer of the epidermis to peel away. The Panel believes these drugs dissolve the "cement" that holds the cells together, rather than the keratin within them (as their name implies). Keratolytics do not prevent scale formation, as cytostatic agents do, but existing scales are loosened so they are easier to wash away.
- *Tar preparations* are widely used to treat dandruff and seborrheic dermatitis, despite the fact that no one knows for sure *how* they are helpful: they may impede cell growth and multiplication or they may penetrate the skin and loosen scales.

- *Antimicrobials (antiseptics)* kill bacteria and other microorganisms that were once thought to cause dandruff. Most contemporary experts doubt that they do cause dandruff, and it is noteworthy that in the reviewers' judgment no antimicrobial agent has been proved effective in relieving dandruff or seborrheic dermatitis.
- *Hydrocortisone preparations* relieve inflammation, so they may have some role to play in alleviating the redness and itchiness of seborrheic dermatitis. They are of no use against ordinary dandruff.
- *Anti-itch preparations* are claimed to relieve itching.

The effectiveness of scale-control drugs depends in part on whether they are formulated with surface-acting agents. Such compounds wet the scalp, emulsify sebum, and loosen scalp scales. But they also may damage the skin in concentrations as low as 1 percent. The surface-acting compounds found in nonprescription medicated shampoos include the following chemicals:

> *quaternary ammonium compounds*
>   benzalkonium chloride
>   cetyl ethyl ammonium chloride
> *anionic surface-acting agents*
>   dioctyl sodium sulfosuccinate
>   sodium lauryl sulfate
> *nonionic wetting agents*
>   propylene glycol
>   spans (sorbitan esters of fatty acids)
>   tweens (polyoxyethylene sorbitan esters of fatty acids)

Three of the five drugs that are safe and effective for treating dandruff are also safe and effective for treating seborrheic dermatitis. The exceptions are selenium sulfide and sulfur preparations, which should not be used for the latter condition (*see* below).

Combination Products

Many shampoos and groomers that are used to treat dandruff and seborrheic dermatitis contain several active ingredients. Evaluators took an extremely dim view of these preparations, noting that very few studies have been conducted to justify their use. Based on the single well-conducted study available, the Panel approved only one combination—and for use only against dandruff: sulfur (2 to 5 percent) + salicylic acid (1.8 to 3 percent).

All other combination products submitted for review were granted conditional approval—unless, of course, they include a disapproved active ingredient, in which case the combination, too, was disapproved. The Panel assessed more than 2 dozen active ingredients formulated into products to treat ordinary dandruff and the greasier variety that is symptomatic of seborrheic dermatitis.

ANTI-FLAKE MEDICATIONS

Approved Active Ingredients

The Panel endorsed five different active ingredients as safe and effective for the control of scales. They represent 3 of 6 types of ingredients found in these products: cytostatic agents, keratolytic agents and tar preparations.

Applications for Approved Over-the-Counter Antiscale Drugs

		To Control	
Approved Ingredient	Scalp Dandruff	Seborrheic Dermatitis of Scalp	Seborrheic Dermatitis of Body
coal-tar preparations	yes	yes	not proved safe
pyrithione zinc	yes	yes	no
salicylic acid	yes	yes	yes
selenium sulfide	yes	no	no
sulfur preparations	yes	no	no

Coal-tar shampoos These messy, black-brown, syrupy substances, extracted from soft coal, have long been mainstays of the skin doctor's trade. In fact, tars of various kinds have been used medicinally for thousands of years and, with sulfur, are the oldest drugs that have won the approval of contemporary medical scientists on the OTC Review Panels.

Coal tar contains, more or less, 2 to 8 percent light oils (principally benzene, toluene, and xylene); 8 to 10 percent middle oils (principally phenols, cresols, and naphthalene); and 8 to 10 percent heavy oils (naphthalene and derivatives), along with 16 to 20 percent anthracine oil and about 50 percent pitch.

Shampoos that contain coal tar may have a disagreeable odor. They can stain hair, skin, and clothing. But they have proved to be remarkably safe when applied to the scalp once or twice weekly and then rinsed off. (Questions have been raised about coal tar's safety when it is applied to body areas other than the scalp, in treating seborrheic dermatitis. *See* COAL-TAR LOTIONS, page 213.)

Coal-tar shampoos are helpful for both dandruff and seborrheic dermatitis of the scalp, although it is not clear how they work. The tar may take oxygen from the skin cells, slowing their reproduction. Or it may penetrate the skin and somehow destroy scales. Alternatively, some tar constituents may react with sulfur-and-hydrogen elements (sulfhydryl groups) in the skin, much as sunlight does, to slow epidermal skin growth and lessen flaking.

Besides its apparent ability to act directly on dandruff flakes, coal tar narrows capillary blood vessels in the skin, kills bacteria, stops itching, and has an astringent effect on the scalp. Thus it would be a highly popular drug if it weren't messy, smelly, and didn't sometimes stain the skin, hair, and clothing.

Despite long use and wide medical acceptance, coal tar has not been studied well in carefully controlled tests. Moreover, the tests that have been done have not all been encouraging. In one, a 5 percent coal-tar shampoo did not produce significantly better results after 8 weeks' use than a dummy shampoo without the tar. However, in another study on patients suffering ordinary dandruff or dandruff associated with seborrheic dermatitis, a 5 percent coal-tar extract shampoo reduced flake counts by one-third to one-half after 4 weeks, compared with only one-tenth to one-quarter in users of a look-alike, nonmedicated dummy shampoo. From this latter study and others, reviewers concluded that coal-tar products are safe and effective for use in shampoos. *See* the APPROVED DOSAGES FOR COAL-TAR SHAMPOO chart.

Approved Dosages for Coal-Tar Shampoo (for Twice-Weekly Shampooing)

Type	Dose
coal-tar extract	2 to 8.75%
coal tar, USP	0.5 to 5%
coal-tar solution	2.5 to 5%
coal-tar distillate	4%

Pyrithione zinc   This is a cytostatic agent, which means that the substance controls ordinary dandruff and seborrheic scaling by slowing cell growth and turnover in the epidermis. It is strikingly different from coal tar, described directly above. Unlike the tar, which is a traditional remedy, pyrithione zinc is a new drug. It was first synthesized in 1950 and chosen as an antidandruff active ingredient through a sophisticated screening test of some 1300 drugs. It is also known as *zinc pyrithione*, *zinc pyridine-2-thiol-1-oxide* and *Zinc Omadine*.

This drug has been demonstrated to be safe in a variety of tests in animals and on humans. It is nonirritating and nonallergenic. Since pyrithione zinc is insoluble in water, it is not absorbed through the skin. A residue of about 1 percent of the applied dose remains on the skin after rinsing—it is this residue that is believed to account for much of the drug's beneficial effect. More than 30 well-controlled studies have been conducted on this ingredient, with excellent results in treating the scaling of dandruff and the effects of seborrheic dermatitis. These preparations continue to be effective after many months of repeated use. They are significantly better than most—if not all—of the single-ingredient and combination drugs that have been tested against them.

The Panel concludes that pyrithione zinc is safe and effective. Approved dosages are 1 to 2 percent pyrithione zinc in shampoos and 0.10 to 0.25 percent pyrithione zinc in hair groomers applied between shampoos.

Salicylic acid   A skin-peeling drug (or keratolytic), salicylic acid is effective against both ordinary dandruff and seborrheic scaling of the scalp. It is also the only approved antiflake agent that reviewers recommend for use in lotions and creams for seborrheic dermatitis on parts of the body other than the scalp.

This drug is, of course, the parent compound of ordinary aspirin. Once obtained from wintergreen leaves and sweet birchbark, it is now manufactured synthetically.

Long-term topical use can be dangerous, because salicylic acid increases the skin's water absorption and eventually softens and weakens the skin, causing it to peel. However, when used twice weekly and then rinsed off, it is safe, as too little will be absorbed through the skin to cause injury.

This ingredient appears to benefit sufferers of dandruff and seborrheic dermatitis by dissolving and removing scales. While widely used, it is less well tested than pyrithione zinc (*see* above). Evaluators could find only two controlled studies in which salicylic acid was assessed alone rather than in combination with other ingredients. In both, 2 percent salicylic acid was more effective than a dummy medication in clearing up dandruff flakes.

Conclusion: salicylic acid is safe and effective in medicated shampoos for treating ordinary dandruff and dandruff caused by seborrheic dermatitis. The approved dosage is 1.8 to 3 percent salicylic acid, applied twice weekly in a shampoo.

Selenium sulfide This is a growth inhibitor (cytostatic agent) that is safe and effective against ordinary dandruff. When used in the 1 percent concentrations that are marketed over-the-counter, it is not effective against the dandruff of seborrheic dermatitis. This disorder requires a 2.5 percent concentration, which is available by prescription.

Selenium sulfide is bright orange in color and is insoluble in water. This insolubility is a saving virtue, for while selenium itself is dangerous —it is a potent poison if taken internally—the sulfide compound is safe because it is not absorbed through unbroken skin. Quite clearly then, it should not be used if one has open scalp wounds or rashes. The substance is also irritating to the eyes and should be rinsed out quickly if some of the shampoo drips there accidentally.

A few individuals who use selenium sulfide will experience a rebound effect—that is, scalp oiliness may increase. They should switch to a different type of medicated shampoo.

Because selenium inhibits growth of *Pityrosporum ovale*, which is found in the hair and scalp, it has been thought to relieve dandruff in this way. More likely, a breakdown product of the selenium sulfide blocks enzyme systems required for the growth of skin tissue. This slows the turnover process in the epidermis (outer layer of skin) and so limits dandruff. Whatever the mechanism, reviewers added, there is no doubt that the drug reduces cell turnover, whether on normal scalps or on itchy, scaly ones.

Several large and carefully conducted comparative studies show that the 1 percent selenium sulfide available over-the-counter is as effective against ordinary dandruff as the 2.5 percent product available by prescription.

While selenium sulfide 1 percent was judged safe and effective for the control of common dandruff, the Panel warns:

"Do not use if you have open sores on your scalp."

Sulfur preparations Scale-removing (keratolytic) substances, these compounds are safe and effective against ordinary dandruff but not against the dandruff produced by seborrheic dermatitis.

Sulfur is an ancient skin remedy, and it continues to be widely used by dermatologists for treating acne and other skin conditions. The most common forms are precipitated sulfur (milk of sulfur), which is a smooth, fine, yellowish-white powder that lacks sulfur's characteristic smell, and colloidal sulfur, which is composed of minute particles of the element suspended in gelatin, egg albumin, or a similar vehicle (base).

In low concentrations, sulfur is not very toxic—although continuing use can produce a reddening and thickening of the skin. Concentrations over 10 percent can be deadly. Basing its judgment largely on sulfur's long use and wide acceptance, the Panel concludes that the chemical is safe for use in dandruff shampoos in the recommended dosages.

Few reliable studies have been conducted on sulfur's dandruff-combating effectiveness as a single ingredient. The findings of those studies conducted suggest acceptable effectiveness, but they are not wholly conclusive in sulfur's favor. Nonetheless, evaluators say that 2 to 5 percent sulfur shampoos are safe and effective in controlling dandruff.

Zinc pyrithione See PYRITHIONE ZINC, above.

Conditionally Approved Active Ingredients

Many of the traditional and present-day drugs formulated into dandruff shampoos and similar products have not been proved to be really useful, although most of them seem to be harmless. Panel findings are summarized below.

Alkyl isoquinolinium bromide This germ-killer has passed the standard animal tests for safety, and some data show that it is not irritating to human skin. When *P. ovale*, which inhabits the hair, and some other microorganisms are exposed to this drug in lab dishes, they are killed. But this action has not been shown to relieve dandruff. So evaluators say it is safe but not proved effective.

Allantoin No adverse effects have ever been reported from the use of this skin-peeling agent. As to its effectiveness, each product submitted for review also contained other active ingredients, so the contribution of allantoin could not be determined. Therefore, pending more specific data, the Panel judges allantoin safe but not proved effective against dandruff and seborrheic dermatitis.

Benzalkonium chloride A widely-used antimicrobial compound, benzalkonium chloride is judged to be safe in low concentrations in antidandruff products. But no studies are available in which the chemical was the sole active ingredient, so reviewers could not assess its particular value. Current conclusion: safe but not proved effective against dandruff.

Benzethonium chloride This surface-acting agent is very similar to benzalkonium chloride. Long use and wide testing indicate that it is safe in the customary low concentrations. However, no studies demonstrate that benzethonium chloride, by itself, may be effective against dandruff. Until there is such evidence, the verdict is: safe but not proved effective.

Captan   An antimicrobial widely used in makeup, shampoos, face masks, and other cosmetic and drug products, captan has been subjected to a variety of challenging toxicity tests. In each case, it was found to be essentially nontoxic. Whether it really works against dandruff is another question. The only results from a double-blind study submitted for review failed to show that a cream shampoo containing captan was significantly more effective than the same shampoo without it. So, captan was assessed safe but not proved effective for the relief of dandruff.

Chloroxylenol (PCMX)   An antimicrobial, choroxylenol is derived from phenol. It may also be called *para-chloro-meta-xylenol* or *PCMX*. This Panel shares the view of one or two others—along with the FDA—that too little is known about chloroxylenol's effect on the skin to say for sure that it is safe.

Coal-tar lotions   These tar preparations are intended for the treatment of seborrheic dermatitis on body areas other than the scalp. They are formulated in many ways. The more refined the tar is, the greater the acceptance it wins from users, but it also appears that the more refined the distillates, liquors, filtrates, and tinctures are, the less they are medicinally effective compared with crude coal tar. Good news is that a recently developed emulsion colloid of coal tar—essentially a "tar gel"—may prove to be as beneficial as crude coal tar, as convenient to apply, and as cosmetically acceptable.

Given the myriad complex petrochemicals that it contains, coal tar has proved to be remarkably free of side effects. Persistent use does raise a mild "tar acne," but this goes away when treatment stops. Coal-tar derivatives also may produce a photosensitivity—high sensitivity to light and a greater chance of getting sunburned. So at least for a day or so after such a product is applied, users should stay pretty much covered up when they venture out of doors.

Evidence exists that coal-tar chemicals can cause skin cancers. Most such cases occur only after many years, or decades, of continued exposure to coal tar. The Panel believes that further testing will absolve mild coal tars from being responsible for such effects, even though at this time it says their safety remains unproved in this regard.

Long clinical usage and some scientific studies suggest that coal-tar lotions and creams are effective against seborrheic dermatitis of the body. But until the safety issue is resolved, the evaluators' decision is that these preparations are effective but not proved safe. Hence approval is only conditional.

The Panel adds this explicit warning:

"Do not use in the anogenital area or in the groin."

Ethohexadiol   An oily liquid, ethohexadiol is sometimes used as an insect repellent. It is classified as safe on the basis of a handful of animal studies, but the compound's effectiveness against dandruff has not been clearly established.

Eucalyptol   This aromatic oil, distilled from eucalyptus leaves, appears to be a relatively safe antimicrobial compound when applied in small quantities to the skin—even though as little as a tenth of an ounce, if swallowed, is dangerous. Panel reviewers decided it is safe for treating dandruff. Effectiveness is something else again. The Panel says that eucalyptol, while safe, has not been proved effective as a dandruff scourge.

Hydrocortisone preparations: hydrocortisone acetate and hydrocortisone alcohol   These and other cortisone preparations have been widely marketed by prescription for more than a quarter of a century. They are generally recognized as safe and effective for the relief of itching and inflammation. A 1 percent hydrocortisone cream, a prescription drug, is widely—and successfully—used to treat seborrheic dermatitis. Weaker concentrations of 0.25 to 0.5 percent hydrocortisone and hydrocortisone acetate have been approved by the FDA for use in nonprescription preparations.

The Panel was asked to approve one combination product containing an antifungal agent, calcium undecylenate 3 percent + hydrocortisone acetate 1 percent—the latter being double the FDA-approved dosage in over-the-counter products. It was also asked to approve a product containing 0.5 percent hydrocortisone acetate, which previously had not been approved for such use.

Reviewers responded cautiously. They believed there were too little data available on hydrocortisone's safety for treating seborrheic dermatitis to give it more than a conditional approval on grounds of safety. As to effectiveness, they concluded that evidence submitted contained insufficient proof of treatment value. So both the safety and the effectiveness of hydrocortisone preparations in treating the scaling of seborrheic dermatitis remain to be proved. The Panel further noted that these preparations are not appropriate therapy for ordinary dandruff, which rarely is accompanied by inflammation or itching.

Juniper tar   An aromatic wood-tar derivative, juniper tar is commonly referred to as *oil of cade* or *cade oil*. It acts as a counterirritant, and so is used as an anti-itch treatment for skin disorders. The present reviewers accept the findings of another Panel (the FDA's Advisory Review Panel on Topical Analgesic, Antirheumatic, Otic, Burn and Sunburn Prevention and Treatment Drug Products) that juniper tar up to 5 percent is safe. But it says it knows of no evidence proving that this tar is effective, by itself, against dandruff.

Lauryl isoquinolinium bromide   This is a quaternary ammonium compound that has been studied thoroughly enough for the Panel to say it is safe to apply it, in low doses, to the skin. However, it is dangerous if swallowed and it can irritate the eyes if it gets into them and is not immediately rinsed out. The chief objection to lauryl isoquinolinium bromide is the lack of data to show that it really combats dandruff. Verdict: safe but not proved effective.

Menthol   A minty alcohol, menthol kills microorganisms. It is generally recognized as safe. But evidence purporting to show that menthol is effective in relieving dandruff and seborrheic dermatitis was found to be seriously inadequate. So, while menthol is safe, its value for use in these conditions remains to be proved.

Methyl salicylate   This fragrant substance is an antimicrobial that is widely used in skin preparations, and the reviewers believe it is safe in low doses. But there are no findings to justify a manufacturer's claim that it is useful against dandruff. So the Panel declared methyl salicylate to be safe but not proved effective when used for this purpose.

Phenol and phenolate sodium   The safety of these chemicals has been exhaustively studied (*see* PHENOL). At the 1 percent concentration recommended by the Panel for treating seborrheic dermatitis, the Panel—like the FDA—judges phenol to be safe. The substance has an anesthetic effect on the skin, which *may* help relieve the itching and inflammation of seborrheic dermatitis. But no controlled studies have been done to prove this. As a treatment for seborrheic dermatitis, therefore, phenol and phenolate sodium are considered safe but yet to be proved effective. The reviewers believe that phenol is ineffective against ordinary dandruff, and do not approve it for this use.

Pine-tar preparations: pine tar and rectified pine tar   These tar formulations have long been used medicinally for treating the skin. Pine tar is also marketed as an expectorant in cough-cold preparations.

There are few if any reports of adverse effects from its use, so it is judged safe. But despite the claims of manufacturers, the Panel could not find any evidence to show that pine tar is effective in relieving dandruff. So the assessment is: safe but not proved effective.

Povidone-iodine   In this antimicrobial preparation, the povidone molecule holds the iodine and then releases it slowly onto the body surface. In extensive tests, povidone-iodine has been shown to be nonirritating to the skin, so the present reviewers judged it to be safe—although another Panel has doubts (*see* FIRST-AID PREPARATIONS FOR SKIN WOUNDS).

On effectiveness, results from 3 controlled tests were submitted in an effort to show that povidone-iodine controls scales. In one, twice-weekly shampooing with a 7.5 percent povidone-iodine preparation reduced flake counts and relieved itching in persons with ordinary dandruff, and did so significantly better than a dummy shampoo that lacked the compound. However, once-weekly shampooing with povidone-iodine was no more effective than once-weekly shampooing with the nonmedicated shampoo. While the Panel was impressed by these results, it decided that they should be confirmed by a second, longer study of twice-a-week shampooing.

In another clinical trial, which was questionable because the control group was too small, povidone-iodine appeared to provide complete control of seborrheic dermatitis. In a third study, povidone-iodine appeared to be as effective as selenium sulfide against seborrheic dermatitis.

Thus tentative approval was granted to povidone-iodine for treating both common dandruff and seborrheic dermatitis. The Panel finds it to be safe, but not proved effective.

Sodium salicylate   This skin-peeling compound increases the skin's water absorption, thereby softening it. But since no adequately controlled scientific study has been conducted to establish how it works or if it is effective, the verdict is: safe but not proved effective.

Thymol   Obtainable from the herb thyme, thymol does not appear to cause serious adverse responses, so the reviewers decided it is safe. As to dandruff-treatment effectiveness, the only submission was of a compound in which thymol was only one of several ingredients labeled for "infectious dandruff." Evidence to support the claims for the combination product, and for thymol, were found inadequate. The Panel considers thymol safe but not proved effective for antidandruff use.

Undecylenate preparations: calcium undecylenate and undecyle-

nate acid monoethanolamide sulfosuccinate sodium salt   These are antifungal substances that also have antibacterial activity. They are not yet marketed in the United States for the control of dandruff or seborrheic dermatitis. Tests performed in animals thus far are inadequate to demonstrate safety. A few studies suggest that these preparations do work against dandruff, but reviewers say that data are needed for confirmation. So both the safety and the effectiveness of undecylenate preparations for treating dandruff and seborrheic dermatitis remain to be proved.

Disapproved Active Ingredients

Of the multiple drugs used to treat dandruff and seborrheic dermatitis, the Panel found a few that appear to be clearly ineffective or unsafe and should be removed from the marketplace unless strong evidence to the contrary is developed through testing.

Benzocaine   The Panel could conceive of no good reason to use this short-acting anesthetic to treat dandruff or seborrheic dermatitis. Also, because it can cause serious side effects (however rare), benzocaine is judged unsafe. Conclusion: not safe and not effective.

Boron compounds: boric acid and sodium borate   These compounds are disapproved because they contain boron, which lately has been identified as a potent poison to body systems. While boric acid and sodium borate are unlikely to be absorbed through intact skin, toxic amounts could enter the body if such preparations were applied over a scalp rash or head sores. In addition, the effectiveness of the borates as single ingredients for dandruff treatments has not been established. The Panel's verdict, then, is that they are unsafe and not proved effective for treating dandruff and seborrheic dermatitis.

Colloidal oatmeal   This suspension of oat grains is a refinement of the time-honored home remedy for itching: a tepid bath laced with oatmeal from the kitchen shelf. Reviewers could not think of any reason why oats might be dangerous, so safety is not the issue. But the Panel could find no data (nor were any submitted) to show that colloidal oatmeal relieves dandruff or seborrheic dermatitis. Conclusion: safe but ineffective.

Inactive Ingredients

A number of inactive ingredients are formulated into the shampoos, grooming aids, lotions, and creams that are used to treat dandruff and seborrheic dermatitis. These substances provide no direct therapeutic benefit, but are included as bulking material, as preservatives, to improve the odor or texture of the product, or for other reasons relating to the manufacturing process.

alcohol
benzoic acid
cetyl alcohol
cholesterol
entsufon sodium
  (entsufon)
glycerin
hydroxypropyl
  methylcellulose

lanolin
lanolin cholesterols
lanolin oil
lead acetate (sugar of
  lead)
mineral oil (liquid
  paraffin oil)
oil of violet
petrolatum

petrolatum, white
polyethylene glycol
  derivatives
polyoxyethylene
  ethers
sodium chloride
stearyl alcohol
vegetable oil
white petrolatum

Safety and Effectiveness: Active Ingredients in Over-the-Counter Dandruff and Seborrheic Dermatitis Shampoos and Other Treatments

Active Ingredient	Type	Panel's Assessment	Effective Against Dandruff	Effective Against Seborrheic Dermatitis
alkyl isoquinolinium bromide	antimicrobial	safe but not proved effective	maybe	no
allantoin	keratolytic	safe but not proved effective	maybe	maybe
benzalkonium chloride	antimicrobial	safe but not proved effective	maybe	no
benzethonium chloride	antimicrobial	safe but not proved effective	maybe	no
benzocaine	anesthetic	not safe or effective	maybe	
boron compounds: boric acid and sodium borate	antimicrobial	not safe		no
captan	antimicrobial	safe but not proved effective	maybe	no
chloroxylenol (PCMX)	antimicrobial	not proved safe or effective	maybe	maybe
coal-tar shampoos	tar	safe and effective	yes	yes*
colloidal oatmeal	anti-itch	safe but not effective		
ethohexadiol	antimicrobial	safe but not proved effective	maybe	no
eucalyptol	antimicrobial	safe but not proved effective	maybe	no
hydrocortisone preparations: hydrocortisone acetate and hydrocortisone alcohol		not proved safe or effective	no	maybe
juniper tar	tar	safe but not proved effective	maybe	no
lauryl isoquinolinium bromide	antimicrobial	safe but not proved effective	maybe	no
menthol	antimicrobial	safe but not proved effective	maybe	maybe
methyl salicylate	antimicrobial	safe but not proved effective	maybe	no
phenol and phenolate sodium	antimicrobial	safe but not proved effective	no	maybe

Safety and Effectiveness: Active Ingredients in Over-the-Counter Dandruff and Seborrheic Dermatitis Shampoos and Other Treatments (continued)

Active Ingredient	Type	Panel's Assessment	Effective Against Dandruff	Effective Against Seborrheic Dermatitis
pine-tar preparations: pine tar and rectified pine tar	tar	safe but not proved effective	maybe	no
povidone-iodine	antimicrobial	safe but not proved effective	maybe	maybe
pyrithione zinc	cytostatic	safe and effective	yes	yes
salicylic acid	keratolytic	safe and effective	yes	yes
selenium sulfide 1 percent	cytostatic	safe and effective	yes	no
sodium salicylate	antimicrobial	safe but not proved effective	maybe	no
sulfur preparations	keratolytic	safe and effective	yes	no
thymol	antimicrobial	safe but not proved effective	maybe	no
undecylenate preparations: calcium undecylenate and undecylenic acid mono-ethanolamide sulfosuccinate sodium salt	antimicrobial	not proved safe or effective	maybe	maybe
zinc pyrithione (see pyrithione zinc)				

*Not proved safe for application to the body in lotions and creams. Avoid use in groin and anogenital area.

Safety and Effectiveness: Combination Products Sold Over-the-Counter to Treat Dandruff and Seborrheic Dermatitis

Safe and Effective

sulfur (2 to 5%) + salicylic acid (1.8 to 3%) (for dandruff only)

Conditionally Safe and Effective

allantoin + phenol (seborrheic dermatitis only)
benzalkonium chloride + alkyl isoquinolinium bromide (dandruff only)
benzalkonium chloride + salicylic acid (dandruff only)
benzalkonium chloride + lauryl isoquinolinium bromide (dandruff only)
benzethonium chloride + captan (dandruff only)
calcium undecylenate + hydrocortisone acetate (seborrheic dermatitis only)
coal tar + benzalkonium chloride + salicylic acid (dandruff only)
coal-tar extract + allantoin (dandruff and seborrheic dermatitis)
coal-tar extract + hydrocortisone alcohol (seborrheic dermatitis only)
coal-tar extract + menthol (dandruff and seborrheic dermatitis)
coal-tar solution + menthol (dandruff and seborrheic dermatitis)
coal tar + pine tar + juniper tar (dandruff and seborrheic dermatitis)
coal tar + salicylic acid (dandruff and seborrheic dermatitis)
phenol + allantoin + salicylic acid + sodium lauryl sulfate (seborrheic dermatitis only)
sulfur + coal tar distillate + salicylic acid (dandruff only)
sulfur + menthol (dandruff only)

Not Safe or Not Effective

a preparation that contains *any* disapproved active ingredient

Dandruff and Seborrheic Shampoos and Hair Dressings: Product Ratings

Single-Ingredient Shampoos

Product and Distributor	Dosage of Active Ingredients	Rating[1] for Dandruff	Rating[1] for Seborrhea	Comment
chloroxylenol (PCMX)				
Metasep (Marion)	**shampoo:** 2%	B	B	not proved safe or effective
coal tar				
DHS Tar (Person & Covey)	**shampoo:** 0.5% coal tar USP equivalent	A	A	for scalp only
Neutrogena T/Gel (Neutrogena)	**shampoo:** 2% crude coal tar equivalent	A	A	for scalp only
Pentrax Tar (Cooper)	**shampoo:** 4.3% crude coal tar	A	A	for scalp only
Tegrin (Block)	**shampoo:** 5% coal tar extract	A	A	for scalp only
pine tar				
Packer's Pine Tar (Cooper)	**shampoo:** 0.82%	B	C	not proved effective against dandruff; not effective against seborrheic scale
povidone-iodine				
Betadine (Purdue Frederick)	**shampoo:** 7.5%	B		effectiveness is the issue
pyrithione zinc				
Danex (Herbert)	**shampoo:** 1%	A	B	effectiveness at this dosage proved for dandruff, not for seborrhea
Zincon (Lederle)		A	B	

Product and Distributor	Dosage of Active Ingredients	Rating¹ for Dandruff	Rating¹ for Seborrhea	Comment
DHS Zinc (Person & Covey)	shampoo: 2%	A	A	
Head & Shoulders (Procter & Gamble)		A	A	
salicylic acid				
Xseb (Baker-Cummins)	shampoo: 4%	C	C	exceeds approved dosage (3%)
selenium sulfide				
selenium sulfide (generic)	lotion: 1%	A	C	not effective for seborrhea
Selsun Blue (Abbott)		A	C	
Sul-Blue (Columbia Med.)		A	C	

Combination Shampoos

Product and Distributor	Dosage of Active Ingredients	Rating¹ for Dandruff	Rating¹ for Seborrhea	Comment
Antiseb (Durel)	shampoo: 2% colloidal sulfur + 2% salicylic acid	A	C	sulfur not effective against seborrheic scale
Sebex (Spencer-Mead)		A	C	
Antiseb-T (Durel)	shampoo: 5% coal-tar solution + 2% salicylic acid + 2% colloidal sulfur	B	C	combination not proved safe and effective against dandruff; sulfur not effective against seborrheic scale
Sebex-T (Spencer-Mead)		B	C	not effective against seborrheic scale
Fostex (Westwood)	shampoo: 2% sulfur + 2% salicylic acid	A	C	sulfur not effective against seborrheic scale
Sebulex Medicated (Westwood)		A	C	
Ionil (Owen)	shampoo: 2% salicylic acid + 0.2% benzalkonium chloride	B	C	combination not proved safe and effective against dandruff; benzalkonium chloride not effective against seborrheic scale

Dandruff and Seborrheic Shampoos and Hair Dressings: Product Ratings *(continued)*

Combination Shampoos

Product and Distributor	Dosage of Active Ingredients	Rating[1] for Dandruff	Rating[1] for Seborrhea	Comment
Mazon (Norcliff-Thayer)	**shampoo:** coal tar + salicylic acid + sulfur + allantoin + disodium undecylenamide MEA sulfosuccinate	B	C	combination not proved safe and effective; sulfur ineffective against seborrheic scale
Sebaquin (Summers)	**shampoo:** 3% diiodohydroxyquin	C	C	ingredient not submitted to or assessed by Panel
Sebisol (C & M Pharm.)	**shampoo:** 2% salicylic acid + 0.1% orthobenzylparachlorophenol + 1% betanaphthol	C	C	latter 2 ingredients not submitted to or assessed by Panel in Over-the-Counter Drug Review

Medicated Hair Dressings

Product and Distributor	Dosage of Active Ingredients	Rating[1] for Dandruff	Rating[1] for Seborrhea	Comment
Drest (Dermik)	**gel:** 0.125% belzalkonium chloride + 0.15% alkyl isoquinolinium bromides	B	C	efficacy is principal issue
Furol (Torch)	**cream:** 5% sulfur ppt + 3% salicylic acid	A	C	sulfur not effective against seborrheic scale
P & S (Baker-Cummins)	**liquid:** less than 1% phenol	C	B	phenol ineffective against ordinary dandruff; not proved effective against seborrheic scale
Sebucare (Westwood)	**lotion:** 1.8% salicylic acid	A	A	

1. Author's interpretation of Panel's criteria. Based on content, not claims.

Daytime Sedatives

See SEDATIVES, DAYTIME

Deodorants for Ostomies and Incontinence

Most body-odor problems can be overcome by adequate personal hygiene, the use of cosmetics, or by antiperspirants, mouthwashes, or other products. But some people face unfortunate situations in which their bodies produce strong, foul odors.

These include persons who are incontinent of urine or feces—which means they do not have control over their bladder or bowels—or who have an opening from the intestinal tract to the outside of their bodies. These openings (enterostomies) are created surgically—usually in the treatment of cancer, ulcerative colitis, or some other serious disease. An estimated 1.1 million Americans are ostomates, and their ranks are increased by 63 thousand each year.

Some people, too, have superficial sores or injuries that do not heal readily and so smell bad. Others feel they are unable to control extremely bad smells emanating from their armpits, crotch, mouth, or feet.

These problems often respond to special hygienic measures suggested by a doctor or rehabilitation counselor. They also may be relieved through the use of deodorant drugs that are taken internally. The Panel evaluated 3 active ingredients used for this purpose. All 3 are safe, and they *appear* to be effective in relieving colostomy and ileostomy odors. One, water-soluble chlorophyllin, may also help conceal the smell of urinary or fecal incontinence—and perhaps other foul body odors as well.

DEODORANTS FOR OSTOMIES AND INCONTINENCE is based on the report "Deodorant/Drug Products for Internal Use" by the FDA's Advisory Review Panel on OTC Miscellaneous Internal Drug Products.

CLAIMS

Accurate
"a colostomy or ileostomy deodorant"
"an aid to reduce odor from colostomies or ileostomies"

False or Misleading
for "the control of breath and body odors"
for "prompt reduction of oral malodors caused by foods, beverages, tobacco, catarrh, and other sources"
"to reduce body [perspiration] or surface lesion odor" (if used for bismuth subgallate or activated charcoal).

Unproved (for chlorphyllin)
for "the control of fecal or urinary odor associated with incontinence not related to faulty hygiene"
"to reduce body [perspiration] or surface lesion odor"

Approved Active Ingredients

None

Conditionally Approved Active Ingredients

Bismuth subgallate   Most people who use this bismuth compound have a surgically created ileostomy or colostomy. Large doses of bismuth salts are quite toxic, but enterostomy experts told the Panel that toxicity rarely if ever occurs when recommended dosages of bismuth salts are taken.

Several authorities on ostomy strongly recommend that bismuth subgallate be taken before meals in order to control urinary and fecal odors. Patients say, too, through a questionnaire study, that they find the drug very effective or even completely effective in controlling odor. However, truly conclusive evidence—from well-controlled scientific tests—is not available to confirm these favorable testimonials. Wanting such evidence, the panelists decided that bismuth subgallate is safe but not proved effective.

Charcoal, activated   This is an inert substance with great adsorptive powers because of its honeycomb structure and enormous surface area. Reviewers say activated charcoal is safe. The Panel does caution that activated charcoal can neutralize other drugs, rendering them ineffective, so it should not be used if one is taking them, except with a doctor's approval.

Activated charcoal is widely used as an adsorbent in industry, in medicine, and in the home. But virtually no data have been reported from acceptable scientific studies to show it acts effectively as an internal deodorant. Despite this, the Panel says that "it is reasonable to assume that the claims are in keeping with [charcoal's] scientifically proven adsorptive capacity." So activated charcoal merits tentative approval: safe but not proved effective.

Chlorophyllin, water-soluble (potassium sodium copper chlorophyllin) This material is harvested from the leaves of food plants. It is evaluated as safe—although it can cause mild diarrhea and will turn one's stools green. No suitable scientific study is available to confirm how well chlorophyllin works in reducing enterostomy odors. But an uncontrolled clinical report indicates that over 95 percent of users obtain marked to total freedom from exuding these smells. Uncontrolled studies also suggest that chlorophyllin can relieve the odor of urinary incontinence, severe body odor, and the smell of superficial sores and injuries—but not the odor of smelly feet. Nonetheless, only conditional approval was granted: safe but not proved effective.

Disapproved Active Ingredients

None

Safety and Effectiveness: Active Ingredients in Over-the-Counter Deodorants for Ostomies and Incontinence

Active Ingredient	Panel's Assessment
bismuth subgallate	safe but not proved effective
charcoal, activated	safe but not proved effective
chlorophyllin, water-soluble (potassium sodium copper chlorophyllin)	safe but not proved effective

Deodorants for Ostomies and Incontinence: Product Ratings

Product and Distributor	Dosage of Active Ingredients	Rating[1]	Comment
bismuth subgallate			
Devrom (Parthenon)	**tablets, chewable:** 200 mg	B	not proved effective

Deodorants for Ostomies and Incontinence: Product Ratings *(continued)*

Product and Distributor	Dosage of Active Ingredients	Rating[1]	Comment
charcoal, activated			
Charcocaps (Requa)	**capsules:** 260 mg	**B**	not proved effective
chlorophyllin, water-soluble derivatives			
Derifil (Rystan)	**tablets:** 100 mg	**B**	not proved effective
	powder: 100 mg per teaspoonful	**B**	not proved effective

1. Author's interpretation of Panel criteria. Based on content, not claims.

Diaper-Rash Medications

Every baby suffers red, sore diaper rash from time to time. Older persons who become incontinent suffer many of the same symptoms—and require similar treatment.

Diaper rash is caused by urine and feces, both of which irritate babies' tender skin. Microorganisms in these body wastes also contribute to the problem. Bacteria metabolize urine to produce ammonia, which of course is highly irritating. The yeast *Candida albicans*, which is often present in a baby's stool, may multiply rapidly and produce a bright red, very irritating rash with sharply delineated edges.

Surrounding heat—as well as body heat trapped by plastic diaper backings or rubber pants—produces angry-looking red marks and itching, stinging, bumpy eruptions where tender wet skin rubs against clothing. This condition—called *prickly heat* or *miliaria*—occurs when the sweat glands become blocked by water or wastes and rupture into the adjacent skin.

The soaps, bleaches, and detergents used to launder reusable cloth diapers can cause or contribute to diaper rash and prickly heat. So does chafing in the baby's skin folds. A red and inflamed diaper area may also be a signal that the baby is allergic to milk or some other food. Diaper

DIAPER-RASH MEDICATIONS is largely based on the unadopted draft report "OTC Diaper-Rash Drug Products" by the FDA's Advisory Review Panel on OTC Miscellaneous External Drug Products.

rash can thus signal an underlying medical problem, and if simple preventive measures and treatment with over-the-counter medicated lotions and powders do not clear the condition in a couple of days, a pediatrician's help should be sought.

SIMPLE REMEDIES

An ordinary, mild diaper rash—in which the skin is reddened (erythematous) but not broken—can often be relieved by frequent diaper changes and simple cleansing with water. Switching to a different kind of diaper may help, too. The Panel suggests changing from plastic-backed disposable diapers to all-cloth washable ones, which allow more air to reach the skin surface. Switching the other way—from cloth to disposable paper—can also help, since disposable diapers, unlike cloth ones, have a highly absorbent inner layer that quickly draws moisture off the skin. Another suggestion is to leave the diaper off while the baby is napping, so the skin is exposed to air.

Types of Medications

If the baby's skin is only mildly irritated, *skin protectants* may relieve the rash. These substances tend to be physically soothing and chemically inactive, so they are safe for regular use. Many people apply them to the baby's skin routinely whenever they change diapers.

Skin protectants that another Panel has approved for use on infants' skin are noted in the chart: SAFE AND EFFECTIVE SKIN PROTECTANTS FOR USE WITHOUT MEDICAL SUPERVISION.

Safe and Effective Skin Protectants for Use Without Medical Supervision

Active Ingredient	Approved Concentrations (%)	For Ages
allantoin	0.5 to 2	all
aluminum hydroxide gel	0.15 to 5	over 6 months
calamine	1 to 25	all
cocoa butter	80 to 100	all
corn starch	10 to 85	all
dimethicone	1 to 30	all
glycerin	20 to 45	over 6 months
petrolatum preparations (petrolatum, white petrolatum)	20 to 100	all

Safe and Effective Skin Protectants for Use Without Medical Supervision
(continued)

Active Ingredient	Approved Concentrations (%)	For Ages
sodium bicarbonate	1 to 100	all
zinc carbonate	0.2 to 2	all
zinc oxide	1 to 25	all

*Based on the report "Skin Protectant Drug Products," by the FDA's Advisory Review Panel on Topical Analgesic, Antirheumatic, Otic, Burn and Sunburn Prevention and Treatment Drug Products. For details, *See* UNGUENTS AND POWDERS FOR THE SKIN.

Skin protectants may contain absorbents, which remove urine from the skin, or adsorbents, which bind, hold, and neutralize irritating and toxic substances. Astringents extract proteins (including bacteria and their breakdown products) from the moisture inside the diaper, and help seal the skin against them. Emollients soften the skin; demulcents soothe it; and lubricants smooth its surface, reducing friction.

Four other classes of drugs are formulated into diapering preparations for the relief of diaper rash and prickly heat:

- *Wound healers* are alleged to speed up the healing process.
- *Itch-pain relievers* act on nerve endings and inflamed tissues to temporarily deaden itching and painful sensations. The Panel particularly recommends 0.5 percent hydrocortisone cream for this purpose.
- *Antimicrobials* inhibit or kill bacteria and other microorganisms that cause irritation, inflammation, and infections.
- *Antifungals* are supposed to act specifically to cure rashes caused by the yeast *C. albicans*.

Unfortunately, the Panel was not able to evaluate the individual active ingredients in these 4 drug categories because it was disbanded before its work was complete. However, before going out of business the group referred the diaper-rash evaluations back to the FDA, noting that many of the ingredients in these products had been assessed by other Panels concerned with different ailments. It suggested that these judgments might be extended to diaper-rash care, but failed to note that in many cases these evaluations specifically excluded the use of certain ingredients by children under age 2, except as recommended by a doctor. Worse, several ingredients that are widely used in baby products were not reviewed for any use that is equivalent to diaper rash —and some were not evaluated at all. For example, mineral oil, lanolin, and topical preparations of vitamin A and vitamin D, to name 3 of the commoner of these ingredients, simply have not been rated for use on infants' tender skins.

A strong warning has been issued by the FDA with regard to phenol, which can damage babies' skin and which also is absorbed through the skin into the body. A baby's liver may not be able to break down and detoxify phenol, which means that it will accumulate in the body. Phenol is a dangerous nerve poison. Covering phenol with a diaper further increases the hazard by increasing the amount of the substance that is absorbed through the skin. The FDA's warning says flatly:

"Do not use phenol for diaper rash."

A number of ingredients formulated into diapering preparations are claimed to counteract yeast infections (*C. albicans*), the Panel says. However, the Antimicrobial II Panel, which evaluated nonprescription antifungal drugs, did not list any of these ingredients as safe and effective "yeast killers."

Safety and Effectiveness: Active Ingredients in Over-the-Counter Diaper Rash Medications†

Active Ingredient	Purpose	Panel's Assessment
alkyldimethyl benzylammonium chloride	antimicrobial	not assessed
allantoin	skin protectant	safe and effective
	wound healer	safe but not proved effective
aluminum acetate	astringent	safe and effective
aluminum dehydroxy allantoinate	skin protectant	not assessed
aluminum hydroxide	skin protectant	safe and effective (for infants under 6 months, use only as recommended by a doctor)
amylum		not assessed
aromatic oils		not assessed
balsam peru oil		not assessed
beeswax		not assessed
benzethonium chloride		
in bar soap	antimicrobial	not safe or effective
as wound cleanser	antimicrobial	safe and effective (for infrequent use on small areas of skin)
as skin antiseptic	antimicrobial	not proved effective
as skin protectant	skin protectant	not proved effective
benzocaine	itch-pain reliever	safe and effective (for children under 2, use only as recommended by a doctor)
bicarbonate of sodium (see sodium bicarbonate)		not assessed
bismuth subcarbonate	skin protectant	not safe
bismuth subnitrate	skin protectant	not safe or effective
boric acid	skin protectant	safe and effective
calamine (prepared calamine)		not assessed
calcium carbonate		

calcium undecylenate	antifungal	safe and effective (for children under 2, use only as recommended by a doctor)
camphor 0.1 to 2.5%	itch-pain reliever	safe and effective (for children under 2, use only as recommended by a doctor)
casein		not assessed
cellulose		not assessed
chloroxylenol (PCMX)	antimicrobial	not proved safe or effective
cocoa butter	skin protectant	safe and effective
cod-liver oil		not assessed
cornstarch	skin protectant	safe and effective
cysteine hydrochloride		not assessed
dexpanthenol		not assessed
dibucaine	itch-pain reliever	safe and effective (for children under 2, use only as recommended by a doctor; not safe for large areas of raw or injured skin)
dimethicone	skin protectant	safe and effective
diperodon hydrochloride		not assessed
glycerin	skin protectant	safe and effective (for infants under 6 months, use only as recommended by a doctor)
hexachlorophene	antimicrobial	unsafe—*banned*
hydrocortisone acetate	itch-reliever	safe and effective (for children under 2, use only as recommended by a doctor)
8-hydroxyquinoline		not assessed
iron oxide		not assessed
lanolin		not assessed
live yeast-cell derivative	wound-healing agent	not proved effective
menthol 1% or less	itch-pain reliever	safe and effective (for children under 2, use only as recommended by a doctor)

Safety and Effectiveness: Active Ingredients in Over-the-Counter Diaper Rash Medications† *(continued)*

Active Ingredient	Purpose	Panel's Assessment
methapyrilene	itch-pain reliever	not safe—withdrawn from the market by manufacturers
methionine		not assessed
dl-methionine		not assessed
methylbenzethonium chloride		
in bar soap	antimicrobial	not safe or effective
in wound cleanser	antimicrobial	safe and effective (for infrequent use on small areas of skin)
as skin antiseptic	antimicrobial	not proved effective
as skin-wound protectant	skin protectant	not proved effective
microporous cellulose		not assessed
mineral oil		not assessed
oil of cade (juniper tar)	itch-pain reliever	safe and effective (for children under 2, use only as recommended by a doctor)
oil of eucalyptus (eucalyptol)		not assessed
oil of lavender		not assessed
oil of peppermint		not assessed
oil of white thyme		not assessed
d-pantothenol		not assessed
para-chloromercuriphenol	antiseptic	not safe or effective
petrolatum	skin protectant	safe and effective
phenol	antimicrobial	not safe
phenylmercuric nitrate	antiseptic	safe but not effective
pramoxine hydrochloride	itch-pain reliever	safe and effective (for children under 2, use only as recommended by a doctor)

Ingredient	Function	Assessment
protein hydrolysate		not assessed
resorcinol (resorcin) 0.5 to 3%	itch-pain reliever	safe and effective (for children under 2, use only as directed by a doctor; do not apply to large areas of body)
salicylic acid	antifungal	not proved effective
shark-liver oil	skin protectant	safe and effective (for children under 2, use only as directed by a doctor)
shark-liver oil	wound healer	safe but not proved effective
silicone		not assessed
sodium bicarbonate	skin protectant	safe and effective
sorbitan monostearate		not assessed
starch (see cornstarch)		
talc		not assessed
tetracaine	itch-pain reliever	safe and effective (for children under 2, use only as recommended by a doctor; do not use in large amounts or on raw or blistered skin surfaces)
vitamin A		not assessed
vitamin A palmitate		not assessed
vitamin D		not assessed
vitamin D$_2$		not assessed
vitamin E		not assessed
zinc carbonate	skin protectant	safe and effective
zinc oxide	skin protectant	safe and effective

†Note: Ingredients for the most part were not specifically assessed for the treatment or prevention of diaper rash. They were assessed more generally for their safety and effectiveness when used to protect the skin, control microorganisms, or for other functions listed in the chart's second column. These assessments were made by the Panels concerned with these functions. For antimicrobials, see SOAPS (ANTIMICROBIAL) and FIRST-AID PREPARATIONS FOR SKIN WOUNDS; for skin protectants see UNGUENTS AND POWDERS FOR THE SKIN; for itch-pain relievers, see ITCH AND PAIN REMEDIES APPLIED TO THE SKIN; for antifungal agents, see "YEAST" KILLERS FOR FEMININE ITCHING and JOCK ITCH, ATHLETE'S FOOT, AND RINGWORM CURES; for antiseptics, see ANTISEPTICS; for the astringent aluminum acetate, see STYPTIC PENCILS AND OTHER ASTRINGENTS.

Diaper-Rash Medications: Product Ratings[1]

Product and Distributor	Dosage of Active Ingredients	Comment
A and D (Schering)	**ointment:** vitamin A + vitamin D + lanolin + petrolatum **cream:** vitamin A + vitamin D + isopropyl myristate + squalane	
Ammorid (Kinney)	**ointment:** benzethonium chloride + zinc oxide + lanolin	
Andoin (Ulmer)	**ointment:** vitamin A + vitamin D + 1% allantoin (in emollient base)	*see* comment above; allantoin also unproved as wound-healer
Desitin (Leeming)	**ointment:** zinc oxide + cod-liver oil + petrolatum + lanolin	vitamins A & D are believed to be active ingredients in cod-liver oil; *see* comment opposite A and D, above
Diaparene (Glenbrook)	**powder:** methylbenzethonium chloride + cornstarch + magnesium carbonate	
Diaparene Peri-Anal Medication (Glenbrook)	**ointment:** 0.1% methylbenzethonium chloride + zinc oxide + vitamin A + vitamin D + starch + casein	*see* comment opposite A and D above
Lobana (Ulmer)	**powder:** methylbenzethonium chloride + sodium bicarbonate + cornstarch	
Methakote (Syntex)	**cream:** benzethonium chloride + protein hydrolysate + cysteine + methionine	
Mexsana Medicated (Plough)	**powder:** triclosan + zinc oxide + kaolin + eucalyptus oil + camphor + cornstarch	
Panthoderm (USV)	**cream:** 2% dexpanthenol **lotion:** 2% dexpanthenol	
RASHanul (Scott-Alison)	**ointment:** 1:5000 methylbenzethonium chloride + zinc oxide + benzocaine + vitamin A + vitamin D + calamine + boric acid + lanolin	boric acid's safety has been strongly questioned

Diaper-Rash Medications: Product Ratings[1] (continued)

Product and Distributor	Dosage of Active Ingredients	Comment
Vaseline Pure Petroleum Jelly (Chesebrough-Pond's)	**ointment:** white petrolatum	if simple is best, then this is best
vitamins A and D (generic)	**ointment:** vitamin A + vitamin D	*see* comment opposite A and D above

1. Because the Panel failed to specifically evaluate active ingredients in over-the-counter diaper-rash medications, no ratings are offered. For skin protectants and wound-healers, *see* product ratings for Unguents and Powders for the Skin, p. 800.

Diarrhea Remedies

Diarrhea, often called "the runs" or "the trots," can be both embarrassing and physically incapacitating. Abdominal cramps, nausea, vomiting, and headache frequently compound the misery it brings. A variety of illnesses, certain parasitic infestations, and unwisely ingested foods and beverages can all cause diarrhea. If the condition is severe—and it may be life-threatening, particularly for infants—or if it continues for longer than 2 days, the Panel recommends: *consult a physician!* Available over-the-counter products offer no more than symptomatic relief and work best for the mildest kinds of diarrhea. Self-treatable cases, the Panel says, are those in which the victim is not feverish and is not passing bloody stools—symptoms requiring a doctor's attention. This mild diarrhea usually goes away by itself in a day or two, but meanwhile a nonprescription antidiarrheal drug may relieve some discomfort.

CLAIMS

Accurate
    for "the treatment of diarrhea"

DIARRHEA REMEDIES is based on the report of the FDA's Advisory Review Panel on OTC Laxative, Antidiarrheal, Emetic, and Antiemetic Drug Products.

REMEDIES AVAILABLE

Given that virtually everyone suffers diarrhea at one time or another, there have been surprisingly few effective nonprescription remedies to treat it. Four agents that the Panel has approved as safe and effective antidiarrheals were in fact not submitted by drug makers for assessment. Three are opiates, derivatives of opium, a narcotic that can become addictive in large doses. Previously such preparations were available only by prescription. In approving them for nonprescription use, evaluators specified certain safeguards: opiates must be formulated in over-the-counter products in very small doses and they must be accompanied by other, nonnarcotic ingredients to discourage abuse. While the change to nonprescription status has been approved at the federal level, state and local governments may forbid over-the-counter opium-product sales within their jurisdiction.

The fourth approved antidiarrheal drug, polycarbophil, was called to the Panel's attention by the FDA; it since has been formulated into a number of nonprescription preparations.

REPLACING LOST BODY SALTS: PRELIMINARY NOTES

The gravest risk of severe diarrhea, particularly in children, is loss of body fluids and, worse, loss of electrolytes—salt substances that are required to maintain the body's fluid, chemical, and physiological balances. Depletion of one or the other of these body salts can be fatal in a surprisingly short time. Infants and toddlers with diarrhea require medical attention.

The Advisory Review Panel on OTC Miscellaneous Internal Drug Products was to have assessed several electrolyte replacements. Specifically, these drugs included: calcium chloride, magnesium chloride, potassium chloride, sodium bicarbonate, sodium chloride (table salt), and sodium lactate. But the group was disbanded before this work could be done. The FDA or another supplemental Panel may complete this effort.

Medically sanctioned preparations are already available. For infants and young children, the World Health Organization endorses an oral hydration solution that is being widely distributed in Third World countries, and now is available without prescription in the United States too, as Infalyte (Pennwalt). Alternatively, the Federal Centers for Disease Control (CDC), in Atlanta, suggest this do-it-yourself regimen:

Prepare 2 separate drinking glasses as follows:

Glass Number 1

Orange, apple, or other fruit juice (rich in potassium)	8 oz.
Honey or corn syrup (contains glucose necessary for absorption of essential salts)	½ tsp.
Table salt (contains sodium and chloride)	1 pinch

Glass Number 2

Water (carbonated or boiled if tap water contaminated)	8 oz.
Baking soda (sodium bicarbonate)	½ tsp.

Drink alternately from each glass. Repeat through the day. Supplement as desired with carbonated beverages, water or tea. Avoid solid foods. It is important that infants continue breastfeeding and receive plain water as desired while receiving these salt solutions. Older persons can take OTC antidiarrheal drugs along with these fluids.

A WORD ABOUT "LOMOTIL"

One of the most popular antidiarrheal drugs, the world around, is diphenoxylate hydrochloride, which is most familiar under its trade name Lomotil (Searle); it is sold under many other names including Loflo (Spencer Mead), L-Trol (Vangard) and Colonaid (Wallace). It is an opiatelike narcotic, although a weak one, and can cause addictive symptoms if taken in large amounts. An overdose could prove fatal. To frustrate abuse, the drug is formulated with a small amount of atropine, which causes dry skin, flushing, rapid heartbeat, and other unpleasant effects.

Diphenoxylate relaxes the colon, which reduces cramping pain. This slows the fecal stream so that more of the water can be reabsorbed before the residue is expelled. The drug thus can provide effective symptomatic relief of diarrhea.

In the United States Lomotil and similar preparations are controlled substances, but since they are considered to have a limited potential for narcotic abuse, they may be obtainable without prescription. In many foreign countries, where American travelers may be most likely to want them, they are nonprescription drugs.

These drugs may do "more harm than good" in treating travelers' diarrhea, experts say, because slowing the bowel's movement may hold back the bacteria that are causing the cramps and diarrhea. The symptoms thus may be "worsened" by taking the drug. The CDC therefore recommends that diphenoxylate—and a similar compound loperamide—be used "with caution" and for not more than 2 or 3 days. The drugs should not be used by persons with fever or blood or mucus in the stools, and they should not be used for children under 2 except under a doctor's supervision.

COMBINATION PRODUCTS

The Panel judged most combination products as useless because they contained too little of one or another drug to contribute significantly to the product's overall effectiveness. Tests are required to show that each ingredient makes a statistically significant contribution to the product's antidiarrheal effect. Evaluators found it difficult to substantiate claims made for many combination products, so they did not designate any of them as safe and effective. Pending submission of data showing the contribution of each ingredient to the product's effectiveness, the Panel granted only *conditional* approval to a half-dozen oral-dosage combinations. It limited to 2 the number of active ingredients allowable in a product (*see* SAFETY AND EFFECTIVENESS: COMBINATION PRODUCTS chart at the end of this unit).

It would make sense, of course, to have combination products of antidiarrheal ingredients with safe and effective drugs to relieve nausea and vomiting. But no such combination has been found. To mix antidiarrheals with other kinds of active ingredients does *not* make sense unless such a mixture would meet the needs of an identifiable group of people. None has. So, for the time being all such combinations are disapproved.

Some substances that are active ingredients in other types of drugs are present—in small amounts—in antidiarrheals. Here they are intended to improve the products' taste or texture, or are included for other pharmacological reasons. They should not be identified as active ingredients, the Panel insists, and claims should not be made for the antidiarrheals based on these added ingredients.

ANTIDIARRHEAL DRUGS

The Panel judged 2 dozen ingredients in terms of their ability to inhibit or control diarrhea in a safe and effective way.

Approved Active Ingredients

Opiates: opium powder, tincture of opium, and paregoric (camphorated tincture of opium)   These opiates are considered to be the most effective and fastest-acting of all antidiarrheal agents, according to the *AMA Drug Evaluations*, 4th Ed., a standard pharmacological guide. They act by increasing the muscle tone of both the large and small intestine, thus slowing the propulsive, outward movement of the contents of the intestines. Because of their well-documented effectiveness, these drugs have been the standard prescription treatment for diarrhea for many decades.

However, when diarrhea is caused by an intestinal parasite, opium may be a poor choice because it can hold the offending bacteria or other organisms in the gut, slowing recovery. Also, because opium causes considerable pressure to build up in the gut, repeated use—particularly in persons with preexisting intestinal disorders—may result in a permanent stretching of the intestinal wall (a condition called diverticular disease). But these problems are uncommon and the opiates are considered to be safe and very effective antidiarrheals.

The doses used to treat diarrhea are said to be too low to cause narcotics addiction. Nevertheless, the Panel recommended that the amended federal regulations stipulate that the preparations "contain one or more nonnarcotic active medicinal ingredients in sufficient proportion to confer upon the preparation valuable medicinal qualities other than those possessed by the narcotic drug alone."

Approved Dosage for Opiates and Polycarbophil in Diarrhea Remedies

Age Group	Approved Dosage of Opium or Its Equivalent	Approved Dosage of Polycarbophil
Adults	15 to 20 mg up to 4 times a day up to 2 days	4 to 6 grams a day
Children		
6 to 12	5 to 10 mg up to 4 times a day up to 2 days	1.5 to 3 grams a day
2 to 5	none	1 to 1.5 grams a day
Infants	none	0.5 to 1 gram a day

Polycarbophil This is an indigestible synthetic resin with an astonishing capacity to hold fluids: it will absorb 60 times its weight in water. For this reason, it is effective as an antidiarrheal. Polycarbophil absorbs free fecal water, forming a gel. This partially dries out the intestine, and allows the fecal matter to solidify into formed stools.

Animal studies indicate that polycarbophil is safe, and clinical studies in human sufferers of acute and chronic diarrhea have demonstrated effectiveness. It is the only over-the-counter antidiarrheal approved for young children.

Conditionally Approved Active Ingredients

Alumina powder, hydrated   This safe and effective antacid sometimes causes constipation. This led to its being sold and promoted as a remedy for diarrhea. No evidence is available that demonstrates this effect or even establishes a dose suitable for testing purposes. So while safe, alumina powder is not proved effective as an antidiarrheal.

Atropine sulfate   This drug blocks nerve impulses that cause propulsive movements in the stomach and intestines. The effective dose of this drug, which is close to the toxic dose, is available only by prescription, and there are no data to show that the tiny doses of atropine sulfate in nonprescription antidiarrheal preparations really work. Nor has safety been proved.

Attapulgite, activated   A natural aluminum magnesium silicate, this substance is inert and has been shown to be nontoxic in animals. So it is presumed to be safe. But no studies were submitted to show that it effectively inhibits diarrhea.

Bismuth salts: bismuth subnitrate and bismuth subsalicylate   Products containing bismuth salts are claimed to coat and protect the digestive tract. But tests with animals, which were studied directly, and with people, who were studied with a special camera, failed to confirm such an action. Also, it seems clear that most people probably use bismuth compounds *after* they get the runs and not before. So a protective coating against infectious agents or other toxic substances may not do them much good. On the other hand, evaluators reviewed some evidence which shows that large and frequent doses of bismuth subsalicylate will control diarrhea in visitors to foreign countries, and more evidence along this line was published after the Panel filed its report.

Bismuth subsalicylate is widely used, and generally regarded as safe. The safety of bismuth subnitrate has not been established. Effectiveness remains to be proved for both of these compounds.

Calcium carbonate   Like alumina powder (*see* above), calcium carbonate may induce constipation in people who take it to relieve acidity. Although safe, there is no evidence that it effectively relieves diarrhea.

Calcium hydroxide   In solution this substance is commonly called *lime water*. It sometimes has a constipating effect when used as an antacid. While it is judged to be safe, its effectiveness as an antidiarrheal needs to be proved.

Carboxymethylcellulose sodium   This soluble, semisynthetic cellulose derivative is an approved bulk-forming laxative ingredient. It well may increase viscosity of the intestine's contents. However, no studies establish this. So, although the Panel says the compound is safe, its effectiveness remains to be proved.

Charcoal, activated   Activated charcoal is obtained by distilling wood pulp, which is then treated to increase its ability to grab and hold on to nearby molecules of chemical substances. Each particle has an enormous surface area available for this purpose—for which reason activated charcoal is a valuable antidote for poisoning. It is considered safe but no studies show that it is an effective antidiarrheal.

Homatropine methylbromide   An extract of deadly nightshade, this drug possesses most of the useful—*and also the hazardous*—properties of atropine sulfate (*see* above). While it is claimed that this drug is less toxic than atropine, this needs to be scientifically established, and the Panel considers homatropine methylbromide not proved either safe or effective.

Hyoscyamine sulfate   This is another drug that acts in the same way as atropine sulfate. But it is twice as potent and may be twice as toxic as atropine sulfate. Neither its safety nor its effectiveness in relieving diarrhea has been proved.

Kaolin   The virtue of this powdered aluminum clay is that it is quite inert—so it is judged to be safe. Proponents claim that it grabs and holds some poisons, bacteria, and viruses, and may solidify (and thus slow) the flow of the fecal stream.

In one study, in which monkeys were fed a diarrhea-inducing diet of oranges, carrots, cabbage, and prune juice, the kaolin firmed up the animals' stools somewhat; but it did not decrease the number of stools. Evaluators accepted these results but questioned their relevance to diarrhea in humans. So kaolin's effectiveness remains unproved.

Lactobacillus acidophilus and Lactobacillus bulgaricus   These are bacteria obtained from milk or from special yogurt cultures. They are administered in the belief that they will multiply in the intestines and displace other bacteria that are causing the diarrhea. Many papers have been written on the use of lactobacilli in treating diarrhea, none of which is very convincing. Apparently one would have to eat a half-pound or more of the sugar lactose, or of dextran—foods in which these bacilli thrive—each day to support a lactobacilli colony large enough to displace other bacteria. Interestingly, consuming the sugars *without* the bacilli preparations would accomplish the same end because there are enough of these organisms naturally present in the gut to flourish and multiply if such a rich diet were presented to them.

These bacteria appear to be safe but proof is lacking concerning their effectiveness as antidiarrheals.

Pectin   Pectin is a plant extract that is used to make jellies gel. The Panel judges it safe when taken in modest amounts. It is not at all clear how the substance may contribute to the relief of diarrhea. In tests in which monkeys were fed diarrhea-inducing diets, pectin, like kaolin (*see* above), firmed up the animals' stools but did not decrease the number of stools. When the diarrhea was induced by disease germs (like those of cholera) or by castor oil or other chemicals, pectin and kaolin both dried up the animals' stools and reduced the number of stools. But clear-cut evidence of pectin's effectiveness in relieving human diarrhea has yet to emerge.

Phenyl salicylate (salol)   Because of questions about safety, this substance has been removed from the 2 principal drug-reference books: *The United States Pharmacopeia* and the *National Formulary*. In the small doses in which it has been used to combat diarrhea, it is safe—according to the Panel. But there is no evidence that it is effective as an antidiarrheal. In fact, the phenol in this compound may be absorbed so rapidly from the digestive tract that little is left when the dose of drug reaches the intestines—where the action is needed. Effectiveness has yet to be proved.

Zinc phenolsulfonate   In the small amounts in which it is used in over-the-counter antidiarrheal products, this phenol compound appears safe. But the Panel could find absolutely no contemporary evidence to show that it is really effective.

Disapproved Ingredients

Aminoacetic acid (glycine)   While approved as an antacid and so safe, this chemical lacks support for any claim of effectiveness as an antidiarrheal product.

Potassium carbonate   This chemical was judged to be safe but not effective as an antidiarrheal because the Panel found it to be an *inactive* —not an active—ingredient.

Rhubarb fluid extract   Reviewers were not altogether clear whether it is Chinese rhubarb (*Rheum officinale*) or American rhubarb (whose Latin name they neglected to provide) that they were assessing.

But in either case they gave this substance the rhubarb: not safe, not effective.

Scopolamine hydrobromide (hyoscine hydrobromide)   Unlike atropine sulfate, which is conditionally approved, this drug acts principally on the central nervous system and various secretory glands rather than on the intestines. So there is little or no rationale for using it in an antidiarrheal, and evaluators pronounced it not effective.

Safety and Effectiveness: Active Ingredients in Over-the-Counter Diarrhea Medications

Active Ingredient	Panel's Assessment
alumina powder, hydrated	safe but not proved effective
aminoacetic acid (glycine)	safe but not effective
atropine sulfate	not proved safe or effective
attapulgite, activated	safe but not proved effective
bismuth subnitrate	not proved safe or effective
bismuth subsalicylate	safe but not proved effective
calcium carbonate	safe but not proved effective
calcium hydroxide	safe but not proved effective
carboxymethylcellulose sodium	safe but not proved effective
charcoal, activated	safe but not proved effective
homatropine methylbromide	not proved safe or effective
hyoscyamine sulfate	not proved safe or effective
kaolin	safe but not proved effective
Lactobacillus acidophilus and *Lactobacillus bulgaricus*	safe but not proved effective
opium powder, combined with nonnarcotic ingredient(s)	safe and effective
opium, tincture of, combined with nonnarcotic ingredient(s)	safe and effective
paregoric, combined with nonnarcotic ingredient(s)	safe and effective
pectin	safe but not proved effective
phenyl salicylate (salol)	safe but not proved effective
polycarbophil	safe and effective
potassium carbonate	safe but not effective
rhubarb fluid extract	not safe or effective
scopolamine hydrobromide (hyoscine hydrobromide)	not effective
zinc phenosulfonate	safe but not proved effective

Safety and Effectiveness: Combination Products
Sold Over-the-Counter to Treat Diarrhea

Safe and Effective

Conditionally Safe and Effective

any combination of 2 approved ingredients in which 1 is present in less than the
minimum dosage set by the Panel
any combination of 2 ingredients in which 1 or both is only conditionally approved
Lactobacillus acidophilus + carboxymethylcellulose sodium
Lactobacillus acidophilus + *Lactobacillus bulgaricus*
activated attapulgite + pectin
kaolin + pectin
tincture of opium + pectin
kaolin + hydrated alumina powder

Unsafe or Ineffective

any combination that contains 3 or more active antidiarrheal active ingredients
any combination in which an ingredient is present at a dosage above the maximum set
by the Panel
any combination containing an antidiarrheal not assessed by the Panel

Diarrhea Remedies: Product Ratings

Single-Ingredient Products

Product and Distributor	Dosage of Active Ingredients	Rating[1]	Comment
attapulgite (activated)			
Quintess (Lilly)	**suspension:** 3 grams + 900 mg colloidal per 2 tablespoonsful	B	not proved effective
Rheaban (Leeming)	**liquid:** 4.2 g per 2 tablespoonsful (colloidal) **tablets:** 600 mg (colloidal)	B	not proved effective
bismuth subgallate			
Devrom (Parthenon)	**tablets, chewable:** 200 mg	C	not submitted to Over-the-Counter Drug Review

Diarrhea Remedies: Product Ratings *(continued)*

Single-Ingredient Products

Product and Distributor	Dosage of Active Ingredients	Rating[1]	Comment
bismuth subsalicylate Pepto-Bismol (Norwich-Eaton)	**suspension:** 525 mg per 30 ml **tablets, chewable:** 300 mg	B	not proved effective The FDA indicates it will say at the next stage of OTC Review that this product effectively *reduces frequency* of bowel movements, and so will qualify for an "A" for this purpose.
charcoal, activated Charcocaps (Requa)	**capsules:** 260 mg	B	not proved effective
Lactobacillus acidophilus DoFUS (Miller)	**capsules:** over 100 million viable *L. acidophilus* organisms	B	not proved effective
polycarbophil Mitrolan (A. H. Robins)	**tablets, chewable:** 500 mg as calcium carbophil	A	

Narcotic Combination Products[2]

Product and Distributor	Dosage of Active Ingredients	Rating[1]	Comment
Corrective Mixture with Paregoric (Beecham Products)	**suspension:** 0.6 ml paregoric + 45 mg pepsin + 10 mg zinc sulfocarbolate + 22 mg phenyl salicylate + 85 mg bismuth subsalicylate per teaspoonful	C	too many active ingredients
Diabismul (O'Neal)	**suspension:** 7 mg opium + 2.5 g kaolin + 80 mg pectin per tablespoonful	C	too many active ingredients

Diarrhea Remedies: Product Ratings *(continued)*

Narcotic Combination Products[2]

Product and Distributor	Dosage of Active Ingredients	Rating[1]	Comment
Kaodene with Codeine (Pfeiffer)	**suspension:** 32.4 mg codeine phosphate + 3888 mg kaolin + 194.4 mg pectin, carboxymethylcellulose sodium and bismuth subsalicylate per 2 tablespoonsful	C	too many active ingredients
Parelixir (Purdue-Frederick)	**liquid:** 0.2 ml tincture of opium + 145 mg pectin per 2 tablespoonsful	B	pectin not proved effective
Parepectolin (Rorer)	**suspension:** 15 mg opium + 5.5 g kaolin + 162 mg pectin per 2 tablespoonsful	C	too many active ingredients

Non-Narcotic Combination Products

Product and Distributor	Dosage of Active Ingredients	Rating[1]	Comment
Bacid (Fisons)	**capsules:** viable *Lactobacillus acidophilus* in high concentration + 100 mg carboxymethylcellulose sodium	B	neither ingredient proved effective
Donnagel (Robins) Quiagel (Rugby)	**suspension:** 6 g kaolin + 142.8 mg pectin + 0.1037 mg hyoscyamine sulfate + 0.0194 mg atropine sulfate + 0.0065 mg hyoscine hydrobromide per 2 tablespoonsful	C	too many active ingredients, several of which not proved safe or not proved effective
kaolin with pectin (generic) K-Pek (Rugby) Kaopectate (Upjohn)	**suspension:** 6 g kaolin + 130 mg pectin per 2 tablespoonsful	B	neither ingredient proved effective

Diarrhea Remedies: Product Ratings *(continued)*

Non-Narcotic Combination Products

Product and Distributor	Dosage of Active Ingredients	Rating[1]	Comment
Lactinex (H., W. & D.)	**granules** and **tablets:** viable mixed cultures of *Lactobacillus acidophilus* + *L. bulgaricus* organisms	B	neither ingredient proved effective
Polymagma Plain (Wyeth)	**tablets:** 500 mg activated attapulgite + 45 mg pectin + 50 mg hydrated alumina powder	C	too many active ingredients; none is proved effective

1. Author's interpretation of Panel criteria. Based on contents, not claims.
2. Not available in all states, or on open shelves. Ask your pharmacist for these products.

Diet Aids

See REDUCING AIDS

Digestive Aids

Almost everybody suffers an occasional stomach ache after eating. Some people suffer these complaints quite frequently. Tutored by ads, they may blame their problem on "gas" and reach for one of the popular over-the-counter drugs that is claimed to relieve "gas distress." While the discomfort certainly is real, the Panel says that "gas" is probably not its cause—and almost certainly is not the cause of distress that comes in the first half-hour after eating. Swallowed air accounts for about 70 percent of the gas in the gut. Everyone swallows air in and with their food when they eat. Between meals, gum chewing and cigarette smok-

DIGESTIVE AIDS is based on the report "Digestive Aid Drug Products for OTC Human Use" by the FDA's Advisory Review Panel on OTC Miscellaneous Internal Drug Products.

ing can cause people to swallow air. Many people also swallow air when they are anxious. Lesser amounts of gas—including hydrogen, carbon dioxide, and methane—are produced by bacterial breakdowns of certain foods, particularly beans and onion, in the large intestine.

A lot of gas is eliminated from the body by belching. Some gas is absorbed into the bloodstream and excreted from the lungs in exhalations. Much is passed from the anus as flatus: one may daily relieve oneself of one-third of a liter to one and a half liters of gas in this way!

Surprisingly, people who complain of "gas" may not have any more gas in their guts than others. In a pathfinding study, gastroenterologists at the Minneapolis Veterans Administration Hospital discovered that "gas-pain" victims had a normal volume of gas but experienced difficulty in moving it outward toward the rectum. They also were more likely than normal persons to suffer movement of gas upward—that is, from the intestines into the stomach. Because of these problems they suffered pain from a volume of gas that would not bother others.

These and related findings convinced the Panel that so-called "excessive gas" is not the cause of distress immediately after eating and may not be the cause of intestinal distress either.

If not gas, then what? Reviewers conceded that they don't know for sure. Perhaps distress after eating may result from eating too much. Intestinal distress may reflect problems in the time it takes food matter to get through the intestines, the nature of the food one eats, and the behavior of intestinal bacteria that share our dinners with us.

TYPES OF DISTRESS

What used to be called "stomach ache after eating" is actually classified two ways. They are explained here because the Panel assessed drugs accordingly.

- *Distress that appears after eating* (postprandial distress). Symptoms arise within a half-hour after a meal. They include feelings of abdominal bloating, distention, fullness, or pressure.
- *Intestinal distress*. Symptoms arise from half an hour to several hours after eating. Because of the longer time interval, they may involve the small and large intestines as well as the stomach. They may also be felt lower in the abdomen—below the belly button—as well as in the stomach. Symptoms of intestinal distress also include bloating, distention, fullness, and pressure, but may include abdominal pain and cramps or anal flatus (breaking wind).

Panel evaluators say that both forms of digestive distress are brief, self-correcting problems, unrelated to any known organic disease. Symptoms that result from swallowing an excess of air—technically called *aerophagia*—are not considered as belonging to either group. Also, digestive distress is different from stomach acidity, constipation, or diarrhea, which produce different symptoms and require different treatments.

Many of the drugs used to treat digestive distress are antacids, which long have been promoted as aids to digestion. In the reviewers' opinion, however, these symptoms are not caused by acidity, and claims that antacids will relieve them have yet to be proved.

How Drugs Might Relieve Digestive Distress

Given the lack of knowledge about what really causes digestive distress, evaluators found it hard to define how nonprescription drugs —or any others—might effectively relieve it. Several possibilities are summarized below.

- The active ingredient lowers surface tension on stomach contents. This facilitates absorption of digestive juices, which in turn speeds up digestion and the passage of food contents out of the stomach and into the small intestine.
- The active ingredient speeds up stomach-emptying by changing the stomach's acidity, or by some similar mechanism.
- The active ingredient works by increasing contractions of the stomach's smooth muscles, hastening stomach-emptying.

The experts remain unconvinced that any of these mechanisms accounts for the beneficial action of ingredients used to relieve distress after eating—if indeed they do act beneficially. If you take a drug for after-meal distress, the Panel says you should wait until you feel the symptoms and *not* take the drug beforehand as a preventive measure. No evidence exists to show that any of these medications is effective when taken in advance of the symptoms.

The Panel says that if intestinal distress persists over days or weeks, one should see a doctor. These symptoms could signal the onset of an organic disease that requires medical care.

COMBINATION PRODUCTS

Reviewers could not find any individual active ingredients that they felt were safe and effective for treating immediate distress after eating or intestinal distress. So, naturally, it follows that no combination of ingredients is wholly approved either.

A few combinations warranted conditional approval pending studies that truly demonstrate effectiveness. Any conditionally approved ingredient for digestive distress may be combined with the safe and effective pain-reliever acetaminophen. A number of combinations that contain disapproved substances are dismissed as unsafe or ineffective (*See* SAFETY AND EFFECTIVENESS: COMBINATION PRODUCTS at the end of this unit).

IMMEDIATE AFTER-MEAL DISTRESS

With the strong doubts that exist about effectiveness, it comes as no suprise that many claims made for these drugs are remarkably vague, misleading, irrelevant, unproved, or unprovable.

CLAIMS

Accurate
for "the relief of upper abdominal distress occurring soon after eating"

for "the relief of upper abdominal bloating, [or] fullness, [or] pressure, [or] distention which occurs soon after eating"

"relieves the over-full feeling in the upper abdomen which occurs soon after eating"

for "the relief of upper abdominal distress which occurs soon after eating, sometimes described as gas"

Unproved
"antigas"

"reduces gaseousness"

"releases entrapped gas"

"relieves discomfort and pain of entrapped gas"

"antiflatulent" (until a manufacturer can prove scientifically his product has this effect)

False or Misleading
for "relief of biliousness"

for "relief of gasid [sic] indigestion"

"stomachic"

"superior to ordinary"

any reference to a drug's *preventing* distress after eating

Approved Active Ingredients

None

Conditionally Approved Active Ingredients

The Panel decided that all of the following ingredients are, generally speaking, safe in the doses recommended for the relief of immediate after-meal distress. The problem, in each case, is lack of proof that the drug is really effective.

Almadrate sulfate   This compound is a combination of aluminum hydroxide and magnesium sulfate, 2 antacids. It has been approved as a safe and effective antacid by the Antacid Panel and by the FDA. Nevertheless, the present Panel could find no reports in the medical literature attesting to this compound's effectiveness for treating either acidity *or* immediate digestive distress. So, while the drug is apparently safe, proof is lacking that it really works.

Almadrate sulfate should not be taken for more than 2 weeks, or by persons with kidney disease, or by persons taking other drugs— except under a doctor's supervision.

Aluminum hydroxide   With moderate usage, aluminum hydroxide is safe for everyone who is not suffering from kidney disease. Reviewers decided that it may have some potential as a treatment for postprandial distress symptoms, but confirming evidence has yet to be developed. The present assessment: safe but not proved effective.

Do not use aluminum hydroxide for longer than 2 weeks or if you are taking other drugs (except if your doctor says otherwise).

Calcium carbonate   The Antacid Panel has ruled that this commonly used antacid is safe in dosages up to 8 grams per day. The present Panel agrees it is safe.

Calcium carbonate releases carbon dioxide gas as it neutralizes acid in the stomach, which may speed gastric emptying. It also has been suggested that the carbon dioxide gas distends the stomach, which also may stimulate emptying of the stomach. Unfortunately, however, no convincing evidence is available to show that moving food more rapidly out of the stomach relieves distress.

In comparative studies, calcium carbonate has been shown to be superior to both simethicone and dummy medication in relieving bloating and other after-meal distress. While these investigations "appeared" to demonstrate effectiveness, the Panel says the tests were "inadequate."

Calcium carbonate should not be used for more than 2 weeks or when one is taking other drugs, unless a doctor is consulted.

Dihydroxyaluminum sodium carbonate (DASC)   In amounts up to 8 grams per day, this antacid is safe for persons who are not on a sodium-restricted diet and who do not have kidney disease. But evidence that it relieves immediate postprandial distress is unconvincing thus far.

Four research reports on DASC's effects on after-meal distress were assessed. One study was rejected because of defects in test methods. A second, which was well designed and well supervised, appears to demonstrate effectiveness. A third test, on 99 subjects, revealed no difference in postprandial relief between DASC and dummy medication; the researchers suggested that menthol used to flavor both the real and the dummy drugs might in fact be the symptom-relieving ingredient rather than the DASC. A fourth study was judged inconclusive. So until these discrepancies can be resolved, DASC has been categorized as safe but not proved effective for immediate postprandial distress.

If you are taking other drugs that DASC might interfere with, or if you have kidney disease, consult your physician. Also, do not take the drug for more than 2 weeks without medical approval.

Magnesium hydroxide   If one's kidneys are working correctly, this anatacid drug is safe when used in the manufacturers' recommended doses. But its effectiveness in relieving abdominal distress has not been documented. In sum: safe but not proved effective for relief of immediate after-meal discomfort.

Magnesium trisilicate   This antacid is safe for use in the recommended dosages if one does not have kidney disease. It reacts with gastric acid in the stomach to make a form of magnesium that has antacid properties. The watery silica gel formed neutralizes some chemicals and also has an antifoaming property.

Two studies submitted for review suggest that magnesium trisilicate relieves distress, but the Panel felt that the test methods were defective. It ruled that the compound is safe but not proved effective.

Magnesium trisilicate should not be taken for more than 2 weeks by persons with kidney disease or by persons using other drugs (unless a doctor approves).

Peppermint oil   Millions of pounds of this substance—distilled from the leaves and stems of the mint plant *Mentha piperita*—are consumed each year in candies and foods. So the Panel believes it is safe. Used medicinally, peppermint oil has been shown to (1) relax the tight muscle between esophagus and stomach, (2) increase gastric secretions and churning in the stomach, and (3) speed up the passage of food from the stomach. These effects strongly suggest that it may help relieve immediate after-meal distress. But until this has been clearly demonstrated, the conclusion is: safe but not proved effective.

Simethicone   An antifoaming substance, simethicone breaks up small, mucus-covered bubbles in the intestine, which hold air back. This action allows the air and other gases to form larger bubbles that are more easily passed as gas, so simethicone is judged safe and effective when used for this purpose (*see* ANTI-GAS AGENTS).

What has *not* been proved is that gas causes distress immediately after eating and that making little gas bubbles into bigger ones will relieve the condition. Lacking such evidence, the reviewers assessed simethicone as safe but not proved effective.

Sodium bicarbonate   This is household baking soda, which releases carbon dioxide as it interacts with acid in the stomach. For many years, it has been used for relieving after-meal distress.

The present Panel considers sodium bicarbonate safe. But, even after all these years of seemingly successful use, scientific evidence could not be found to clearly establish its effectiveness. Pending such evidence, the verdict remains: safe but not proved effective.

If you are over 60, use no more than 1 heaping teaspoonful daily. If you are on a sodium-restricted diet, check with your doctor beforehand. Finally, do not use for more than 2 weeks without getting medical approval.

Sodium citrate   This compound—containing a form of sodium with citric acid—is approved as an antacid. It is safe in dosages of up to 8 grams a day for people who are not on sodium-restricted diets. Sodium citrate is commonly combined with sodium bicarbonate in digestive aids. When this combination is dissolved in water, it produces an antacid active ingredient, buffered sodium citrate, and bubbles of carbon dioxide gas. While sodium citrate is effective as an antacid, the present Panel says it has not seen convincing evidence that it effectively relieves immediate after-meal distress. Therefore: safe but not proved effective.

As is true for those on sodium-restricted diets, older people and individuals with kidney problems should use sodium citrate with care.

Disapproved Active Ingredients

The panel dismissed many ingredients that are or have been used to relieve distress immediately following eating. It divided these ingredients into 2 groups. The first represents those that manufacturers failed to submit for evaluation or for which the ingredient's name was submitted without supporting test results. This group has been summarily disapproved by evaluators. (*See* the first SAFETY AND EFFECTIVE-NESS chart at the end of this unit.)

The second group of disapproved active ingredients consists of chemicals for which at least some supportive material was forwarded by manufacturers to the FDA and the Panel. All of them, it is worth noting, were judged to be safe in the dosages customarily recommended for relief of after-eating distress. But none of them was found to be effective. They are described below.

Cellulase A substance obtained from molds and other sources, cellulase will break down vegetable matter. It has been used as a digestive aid for a long time and reviewers agree it is safe. But no adequate and well-controlled scientific studies appear to have been conducted to show effectiveness. Verdict: safe but not effective.

Dehydrocholic acid This drug has been approved as a safe and effective stimulant laxative. It is a derivative of cholic acid, a natural bile acid that is one of the principal digestive juices. But evaluators concur with the Laxative Panel that there is no evidence to support the claim that dehydrocholic acid relieves bloating, fullness, or other symptoms of immediate postprandial distress. The present Panel's conclusion: safe but not effective.

Garlic, dehydrated This aromatic ingredient is a major food item the world over, so it can be considered safe. Garlic has been used to relieve stomach ache and intestinal gas, and some supportive data were submitted for review. But there was not enough of it, nor was it of high scientific caliber. So the Panel concluded that dehydrated garlic, while safe, is not effective in relieving after-meal bloating, distention, and related symptoms.

Glutamic acid hydrochloride This is a water-soluble compound derived from glutamic acid, an amino acid that is common in food. When eaten, it releases hydrochloric acid in the stomach, and so is alleged to speed up digestion. But this action has not been clearly established, so the ingredient cannot be said to be effective even though it is safe.

Homatropine methylbromide This drug relaxes smooth muscles in the intestinal tract and other organs. In this way it allegedly slows the passage of food matter. Since the dosages customarily used are quite small, reviewers give this compound the nod for safety. But in the absence of careful and controlled scientific studies in humans, the Panel concludes that homatropine methylbromide is not effective in treating immediate after-meal distress.

Ox-bile extract Manufacturers apparently reason that consuming some of this mixture of digestive enzymes—taken from slaughtered cattle—will aid people in digesting their own food. This has not been proved. Neither has it been shown that ox-bile extract relieves the symptoms of abdominal distress that occur immediately following a meal. In fact, ox-bile extract reportedly can cause stomach pain and diarrhea if taken in large doses. But in the usual amounts, it is considered safe—albeit not effective for the intended purpose.

Pancreatic preparations: pancreatin and pancrelipase These drugs are mixtures of digestive enzymes (*see* PANCREATIC ENZYME SUPPLEMENTS). These substances are recognized as useful for some people who have medically diagnosed pancreatic insufficiency as might occur when the pancreas has been injured or removed surgically. But they have *not* been shown to relieve fullness or bloating following meals in otherwise normal individuals. Verdict: safe but not effective.

Pepsin A natural digestive enzyme, pepsin breaks down proteins. The hog pepsin used for medicinal purposes is chemically quite similar to human pepsin, so it is judged safe. But in the absence of acceptable data showing that it relieves stomach ache or other symptoms of immediate after-meal distress, the Panel decided pepsin is not effective.

Sorbitol This alcohol, obtained from sugar, has been approved as a laxative. Sorbitol may set the stomach to rumbling, but the Panel believes that available studies show it is safe. As to the effectiveness, adequate and well-controlled studies do not exist at present. Therefore, the Panel concluded that sorbitol is safe but not effective for after-meal distress.

INTESTINAL DISTRESS

Many drugs are marketed for the relief of intestinal distress. Again, to differentiate intestinal distress from distress immediately after eating, the present condition is defined as abdominal discomfort that occurs *30 minutes to several hours* after a meal. The symptoms may include feelings of bloating, abdominal distention, fullness, pressure, excess flatus (passing of gas from the anus), and abdominal pain or cramps. Here, too, none of the active ingredients was judged to be both safe and effective. A few are considered safe but of unproven therapeutic value. Many others are categorized as unsafe and ineffective.

Overblown medicinal claims are often printed on the labels of ineffective drugs, and intestinal-distress products are a textbook example. Examining product bottles and boxes, the Panel found more than 2 dozen claims that it rejects as vague, misleading, unrelated to the symptoms of intestinal distress, unproven, unprovable, or unreasonable. The Panel specifically rejects all claims for "prevention" of intestinal distress because no ingredient has been shown to do this. Moreover, using these drugs on a preventive basis could lead to overdosing.

CLAIMS

Accurate

for "relief of intestinal distress occurring 30 minutes to several hours after eating and often accompanied by complaints of bloating, distention, fullness, pressure, pain, cramps, or excess anal flatus"

for "the relief of fullness, [or] pressure, [or] cramps, sometimes decribed as 'gas,' and/or excess anal flatus which occurs 30 minutes to several hours after eating"

Note: Consumers should bear in mind, however, that while these circumspect claims are approved, no over-the-counter active ingredient has as yet been shown to fulfill them.

Unproved

Several claims won tentative approval, meaning that manufacturers can use them for now but not in the future unless they are proved true.

for "gas"

for "gas distress"

"digestive aid"

"assists digestion"

for "relief of indigestion"

"improved digestion and relief of the discomfort due to excess intestinal gas"

False or Misleading

"stimulates the cells of the stomach to help increase the amount of gastric juice and thus improve digestion and nutrition"

"helps create a healthy intestinal environment for more normal digestion"

"stomachic"

for "relief of biliary indigestion"

"helps to improve poor appetite"

for "gastrointestinal distress due to irritation and inflammation of the intestinal tract"

"aids digestion of hard-to-digest foods"

for "temporary relief of indigestion due to overeating"
for "expelling gas from the stomach and intestine"
"helps to relieve heartburn due to indigestion"
"relieves discomfort and pain caused by constipation"
"an adsorbent to arrest toxins and/or gas in the digestive tract which may cause discomfort, cramping, flatulence, or diarrhea"
to correct "abdominal rumblings"

Approved Active Ingredients

None

Conditionally Approved Active Ingredients

The situation here duplicates the one described for after-meal distress. Active ingredients conditionally approved for intestinal distress were all evaluated as safe. What is lacking is convincing scientific evidence that they really work.

Cellulase and hemicellulase   These enzymes are not normal constituents of the human gut. They are obtained from molds. They have been used for years as digestive aids, for breaking down cellulose, hemicellulose, and other plant roughage in the stomach.

No data were submitted to show that these enzymes are safe, but because of long use they are considered harmless in the doses usually recommended for intestinal distress. The Panel even believes that these preparations might be confirmed as useful in relieving intestinal distress and recommends further testing. However, in the meantime, cellulase and hemicellulase are listed as safe, but not proved effective.

Charcoal preparations: activated charcoal and wood charcoal
These preparations appear to be safe. But charcoal can bind and hold any number of drugs, inactivating them, and its safety when used over long periods has not been clearly established. So reviewers say charcoal can be regarded as safe only when taken in dosages of no more than 10 grams per day, for up to 7 days. The full 10-gram daily dose should be divided into several smaller doses and taken at different times during the day. Also, persons taking other drugs should ask their doctors whether they can safely use nonprescription charcoal medications.

The binding and inactivating properties mentioned above are termed *adsorption*. Many noxious substances can be neutralized by adsorption—so there is justification for believing that the process may be effective in relieving bloating and other intestinal distress symptoms. Further, because activated charcoal is one-third more effective in this regard than wood charcoal, the Panel recommends that the former be used for intestinal-distress products.

Nonetheless, until definitive proof of effectiveness is established, the evaluators granted only conditional approval.

Homatropine methylbromide   This is the same drug described under Disapproved Ingredients intended for relief of after-meal distress. It acts to relax and quiet the gut. Does this action relieve intestinal distress? No one knows for sure because tests to answer this question have not been done. So reviewers assessed the drug as not proved effective for intestinal distress, even though it is safe.

Magnesium hydroxide   Safe and effective as an antacid, it remains to be shown whether magnesium hydroxide actually works against intestinal distress. In any event, it should be used cautiously by persons who are on sodium-restricted diets or who are suffering kidney disorders. Also, if one is using other drugs, a doctor should be consulted about whether it is safe to use magnesium hydroxide as a digestive aid. The drug should never be taken for more than 2 weeks without medical supervision. Panel's verdict: safe but not proved effective for intestinal distress.

Pancreatic preparations: pancreatin and pancrelipase   These hog pancreas extracts are safe in the doses usually recommended for self-medication for the rare individual who suffers decreased pancreatic function (*see* PANCREATIC ENZYME SUPPLEMENTS). Their value for relieving intestinal distress is far less certain. Evaluators say that the many reports attesting to the value of the preparations in relieving fullness, bloating, and other symptoms were for the most part poorly structured and the results, therefore, not conclusive. More and better studies are needed. Pending such evidence, pancreatic preparations are deemed safe but not proved effective.

Simethicone   Both the Antacid Panel and the FDA say that up to 500 mg of this substance daily is safe and effective in relieving symptoms of intestinal gas (*see* ANTI-GAS AGENTS). The present Panel is less convinced of its value for this purpose, or, more generally, as a digestive aid for relieving intestinal distress. Granting that some favorable evidence exists, evaluators were able to grant only conditional approval on grounds of unproved effectiveness.

Sodium bicarbonate   This substance—baking soda—is widely used as an antacid and digestive aid. Sodium bicarbonate's long use as a cooking aid and household remedy persuades reviewers that it is safe. But whether it acts on the gut—and, if so, *how*—has not been established. Older persons, individuals who must restrict sodium intake, or those with kidney problems should limit their use of sodium bicarbonate. In sum, the present verdict on sodium bicarbonate as an intestinal distress reliever is: safe, but not proved effective.

Sodium citrate   This sodium citric acid compound is often combined with sodium bicarbonate in effervescent preparations. Evaluators say it is safe in the usual dosage of 1 to 4 grams, up to 4 times daily. But the question of whether sodium citrate is effective—alone or in combination with sodium bicarbonate—remains to be answered. Panel members also note some special warnings: (1) if you are over age 60, the maximum daily dose should not exceed 8 grams; (2) do not take for more than 2 weeks or in greater than the recommended amounts except under the advice of a physician; and (3) if the product contains more than 5 mg of sodium—the label should indicate if it does—you should not use it if you are on a sodium-restricted or salt-restricted diet, except under a doctor's supervision.

Disapproved Active Ingredients

As is the case with medications for after-meal distress, many drugs promoted for the relief of intestinal distress are of no proven value. Here, too, the Panel divided these disapproved active ingredients into 2 groups. The first contains ingredients that either were not submitted to the Panel by manufacturers or were submitted in name only—without scientific data to indicate that they are safe and effective. The Panel summarily dismissed these ingredients (*see* the second SAFETY AND EFFECTIVENESS chart at the end of this unit).

The second group of disapproved intestinal relief drugs consists of ingredients for which at least some data were provided by manufacturers, or for which some information could be unearthed from the medical records. For 2 of these—bismuth sodium tartrate and duodenal substance—evaluators felt there was a safety problem. For all of the rest, lack of effectiveness wholly accounts for the Panel's disapproval.

Bismuth sodium tartrate (sodium bismuthyltartrate)   This compound is derived from the metal bismuth. In recent years bismuth has been shown to be a potent—and, indeed, potentially lethal—nerve poison. Furthermore, no studies have been published which demonstrate that the compound relieves intestinal distress. So the Panel's judgment is: unsafe and ineffective.

The combination of blessed thistle + golden seal   This is a combination preparation that contains the extract of the whole blessed thistle plant (*Cnicus benedictus*) and the roots and tubers of golden seal

(*Hydrastis canadensis*). These are bitter-tasting traditional herbal remedies, and evaluators judge the combination safe in the doses usually recommended for intestinal distress. But manufacturers' data are unconvincing that it is effective for the intended purpose. Verdict: safe but not effective.

Dehydrocholic acid This drug has been approved as a safe and effective laxative. The present Panel agrees that it is safe, but also shares the other Panel's view that there is no evidence that dehydrocholic acid will relieve indigestion, belching, or intestinal distress. In short: not effective.

Duodenal substance Presumably this compound is a mixture of digestive enzymes from the duodenum, or small intestine, obtained from slaughtered animals. The Panel says there is no definition in the drug or medical literature that says precisely what it is, and it knows of no therapeutic uses for these substances. Therefore duodenal substance was branded not safe or effective.

Garlic, dehydrated There is no more evidence that this substance relieves late feelings of digestive distress after a meal than that it relieves immediate ones. Worldwide use indicates that it's safe, but the substance has been proved ineffective.

Glutamic acid hydrochloride This drug may well increase the stomach's acidity (*see* STOMACH ACIDIFIERS), but there is no evidence that this action relieves intestinal distress. So the evaluators say that, while safe, the compound is not effective.

Ox-bile extract While commercial preparations of ox-bile may cause diarrhea or stomach ache, the Panel believes that currently recommended dosages are safe. But it finds no evidence to show that ox-bile extract effectively relieves intestinal distress.

Papain An extract of papaya, papain is used in table-top meat tenderizers. Except for an occasional case of allergic reaction, no side effects have been reported—so evaluators decided that papain is safe. But no data supporting its effectiveness for treating intestinal distress were submitted to the Panel. Conclusion: papain is not effective.

Pepsin This is a natural digestive enzyme that is obtained for medicinal use from hog stomachs. Its long use and its inclusion in drug-reference guides like the *National Formulary XII* persuade experts that pepsin is safe. But most people can function without pepsin, and the Panel doubts the substance has any therapeutic value. Nor were any studies submitted to support its worth. Verdict: safe but not effective.

Sorbitol An approved laxative, sorbitol was submitted for review without convincing evidence to show that it relieves pain, cramping, feelings of fullness, or other symptoms of intestinal distress. So it was assessed as safe but ineffective.

Safety and Effectiveness: Active Ingredients in Over-the-Counter Products Used to Treat Distress Appearing Within One-Half Hour After Eating

Active Ingredient	Panel's Assessment
alcohol	summarily disapproved
almadrate sulfate	safe but not proved effective
aluminum hydroxide	safe but not proved effective
anise seed	summarily disapproved
aromatic powder	summarily disapproved
asafetida	summarily disapproved
bean	summarily disapproved
belladonna alkaloids (except homatropine methylbromide)	summarily disapproved
belladonna leaves, powdered extract	summarily disapproved
bismuth subcarbonate	summarily disapproved
bismuth subgallate	summarily disapproved
calcium carbonate	safe but not proved effective
capsicum	summarily disapproved
capsicum, fluid extract	summarily disapproved
carbon	summarily disapproved
cascara sagrada extract	summarily disapproved
catechu, tincture	summarily disapproved
catnip	summarily disapproved
cellulase	safe but not effective
chamomile flowers	summarily disapproved
charcoal, activated	summarily disapproved
chloroform	summarily disapproved
cinnamon tincture	summarily disapproved
dehydrocholic acid	safe but not effective
diatase	summarily disapproved
dihydroxyaluminum sodium carbonate (DASC)	safe but not proved effective
dog grass	summarily disapproved
elecampane	summarily disapproved
ether	summarily disapproved
galega	summarily disapproved
garlic, dehydrated	safe but not effective
ginger	summarily disapproved
glutamic acid hydrochloride	safe but not effective
glycine	summarily disapproved
homatropine methylbromide	safe but not effective
horsetail	summarily disapproved

Safety and Effectiveness: Active Ingredients in Over-the-Counter Products Used to Treat Distress Appearing Within One-Half Hour After Eating *(continued)*

Active Ingredient	Panel's Assessment
huckleberry	summarily disapproved
hydrastis fluid extract	summarily disapproved
hydrochloric acid	summarily disapproved
iodine	summarily disapproved
johnswort	summarily disapproved
kaolin, colloidal	summarily disapproved
lactic acid	summarily disapproved
lavender compound, tincture	summarily disapproved
linden	summarily disapproved
magnesium hydroxide	safe but not proved effective
magnesium trisilicate	safe but not proved effective
mannitol	summarily disapproved
myrrh, fluid extract	summarily disapproved
nettle	summarily disapproved
nux vomica extract	summarily disapproved
orthophosphoric acid	summarily disapproved
ox-bile extract	safe, but not effective
pancreatic preparations: pancreatin and pancrelipase	safe but not effective
pectin	summarily disapproved
peppermint oil	safe but not proved effective
peppermint spirit	summarily disapproved
pepsin	safe but not effective
potassium bicarbonate	summarily disapproved
potassium carbonate	summarily disapproved
rhubarb fluid extract	summarily disapproved
simethicone	safe but not proved effective
sodium bicarbonate	safe but not proved effective
sodium citrate	safe but not proved effective
sodium salicylate	summarily disapproved
sorbitol	safe but not effective
strawberry	summarily disapproved
strychnine	summarily disapproved
tannic acid	summarily disapproved

Safety and Effectiveness: Active Ingredients in Over-the-Counter Products Used to Relieve Intestinal Distress Appearing from One-Half Hour to Several Hours After Eating

Active Ingredient	Panel's Assessment
amylase	summarily disapproved
aspergillus oryza enzymes	summarily disapproved
betaine hydrochloride	summarily disapproved
bismuth sodium tartrate (sodium bismuthyltartrate)	not safe or effective
black radish powder	summarily disapproved
blessed thistle + golden seal	safe but not proved effective
buckthorn	summarily disapproved
calcium gluconate	summarily disapproved
catechu, tincture	summarily disapproved
cellulase and hemicellulase	safe but not proved effective
charcoal preparations: activated charcoal and wood charcoal	safe but not proved effective
cinnamon oil	summarily disapproved
citrus pectin	summarily disapproved
dehydrocholic acid	safe but not effective
diastase malt	summarily disapproved
duodenal substance	not safe or effective
fennel acid	summarily disapproved
garlic, dehydrated	safe but not effective
glutamic acid hydrochloride	safe but not effective
glycine	summarily disapproved
hectorite	summarily disapproved
homatropine methylbromide	safe but not proved effective
iron ox bile	summarily disapproved
johnswort	summarily disapproved
juniper	summarily disapproved
knotgrass	summarily disapproved
Lactobacillus acidophilus	summarily disapproved
lactose (lipase)	summarily disapproved
lysine hydrochloride	summarily disapproved
magnesium hydroxide	safe but not proved effective
mycozyme	summarily disapproved
nickel-pectin	summarily disapproved
orthophosphoric acid	summarily disapproved
ox-bile extract	safe but not proved effective
pancreatic preparations: pancreatin and pancrelipase	safe but not proved effective
papain	safe but not effective
papaya, natural	summarily disapproved
peppermint	summarily disapproved
peppermint oil	summarily disapproved

Safety and Effectiveness: Active Ingredients in Over-the-Counter Products Used to Relieve Intestinal Distress Appearing from One-Half Hour to Several Hours After Eating *(continued)*

Active Ingredient	Panel's Assessment
pepsin	safe but not effective
phenacetin	summarily disapproved
prolase	summarily disapproved
senna	summarily disapproved
simethicone	safe but not proved effective
sodium bicarbonate	safe but not proved effective
sodium chloride	summarily disapproved
sodium citrate	safe but not proved effective
sorbitol	safe but not effective
stem bromelains	summarily disapproved
tannic acid	summarily disapproved
trillium	summarily disapproved
woodruff	summarily disapproved

Safety and Effectiveness: Combination Products Sold Over-the-Counter to Relieve Digestive Distress

Safe and Effective

None

Conditionally Safe and Effective

for intestinal distress: pancreatin + simethicone
for immediate postprandial distress: aluminum hydroxide + magnesium trisilicate
for immediate postprandial distress or for intestinal distress: magnesium hydroxide + simethicone
for intestinal distress: pancreatin or pancrelipase + hemicellulase
for immediate postprandial relief or for intestinal distress: acetaminophen + 1 conditionally approved aid for digestive distress

Unsafe or Ineffective*

cellulase + pancreatin + glutamic acid hydrochloride + ox-bile extract + pepsin
cellulase + dehydrocholic acid + pancreatic enzyme concentrate + pepsin
alcohol + peppermint oil + cinnamon oil + tannic acid + tincture of catechu
sorbitol + homatropine methylbromide
for immediate postprandial distress: pancreatin + simethicone
for immediate postprandial distress: bean + dog grass + elecampane + galega + horsetail + huckleberry + johnswort + nettle + linden + strawberry
for immediate postprandial distress: peppermint spirit + orthophosphoric acid

Safety and Effectiveness: Combination Products Sold Over-the-Counter to Relieve Digestive Distress *(continued)*

---

*Unsafe or Ineffective**

for intestinal distress: blessed thistle + golden seal

for intestinal distress: ox-bile extract + papain + pepsin + pancreatin + duodenal substance + dehydrocholic acid + activated charcoal

for intestinal distress: pancreatin + hemicellulase + ox-bile extract

for intestinal distress: senna + buckthorn + johnswort + woodruff + juniper + peppermint + knotgrass

---

*Except where specified, these combinations were judged "unsafe or ineffective" for both categories of distress.

Digestive Aids: Product Ratings

Single-Ingredient Products[1]

Product and Distributor	Dosage of Active Ingredients	Rating[2] for Distress Immediately After Meals	Rating[2] for Intestinal Distress	Comment
bismuth subgallate				
Devrom (Parthenon)	**tablets, chewable:** 200 mg	C		not safe or effective
charcoal preparations				
Charcoal (Paddock)	**tablets:** 325 mg		B	not proved effective
Charcocaps (Requa)	**capsules; activated:** 260 mg	C	B	not safe or effective for first use; not proved effective for second use
dehydrocholic acid				
dehydrocholic acid (generic)	**tablets:** 250 mg	C	C	not effective
dihydroxyaluminum sodium carbonate				
Rolaids (Warner-Lambert)	**tablets, chewable:** 334 mg	B		not proved effective
glutamic acid hydrochloride				
Acidulin Pulvules (Lilly)	**capsules:** 340 mg	C	C	not effective
iron ox bile				
Bilron Pulvules (Lilly)	**capsules:** bile acids + iron		C	not safe or effective
Lactobacillus acidophilus				
DoFUS (Miller)	**capsules:** at least 100 million viable *L. acidophilus* organisms		C	not safe or effective

		Rating² for Distress Immediately After Meals	Rating² for Intestinal Distress	Comment
magnesium hydroxide milk of magnesia (generic)	**tablets:** 325 mg	B	B	not proved effective
ox-bile extract Ox Bile Extract Enseals (Lilly)	**tablets, enteric coated:** 325 mg	C		not effective
pancreatic preparations Pancreatin (Lilly)	**tablets:** 325 mg USP	C	B	efficacy is the issue
simethicone Mylicon (Stuart)	**tablets, chewable:** 40 mg	B	B	not proved effective
sodium bicarbonate Arm & Hammer Baking Soda (Church & Dwight)	**powder**	B	B	not proved effective
sodium bicarbonate (generic)	**tablets:** 325 mg, 650 mg	B	B	not proved effective
sodium salicylate sodium salicylate (generic)	**tablets:** 325 mg	C		not safe or effective

Combination Products

Product and Distributor	Dosage of Active Ingredients	Rating² for Distress Immediately After Meals	Rating² for Intestinal Distress	Comment
Accelerase (Organon)	**capsules:** 4,000 units lipase + 15,000 units amylase + 15,000 units protase + 2 mg cellulase + 65 mg mixed conjugated bile salts + 20 mg calcium carbonate		B	not proved effective

Digestive Aids: Product Ratings *(continued)*

Combination Products

Product and Distributor	Dosage of Active Ingredients	Rating[2] for Distress Immediately After Meals	Rating[2] for Intestinal Distress	Comment
Bilogen (Organon)	**tablets:** 250 mg pancreatin + 120 mg ox-bile extract + 75 mg oxidized mixed ox-bile acids + 30 mg desoxycholic acid		C	unassessed combination
Bromo Seltzer (Warner Lambert)	**effervescent granules:** 325 mg acetaminophen + 2.781 g sodium bicarbonate + 2.224 g citric acid per dosage measure	B	B	the latter 2 ingredients form sodium citrate in the stomach, which is not proved effective; hence the combination is not proved effective
Controflex (Bowman)	**syrup:** orthophosphoric acid + sucrose + peppermint	C		not effective
Digestalin (Vortech)	**tablets:** 0.4 mg pancreatin + 1.2 mg papain + 2 mg pepsin + 5.3 mg activated charcoal + 3.8 mg bismuth subgallate + 1.2 mg berberis + 0.08 mg hydrastis		C	papain not effective
Festal (Hoechst-Roussel)	**Tablets, enteric coated:** 20,000 units protease + 30,000 units amylase + 6,000 units lipase + 25 mg bile constituents + 50 mg hemicellulase		C	disapproved combination

Product	Contents	Rating	Comment
PAMA Tablets (North American)	**tablets:** 420 mg calcium carbonate + 180 mg glycine	C	glycine not safe and/or not effective
Phazyme (Reed & Carnrick)	**tablets:** 3,000 units protease + 240 units lipase + 2,000 units amylase + 60 mg simethicone	B	not proved effective
ProBilagol (Purdue-Frederick)	**liquid:** 45 g d-sorbitol + 1 mg homatropine MBr per teaspoonful	C	not effective
Tri-Cone (Glaxo)	**capsules:** 10 mg amylase + 10 mg prolase + 10 mg lipase + 40 mg simethicone	B	not proved effective

1. For products containing aluminum hydroxide or calcium carbonate, *see* product ratings for Antacids, pages 39–44.
2. Author's interpretation of Panel criteria. Based on contents, not claims.

Douches and Other Vaginal Applications

Women douche for a variety of reasons, many of which make sense, a few of which do not. Douching may help a woman feel cleaner and fresher. It may relieve itching and minor vaginal irritation. But douching before making love has not been proved to increase the likelihood of conceiving a boy, as some doctors say it may; and douching after making love certainly will not prevent pregnancy—as more than a few women have learned to their regret. The Panel defined *vaginal douche* as a liquid preparation used to irrigate the vagina over an indeterminate period of time for one or more of the purposes listed below:

> cleansing
> soothing and refreshing
> deodorizing
> relieving minor vaginal irritations
> reducing the number of pathogenic organisms
> changing the vagina's acidity to encourage the growth of
>   normal vaginal flora (microorganisms)
> producing an astringent effect
> lowering surface tension
> dissolving vaginal discharge and debris

Douching products are sold as premixed liquids, as concentrates, and as powders that must be diluted for use. They may be directed into the vagina from rubber or plastic douche bags, from single-use disposable containers, or from bulb syringes. Alternatively, they can be introduced into the vagina as suppositories that melt when heated to body temperature, releasing their active ingredients. A few vaginal self-treatment drugs are available as ointments or gels.

CLAIMS

False, Misleading, or Unproved
"intimately understood"
"contains only the mildest of ingredients"

DOUCHES AND OTHER VAGINAL APPLICATIONS is based on the unapproved draft report of the FDA's Advisory Review Panel on OTC Contraceptives and Other Vaginal Drug Products.

"completely refreshed"

"complete feminine hygiene"

"intended for all women who want to enjoy extra confidence in meeting people"

"complete feminine daintiness"

"intimate cleanliness"

"gentle"

"safe"

"removes contraceptive jellies and creams"

"safe for delicate membranes"

for "relief of minor vaginal soreness"

References to "cleansing," "refreshing," "soothing," or "deodorizing" are *cosmetic* claims which need not be proved and which are outside the Panel's jurisdiction.

COSMETICS OR DRUGS?

The FDA previously has treated douches as cosmetics, requiring them to carry one of these notices:

for "cleansing purposes only, after menstruation and after marital relations"

for "cleansing purposes only. Do not use more than twice weekly unless directed by a physician"

More recently, the FDA and the Panel have decided—on the basis of recent revisions in the Federal Food, Drug, and Cosmetic Act—that douches may be cosmetics, or drugs, or both. The first 3 purposes of douching—cleansing, soothing and freshening, and deodorizing—for the most part are cosmetic effects. So they are outside the review's jurisdiction. If, however, a douche contains medicinal amounts of any active drug ingredient—or if the label claims that it may prevent, mitigate, or be otherwise useful for treating any illness, injury, or disease condition—then it is considered a drug.

These distinctions are sometimes quite fine. Insofar as a product kills bacteria or inhibits their growth, thereby reducing vaginal odor, it is a drug. These distinctions, however, are important for consumers to understand. Cosmetic ingredients are not required to meet scientific standards for effectiveness. Drug ingredients are. So a buyer can have greater confidence in the effectiveness of a drug—particularly one that evaluators have assessed as safe and effective—than one can in a cosmetic ingredient, for which no proofs are asked.

DOUCHING AND CONTRACEPTION

Many women have become mothers because of their belief that douching after sexual intercourse is an effective contraceptive method. *It is not!* Sperm cells enter the uterus too quickly to be washed away by water or other douching solutions. In fact, they may reach the cervical opening within 30 seconds after ejaculation. Within 90 to 180 seconds, they are inside the uterus—safe from spermicides. The cells then reach the fallopian tubes—where conception occurs if the ovum (egg) is ready—within half an hour. As the *Handbook of Nonprescription Drugs*, 6th Ed., puts it: "It is highly improbable that douching can be initiated quickly or thoroughly enough to remove all traces of semen, and therefore of sperm, from the vagina." The Panel, concurring in this judgment, recommends that all douching product labels state explicitly that the products are not intended to prevent pregnancy.

Some women douche after intercourse whether or not they are protected by a contraceptive. This may be a mistake for women who use spermicides, for if they douche too soon they may wash the contraceptive out while viable sperm cells remain in the vagina. The panel suggests: wait at least 6 hours before douching.

DOES A WOMAN NEED TO DOUCHE?

The answer is: probably no. In the Panelists' opinion there is widespread overindulgence in a practice for which there is no clear-cut scientific support, and they cited "tradition, ignorance, and commercial advertising" as major contributors to the persistence of this practice.

The other side of the coin: there is no good reason *not* to douche. The same reviewers also say that for the normal, healthy, nonpregnant woman who believes she derives some benefit from the practice, there is no medical reason not to. (Douching during pregnancy is discussed below.)

Vaginal Hygiene

The vagina is naturally self-cleansing. It is a 3-to 4-inch-long tissue sheath lined on the inside by a unique and relatively thick mucous membrane that is highly responsive to cyclical changes in blood levels of female sex hormones (estrogen and progesterone). A thin superficial layer develops only at menarche (when a girl begins to menstruate). It is shed into the vagina itself each month—under the influence of estrogen—and then regrows. After menopause, this layer vanishes.

The vaginal mucosa is naturally bathed by a variety of secretions —mucus, water, proteins, and salt. Vaginal fluids also include sloughed-off superficial cells from the uterine cavity and vaginal walls, blood, microorganisms and the debris they produce, possibly seminal fluid, and debris from contraceptive and other drugs that have been introduced into the vagina or from tampons.

During menstruation, and throughout the month as well, vaginal secretions gravitate downward and outward. Douching may enhance this natural self-cleansing process.

The Vaginal Flora

The vagina is naturally inhabited by large numbers of microorganisms that together are called the *vaginal flora*. Major components are:

cocci	fungi (including *Candida albicans*)
coliforms	lactobacilli (Doederlein's bacilli)
diphtheroids	micrococcacae
facultative anaerobes	trichomonas

The normal acidity of the vagina (pH 4.0), sustained by lactic acid secretions from the resident lactobacilli, is required for maintenance of the normal vaginal flora. It also helps protect against overgrowth by resident bacteria or other organisms from outside sources.

Under abnormal conditions, some microorganisms that normally are present in the vagina overgrow. This results in vaginal discharge, itching and irritation, and vaginal malodor—the symptoms of vaginitis. The symptoms may also be produced by microorganisms invading from the outside.

It may be impossible for a woman to decide for herself which kind of organisms are causing a vaginitis. This may make it difficult for her to self-treat it effectively, since different microorganisms respond to treatment by different drugs. At the same time, many women come to recognize 2 of the commonest types of vaginitis—those caused by *Candida albicans* and related yeasts and those caused by the flagella *Trichomonas vaginalis*. Both "yeast" and "tric," as they have come to be called, produce intense itching, inflammation, and malodorous vaginal discharge, which in the case of yeast tends to be whitish in color. The present Panel believes that these infections should be diagnosed by a doctor, who then should supervise their treatment. But the Antimicrobial II Panel believes that there is place for first aid, in the form of nonprescription drugs, to relieve the "extreme itching" that yeast infection particularly may provoke. So it has recommended that 3 safe and effective prescription drugs be switched to nonprescription status for this purpose (see "YEAST" KILLERS FOR FEMININE ITCHING).

Changes in the vaginal flora will alter a woman's vaginal odor, and infectious microorganisms can produce unpleasant smells as well as itching and other symptoms. If douching successfully eliminates an unpleasant or unaccustomed odor, and clears up itching, irritation, or other symptoms that accompany it, then a woman has no further cause for concern. But if these symptoms persist for several days, experts advise consulting a doctor.

Risks for Pregnant Women

Some douche ingredients are irritating or cause allergic reactions. A woman who notices redness, swelling, itching, or other symptoms after douching should stop using the product temporarily and consider changing to a different brand. A more insidious hazard, in the Panel's view, is systemic poisoning resulting from the absorption of douche ingredients across the vaginal wall and into the bloodstream.

Many factors influence vaginal absorption of drugs, including the type of drug and its base, the user's age, and the stage of her menstrual cycle. What is certain is that absorbed drugs can be directly injurious to the woman herself and may cross the placenta and damage her fetus if she is pregnant.

Evaluators have taken one step to reduce this risk: they have identified as "unsafe" a number of douche ingredients that are general poisons. A second step is up to women: don't douche if you are pregnant, the Panel says, except with the approval of your physician.

The risk of drug absorption is not the only reason for pregnant women to avoid douching. Panel members report from their own experiences with pregnant patients, as well as from reports in medical literature, that the proliferation of blood vessels in the placenta and uterine wall, as well as in the vaginal wall, can set the stage for serious douching mishaps. The worst possible risk is the introduction of an air bubble into one of the uterine blood vessels. In one reported case, when the air reached the woman's brain, she died.

Douching solutions that enter the uterus can induce abortion. If they pass up through the fallopian tubes, they may carry microorganisms into the abdominal cavity—seeding a severe, possibly life-threatening infection. While these are uncommon risks, experts urge that pregnant women douche only after consulting their doctors.

For nonpregnant women, the risk is much less. In fact, the Panel could not see the wisdom or need for the FDA-inspired label warning that a woman douche no more often than twice a week. No scientific basis could be found for this limitation, and in the evaluators' view a healthy nonpregnant woman can douche as often as she likes—even once daily if she wishes. Women who have been warned against douching but wish to do it will be heartened by the Panel's conclusion that no valid evidence indicates that frequent douching affects natural flora or induces irritation or injury.

COMBINATION PRODUCTS

No combination douching product now marketed warranted approval as safe and effective. Conditional approval was granted to 8 combinations that were submitted for Panel assessment. The balance were rejected as unsafe or ineffective (*see* SAFETY AND EFFECTIVENESS: COMBINATION PRODUCTS chart at the end of this unit).

CATEGORIES OF PRODUCTS

The Panel divided the active drug ingredients in douches into 4 groups:

- *Anti-irritants* relieve minor itching and irritation, principally by killing or inhibiting the microorganisms that cause these conditions.
- *Acidifiers* are alleged to encourage normal flora—which discourages infectious microorganisms—by enhancing the acidity of vaginal secretions. A few active ingredients have the opposite, or alkalizing effect.
- *Astringents* pucker the vaginal mucosa and pull protein-type substances out of the vaginal secretions. This may *feel* good, but the evaluators' draft report offers no explanation of how or why this is a medicinal benefit.
- *Detergents* lower surface tension on the walls of the vagina and soften, loosen, and help remove mucus and other secretions.

The active ingredients that actually or allegedly provide these benefits are described under their respective headings below. Because some ingredients are said to provide two or more of these actions, they are assessed separately under each appropriate heading.

ANTI-IRRITANTS

Perhaps the commonest medicinal claim made for douches is that they relieve minor vaginal itching, irritation, and soreness. Two dozen ingredients for which this claim is made were submitted for assessment, and it is interesting that only one—potassium sorbate—warranted unqualified approval. Perhaps this disappointing outcome prompted Panel members to vote to reclassify as nonprescription drugs 2 anti-irritants that have been used successfully as prescription drugs for over 3 decades. They are calcium propionate and sodium propionate, which are available as vaginal gels, not as douches. The 3 approved anti-irritants all act to inhibit the growth of infectious microorganisms.

Given this poor rate of proven effectiveness, some of the claims made for products seem particularly immodest.

CLAIMS

Accurate

for "temporary [or] symptomatic relief of minor vaginal irritations, [or] itching"

for "relief of minor vaginal soreness"

Unproved, False or Misleading

"complete feminine hygiene"

"reduces the number of pathogenic organisms"

WARNING If redness, swelling, or pain develop, discontinue douching or using. Consult your physician if symptoms persist.

Approved Active Ingredients

Calcium propionate and sodium propionate These 2 chemicals are assessed together because they are formulated together in one prescription product—a vaginal gel—that impressed the Panel as safe enough and effective enough to recommend that it be switched to nonprescription status. These propionates have for many years been used by bakers and dairy operators as mold retardants. They also are widely used by veterinary doctors and by physicians for treating conjunctivitis, vaginitis, and other infections. Evaluators say their safety has been well established in the medical literature.

Calcium and sodium propionate stop the growth of fungal organisms and a number of bacteria. Clinical data from 30 years of use show that these substances cure 80 percent of cases of fungal vaginitis in nonpregnant women. The Panel feels these ingredients would benefit women with minor vaginal irritations and should be available over-the-counter. The drugs are also suitable for treating the "yeast" infections caused by *Candida albicans*, once the infection has been diagnosed by a physician who then supervises treatment.

The safe and effective total dosage of calcium and sodium propionate is 0.6 grams, applied intravaginally twice daily.

Potassium sorbate   This is the one "old-timer" douche ingredient that the reviewers say will safely and effectively relieve minor vaginal irritation. Sorbates are widely used to inhibit mold on foods, and their lack of toxicity has been carefully established. Their use in treating vaginal itch and irritation poses no safety problem. As to effectiveness, in many cases symptoms subside after the first treatment and remain in abeyance months or years later. Many studies have demonstrated that potassium sorbate is also effective against yeast vaginitis, or a combination of yeast and *Trichomonas vaginalis* ("tric"). The symptoms disappear gradually over a period of a week or so.

Potassium sorbate is listed as safe and effective in concentrations of 1 to 3 percent as a douche solution or vaginal suppository. In solution, the 3 percent may work better than the 1 percent.

Sodium propionate   See CALCIUM PROPIONATE AND SODIUM PROPIONATE, above.

Conditionally Approved Active Ingredients

Allantoin   No report has ever appeared in the medical literature suggesting that this ingredient causes side effects, so the Panel grants that it is safe. But evaluators were given no data to show that allantoin relieves minor vaginal irritations. Conclusion: safe but not proved effective.

Aloe vera, stabilized gel   This leaf substance from the aloe vera plant has been used medicinally since ancient times. The crude plant extract deteriorates within hours, but one manufacturer claims to have stabilized the active substance in a medicinal gel. Standard animal tests have demonstrated the basic safety of stabilized aloe vera, and in the hundred reports submitted to the present Panel not one adverse effect was reported. Clearly the substance is safe.

Effectiveness is another matter. Tests in the laboratory demonstrated that aloe vera kills a number of microorganisms that cause vaginal itching and irritation. These include *Candida albicans*, *Staphylococcus aureus*, *Streptococcus viridans*, and *Trichomonas vaginalis*. But clinical reports on the use of aloe vera in treating women were found wanting. So the Panel says its effectiveness remains to be proved, even though aloe vera is safe.

Benzalkonium chloride and benzethonium chloride These compounds, assessed together, have long been used in douches and vaginal compounds. Practically no complaints have been received from women saying the products were ineffective or caused adverse reactions. But the Panel says the medical and scientific view of these drugs —once highly favorable—has now changed. There is concern that while the compounds effectively kill microorganisms in the test tube, they may be far less serviceable in actual use. They are, for example, inactivated by many natural and manufactured substances including soaps, human tissue, proteins, and even the containers in which they are packaged. Also, some bacterial organisms resist these drugs and, in fact, may actually grow more rapidly in their presence—a risk evaluators believe must be assessed.

On top of the new questions that have arisen about the safety of benzalkonium chloride and benzethonium chloride, reviewers received no data which clearly show that the drugs really work in treating minor vaginal irritation. So the Panel concludes that both the safety and effectiveness of these ingredients need to be proved if they are to be granted better than conditional approval.

Benzocaine A highly effective anesthetic, benzocaine has an impressive safety record; because of this the present Panel rates benzocaine safe, despite a paucity of data on its use in the vagina. The effective concentration of benzocaine is generally recognized as being between 5 and 20 percent. The concentrations in currently marketed vaginal suppositories are much lower—between 0.2 and 0.65 percent —and the Panel doubts that they are strong enough to effectively relieve vaginal itching and irritation. So if manufacturers wish to continue to market such low doses of this anesthetic, evaluators say they must demonstrate through scientific studies that they are actually effective.

Edetate disodium and edetate sodium The edetates hold (bind) mineral particles—including calcium and zinc. Theoretically this action would prevent these essential "nutrients" from being eaten by microorganisms that are causing vaginal complaints.

Edetates are widely used in food processing, and have been assumed to be safe. But the Panel notes that loss of zinc in the early stage of human embryonic development can lead to serious birth defects—

so it questions the safety of the edetates and strongly warns pregnant women not to use them.

If the safety issue were clearly resolved, the evaluators believe these compounds might win a permanent place as safe and effective anti-irritants: they do appear to be effective against the class of microorganisms called *flagella*—which includes *Trichomonas vaginalis* ("tric"). But further studies are still needed to establish this effectiveness when the drugs are used in self-treatment. In sum, at this time both the safety and effectiveness of edetate disodium and edetate sodium remain to be proved. However, these compounds may be recommended by a doctor for treating "tric" once it has been determined that this organism is responsible for the itching, irritation, or other vaginal symptoms. This treatment should be under the doctor's supervision.

Nonoxynol 9 and octoxynol 9 These compounds, described under APPROVED SPERMICIDES, in CONTRACEPTIVES, are considered safe. The Panel reviewed studies which suggest that when one of these two closely related compounds is used in a douche, it will reduce the count of microorganisms responsible for vaginal irritation. Studies in culture dishes indicate that the flagella *Trichomonas vaginalis*—the cause of "tric"—is inhibited by the oxynol drugs. Reviewers were impressed by this evidence, but not convinced. They call for testing to see if effectivess can be clearly demonstrated. Verdict: safe but not proved effective.

Oxyquinoline citrate and oxyquinoline sulfate Both compounds were once used to treat gonorrhea and other infections. No adverse effects were reported. In recent years, however, it has been suggested that they might cause cancer and genetic damage. Until such questions are settled, safety remains in doubt.

As to whether they really work, the Panel received no data to show that these drugs are effective in relieving minor vaginal irritation—despite their long use as antimicrobial agents. So both safety and effectiveness need to be proved.

Phenol and phenolate sodium (under 1.5 percent) Phenol is the antiseptic ingredient that has that characteristic "medicinal" smell. Phenol is the active ingredient in phenolate sodium. In recent years, phenol has been shown to be extremely toxic. The present Panel concurs with the Antimicrobial I Panel that in concentrations above 1.5 percent it is too dangerous to use (*see* PHENOL under 1.5 percent aqueous/alcoholic, page 615). In addition to considering 1.5 percent phenol safe, reviewers believe it may effectively relieve vaginal irritation. But studies to prove these propositions have not yet been done.

At present, phenol at 1.5 percent concentration or less is listed as not proved safe or effective.

Note: An FDA summary document suggests that the Panel will disapprove even mild phenol preparations as unsafe in its final published report.

Sodium edetate   See EDETATE DISODIUM AND EDETATE SODIUM, above.

Vitamins A and D   These vitamins appear to be safe, the Panel says. They are claimed to have a soothing, healing property when applied to burned and irritated body surfaces. But Panel evaluators found no data to justify the use of these substances in a vaginal drug product. Conclusion: safe but not proved effective for relieving irritation of the vagina.

Disapproved Active Ingredients

Boron compounds: boric acid, boroglycerin, sodium borate, and sodium perborate   These compounds have been widely used medicinally, and they do kill some microorganisms. But they also have been discovered to be extremely potent poisons, so that their use as drugs has fallen off rapidly in recent years. The Panel claims that "a serious question of safety exists" when these compounds are used in concentrations over 1 percent. Added to questionable safety is the fact that no evidence was presented to show that boric acid and related compounds are effective in treating self-diagnosable, minor vaginal irritations. The Panel concluded that boric acid and related compounds are not safe or effective.

Hexachlorophene   This detergent is absorbed through the skin and undoubtedly is absorbed through the vaginal mucosa, too. It causes nerve damage. The FDA has already banned it as an active ingredient in nonprescription products. Not only is it unsafe, but evaluators could find no support for claims that it is effective against vaginal microorganisms or that it will relieve minor irritations. So it was judged not safe and not effective.

Phenol and the phenol compounds: phenolate sodium and sodium salicylic acid phenolate (over 1.5 percent phenol)   These compounds are hazardous because phenol is a potent nerve poison. There is little doubt that it will be absorbed through the vaginal wall and into the bloodstream when these compounds are applied to the vagina in douches or other over-the-counter medications. Although, generally speaking, phenol is mildly effective as a topical antimicrobial agent,

Panel reviewers said that studies submitted on its behalf as a vaginal drug were inadequate. Conclusion: phenol and its derivatives are unsafe and ineffective when used in concentrations over 1.5 percent phenol in douches and nonprescription vaginal drug products.

Sodium borate   *See* BORON COMPOUNDS, above.

Sodium perborate   *See* BORON COMPOUNDS, above.

Sodium salicylate   The Panel says it is not aware of any data to show that sodium salicylate is either safe or effective when used intravaginally. In sum: not safe and not effective.

Sodium salicylic acid phenolate   *See* PHENOL AND THE PHENOL COMPOUNDS, above.

VAGINAL ACIDIFIERS OR ALKALIZERS

Vaginal secretions are somewhat acidic; they have a pH of about 4.0. This acidness is maintained by bacteria—sometimes called Doederlein's bacilli—which secrete lactic acid. Vaginal acidity helps prevent overgrowth of invasive, irritating, disease-producing bacteria, most of which cannot thrive in an acid milieu. The acidic nature of this region also appears to prevent these dangerous bacteria from migrating upward through the cervix, where they could cause infections in the uterus and abdominal cavity.

Women have apparently long understood the hygienic value of maintaining vaginal acidity—how else can one explain the wide use of vinegar for douching! Other acids are included in commercial preparations. What remains unclear is whether douching adds enough acid—and for a long enough period of time—to stimulate the normal flora (microorganisms). It also is unclear whether this would help relieve vaginal symptoms.

CLAIMS

Accurate
   "helps keep vagina in its normal acid state"

Unproved, False or Misleading
   "completely compatible with normal vaginal environment"
   "formula like the natural environment in your own body"
   "buffered to control a normal vagina pH"
   "pH 3.5"
   "alters vaginal pH"

The claim is made by some manufacturers that *reducing* the vaginal acidity —by using an alkalizing or neutralizing agent—will help restore the natural vaginal flora. Evaluators have the same doubts about this claim as they do about those made for acidifiers. A few of the ingredients assessed below are alkalizers and are identified as such.

WARNING   If vaginal itching, redness, swelling, or pain develops, the douching should be discontinued. If the symptoms persist, consult a physician.

Approved Active Ingredients

None. The Panel evaluated a number of mild acids used for douching. It could not find any one of them that it could say, with confidence, is safe and effective.

Conditionally Approved Active Ingredients

The Panel gave tentative assent to most of the acidifiers and alkalizers it considered. Its principal findings are summarized below.

Acetic acid   This is the acid in household vingegar, which has a venerable history of use for douching; it contains 4 to 6 percent acetic acid. The usual dose is 1 ½ teaspoonful of vinegar in a quart or a liter of water. Reviewers believe this dosage is safe. Vinegar may also be effective in encouraging the growth of normal vaginal flora, but studies that could clearly establish this remain to be done. Therefore the verdict is: safe but not proved effective.

Citric acid   Like vinegar, this is a douche material with long years of use. With no reports of toxicity or irritation, evaluators judge citric acid safe. No hard data were present to prove that citric acid douches in fact change the vaginal acidity or have a beneficial effect on the vaginal flora. In short: as a douche ingredient citric acid is safe in the currently marketed concentration of 0.1 to 0.5 percent—but proof of effectiveness is lacking.

Lactic acid and the combination of lactic acid + sodium lactate These ingredients have for a long time been used for douching and they have the theoretical advantage that lactic acid is the principal *natural* acid in the vagina. Concentrated lactic acid can be quite corrosive, but the weak concentrations found in douches (0.4 to 1.3 percent) were judged safe. Sodium lactate is neutral and nontoxic, and there are no reports of serious toxic consequences despite a long history of use in douches.

While there is every reason to believe that lactic acid and lactic acid combined with sodium lactate will help maintain the normal, acidic atmosphere of the vagina, it has not been satisfactorily demonstrated that these chemicals remain there long enough to do very much good. So, pending studies that clarify this question, the Panel's assessment of lactic acid—alone or in combination with sodium lactate—is that it is safe but not proved effective.

Sodium bicarbonate   A common household chemical better known as *baking soda*, sodium bicarbonate does not acidify the vagina. On the contrary, it alkalizes, or neutralizes, it—at least briefly. Although evaluators could find no evidence to substantiate sodium bicarbonate's safety when used in douching, the compound is so widely used in food and as a home remedy that the Panel accepts it as safe.

But the reviewers claimed to have no idea of how neutralizing the vaginal secretions might enhance the growth of normal bacterial flora. In fact, no studies submitted show that brief treatment with sodium bicarbonate has any lasting effect whatsoever. So, while safe, the chemical's effectiveness remains in doubt.

Sodium carbonate   Like sodium bicarbonate, this compound has an alkalizing effect. It is quite corrosive at high concentrations. Even in the extreme dilutions in which it is formulated into douches its safety has not been well established. Neither is it clear to reviewers what, if any, effect its use has on the normal microorganisms of the vagina. Conclusion: both safety and effectiveness need to be proved.

Tartaric acid   This weak acid is a byproduct of grape fermentation in the production of wine. At low concentrations, it is considered safe. But the Panel received no data from manufacturers to show that adding tartaric acid to a douche will enhance vaginal acidity or that this will encourage the growth of normal vaginal flora. So, while safe, tartaric acid is yet to be shown effective as a vaginal acidifier.

Vinegar   *See* ACETIC ACID, above.

Disapproved Active Ingredients

In step with findings reported elsewhere in several sections of this book, the Panel rejected 4 douche ingredients because of boron content.

Boron compounds: boric acid, borogylcerin, sodium borate, and sodium perborate   These compounds are potent toxins (poisons) that reviewers say are unsafe for use in the vagina. Besides the issue of safety, no data were presented to show that boron compounds effectively alter the acidity of the vagina. Verdict: unsafe and ineffective.

ASTRINGENTS

The Panel has virtually nothing to say about whether an astringent is pharmacologically useful—and, if so, how—in a douche or other vaginal preparation. Generally speaking, astringents create a puckery sensation when applied to the skin or mucous membranes. They also pull proteins—including cellular debris and microorganisms—out of solution, and concentrate them. This may facilitate their removal from the body.

Approved Active Ingredients

None

Conditionally Approved Active Ingredients

Alum   This is a widely used astringent that may consist of ammonium aluminum sulfate or potassium aluminum sulfate, both of which are aluminum salts. Alum has a long medicinal history in the treatment of animals and humans, and while it is mildly toxic in high concentrations, the Panel says that the doses used in vaginal products —between 0.03 and 0.06 percent—appear to be safe. These doses are, however, far below the concentrations at which alum is usually regarded as being effectively astringent; the effectiveness of these low concentrations needs to be proved. Also, if alum is to be used at concentrations of 0.5 to 5 percent—doses generally recognized as effective— then its safety will have to be proved. At present no data are available to show that these concentrations are safe for intravaginal application. Here the Panel's verdict is twofold. Alum can be considered not proved safe *or* not proved effective, depending on the dosage.

Zinc sulfate   The dose of zinc sulfate currently used in douches, 0.02 percent, is low enough to be safe, but it is far below what are considered to be effective astringent levels. So if the currently used dose is maintained, it will have to be proved to be effective. And if the dose generally accepted as effective is used, it will have to be proved safe for use in the vagina. In short, depending on the concentration in which it is used, zinc sulfate is assessed as either not proved safe *or* not proved effective for use in the vagina.

Disapproved Active Ingredients

Boron compounds: boric acid, borogylcerin, sodium borate, and sodium perborate   As noted above and in other sections of this book, compounds derived from boron are unsafe because of its toxicity. Furthermore, no evidence was submitted to show that these substances effectively act as an astringent.

DETERGENTS

Many douche products contain ingredients that lower surface tension on the vaginal wall. This action facilitates removal of vaginal secretions, discharge, and debris—so such preparations are said to have a cleansing or detergent effect.

CLAIMS

Accurate
"removes vaginal debris, discharge"
"removes vaginal secretions"
"mild detergent action"
"thins out vaginal mucus, discharge"

Approved Active Ingredients

The 4 vaginal detergents considered safe were assessed in pairs. So they are listed this way in the discussion that follows.

Dioctyl sodium sulfosuccinate and sodium lauryl sulfate Pharmacologically, these are similar compounds that are generally recognized as wetting, solubilizing, mucus-removing agents. Although toxic in high doses, they are judged safe at the levels used in douches: 25.3 mg of dioctyl sodium sulfosuccinate per dose; 98 to 200 mg of sodium lauryl sulfate per dose.

The Panel cites no data to show that these ingredients are specifically useful. Nevertheless, on the basis of the compounds' recognized detergent properties and wide use in various drugs, they were judged as effective as well as safe for vaginal application as long as the above-noted dose levels are maintained.

These drugs are also safe and effective for the treatment of *Trichomonas vaginalis* ("tric") when that condition has been diagnosed by a physician, who then supervises their use in treating the infection.

Nonoxynol 9 and octoxynol 9 When used in spermicides these surface-acting compounds were found to be safe. The Panel's report does not mention any specific evidence of how well these compounds work to soften and loosen discharge and debris from the vagina. The vote for a rating of "effective" is based on how well they perform in other drugs used for wetting, solubilizing, and mucus removal.

The safe and effective dose for products that contain nonoxynol 9 is 1.765 grams per vaginal dose. The safe and effective dose of octoxynol 9 is 0.866 grams per vaginal dose. Both these doses work out to less than $\frac{1}{10}$ of 1 percent of the douche itself.

Conditionally Approved Active Ingredients

The Panel was able to grant only conditional approval to several drugs that are alleged to help remove mucus and other debris from the vaginal wall. In most instances it is effectiveness rather than safety that remains in doubt.

Alkyl aryl sulfonate   Animal studies confirm that this substance, commercially used as an insecticide, is safe. But no studies were submitted to show that alkyl aryl sulfonate removes mucus from the vagina. The Panel has doubts about its effectiveness. While categorizing the compound as safe, reviewers stipulate that its effectiveness must be established through testing if this preparation is to remain on the market.

Lactic acid   Although rated as safe, the Panel noted that no data have been presented showing that lactic acid has mucus-removing properties that would subtantiate its usefulness in a vaginal douche. So while safe, lactic acid is granted only tentative approval for want of evidence that it is effective as a vaginal detergent.

Papain   This protein-dissolving enzyme from the papaya tree is the principal ingredient in meat tenderizers. Papain has seen long-term use for the treatment of open wounds. Since no adverse effects have been reported, the present Panel feels that papain is safe for use in the vagina—even though no *specific* toxicity studies were submitted. No data were submitted to show that this enzyme effectively removes secretions from the vaginal wall when used in a douche. Conclusion: safe but not proved effective.

Povidone-iodine   The Panel considered this a detergent whose safety and effectiveness remain in doubt.
Note: An FDA summary document indicates that the Panel recategorized and reevaluated povidone-iodine and will list it as approved—that is to say, safe and effective—as a *vaginal anti-irritant* in its final published report.

Sodium bicarbonate   The Panel lists this substance (household baking soda) as safe but not proved effective as a detergent-type drug for use in the vagina.

Sodium lactate This substance, too, was listed as safe but not proved effective as a vaginal detergent.

Disapproved Active Ingredients

Boron compounds: boric acid, borogylcerin, sodium borate, sodium perborate The potent toxin boron makes these substances unsafe for vaginal use. In addition, no evidence was presented to show that boron derivatives actually work to soften, loosen, or remove mucus or other secretions and debris. The Panel's decision: not safe and not effective.

Inactive Ingredients

A variety of inactive ingredients are put into douches and other vaginal self-treatments for cosmetic or formulation purposes.

For the most part they are harmless, but the Panel expresses concern about the safety of 2 of them. Silica (fine) is abrasive and potentially dangerous to the soft tissues of the vagina. Camphor is readily absorbed through mucosal tissues and is highly toxic (*see* CAMPHOR). Inactive ingredients are:

alcohol	lactose	purified water
amerchol L 101	menthol	silica, fine
aromatic oils	methylparaben	sodium chloride
camphor	methyl salicylate	stearic acid
cetyl alcohol	oil of eucalyptus	sodium sulfate
chlorothymol	oil of peppermint	thymol
eucalyptol	polysorbate 20	tragacanth
fragrance	potassium hydroxide	water-soluble
glycerin	propylene glycol	ingredients of
isopropyl myristate	propylparaben	chlorophyll

Safety and Effectiveness: Active Ingredients
in Over-the-Counter Douches and Other Vaginal Applications

Panel's Tentative Assessment

Active Ingredient	As Anti-irritant	As Acidifier or Alkalinizer	As Astringent	As Detergent
acetic acid		safe but not proved effective		
alkyl aryl sulfonate				safe but not proved effective
allantoin	safe but not proved effective			
aloe vera, stabilized gel	safe but not proved effective			
alum			not proved safe (high dose); safe but not proved effective (low dose)	
ammonium aluminum sulfate (*see* alum)				
benzalkonium chloride	not proved safe or effective			
benzethonium chloride	not proved safe or effective			
benzocaine	safe but not proved effective			
boric acid	not safe or effective	not safe or effective	not safe or effective	not safe or effective
boroglycerin	not safe or effective	not safe or effective	nor safe or effective	not safe or effective
calcium propionate	safe and effective			
citric acid		safe but not proved effective		
dioctyl sodium sulfosuccinate				safe and effective
edetate disodium	not proved safe or effective			
edetate sodium	not proved safe or effective			
hexachlorophene	not safe or effective			
lactic acid		safe but not proved effective		safe but not proved effective
lactic acid + sodium lactate	safe but not proved effective	safe but not proved effective		
nonoxynol 9	safe but not proved effective			safe and effective
octoxynol 9	safe but not proved effective			safe and effective

oxyquinoline citrate	not proved safe or effective	
oxyquinoline sulfate	not proved safe or effective	
papain		safe but not proved effective
phenol (under 1.5%)*	not proved safe or effective	
phenol (over 1.5%)	not safe or effective	
phenolate sodium (under 1.5% phenol)	not proved safe or effective	
phenolate sodium (over 1.5% phenol)	not safe or effective	
potassium aluminum sulfate (see alum)		
potassium sorbate	safe and effective	
povidone-iodine†	not proved safe or effective	safe but not proved effective
sodium bicarbonate (alkalizer)	safe but not proved effective	
sodium borate	not safe or effective	not safe or effective
sodium carbonate (alkalizer)	not proved safe or effective	
sodium lactate		safe but not proved effective
sodium lauryl sulfate		safe and effective
sodium perborate	not safe or effective	not safe or effective
sodium propionate	safe and effective	
sodium salicylate	not safe or effective	
sodium salicylic acid	not safe or effective	
sodium salicylic acid phenolate (over 1.5%)		safe but not proved effective
tartaric acid	safe but not proved effective	
vinegar (see acetic acid)	safe but not proved effective	
vitamin A		not proved safe (high dose); safe but not proved effective (low dose)
vitamin D		
zinc sulfate		

*An FDA summary document indicates that phenol ingredients will be downgraded to unsafe and ineffective in the Panel's final published report.

†An FDA summary document indicates that this ingredient may be recategorized and upgraded to a safe and effective *vaginal anti-irritant* in the Panel's final published report.

Safety and Effectiveness: Combination Products Sold Over-the-Counter for Douching and Other Vaginal Self-Treatment

Safe and Effective

Conditionally Safe and Effective

citric acid + papain
oxyquinoline sulfate + alkyl aryl sulfonate + disodium edetate
nonoxynol 9 + sodium edetate
alum + zinc sulfate
benzalkonium chloride + disodium edetate
sodium lactate + lactic acid + octoxynol 9
sodium lauryl sulfate + sodium bicarbonate + sodium carbonate
stabilized aloe vera gel + allantoin + vitamin A + vitamin D

Not Safe or Not Effective

hexachlorophene + boric acid + zinc sulfate + alum + tartaric acid +
 camphor + phenol + octoxynol 9
phenol (greater than 1.5%) + sodium borate + sodium salicylate
sodium salicylic acid phenolate (phenol greater than 1.5%) + boroglycerin +
 benzocaine
sodium salicylic acid phenolate (phenol greater than 1.5%) + boroglycerin +
 benzocaine + povidone-iodine
phenol + sodium phenolate (phenol greater than 1.5%)
sodium perborate + sodium borate + sodium lauryl sulfate
oxyquinoline citrate + boric acid + alum + zinc sulfate
calcium propionate + sodium propionate + boric acid
sodium borate + sodium lauryl sulfate

Douches: Product Ratings

Single-Ingredient Products

Product and Distributor	Dosage of Active Ingredients	Rating[1]	Comment
acetic acid (vinegar)			
New Freshness (Fleet)	**liquid**	**B**	not proved effective
Summer's Eve Disposable (Fleet)		**B**	
benzethonium chloride monohydrate			
Phemithyn (Scrip)	**solution: 3.17%**	**B**	not proved safe or effective

Douches: Product Ratings *(continued)*

Single-Ingredient Products

Product and Distributor	Dosage of Active Ingredients	Rating[1]	Comment
potassium sorbate Summer's Eve Medicated Disposable (Fleet)	**solution:** 1%	**A**	
povidone-iodine Betadine (Purdue Frederick)	**solution**	**B**	not proved safe or effective; an FDA summary document indicates that Betadine will be safe and effective in Panel's published report, in which case this product would be rated "A"

Combination Products

Product and Distributor	Dosage of Active Ingredients	Rating[1]	Comment
Bo-Car-Al (Beecham Products)	**powder:** boric acid + ammonium alum	**C**	not safe or effective
Gentle Spring Disposable (Block Drug)	**powder:** edetate sodium + sodium lauryl sulfate + sodium phosphate	**C**	sodium phosphate not submitted to or assessed by Panel
Massengill (Beecham Products)	**liquid concentrate:** lactic acid + sodium bicarbonate + octoxynol 9	**B**	first two ingredients not proved effective
	powder: boric acid + ammonium alum	**C**	boric acid not safe or effective
Triva (Boyle)	**powder:** 2% oxyquinoline sulfate + 35% alkyl aryl sulfonate + 0.33% edetate sodium	**B**	not proved effective
trichotene (Reed & Carnrick)	**liquid:** sodium lauryl sulfate + sodium borate	**C**	borate not safe or effective

1. Author's interpretation of Panel criteria. Based on contents, not claims.

Ear-Care Aids

Ear disorders are difficult to self-diagnose; they usually require medical attention and prescription drugs. For these reasons the Panel approves only one type of nonprescription self-treatment of the ear: agents that soften and loosen ear wax. Ear ache, drainage of fluid from the ear, itching, any hearing impairment, and ringing in the ears or other unusual sensations all require medical attention. (Specialists in ear care are called otologists or otolaryngologists.)

Heat is a popular remedy for ear ache. The Panel does not object to the hot-water bottle approach to pain, but it recommended that pain-relieving ingredients be banned from ear-care aids, such as ear-drops. If you have an ear ache, see a doctor.

EAR WAX

Cerumen, the technical name for ear wax, is a yellowish-brown material composed of several substances secreted from glands in the outer part of the ear canal. Ear wax is water-repellent and it plays a role in protecting the ear from moisture, injury, and infection.

The ear canal is self-cleansing: when one chews food slowly ear wax is moved, and sloughed-off cells and other debris are gently forced outward. Swimmers and divers, whose ears are constantly flushed out by water, have reduced amounts of wax in their ears—which may be why they are prone to the itchy disorder called "swimmer's ear," as well as other infectious ear conditions. The protective action of ear wax may also be lost as the result of overzealous cleansing or picking at one's ear.

Panel reviewers say that the best thing to do about ear wax is to leave it alone. If something *must* be inserted to remove some of it, the object of choice is the tip of a finger. The evaluators frown on sticks and hairpins, but reserve their greatest scorn for cotton-tipped wooden applicators. These devices push the wax inward rather than pull it outward and may even injure or puncture the eardrum.

Many people have misconceptions about ear wax. Experts explain that:

EAR-CARE AIDS is based on the report "OTC Topical Otic Drugs" by the FDA's Advisory Review Panel on OTC Topical Analgesic, Antirheumatic, Otic Burn, and Sunburn Prevention and Treatment Drug Products, and the FDA's Tentative Final Order on these drugs.

- it does not cause deafness
- it does not cause the normal loss of hearing that occurs with age
- it does not imply poor hygiene
- it does not require daily removal with cotton applicators or other instruments

For most people, occasionally wiping off the outer ear with a wash-cloth is treatment enough for removal of excess ear wax. But a minority of individuals have a tendency—and this may be inherited—to accumulate this wax, which from time to time must be removed by other means. These people characteristically may feel the buildup of wax as a sense of fullness in the ear. To relieve the condition, self-treatment with nonprescription ear-wax softening agents is judged to be safe and effective. These substances infiltrate, soften and loosen the wax so that it can be gently flushed out with warm water. If the wax has become hard-packed, however, its removal should be left to a doctor.

CLAIMS

Accurate
"for occasional use as an aid in the removal of excessive ear wax"
"softens and loosens excessive ear wax"
"aids in the removal of accumulated ear wax"

False or Misleading
promotes "ear hygiene" (the ears are clean)
"wax prevention" (wax is protective and should be present)
"aids healing"
for "itching," "pain" "raw, inflamed tissues," "relief of swimmer's ear"

DRUGS FOR EAR-WAX REMOVAL

Softening agents—approved for nonprescription use—infiltrate, soften, and loosen the wax mechanically so that it can be gently flushed out with warm water from an ear syringe. (An NIH specialist notes, however, that a jet of water from an ear syringe can injure the ear—particularly if the eardrum has been perforated.) Cerumnolytic agents are solvents that melt the wax. They are stronger, and they are *not safe* for nonprescription use.

If symptoms of fullness persist following self-removal of ear wax, or the maneuver causes pain or dizziness, it is recommended that a doctor's help be sought. One should not attempt to remove wax accumulations if one has an ear ache, ear drainage, or perforated eardrum. Also, wax softeners should not be used on children under 12 except as specified by a doctor.

Approved Active Ingredient

Carbamide peroxide, in glycerin   The substance carbamide peroxide—which also is known as *urea hydrogen peroxide*—effervesces when brought in contact with body tissue in the ear. The hydrogen peroxide releases its oxygen component, which in turn loosens tissue debris and wax. The urea also acts to remove loose, dead bits of tissue.

Experts specify that 6.5 percent by weight is the safe concentration of carbamide peroxide, dissolved in anhydrous glycerol. The mixture's safety and effectiveness in softening ear wax has been established by long clinical use, but there are no acceptable studies to confirm this action.

Directions for use are the same as for glycerin (*see* below).

Conditionally Approved Active Ingredient

Glycerin   Discovered 2 centuries ago, this is a viscous substance that stays in one place in the ear and appears to slowly soften ear wax. But there are no scientifically controlled studies to show this is so or how it works. Glycerin is extremely safe, except that it may irritate broken skin. Glycerin may be called glycerol or glycerine; when it is formulated without water it is called anhydrous glycerol.

The reviewers approve a 95 percent glycerin solution in water and recommend that it be put into the ear with a dropper and kept there by tilting the head. After 15 minutes, the glycerin and ear-wax debris can be removed with lukewarm water injected from an ear syringe. This treatment can be repeated once, if necessary, for each ear. By whatever name, the FDA says glycerin, while safe, has not been proved effective for loosening ear wax for removal.

Disapproved Active Ingredients

None

OTHER EAR-CARE PRODUCTS

The Panel did not approve for self-treatment any product other than those for softening and loosening wax. Two pain-relieving agents that have been included in over-the-counter ear products are judged by the Panel to be unsafe and ineffective.

Disapproved Active Ingredients

Antipyrine   Nominally speaking this is a pain-relieving agent, but in fact it is an irritant and may cause pain when used in ear drops. It has no effect on ear wax. Antipyrine is not safe, nor is it effective as an ingredient for over-the-counter ear medications.

Benzocaine   This is a widely used anesthetic that sometimes is present in ear drops available by prescription. The Panel says it is dangerous in nonprescription preparations because its numbing effect can mask painful symptoms of infection that requires medical care. Moreover, since the tissues of the ear canal and eardrum are not highly absorbent, it is not clear how much pain relief benzocaine can in fact provide.

Finally, benzocaine does not facilitate ear-wax removal—so it was evaluated as unsafe and ineffective for nonprescription use in the ears.

Safety and Effectiveness: Active Ingredients in Over-the-Counter Ear-Care Products

Active Ingredient	Action	Panel's Assessment
antipyrine	pain reliever	not safe or effective
benzocaine	pain reliever	not safe or effective
glycerin (glycerol and anhydrous glycerol)	ear-wax softener	not proved effective
carbamide peroxide, in glycerin (urea hydrogen peroxide)	ear-wax softener	safe and effective

Ear-Care Aids: Product Ratings

Product and Distributor	Dosage of Active Ingredients	Rating[1]	Comment
Benadyne Ear Drops, Improved (Rugby)	**ear drops:** 6.5% carbamide peroxide in anhydrous glycerin	A	
Debrox (Marion)		A	
Murine Ear Drops (Abbott)		A	

Ear-Care Aids: Product Ratings *(continued)*

Product and Distributor	Dosage of Active Ingredients	Rating[1]	Comment
Dri-Ear (Pfeiffer)	**ear drops:** 2.75% boric acid	C	drugs to dry swimmer's ear not approved by Panel for use without prescription
E.R.O. (Scherer)	**ear drops:** 95% glycerin	B	not proved effective

1. Author's interpretation of Panel/FDA criteria. Based on contents, not claims.

Eye Drops and Ointments

The eye is one of the most sensitive organs that people self-treat with nonprescription drugs. Structurally, the eyes are well protected from disease and injurious objects. They are tough. But they are also vulnerable and may easily sustain serious damage. A principal hazard of self-care with nonprescription eye drops and ointments is that diagnosis, frequently based on guesswork, can lead to incorrect self-treatment that, in turn, can worsen the symptoms or the disease itself. The Panel warns that the drugs described in this unit should not be used for more than 72 hours without a doctor's diagnosis and supervision. Ophthalmologists (medical doctors who care for eyes) are the specialists to consult when something is wrong with one's eyes.

"There are very few disorders of the eye which are amenable to treatment with OTC ocular preparations," the Panel says. These drugs for the most part only "relieve symptoms." They "do not have any truly curative effect."

The safety of eye drugs is easier to test than most other drugs, because of a very responsive—but now quite controversial—method called the Draize test. Chemicals are put into the eyes of rabbits, which are held in stockades so they cannot remove the drugs with their feet or by rubbing their eyes against their cages. Rabbits' eyes are considered to be more sensitive than people's, and irritation, inflammation,

EYE DROPS AND OINTMENTS is based on the report of the FDA's Advisory Review Panel on OTC Ophthalmic Drug Products.

and other adverse changes caused by the material being tested are easy to detect. The problem, animal lovers say, is that the Draize test is cruel. Advocates reply that it is better to discover that a drug is harmful in rabbits' eyes than in those of people.

Data on the effectiveness of nonprescription eye drugs, as with many other groups of over-the-counter drugs, is scanter than one might wish. Because of the limited number of well-controlled, well-executed studies, the Panel had to rely on less scientific data—such as long use, acceptance by doctors, and manufacturers' marketing data on user satisfaction.

CLAIMS

Accurate

for "temporary relief" of "minor" eye problems
for "discomfort from minor irritations"
for "dryness," "redness," or "external infections"

False or Misleading

for "tired eyes," "fatigue," or "eyes over forty"
for "continuous everyday use"
for "improvement of tired eyes"
for "use before putting on makeup"
produces "sparkling," "bright," "diamond," or "bedroom" eyes

It is wrong to suggest that cosmetic benefits result from use of these drugs. The Panel wants to ban all references to eye appearance in labeling claims, on the grounds that they promote continuing use of eye drugs—which could be dangerous. No eye product is particularly suitable or helpful for people of any particular age group, demographic group, or gender.

WHICH EYE CONDITIONS ARE SELF-TREATABLE?

The evaluators' conservatism prompted them to define far more specifically than most other Panels the disorders it believes should—and should not—be self-treated.

Self-Treatable Conditions

Tear insufficiency This condition, sometimes called "dry eye," is caused by sun, wind, and chemical irritants and also by aging and several serious eye diseases. The over-the-counter drugs that relieve the symptoms of tear insufficiency are called *ocular demulcents* (soothers). They moisten the eye, lubricate it, and guard and enhance its protective tear-fluid (*see* EYES: ARTIFICIAL TEARS). Some contact-lens wearers use them to maintain a moist, protective environment where the plastic lenses meet eye surfaces. However, this use falls outside the purview of the FDA's over-the-counter drug review and will not be considered in this book.

Corneal edema   This is a serious condition, in which the cornea swells with fluid. It can cause excruciating pain and dim the vision. Corneal edema *can* be treated with nonprescription drugs—*but only under a doctor's supervision*. (The disease and its treatment are described more fully in EYES: CORNEAL EDEMA.)

Foreign bodies in the eye   When acid or some other chemical splashes into the eye, emergency care is required. Treatment is also needed—albeit less urgently—for pollen, dust, smog, and other solid, liquid, and gaseous pollutants that enter and irritate the eye. Eyewashes, lotions, and eye-irrigating solutions are available for diluting these substances and washing them out. Their emergency and first-aid uses are described under EYEWASH.

All chemical burns of the eye require medical attention after emergency measures have been taken. If a foreign body cannot be removed, one should see a doctor without delay.

Irritation and inflammation   If mild, these conditions can be self-treated. They principally affect the transparent, front part of the eyeball (the cornea); the "whites" of the eyes; and the pinkish-white areas called the conjunctiva. These surfaces need to be slippery and moist. Normally moisture is provided by tear-fluid.

When the conjunctiva are irritated (conjunctivitis), the eye responds by tearing copiously. If this fails to remove the irritant, the eye tissue absorbs fluids and swells up, blood vessels dilate (widen) and fill with blood, creating what is called "red eye" or, more commonly, "bloodshot eyes." When this occurs the eyes may itch, smart, burn, and continue to tear. If the pain is intense, a doctor's help should be sought —in a hospital emergency room if need be. (*See* EYEWASH for emergency treatment of chemical burns.)

Red eye is not always caused by environmental pollutants. Eye drugs, even those prescribed by a doctor, can also cause it. So can trauma—for example, being hit on or near the eye—and allergic reactions, infections, and increased pressure inside the eyeball (which can occur with a serious underlying disease like glaucoma). Since there is often no way for a person to know what is causing the inflammation and irritation, self-treatment with over-the-counter drugs should not continue for more than 3 days. If the symptoms get worse in this time, one should consult a doctor at once. Persons who know they have glaucoma should *never* self-treat their eyes except under their doctors' supervision, because doing so may worsen an already serious condition or delay getting urgently needed prescription drugs or other treatment.

The Panel approves self-treatment for red eye that results when a foreign object has been successfully removed from the eye. It also approves self-treatment for inflammation and irritation caused by gases, smoke, and other air pollutants, and from the water in chlorinated swimming pools. Reddening of the eyes is very often an allergic response. Cold compresses over the eye may bring relief or the redness, itching, and tearing may be safely relieved by over-the-counter drugs. If self-treatment fails to relieve the irritation, inflammation, and swelling, a doctor's help should be sought.

Conditions Possibly Self-Treatable

Evaluators say several types of minor infections might suitably be self-treated with over-the-counter drugs—*if* safe and effective drugs were available for the purpose. But it says no such products exist at present.

The FDA takes an even tougher stance than the Panel on self-treatment of eye infections. It says there is often a similarity between the symptoms of minor infections and serious infections so that the ordinary lay person has no way of distinguishing between them. The FDA therefore has decided that the risks of self-treating minor infections outweigh the benefits. It has tentatively decided to announce, at the next stage of the OTC Drug Review of Ophthalmic Products, that the use of nonprescription drugs to self-treat eye infections is unsafe and that such products should be banned.

The minor infections that the Panel—but not the FDA—would allow to be self-treated are:

Stye This condition, technically called *hordeolum*, is a staphylococcal abscess that develops in skin glands on the edge of the eyelid. A stye on the eye looks red and swollen and may be quite sore. Warm, moist compresses and anti-infective drugs—whether nonprescription or prescription—are the usual treatments. These infections tend to recur.

Granulated eyelids Redness, itching, burning, and crusting along the eyelid margins is called blepharitis: *blepharo*-means "eyelid"; -*itis* means "inflammation." The cause is likely to be a staph infection, or dandruff, or the two together. When staph is the principal cause, the scales that form on the lids tend to be small and dry; when dandruff is principally to blame, they are oily. Persons affected by the latter variety usually have scalp dandruff.

The treatment for granulated eyelids is control of head dandruff, removing scales on the eyelid margin by using a cotton applicator, and treatment with an anti-infective ophthalmic ointment.

Pink eye   The Panel draws a not-altogether-clear distinction between red eye, which is mild conjunctivitis due to allergic response (and which is unquestionably self-treatable) and pink eye, which is a more serious conjunctivitis that may be allergic but also may be caused by bacterial or viral infections. So "pink" is worse than "red." Evaluators were cautious, although not wholly opposed to attempts to self-treat the condition as long as an individual sees a doctor if the eye does not clear up within 3 days.

Two signs of pink eye are redness and discharge. The main symptom is a feeling that sand is in the eye. Vision is not impaired and there is little pain. If the pink eye is bacterial in origin, the cause is likely to be pneumococcus, *Staphylococcus aureus*, hemophilus bacteria, or hemolytic streptococci. On the one hand, the Panel says that medical help should be sought to identify the infectious organism and propose or prescribe a suitable broad-spectrum antibiotic or sulfonamide for treatment. On the other hand, it permits self-treatment.

The risk of treatment with nonprescription drugs, of course, is that secondary infections may arise in the cornea, injuring its light-transmitting surface. Evaluators nevertheless believe that self-treatment can be attempted for up to 3 days without undue hazard. But the FDA, as noted above, disagrees, and recommends that all eye infections be treated by a doctor.

Conditions Not Self-Treatable

A number of eye problems clearly require medical assistance; they are:

Embedded foreign body   If an eyewash will not clear a foreign body from the eye, help must be sought from a doctor or other qualified health professional.

Uveitis   This is inflammation that affects the iris—the tissue that makes one blue-, brown- or green-eyed—or related structures inside the eyeball. Uveitis is a serious disease and medical care is necessary.

Glaucoma   The increased pressure inside the eyeball that characterizes this disease often leads to blindness. The eyes may appear red, prompting attempts at self-treatment with nonprescription vasocon-strictors (preparations that constrict blood vessels). This is a mistake. Only a doctor can decide what drug is needed—and a vasoconstrictor is unlikely to be it.

Flash burns   The ultraviolet rays emitted by welding torches can cause flash burns that redden the eye. These burns will heal, but medical attention is a must.

Tear-duct infections   In these rare infections the inner corner of the eye becomes swollen, sore, and red. Pus appears. It is essential that a doctor provide the treatment.

Corneal ulcers   Besides being quite painful, these sores—which may be caused by microorganisms or other factors—endanger one's vision. Medical treatment is the only answer.

SPECIAL NEEDS OF EYE MEDICATIONS

Treating the eye with drugs is harder than it may seem. For one thing, the drugs do not stay put: the normal turnover time for tear-fluid in the eye is 16 percent per minute. This means that at the end of 3 minutes, half of a drug dose already will have vanished down the tiny drainage holes in the corners of the eyes, through which tears drain into the nostrils. Ointments applied under the lower lid may stay in place longer than liquid eye drops.

INACTIVE INGREDIENTS

Because the eye is so sensitive, drugs for use in it must be formulated very carefully. This means, for one thing, that a variety of inactive ingredients are required to make the final product suitable for the eye: Preservatives are required to prevent bacterial contamination of products before use. Buffering agents are needed to stabilize the products chemically while keeping them close to the acidity of tear fluid. Tonicity agents are required to keep the preparations close to tear fluid in salinity (saltiness) and thereby in osmotic pressure. Ointment bases and chemical stabilizers also may be required. And soothers (demulcents) may be included as viscosity agents that briefly thicken the tear-fluid or slow its drainage from the eye by other means. The only acceptable solvent for eye drugs is sterile water.

Reviewers also assessed the following inactive ingredients used in nonprescription eye drugs.

Suitable buffering agents

acetic acid
boric acid
hydrochloric acid
phosphoric acid
potassium bicarbonate
potassium carbonate
potassium citrate

potassium phosphates
    (monobasic, dibasic,
    or tribasic)
potassium tetraborate
sodium acetate
sodium bicarbonate
sodium biphosphate

sodium borate
sodium carbonate
sodium citrate
sodium hydroxide
sodium phosphate

Suitable ointment bases

lanolin preparations (including
    anhydrous lanolin and nonionic
    lanolin derivatives)
light mineral oil
mineral oil

paraffin
white ointment
white petrolatum
white wax

Unsuitable ointment bases

cod-liver oil
corn oil
cottonseed oil
peanut oil

Suitable preservative agents

benzalkonium chloride
benzethonium chloride
cetylpyridinium chloride
chlorhexidine gluconate
chlorhexidine hydrochloride
chlorobutanol
methylparaben in combination with
    other approved preservatives
phenylethyl alcohol
phenylmercuric acetate

phenylmercuric nitrate
propylparaben in combination with
    other approved preservatives
sodium benzoate in combination
    with other approved
    preservatives
sodium propionate
sorbic acid in combination with
    other approved preservatives
thimerosal

Unsuitable preservative agents

methylparaben
propylparaben
sodium benzoate
sorbic acid

Suitable stabilizing agents and antioxidants

edetate calcium disodium
edetate disodium (EDTA)

edetate sodium
edetate trisodium

edetic acid
ethylendiaminetetraacetic acid
 (EDTA) (max. 0.1%)
sodium bisulfate (max. 0.1%)

sodium metabisulfate (max. 0.1%)
sodium thiosulfate (max. 0.2%)
thiourea (max. 0.1%)

Suitable viscosity agents

carboxymethylcellulose sodium
dextran 70
gelatin
glycerin
hydroxyethylcellulose
hydroxypropylmethylcellulose

polyethylene glycol 300
polyethylene glycol 400
polysorbate 80
polyvinyl alcohol
povidone
propylene glycol

Unsuitable colorants

berbine bisulfate
berbine hydrochloride
berbine sulfate
hydratine hydrochloride

Unsuitable odorants

camphor
camphor water
geranium oil, Algerian
peppermint oil

peppermint water
rose and camphor water
rosewater
witch hazel

COMBINATION PRODUCTS

This Panel, like others, took a dim view of combination products. Single-ingredient products are safer. But it approved a few combinations, particularly of 2 or 3 demulcents and the one approved astringent plus a vasoconstrictor. Two or more emollient ingredients also may be combined.

The Panel dealt with what might appear to be a bewildering array of eye-drug ingredients. But for consumers who wish to restrict themselves to safe and effective single-ingredient products or combinations, the choice is narrower—and thus simpler—than it may seem.

For two classes of drugs—*ocular anesthetics* and *ocular anti-infectives*—there is no safe and effective ingredient.

There is only a single safe and effective *ocular astringent*, zinc sulfate.

Reviewers approved 4 *ocular vasoconstrictors*, but only 1 per product.

The remainder of the approved ingredients, *demulcents* and *emollients*, are principally useful for their physical properties, rather than chemical activity—which is minimal at most. The only approved combinations of chemically active ingredients are: demulcents + an approved vasoconstrictor, or zinc sulfate, or both.

ANESTHETICS

An anesthetic masks pain, so the Advisory Panel believes it is extremely dangerous to self-treat an eye with an anesthetic.

Pain relief may dangerously delay medical help for a rapidly deteriorating problem caused by corneal abrasion (a wearing away of the eyeball's outer layer), an embedded foreign body, or serious eye disease. Worse, anesthetic agents used in the drugs can themselves cause serious damage to the eye, even with one application. So the judgment of *whether*, *when*, and *how* to use anesthetics must be made by a doctor. Accordingly, the Panel wants all anesthetics removed from nonprescription eye drugs, and all claims made for them dropped from product labels and ads.

Approved Active Ingredients

None

Conditionally Approved Active Ingredients

None

Disapproved Active Ingredients

Two specific nonprescription ingredients that are claimed to be anesthetics were assessed.

Antipyrine This is not an anesthetic, as one manufacturer claims, but rather is a pain-reliever. The 0.4 percent antipyrine solution in the product submitted was found to have only slight anesthetic effect—so it is ineffective as well as unsafe.

Piperocaine hydrochloride An effective ocular anesthetic in 2 percent solutions or 4 percent ointments, this substance may be appropriate for prescription use. But because it can effectively curb pain that really signals the need to see a doctor, the substance was judged unsafe for use in over-the-counter medications.

ANTI-INFECTIVES

An anti-infective kills or limits the growth and multiplication of bacteria and other microorganisms. Self-treatment of eye infections with nonprescription anti-infectives is a controversial subject. The Panel points out that minor infections on the *external* surfaces of the eye—that is, *not* on or in the eyeball—usually are not dangerous. They will heal of their own accord rather quickly. So self-treatment could be recommended if safe and effective drugs were available for the purpose. But none of the anti-infectives in over-the-counter products is considered safe and effective. One prescription anti-infective, sulfacetamide sodium, was evaluated in the hope that it could be recommended for availability over-the-counter. It turned out to be too irritating for self-treatment use.

The infectious conditions that *may* be self-treatable include stye, granulated eyelids, and pink eye, or conjunctivitis.

CLAIMS FOR ANTI-INFECTIVES

Accurate

for "the treatment of minor external infections of the eye"

Approved Active Ingredients

None

Conditionally Approved Active Ingredients

Boric acid   Eye drops and ointments that contain this anti-infective agent—which is also called *boracic acid* and *orthoboric acid*—have been widely used for years. In low concentrations of around 1 percent, it may be useful in adjusting a product's acidity. But boric acid's anti-infective potency when put into the eye has not been proved, although it has been a standard eye-product ingredient for decades.

Without any doubt, boric acid will kill bacteria. But one investigator discovered that in order to be truly effective at this task, it must remain in contact with the bacteria for at least 24 hours. Within a matter of minutes, liquid ingredients put into the eye are diluted 10 times by tear-fluid. Ointments may keep the active drug in contact with the eye for a while longer. Even so, the Panel finds no data to support the notion that boric acid in an ointment reaches a concentration that will adequately stop bacterial growth.

Much has been said by other Panels about the growing evidence that boric acid is unsafe as well as of dubious effectiveness. This ingredient is used in a variety of products. To locate additional discussions on boric acid consult the index. The present Panel says that the tiny amounts present in over-the-counter eye products pose no risk. But its effectiveness—now much in question—remains to be proved.

Mercuric oxide, yellow   Recent reports from ophthalmologists indicate that some patients delay seeking care for eye infections while they self-treat with mercuric oxide, which has been used in eye drugs for a century. This sometimes causes serious consequences. The other side of the coin is that one manufacturer reports that he sold more than 1 million units of a yellow mercuric oxide preparation, yet received only a few minor complaints about it. However, the Panel thinks that the safety question is unresolved. It adds that there is insufficient evidence to show that the mercury present in these products effectively inhibits bacterial growth. So safety and effectiveness both remain unestablished.

Silver protein, mild   There is no question that silver can inhibit bacterial growth. But there is considerable doubt about the effectiveness of currently marketed nonprescription eye preparations that contain 20 to 40 mg of silver per milliliter of solution. While continuing use of silver could stain the eyes and adjacent skin gray or brown, evaluators found no risk of this (or other complications) from 2 or 3 days' use of these products. So the substances are safe, but their effectiveness remains to be proved.

Disapproved Active Ingredients

None

VASOCONSTRICTORS

Ocular vasoconstrictors constrict blood vessels in the eye. Those approved are all sympathomimetic amines. They mimic the natural action of the involuntary nervous system, acting by tightening smooth muscle, thus constricting or making blood vessels in the eye narrow. Bloodshot eyes are "whitened" in this way.

However, most of these preparations can provoke a rebound effect, in which the blood vessels dilate again and the eyes again appear red.

The treatment then is to stop using the drug and not to use more of it (which, unfortunately, is what some users are tempted to do).

Vasoconstrictors may also dilate the pupil. This is a particular risk for persons who wear contact lenses or whose corneas may have been scratched by other objects. Pupillary dilation can even lead to glaucoma, a very serious eye condition.

However, in view of the low concentrations used in over-the-counter products, these risks are slight enough that the evaluators say vasoconstrictors are safe. But the Panel warns that persons with diagnosed glaucoma, which could be made worse, should not use them.

CLAIMS FOR VASOCONSTRICTORS

Accurate
for "the relief of redness of the eye due to minor eye irritations"

False or Misleading
for "tired eyes" (an eye examination and glasses or stronger lenses are indicated)

Approved Active Ingredients

Ephedrine hydrochloride   This substance occurs naturally in the MaHuang plant, and the Chinese used it medicinally over 5,000 years ago. It was introduced into Western medicine in 1924, and now is usually produced synthetically. A 0.123 percent concentration of ephedrine has been used for years to treat minor eye irritation; it may be particularly valuable when the eyes are swollen by allergic reactions. The drug is safe and effective for adults and children. Correct dosage is 1 to 2 drops of a 0.123 percent concentration of ephedrine hydrochloride per eye, up to 4 times daily.

Naphazoline hydrochloride   In the low concentrations of 0.01 to 0.03 percent for which it is approved in nonprescription eye products, this vasoconstrictor is safe and effective. At higher dosages, however, it can dilate the pupils.

Tests show that naphazoline hydrochloride will correct—and may prevent—the red eyes that some people suffer when they swim in chlorinated swimming pools. For adults and for children, the approved dosage is 1 to 2 drops per affected eye of a 0.01 to 0.03 percent concentration of naphazoline hydrochloride, up to 4 times each day.

Phenylephrine hydrochloride (0.08 to 0.2 percent)   This vasoconstrictor has been a standard ingredient in over-the-counter eye products for a long time. Studies in animals and in humans show that it effectively rewhitens eyes that have been reddened for experimental purposes with irritating substances. In several tests, for example, phenylephrine hydrochloride was compared to eye-soothing artificial tears that did not contain a vasoconstrictor. Subjects were humans whose eyes had been reddened by exposure to the irritating body chemical *histamine* or to chlorinated water like that found in swimming pools. In all tests, the phenylephrine hydrochloride, in a 0.12 percent solution, was more effective than the tear substitute that lacked it. So this drug is judged safe and effective in dosage of 1 to 2 drops of 0.08 to 0.2 percent phenylephrine hydrochloride, used no more than 4 times per day.

Tetrahydrozoline hydrochloride   This drug has been shown to be effective in relieving conjunctivitis caused by allergies and chemical and physical irritants. In one study of 348 patients, an investigator reported that 96 percent obtained relief from the drug. In another study of 808 patients, relief was obtained by 87 percent of the participants.

Tetrahydrozoline hydrochloride has the advantage that it rarely if ever dilates the pupil of a healthy eye. No cases of rebound conjunctivitis have been reported either. Thus, this ingredient is assessed as safe and effective. The approved dosage is 1 to 2 drops of a 0.01 to 0.05 percent solution of tetrahydrozoline hydrochloride in each affected eye, up to 4 times daily.

Conditionally Approved Active Ingredient

Phenylephrine hydrochloride (under 0.08 percent)   In this lower concentration the drug is undoubtedly safe. But evaluators could find no data to show that concentrations below 0.08 percent are effective. Thus the preparation was only conditionally approved.

Disapproved Active Ingredients

None

ASTRINGENTS

An astringent is a substance that "pulls" particles out of solution, holding and solidifying them. For the most part astringents do not enter body cells; they act on their outer layers or between individual cells.

These substances will draw the surface molecules of cells together, puckering the skin and mucosal surfaces. Only very weak astringent concentrations are found in nonprescription ophthalmic preparations. Reviewers believe they act mainly to clear mucin and perhaps other substances from the surface of the eye, and do not otherwise act on the outer layers of the cornea or conjunctiva (inner eyelid)—which could be dangerous.

Manufacturers have made inflated claims for eye astringents—suggesting that they will cure hay fever and styes. They will not, although they may relieve some symptoms of hay fever, such as itchiness and irritation.

CLAIMS FOR ASTRINGENTS

Accurate
> for "the temporary relief of discomfort from minor eye irritations"

False or Misleading
> relieves "congestion"
> "relief from tired eyes"
> "relief from most forms of minor eye distress"

Approved Active Ingredient

Zinc sulfate Some eye preparations contain zinc sulfate as their single active ingredient, but it is usually combined with a vasoconstrictor and sometimes other ingredients as well. Zinc sulfate's safety is attested to by the sale of millions of bottles of these products over several decades, with only very few adverse effects having been reported. In a 20-day Draize test, rabbits' left eyes, treated with zinc sulfate, showed no greater irritation than their right eyes, which were not treated.

Evaluators conclude from the available evidence that zinc sulfate is both safe and effective. The dosage is 1 to 2 drops of a 0.25 percent solution in the affected eye(s), up to 4 times daily.

Conditionally Approved Active Ingredient

Rose petals, infusion This substance is an extract from rosebud petals that contains volatile oils and other chemicals in undefined concentrations. Reviewers were not able to determine which was the astringent ingredient or how it works—if it does.

Safety testing in rabbits' eyes and clinical studies in human subjects indicate that this preparation is safe, however. The manufacturer of the product assessed by the Panel reported few complaints.

This preparation has been shown to relieve irritation in new users of contact lenses. The Panel judges this substance safe, but says more studies are required to prove that it is effective; otherwise, it should be removed from the market.

Disapproved Active Ingredients

None

DEMULCENTS

A demulcent is a substance that coats and protects mucous membrane surfaces. These compounds for the most part are chemically inert and provide beneficial effects through their protective physical properties. They help the tissues retain moisture and insulate them from sun, wind, and other environmental forces. They also slow the turnover of tear-fluid, or serve by other means to increase the water that is present on the eye surfaces. So they are sometimes called *artificial tears*. Demulcents are also used as wetting agents for contact lenses.

The Panel assessed the demulcent ingredients listed below. All of them were judged both safe and effective.

> cellulose derivatives
>> carboxymethylcellulose sodium
>> hydroxyethylcellulose
>> hydroxypropyl methylcellulose
>> methylcellulose
> dextran 70
> gelatin
> liquid polyols
>> glycerin
>> polyethylene glycol 300
>> polyethylene glycol 400
>> polysorbate 80
>> propylene glycol
>> polyvinyl alcohol
> povidone

For a more detailed discussion of these compounds and their use in relieving tear insufficiency ("dry eye"), *see* EYES: ARTIFICIAL TEARS. Demulcents are also formulated into safe and effective combination products that contain a vasoconstrictor and/or an astringent.

EMOLLIENTS

The emollients, like the demulcents, are inert, bland, soothing substances—with the difference that they are oily and therefore are less readily washed away by tear fluids. They soften the skin and hold in moisture, so they are useful for treating teary and irritated eyes. They also cover skin and mucosal surfaces, keeping out water-soluble irritants, air, and airborne bacteria. Emollients lubricate tissue—for example, the surfaces of the eyeball and the eyelids—and are also widely used as bases for other drugs for eye care.

Emollients are usually formulated as ointments. To apply them, one gently pulls down the lower eyelid and applies a ¼-inch-long ribbon of the product to the inside of the lid.

CLAIMS FOR EMOLLIENTS

Accurate

for "the temporary relief of discomfort due to minor irritations of the eye or to exposure to wind or sun"

for "use as a protectant against further irritation or to relieve dryness of the eye"

for "use as a lubricant to prevent further irritation or to relieve dryness of the eye"

Approved Active Ingredients

The Panel assessed 9 emollients in 2 categories, as grouped below. It approved all of them as safe and effective.

Lanolin preparations: anhydrous lanolin, lanolin, and nonionic lanolin derivatives   These substances are obtained from sheep-skin secretions that are extracted from wool. Lanolin contains about 25 percent water; anhydrous lanolin is lanolin with the water removed. Lanolin is a yellowish semisolid fat with little or no odor. A fair number of people are allergic to it, but the reviewers believe that the small amounts in ophthalmic drugs are unlikely to cause allergic reactions.

The more refined and purified nonionic lanolin derivatives are less likely to cause this problem. One such product has been marketed for years and no serious adverse effects have been reported as the result of its use.

Vision may blur briefly when lanolin preparations are first put in the eyes; this is not harmful. In most emollient products intended for use in the eye, lanolin is present in concentrations of 1 to 10 percent in white petrolatum or mineral oil.

Basing their assessment on wide usage and the protective and lubricating qualities of these preparations, the Panel judges lanolins to be safe and effective emollients and lubricants. The dosage for adults and children is a ¼-inch-long streak of ointment applied to the inside of the eyelid.

Oily ingredients: light mineral oil, mineral oil, paraffin, white ointment, white petrolatum, and white wax These are bland and essentially inert substances that are the bases—with or without lanolin —for virtually all ophthalmic ointments. All are derived from petrolatum—except white wax, which is made by bees and has a honeylike odor. White wax and paraffin are harder than the other oily ingredients listed here, and are used to increase the consistency of ointment products; they are not used alone as emollients.

Long use attests to the safety of these substances. An eye surgeon reported using ointments made with these substances on more than 20,000 surgical patients—with no ill effects as the result. The safe and effective dosage for these emollient preparations is a ¼-inch-long streak applied to the inner side of the lower eyelid.

Conditionally Approved Active Ingredients

None

Disapproved Active Ingredients

None

Safety and Effectiveness: Active Ingredients in Over-the-Counter Eye-Care Products

Active Ingredient	Drug Group*	Panel's Assessment
anhydrous lanolin	emollient	safe and effective
antipyrine	anesthetic	not safe or effective
boric acid	anti-infective	safe but not proved effective

Safety and Effectiveness: Active Ingredients in Over-the-Counter Eye-Care Products *(continued)*

Active Ingredient	Drug Group*	Panel's Assessment
carboxymethylcellulose sodium	demulcent	safe and effective
dextran 70	demulcent	safe and effective
ephedrine hydrochloride	vasoconstrictor	safe and effective
gelatin	demulcent	safe and effective
glycerin	demulcent	safe and effective
hydroxyethylcellulose	demulcent	safe and effective
hydroxypropyl methylcellulose	demulcent	safe and effective
lanolin	emollient	safe and effective
lanolin, anhydrous	emollient	safe and effective
lanolin, nonionic derivatives	emollient	safe and effective
mercuric oxide, yellow	anti-infective	not proved safe or effective
methylcellulose	demulcent	safe and effective
mineral oil	emollient	safe and effective
mineral oil, light	emollient	safe and effective
naphazoline hydrochloride	vasoconstrictor	safe and effective
paraffin	emollient	safe and effective
petrolatum, white (*see* white petrolatum)		
phenylephrine hydrochloride (0.08 to 0.2%)	vasoconstrictor	safe and effective
phenylephrine hydrochloride (under 0.08%)	vasoconstrictor	safe but not proved effective
piperocaine hydrochloride	anesthetic	not safe
polyethylene glycol 300	demulcent	safe and effective
polyethylene glycol 400	demulcent	safe and effective
polysorbate 80	demulcent	safe and effective
propylene glycol	demulcent	safe and effective
polyvinyl alcohol	demulcent	safe and effective
povidone	demulcent	safe and effective
rose petals infusion	astringent	safe but not proved effective
silver protein, mild	anti-infective	safe but not proved effective
tetrahydrozoline hydrochloride	vasoconstrictor	safe and effective
white ointment	emollient	safe and effective
white petrolatum	emollient	safe and effective
white wax	emollient	safe and effective
zinc sulfate	astringent	safe and effective

*These terms are explained in the text.

Safety and Effectiveness: Combination Products Sold Over-the-Counter for the Care of the Eyes

Safe and Effective

Each ingredient must be approved, must be present in an approved dosage, and the final marketed product must be shown to be safe and effective.

zinc sulfate (astringent) + vasoconstrictor
any 2 or 3 demulcents
2 or 3 demulcents + 1 vasoconstrictor
zinc sulfate + 1 vasoconstrictor + 1, 2, or 3 demulcents
2, 3, or more emollients

Conditionally Safe and Effective

when any approved ingredient is present in less than the established minimum dose
when one or more ingredients are only conditionally approved

Unsafe or Ineffective

contains 2 vasoconstrictors
contains any other combination of 2 approved ingredients that would not be safe or effective together
contains any disapproved ingredient
contains any ingredient at a higher-than-approved dosage
contains an active eye drug not reviewed by the Panel

Eye Drops and Ointments: Product Ratings

Single-Ingredient Products

Product and Distributor	Dosage of Active Ingredients	Rating[1]	Comment
Anesthetics			
antipyrine			
Collyrium Eye Lotion (Wyeth)	**solution:** 0.4% antipyrine	**C**	not safe or effective
Anti-Infectives			
boric acid			
boric acid (generic)	**ointment:** 5%	**B**	not proved effective
Boric Acid (Lilly)	**ointment:** 5%	**B**	not proved effective
	10%	**B**	not proved effective
mercuric oxide, yellow			
yellow mercuric oxide (generic)	**ointment:** 1% and 2%	**B**	not proved safe or effective
Yellow Mercuric Oxide (Lilly)	**ointment:** 1%	**B**	not proved safe or effective

Eye Drops and Ointments: Product Ratings *(continued)*

Single-Ingredient Products

Product and Distributor	Dosage of Active Ingredients	Rating[1]	Comment
Anti-Infectives			
Yellow Mercuric Oxide (Lilly)	2%	B	not proved safe or effective
silver protein, mild			
Argyrol S.S. 10% (CooperVision)	**solution:** 10%	B	not proved effective
silver protein, mild (generic)	**powder for solution**	B	not proved effective
thimerosal			
Merthiolate Ophthalmic (Lilly)	**ointment:** 1:5000	C	not submitted to or assessed by Panel as active ingredient
Vasoconstrictors			
naphazoline hydrochloride			
Allerest Eye Drops (Pharmacraft)	**solution:** 0.012%	A	
Clear Eyes (Abbott)		A	
Naphcon (Alcon)		A	
VasoClear (SMP)	**solution:** 0.02%	A	
phenylephrine hydrochloride			
Optigene II Eye Drops (Pfeiffer)	**solution:** 0.12%	A	
Prefrin Liquifilm (Allergan)		A	
Tear-Efrin Eye Drops (SMP)		A	
tetrahydrozoline hydrochloride			
Clear & Brite (Hudson)	**solution:** 0.05%	A	
Murine Plus Eye Drops (Abbott)		A	
Soothe Eye Drops (Alcon)		A	
Tetrasine (Steri-Med)		A	
Astringents			
rose petals (infusion of)			
Estivin (Alcon)	**solution:** aqueous infusion of rose petals	B	not proved effective

Eye Drops and Ointments: Product Ratings *(continued)*

Single-Ingredient Products

Product and Distributor	Dosage of Active Ingredients	Rating[1]	Comment
Astringents			
zinc sulfate solution			
BufOpto Zinc Sulfate (Professional Pharmacal)	**solution:** 0.25%	A	
Eye-Sed (Scherer)	**solution:** 0.217% + 2.17% boric acid	B	boric acid not proved effective
Op-Thal-Zin (Alcon)	**solution:** 0.25%	A	
Demulcents			
Adapettes (Alcon)	**solution:** 1.67% povidone + other water-soluble polymers	A	
Pre-Sert (Allergan)	**solution:** 3% polyvinyl alcohol	A	
Emollients			
Duraters Lubricant Ointment (Alcon)	**ointment:** white petrolatum + anhydrous lanolin + mineral oil	A	
Lacri-Lube S.O.P. Ointment (Allergan)	**ointment:** 55% white petrolatum + 42% mineral oil + 2% nonionic lanolin derivatives	A	

Combination Products

Product & Distributor	Dosage of Active Ingredients	Rating[1]	Comment
Collyrium with Ephedrine (Wyeth)	**solution:** 0.1% ephedrine + 0.4% antipyrine	C	antipyrine not safe or effective
Neozin Ophthalmic (A.O.C.)	**solution:** 0.125% phenylephrine HCl + 0.25% zinc sulfate	A	
optised ophthalmic (generic)	**solution:** 0.12% phenylephrine HCl + 0.25% zinc sulfate	A	
Zincfrin (Alcon)		A	

1. Author's interpretation of Panel criteria. Based on contents, not claims.

Eyes: Artificial Tears

Our eyes must remain moist. Dry eyes quickly become excruciatingly painful. Severe and permanent damage, including blindness, may follow.

Fortunately, effective over-the-counter drugs are available to relieve dryness—whether due to sun or wind exposure, illness, the effects of old age, or serious eye disease. These medications are called *ocular demulcents* (eye soothers) and the Panel that assessed them says they are one of the very few kinds of eye preparations safe and effective for people to use as self-treatment.

Most of these medications can absorb large amounts of water. Administered by dropper, they coat dry mucous membranes and other raw surfaces—protecting them from environmental irritants (including the air itself). They lubricate these surfaces and hold in their natural moisture. Some act by thickening and retaining the tear-fluid in the eye. Most of these preparations are formulated as sterile-water solutions that have about the same saltiness and acidity as natural eye secretions. These drugs are popularly called "artificial tears."

CLAIMS

Accurate

for "the temporary relief of burning and irritation due to dryness of the eye"

for "the temporary relief of discomfort due to minor irritations of the eye or to exposure to wind or sun"

for "use as a protectant against further irritation to relieve dryness of the eye"

for "use as a lubricant to prevent further irritation or relieve dryness of the eye"

DRY EYE

When exposure to sun, wind, chemicals, or other drying environmental influences produces what is technically called tear insufficiency, a person experiences dry eye. This may be felt as a burning sensation

EYES: ARTIFICIAL TEARS is based on the report of the FDA's Advisory Review Panel on OTC Ophthalmic Drug Products.

or the feeling that a foreign body is caught in the eye. The eye itself may become red.

Dry eye is common in older people and causes them greater suffering during waking hours than at night, when closed lids retain the eyes' moisture. The flow of tears from the lacrimal glands may also be reduced by any of several diseases, including a condition called by the jaw-breaker medical term *keratoconjunctivitis sicca*. Scarring or damage to the tear-fluid system is one of this disorder's main causes.

DEMULCENTS

Artificial-tear products principally consist of water. But their action goes beyond the replacement of tear-fluid—which would be of brief benefit at best since it is washed away so quickly. Demulcents (soothers) thicken and hold water and natural tear secretions so that they flow more slowly across and out of the eye. They may double the turnover time of tears. Some demulcents also coat dry eye-surfaces, postponing evaporation of leftover moisture. By holding moisture in contact with the eye and lubricating dry surfaces (as tears normally do) they reduce friction and irritation.

The active demulcent ingredient(s) may constitute only 1 percent or so of the product. Panel reviewers say that such a product also should contain a preservative to prevent bacterial contamination, along with buffers that would approximate the acid and salt content of normal tears and tonicity ingredients to aid in maintaining normal tone and tension. (Evaluations of the suitability of these agents appear in the unit EYE DROPS AND OINTMENTS, beginning on page 312).

Demulcents do not react with the eye tissue or with each other. For these reasons, reviewers approved combinations of 2 or 3 safe and effective demulcents—but no more. They also would permit demulcents to be combined with ocular astringents and vasoconstrictors to relieve irritation and slow down the passage of the other ingredients from the eye (*see* COMBINATION PRODUCTS in EYE DROPS AND OINTMENTS, page 305).

The same artificial-tear products used for temporary relief of dry eye—for example, after a day of hang-gliding, boat racing, or suntanning on the beach—are also used routinely by older people and others with chronic tear insufficiency. But the experts warn that self-treatment of a self-diagnosed dry-eye condition for more than 72 hours is potentially a very dangerous mistake. One should consult a doctor.

For persons with severe dry-eye conditions, the moisture provided by nonprescription artificial tears may disappear too quickly to provide ongoing relief and a prescription product may be needed.

Approved Active Ingredients

These substances appear to be among the safest and most effective of any assessed in the review of over-the-counter drugs; the Panel evaluated 13 demulcent ingredients and judged all of them to be safe and effective. The descriptions below follow the reviewers' practice of evaluating some ingredients individually and others (cellulose derivatives and liquid polyols) in groups.

Cellulose derivatives: carboxymethylcellulose sodium, hydroxymethylcellulose, hydroxypropyl methylcellulose, and methylcellulose Cellulose derivatives have been used in the eye for 40 years; they are the bulk-providing ingredients in half of all prescription eye drugs. Most studies on safety and effectiveness of cellulose derivatives have been based on methylcellulose, a drug that was one of the first used in eye drugs. There is no reason to believe the others are less safe or less effective. Reviewers concluded that there are no known adverse reactions from the use of cellulose derivatives. The dry crusts of this material that may form on the eyelids are harmless and can be easily wiped off.

The cellulose derivatives have been shown to remain in the eye 2 to 4 minutes after use. One report says that a solution of 1 percent hydroxypropyl methylcellulose remained in the eye for an average of 6½ minutes—a remarkably long time.

Dosage for adults and children is 1 to 2 drops of an aqueous solution containing 0.2 to 2.5 percent of total cellulose derivatives.

Dextran 70 This is a grouping of sugary subunits produced by bacteria that grow on table sugar. This type of long-chained molecular structure, made up of many similar or identical subunits, is called a *polymer*. One of the polymers' most useful traits is that they are chemically inert (inactive).

For a long time, dextran has been used as a volume expander for plasma used in blood transfusions. When it is applied to the skin, it can cause hives, swelling, and other intense allergic reactions. But when put into rabbits' eyes in the low concentrations used in artificial-tear preparations, no significant reactions occurred. In one of the few tests on human subjects, the only adverse reactions were brief periods of stinging and blurred vision. Though dextran has not been extensively studied as an eye drop, reviewers believe that the approved dose—0.1

percent dextran 70—is safe and effective, though the substance must be combined with another approved polymer-type demulcent ingredient to reach an effective dosage level.

Gelatin A polymer (*see* above), gelatin is widely used in foods. It is colorless or faintly yellow, transparent, brittle, practically odorless, and has no taste of its own. Before cellulose derivatives became available gelatin was widely used in formulating ophthalmic (eye) drugs as a substitute for the natural, water-soluble proteins in tear fluid.

The effectiveness of gelatin in artificial-tear products has not been studied, but the Panel nevertheless evaluates it as effective, as well as safe, in concentrations of 0.01 percent ($\frac{1}{100}$ of 1 percent) if it is combined with other polymeric demulcents.

The safe dosage for adults and children is 1 to 2 drops of a 0.01 percent gelatin concentration in a water solution with another approved polymer-type demulcent.

Glycerin *See* LIQUID POLYOLS, below.

Hydroxyethylcellulose *See* CELLULOSE DERIVATIVES, above.

Hydroxypropyl methylcellulose *See* CELLULOSE DERIVATIVES, above.

Liquid polyols: glycerin, polyethylene glycol 300, polyethylene glycol 400, polysorbate 80, and propylene glycol These substances are all gooey, clear, water-soluble fluids that tend to be bland, stable, and nontoxic. They are widely used as vehicles (bases) and solvents for other active drugs, as well as in moisturizers and other cosmetics. Although their safety and effectiveness as eye-drug ingredients have not been well studied, their few side effects and their ability to "coat" tissue surfaces led evaluators to deem these ingredients effective and safe as demulcents and eye lubricants.

For adults and children dosage is 1 to 2 drops of 0.2 to 1 percent concentration in water solution, applied as needed.

Methylcellulose *See* CELLULOSE DERIVATIVES, above.

Polyethylene glycol 300 and polyethylene glycol 400 *See* LIQUID POLYOLS, above.

Polysorbate 80 *See* LIQUID POLYOLS, above.

Propylene glycol *See* LIQUID POLYOLS, above.

Polyvinyl alcohol This alcohol has been widely used as a base for prescription eye medications. It has been carefully tested. Serious side effects have not been found and minor ones have been uncommon, even though millions of product units of polyvinyl-alcohol eye preparations have been sold.

Polyvinyl alcohol is less syrupy than methylcellulose and other artificial tear substances, so evaluators guess that it acts by forming a protective film which lubricates eye surfaces and holds in moisture. It is formulated into products that wearers of hard contact lenses use to reduce eye irritation.

The safe and effective dosage for children and adults is 1 to 2 drops of water solution containing 0.1 to 4 percent polyvinyl alcohol, administered as needed.

Povidone   This substance is essentially inert, so it is widely used as an inactive ingredient in the manufacture of drugs. While less well studied as an eye drug than polyvinyl alcohol (*see* directly above), a 1968 report from the National Academy of Sciences indicates that a 3 percent povidone product probably is safe and effective for use in soothing and lubricating dry eyes, and for enhancing the comfort of contact lenses. The Panel concurs with this judgment of safety and effectiveness.

For adults and children, approved dosages are 1 to 2 drops of 0.1 to 2 percent povidone, used as needed.

Safety and Effectiveness: Active Ingredients in Over-the-Counter Eye Soothers (Demulcents)

Active Ingredient	Panel's Assessment
carboxymethylcellulose sodium	safe and effective
dextran 70	safe and effective
gelatin	safe and effective
glycerin	safe and effective
hydroxymethylcellulose	safe and effective
hydroxypropyl methylcellulose	safe and effective
methylcellulose	safe and effective
polyethylene glycol 300	safe and effective
polyethylene glycol 400	safe and effective
polysorbate 80	safe and effective
propylene glycol	safe and effective
polyvinyl alcohol	safe and effective
povidone	safe and effective

Artificial Tears: Product Ratings

Product and Distributor	Dosage of Active Ingredients	Rating[1]
Adsorbotear (Alcon)	0.44% hydroxyethylcellulose + 1.67% povidone	A
Isopto Tears (Alcon)	0.5% hydroxypropyl methylcellulose	A

Artificial Tears: Product Ratings *(continued)*

Product and Distributor	Dosage of Active Ingredients	Rating[1]
Liquifilm Forte (Allergan)	3% polyvinyl alcohol	A
Liquifilm Tears (Allergan)	1.4% polyvinyl alcohol	A
Methopto ¼% (Professional Pharmacal)	0.25% methylcellulose	A
Methopto-Forte ½% (Professional Pharmacal)	0.5% methylcellulose	A
Methopto-Forte 1% (Professional Pharmacal)	1% methylcellulose	A
Visculose-1% (A.O.C. Soft Contact Lens Div.)	1% methylcellulose	A

1. Author's interpretation of Panel criteria. Based on contents, not claims.

Eyes: Corneal Edema

The eye's cornea, that clear window through which we see, may become swollen because it has absorbed too much fluid. This condition is called *corneal edema*. Vision becomes blurred or foggy. Lights appear to be surrounded by halos. In some cases the eye may become quite irritated, even excruciatingly painful, so that the sufferer cannot tolerate light.

Experts say that corneal edema can be at least partially corrected with sterile salt water available over-the-counter. But since the swelling is usually the symptom of a more serious underlying disorder that requires medical diagnosis and care, the panel stipulates that this sterile salt water be used only under a doctor's supervision.

CLAIMS

Accurate
for "the temporary relief of corneal edema"

EYES: CORNEAL EDEMA is based on the report of the FDA's Advisory Review Panel on OTC Ophthalmic Drug Products.

WARNING   Two to 5 percent salt solutions should *not* be used as an eyewash or to treat the eyes for problems other than corneal edema.

CORNEAL EDEMA

Causes and Treatment

A variety of problems can cause this condition. Contact lenses that fit badly or are not removed often enough to rest the eye can injure the cornea, causing it to absorb tear-fluid and swell. Inflammatory reactions and infection can also produce this effect. Finally, the serious eye disease glaucoma can result in corneal edema, as can iritis, which is an inflammation of the colored part of the eye.

The sterile salt water (saline solutions) that can be safely used to treat this condition ranges from 2 to 5 percent salt. When put into the eye every 3 or 4 hours—as directed by a doctor—these solutions (called *ocular hypertonicity agents*) will draw water out of the cornea. This reduces the swelling. A demulcent to help hold the salt water is also allowed.

HYPERTONICITY AGENT

Approved Active Ingredient

Sodium chloride   Ordinary salt (in sterile water) is the one substance judged to be safe and effective in reducing corneal edema—providing the patient is under medical supervision. The safe and effective concentrations are from 2 to 5 percent.

These preparations—which are formulated as eye drops or as an ointment—may cause stinging, redness, and temporary discomfort in the eye. The reactions are not dangerous, but this mild discomfort should serve to prevent overdosing or use by persons who do not really need the medication.

Tests in rabbits and in humans indicate that such salt solutions will produce a 10 to 20 percent reduction in corneal swelling. The likelihood is that one's vision will sharpen and improve as a result.

The approved dosage for adults and children is 1 to 2 drops of a 2 to 5 percent concentration of salt water in the affected eye(s) every 3 or 4 hours, as directed by a physician.

**Safety and Effectiveness: Active Ingredients in
Solutions Sold Over-the-Counter for Corneal Edema**

Active Ingredient	Panel's Assessment
sterile salt water (2 to 5%)	safe and effective

Saltwater Preparation for Corneal Edema: Product Ratings

Product and Distributor	Dosage of Active Ingredients	Rating[1]
Adsorbonac Ophthalmic (Alcon)	**solution:** 2% sodium chloride + 1.67% povidone	A
	solution: 5% sodium chloride + 1.67% povidone	A
Hypersal Ophthalmic (A.O.C. Soft Contact Lens Division)	**solution:** 5% sodium chloride	A

1. Author's interpretation of Panel criteria. Based on contents, not claims.

Eyewash

An eyewash is a sterile water solution that can be used to bathe the eye or to dilute and flush out irritating foreign matter. Dust, pollen, and airborne pollutant gases and liquids—including smog and swimming-pool chlorine—that have dissolved in the eye's tear-fluid can be removed with eyewash. Experts say that these washes (also called *eye lotions* and *eye-irrigating solutions*) should be present in sealed, sterile containers in home and workplace first-aid and emergency kits.

Eyewash products differ from all other over-the-counter preparations in that the reviewing Panel insists they must not contain any active drug ingredients. This might worsen the irritation and pain. Only sterile water and inactive ingredients that approximate ordinary tear-fluid's saltiness and acidity are allowed.

EYEWASH is based on the report of the FDA's Advisory Review Panel on OTC Ophthalmic Drug Products.

CLAIMS

Accurate

for "flushing or irrigating the eye to remove loose foreign material, air pollutants, or chlorinated water"

EMERGENCY TREATMENT: CHEMICAL BURNS

When acid or a caustic substance like lye (or any other potent chemical) splashes into the eye, definite steps must be taken at once to neutralize and remove the substance. The eye must be flushed out immediately by using large amounts of an eyewash or irrigating solution, or warm clean tap water, or both. The National Poison Center Network warns that a delay of only seconds may greatly increase the extent of injury. The center offers these emergency instructions:

Forcibly hold eyelids open and immediately rinse eyes and face with gentle stream of warm running water from tap or pitcher for at least 15 minutes. Then take victim to the emergency department of a hospital or to an eye doctor (ophthalmologist).

The Panel concurs that in the absence of adequate amounts of prepackaged eyewash, copious flushing with water is a must—followed by medical care. It adds this urgent warning:

If you experience severe eye pain, headache, rapid change in vision (side or straight ahead), sudden appearance of floating spots, acute redness of the eyes, pain on exposure to light, or double vision, consult a physician at once.

If symptoms persist or worsen after use of (an eyewash), consult a physician.

The clear message in treating chemical burns—or for that matter any massive infiltration of alien material into the eye—is: Don't take chances. Don't wait. Give emergency care with eyewash or water. Get medical help.

NATURAL AND ASSISTED EYE IRRIGATIONS

The tears are the eyes' first line of defense against noxious gases, liquids, and solid particles from the environment. They dilute and carry away these substances when they enter and irritate the sensitive whites of the eyes, the clear visual windows (the corneas), and the eyes' inner lids. Even very tiny foreign particles and liquid droplets can create a sand-in-the-eye sensation. Their presence can also redden the eye, cause it to swell, and produce uncontrollable blinking. Burning, smarting, stinging, and itching may be felt.

The irritants' presence quickly stimulates increased tear secretion as the eye attempts to cleanse itself. Keeping the eye closed may facilitate this effort and help control pain. But an eyewash—to dilute and flush out the foreign matter—is the next thing to try.

Some eyewash products come with a sterile eye cup. To use: Rinse the eye cup. Fill halfway up with the liquid and press tightly against the eye to avoid spillage. Tilt the head back, open the eyelids wide, and rotate the eyeball by tracking visual circles (i.e., as if following circles around the head). This helps ensure that all eye surfaces will be bathed by the fluid.

Eyewash products may also be packaged in a container that can be gently pressed to let a stream of the liquid go into the eye.

If these first-aid measures fail, a doctor's help should be sought. While the eye usually reacts sensitively to foreign bodies, it also may accommodate quickly to them so that the pain largely subsides. An embedded particle, however, can cause both physical and chemical damage; it must be removed by a doctor or other qualified health-care professional.

EYEWASH INGREDIENTS

No active medicinal ingredients should be present in eyewash products. Thus none was approved and any eyewash that includes an active ingredient would be disapproved as unsafe and misbranded. None of the active ingredients that are rated safe or effective in eye drops or ointments should be found in eyewashes. For a list of such substances *see* SAFETY AND EFFECTIVENESS chart on page 314.

The principal *inactive* ingredient in all eyewashes is sterile water. Also included should be tiny amounts of one or more suitable preservatives—for example, benzalkonium chloride 0.01 percent; appropriate buffers, like weak concentrations of boric acid to establish an acidity to match that of normal tear-fluid; and compounds like sodium chloride (common table salt) to allow for a tearlike salinity (saltiness) of about 1 percent. For suitable and unsuitable inactive ingredients found in eye-care products *see* lists on pages 303–305.

Eyewash: Product Ratings

Product and Distributor	Dosage of Active Ingredients	Rating[1]	Comment
A/K/Rinse (Akorn)	none	A	
Blinx (Barnes-Hind)	none	A	

Eyewash: Product Ratings *(continued)*

Product and Distributor	Dosage of Active Ingredients	Rating[1]	Comment
Collyrium Eye Lotion (Wyeth)	0.4% antipyrine	**C**	antipyrine is not safe or effective
Lauro (Otis Clapp)	none	**A**	
Lavoptik Eye Wash (Lavoptik)	none; comes with eyecup	**A**	
M/Rinse (Danker)	none	**A**	

1. Author's interpretation of Panel criteria. Based on contents, not claims.

Fever Remedies

See PAIN, FEVER, AND ANTI-INFLAMMATORY DRUGS TAKEN INTERNALLY

First-Aid Preparations for Skin Wounds

Cuts, scrapes, burns, and other small skin wounds are common events in most families—particularly those with active children. Given minimal care, these injuries usually will heal by themselves within a week. If they fail to heal, a doctor should be consulted.

The first-aider's first task, particularly with children, is to deal with the situation in a reassuring manner. Inspect the wound to see if it requires medical attention. If it is deep, wide, ragged, or if dirt, wood,

FIRST-AID PREPARATIONS FOR SKIN WOUNDS is based on the report "OTC Topical Antimicrobial Products" by the FDA's Advisory Review Panel on OTC Antimicrobial Drug Products for Repeated Daily Human Use (Antimicrobial I Panel); the FDA's initial Tentative Final Order on these drugs plus official addenda; the report "Topical Antibiotic Products" by the FDA's Advisory Review Panel on OTC Microbial Drug Products (Antimicrobial II Panel) and the FDA's Tentative Final Order on these drugs; and reports by the FDA's Advisory Review Panel on Miscellaneous External Drug Products.

or other debris is deeply embedded in it, seek professional help. Deep wounds, particularly if caused by metal or dirty out-of-doors objects, definitely should be shown or described to a physician, since a shot to prevent tetanus ("lockjaw")—a dangerous illness caused by microorganisms in the soil—may be needed. Animal bites also require medical attention.

FIRST-AID TREATMENT APPROACHES

Debris and dirt should be washed out of small wounds, and off surrounding skin. An effort should be made to destroy "germs" or microorganisms in and around the injury to forestall infection. Ways to do this are described below.

Antiseptics   An antiseptic kills germs. The only 2 safe and effective antiseptics are ethyl alcohol (60 to 95 percent) and isopropyl alcohol (65 to 91.3 percent), which kill significant numbers of bacteria within seconds when applied to the skin. Since they also sting, however, they may not be appropriate for cleaning and degerming skinned knees and other large, raw areas (*see* ANTISEPTICS).

Skin-wound cleansers   A skin-wound cleanser is defined as a nonirritating liquid preparation (or product to be used with water) that assists in the removal of foreign material from small superficial wounds. It may contain a germ-killing ingredient.

Such a cleanser might well be the *first* first-aid product one would use—particularly since the Antimicrobial I Panel says that several active ingredients are safe and effective for this purpose. The value of these products, however, is not clear-cut. A cleanser is not required to show effectiveness in the prevention of infection. "It is obvious," the Antimicrobial I Panel tartly remarks, "that products such as [an ordinary] bar soap, with water, could serve as a skin-wound cleanser." Besides, cool or cold running water washes away dirt, dried blood, and other debris and helps staunch blood flow (blood vessels contract in response to cold).

Skin-wound protectants   Once the wound is clean, skin-wound protectants may be helpful. A skin-wound protectant is a nonirritating preparation that can be applied to small cleansed wounds. It provides a physical and chemical barrier against germs, to protect the wound so it can heal normally. The "physical barrier" is the ointment, cream, or other base with which the product is formulated. The "chemical barrier" is an antimicrobial ingredient.

First-aid antibiotics   These preparations contain special, potent, germ-killing substances called antibiotics (defined below) which help to prevent infections. Most first-aid antibiotics are formulated as ointments, with petrolatum as their vehicle (base)—although the Antimicrobial II Panel says that antibiotics in solution or cream bases are more effective. Antibiotics do not dissolve in a greasy, viscous, ointment base, so only the antibiotic that is right at the barrier-wound interface is in a position to help fight infection in this type of preparation. Antibiotics used in water-based creams, however, are water-soluble; they readily diffuse through the cream toward the wound interface. So consumers should consider purchasing first-aid antibiotic products as creams rather than as ointments—if they can find them.

Must a first-aider use *both* an antimicrobial skin-wound cleanser and an antimicrobial wound protectant? The FDA says *no*. One should be free to choose between a two-step method (first cleansing a wound and then applying the germ killer) and a one-step method (applying a cleanser combined with an antimicrobial). Wounds should be cleansed before a first-aid antibiotic is applied.

GERM-FIGHTERS DEFINED

Consumers may well be confused by the similarities and differences between the several germ-fighting types of drugs that are used to prevent infections. An *antimicrobial* is a drug that "kills or inhibits the growth and reproduction of micro-organisms," the FDA says. Antimicrobials usually are synthetically created chemicals that must be used in relatively high concentrations in order to be effective. *Antiseptics* are defined as "germ-killers," and generally are considered to be antimicrobials. They may be derived from natural sources; ethyl alcohol, for example, can be distilled from grain or fruit.

Antibiotics are essentially germ products that fights other germs, or, as the Antimicrobial II Panel defines them: "chemical substances produced by a microorganism and having the capacity, in dilute solutions, to kill or inhibit the growth of other micro-organisms." While antibiotics originally were derived from living microorganisms—the well-known antibiotic penicillin came from the bread mold *Penicillium notatum,* for example—they are now for the most part manufactured synthetically. Generally speaking, antibiotics are extremely powerful drugs, particularly when injected or ingested. But their value in combating infections when they are applied directly to the skin in over-the-counter first-aid products has been questioned by the Antimicrobial II Panel and the FDA.

CLAIMS

Accurate for antiseptics

for "first-aid use to decrease germs in minor cuts and scrapes"
"to decrease germs on the skin prior to removing a splinter or other foreign objects"

Accurate for skin-wound cleansers

"to clean superficial wounds"
"aids in removal of foreign material such as dirt and debris"

Accurate for skin-wound protectants

"protects wounds"
"first aid for small [minor] cuts, abrasions and burns"
"protects against wound contamination"

Accurate for first-aid antibiotics

"first aid to help prevent infection in minor cuts, scrapes, and burns"
"decreases [or] helps reduce the number of bacteria on the treated area"
"helps reduce the risk [or] chance of skin infection"
"helps prevent bacterial contamination"

False or Misleading

"speeds," "promotes," or "aids" healing
"heals wounds"

The FDA says these vague, false, and misleading claims imply a primary function in healing while "their only action is to remove . . . microorganisms that might slow the healing process" so that the healing can occur in a normal period of time.

WARNING   The Panels and the FDA warn that these products should not be used on large or deep wounds. Neither should they be used for chronic conditions such as leg ulcers, diaper rash, and eczema of the hands. If the wounds become red, swollen, or painful, stop applying the first-aid preparation and consult a doctor. Further, these products should not be used on animal bites —whether from pets or other animals, domestic or wild—which should be examined by a doctor at once.

COMBINATION PRODUCTS

First-aid preparations with antibiotics often contain more than one antibiotic and are usually not combined with other types of active ingredients. Reviewers say 2 or 3 safe and effective antibiotics may yield a safe and effective combination, and it specifies that polymyxin *must* be combined with bacitracin or a tetracycline.

The following pain-relieving ingredients, often found in the first-aid preparations that do not contain antibiotics, have been assessed as safe and effective as topical analgesics:

> benzocaine
> camphor (*Note*: Other Panels question the safety of camphor.)
> lidocaine hydrochloride
> menthol
> methyl salicylate
> tetracaine hydrochloride

Many first-aid products are formulated in convenient aerosol sprays that contain benzocaine and an antimicrobial. In shopping for these heavily promoted first-aid aids, it is worth keeping in mind that the approved concentration of benzocaine is 5 percent to 20 percent.

SKIN-WOUND CLEANSING INGREDIENTS

The Antimicrobial I Panel evaluated close to 2 dozen active ingredients that are used to cleanse superficial burns, cuts, scrapes, and other minor skin injuries. Over half of these ingredients are either fully or conditionally approved for this purpose.

Approved Active Ingredients

The Panel approved several antimicrobial agents as safe and effective for cleansing small wounds. The FDA added another, poloxamer 188.

Benzalkonium chloride See QUATERNARY AMMONIUM COMPOUNDS, below.

Benzethonium chloride See QUATERNARY AMMONIUM COMPOUNDS, below.

Hexylresorcinol For decades, this substance has been used for a variety of medicinal purposes. In concentrations of $\frac{1}{1000}$ or less it undoubtedly is safe, and it is effective in cleansing small wounds. Beyond this bare-bones assessment, neither the Antimicrobial I Panel nor the FDA has much to add about hexylresorcinol's use in cleansing wounds.

Methylbenzethonium chloride See QUATERNARY AMMONIUM COMPOUNDS, below.

Poloxamer 188 This detergent substance does not kill microbes, but it is nonirritating and efficient for cleansing minor wounds when dissolved in water in concentrations of 20 to 40 percent. It is not broken down in the body, is rapidly excreted, and is generally regarded as nontoxic. So it is approved as safe and effective as a skin-wound cleanser.

Quaternary ammonium compounds Three compounds in this group, called "quats," are safe and effective for use as wound cleansers: benzalkonium chloride, benzethonium chloride, and methylbenzethonium chloride.

Quats act as detergents in the removal of foreign matter from small wounds. They also kill gram-positive bacteria (albeit less effectively than was thought when they were introduced a half-century ago). But these drugs have the disadvantage of being inactive against dangerous *Pseuodomonas* species of gram-negative bacteria. Too, they are relatively ineffective against fungi and viruses. But, as the Antimicrobial I Panel notes, the ability to kill germs need not be proved—and, in fact, is not required—in order for a substance to be an effective wound cleanser. (For explanation of terms "gram-positive" and "gram-negative," *see* page 47.)

Quats may sting and irritate the skin. This effect can delay wound healing if the substances are used repeatedly. The Panel specifies, therefore, that they be used only on small and superficial wounds—and then only infrequently and in concentrations of under $1/750$. With these precautions, the Panel concludes, the 3 approved quats are "reasonable" choices for cleansing wounds.

Conditionally Approved Active Ingredients

Chloroxylenol (PCMX) Little usable data were submitted to the Panel or the FDA on this substance's value or its effects on human skin.

Cloflucarban This substance is widely used as an antimicrobial ingredient in bar soaps. In this form—and in this form only—it is conditionally approved for washing dirt and debris out of superficial wounds.

Iodine complexed with phosphate ester of alkylaryloxy poly-ethylene glycol (*see* IODOPHORS, below.)

Iodophors Iodophors are the class of compounds that include tincture of iodine and iodine or iodide chemically combined with other substances intended to bind, hold, and release the iodine *slowly*, thus enhancing its safety.

Most older people remember tincture of iodine from their childhood, since it was—and in some families may still be—the standard first-aid preparation for superficial wounds. The trouble is that it *stings*. Iodine is so irritating, in fact, that it actually may *inhibit* the healing of small wounds, so that its use could be counterproductive. Tincture of iodine thus is granted only conditional approval, on grounds of safety. The FDA warns:

"Do not apply this product with a tight bandage, as a burn may result."

While irritating to human skin cells, iodine has the unquestionable advantage of being lethal to a broad spectrum of microorganisms, including both gram-positive and more hazardous gram-negative bacteria, as well as fungi and viruses. This has prompted drug makers to try to formulate it in a safer way, attached to "carrier" molecules, as the FDA calls them. This reduces the amount of "free" iodine that reaches the wound surface at any given time. These products sting less and stain less than elemental iodine preparations, and they can be used under bandages without causing burns. This significant advantage, the FDA says, may be negated since the iodine may be released *too* slowly to be effective.

Because insufficient data were presented about the release of iodine, all the iodophor complexes were given only conditional approval (pending new data to demonstrate they are effective, stable, and also safe). These complexes include iodine joined with phosphate ester of alkylaryloxy polyethylene glycol, nonylphenoxypoly (ethyleneoxy) ethanoliodine, poloxamer-iodine complex, povidone-iodine complex, and undecoylium chloride-iodine complex.

A new problem has been discovered in recent years: Iodophors, and particularly povidone-iodine, have been shown to profoundly depress the body's protective immune system. This has been demonstrated in laboratory animals and in patients who have been badly burned. The significance of these findings for those who use povidone-iodine and other iodophors to treat minor injuries also still is unclear.

Nonylphenoxypoly (ethyleneoxy) ethanoliodine *See* IODO-PHORS, above.

Phenol (under 1.5 percent aqueous/alcoholic) While the Panel says phenol (carbolic acid) is a hazardous substance, it believes it may be safe at these low concentrations. But, phenol at these concentrations may not be effective in killing microorganisms. The FDA warns:

"Do not use for diaper rash or over large areas of the body or cover the treated area with a bandage or dressing."

Poloxamer-iodine *See* IODOPHORS, above.

Povidone-iodine *See* IODOPHORS, above.

Tincture of iodine *See* IODOPHORS, above.

Triclocarban This ingredient is widely used in antimicrobial bar soaps. Only in this form is it conditionally approved for use in washing dirt and debris out of superficial skin wounds.

Triclosan Although there are no known hazards to the general public from use the of products with 1 percent or lower concentrations of triclosan, the FDA says data to confirm its effectiveness and safety as a skin-wound cleanser still are wanting.

Disapproved Active Ingredients

Some substances that the Panel disapproves as hazardous or ineffective for cleaning small wounds have already been removed from the United States over-the-counter market by the FDA. The banned ingredients are indicated below.

Cloflucarban This substance is conditionally approved as a wound cleanser when formulated in a bar soap. This is the only way it has been marketed in the United States; there are no data to show that it is either safe or effective as a wound cleanser when formulated in other ways.

Fluorosalan Several closely related salicylanilide compounds have been shown to cause serious skin reactions. Like them, fluorosalan may be dangerous and has been banned.

Hexachlorophene This is a potent but dangerous antimicrobial, once widely used, that was involved in the death of a number of babies and injured many others. It is considered too dangerous for nonprescription marketing and has been banned—though it remains available as a prescription product.

Phenol (over 1.5 percent aqueous/alcoholic)   This potent germ killer can cause painful skin burns and other damage to human tissue (*see* PHENOL).

Tribromsalan   This banned ingredient can cause serious skin reactions.

Triclocarban   Triclocarban has not been marketed as a skin-wound protectant in the United States and there are no data to show it is safe or effective.

The above ingredients are used in a variety of products. To locate where these ingredients are discussed elsewhere in this book, consult the index.

SKIN-WOUND PROTECTING INGREDIENTS

Approved Active Ingredients

None.

Conditionally Approved Active Ingredients

Over a dozen germ killers are conditionally approved as skin-wound protectants.

Benzalkonium chloride   This compound is considered safe and effective for occasional use in cleansing small skin wounds, but convincing data on effectiveness when used as a wound protectant remain to be gathered. Some minor safety questions remain, too: benzalkonium and other "quats" are irritating to the skin, which may delay healing. The risk, if any, of their precipitating skin eruptions—whether on contact or through allergic sensitization—also needs to be explored.

Benzalkonium chloride and related drugs are more effective against gram-positive organisms than they are against some of the more dangerous gram-negative ones. Their germicidal activity is diluted by blood serum and by soap, and they are absorbed off wound surfaces by bandages or clothing, and so may become less useful than they are believed to be.

Benzethonium chloride   This substance is closely related to benzalkonium chloride. Its approval as a protectant is only conditional.

Chloroxylenol (PCMX)   Little conclusive data were submitted to the Antimicrobial I Panel and the FDA on the value of this substance, or its effect on the skin when used as a wound protectant.

Hexylresorcinol   This substance is used for a variety of medicinal purposes, and the Panel says its use on the skin does not represent a known hazard to the general public. What is wanting are data to show the agent's actual effectiveness as a skin-wound protectant.

Iodine complexed with phosphate ester of alkylaryloxy polyethylene glycol   This molecular complex is intended to bind and hold iodine so that it is released slowly onto the wound, and thus not irritate the skin and delay healing. (*See* IODOPHORS, page 335.)

Methylbenzethonium chloride   This is another quaternary ammonium compound (*see* QUATERNARY AMMONIUM COMPOUNDS, page 334) the approval of which remains conditional in the present context.

Nonylphenoxypoly (ethyleneoxy) ethanoliodine   This iodine molecular complex is assessed by the Antimicrobial I Panel and the FDA as an iodophor (*see* IODOPHORS, page 335); as a skin-wound protectant, its approval is conditional.

Phenol (under 1.5 percent aqueous/alcoholic)   This medicinal-smelling substance, better known as carbolic acid, is a potent germicidal agent at higher concentrations. However, even at lower concentrations it can be extremely dangerous because phenol burns the skin; it is also absorbed into the body, where it may injure internal organs.

Phenol's effectiveness at relatively safe, low concentrations of 1.5 percent or less remains to be proved, and when it is covered up and pressed against the skin it may be considerably more dangerous than when left uncovered. So the Panel and the FDA warn: "Do not use for diaper rash or over large areas of the body or cover the treated area with a bandage or dressing."

Poloxamer-iodine   This molecular complex is intended to bind and hold iodine so that it is released only slowly onto the wound. The aim is to reduce the iodine's irritancy to the skin and so facilitate healing.

Povidone-iodine   See IODOPHORS, page 335.

Tincture of iodine   It was in this form that iodine—a potent germicidal—was formerly sold and used. But in this form iodine is extremely irritating to the skin. This irritation, felt as the familiar painful sting of iodine when applied, may delay healing, and thus its use may not be safe.

Triclosan   Widely used as an antimicrobial agent, triclosan poses no known hazard to the general public. But the Panel and the FDA say that data on its safety and effectiveness as a skin protectant are wanting.

Undecoylium chloride-iodine complex   See IODOPHORS, page 335.

Disapproved Active Ingredients

The substances listed below are generally recognized as unsafe as wound protectants. Several no longer are sold over-the-counter in the United States as wound protectants.

Cloflucarban This agent principally appears in special soaps. No data were submitted to the FDA on its use as a wound protectant.

Fluorosalan A number of chemically related salicylanilide compounds have been shown to cause serious skin reactions. This one also may be dangerous; thus it was banned.

Phenol (over 1.5 percent aqueous/alcoholic) In higher concentrations, phenol is a potent germ killer—but it is also a potent destroyer of human tissue. It burns the skin, is absorbed, and can cause internal injury (*see* PHENOL).

Tribromsalan This ingredient was banned because it can cause serious skin reactions.

Triclocarban This antimicrobial has not been marketed as a skin-wound protectant in the United States and there are no data to show it is safe or effective.

The above ingredients are used in a variety of other products. To locate where these ingredients are discussed elsewhere in this book, consult the index.

ANTISEPTICS

See ANTISEPTICS, page 68.

FIRST-AID ANTIBIOTICS

Millions of tubes of these products have been sold over-the-counter in the last 30 years. Yet the Antimicrobial II Panel declared: "No data from well-controlled studies were presented to [us] concerning either the therapeutic or preventive effects of OTC use of topical antibiotics on minor cuts, abrasions, or burns. The Panel concludes that no such data presently exist."

Five years later, in 1982, the FDA could find little more convincing data on these products' value. It decided that it is "inappropriate" for consumers to select and use over-the-counter antibiotics to *treat* skin infections once they have arisen. The reasons? They have no way to know which drug will work against which infection, and this form of self-treatment has not been shown to be effective (*see* ANTIBIOTICS FOR SKIN INFECTIONS).

The FDA was more generous in assessing antibiotics' role in *preventing* infections, based on two developments that followed publication of the Panel's report:

- The American Academy of Pediatrics published an extensive review of the medical literature on these drugs, and concluded—in an official position paper—that topical antibiotics may prevent infection after minor cuts, abrasions, and burns, and therefore may be appropriate as an "adjunct" to careful washing of the wound.
- A report was published on a 15-week study of 59 toddlers at a rural day-care center. The youngsters were examined daily, and half had their minor skin injuries and insect bites treated with an antibiotic ointment containing neomycin sulfate + zinc bacitracin + polymyxin B sulfate. The others were treated with a drug-free ointment. Only 15 percent of the kids treated with the active drugs suffered streptococcal skin infections, and none had a recurrence; only 1 needed treatment with an oral antibiotic. By contrast, 47 percent of the children who received the dummy medication suffered infections, and 5 had recurrences; 12 required oral antibiotic therapy. The antibiotic combination thus provided statistically significant advantage over the dummy medication.

Different antibiotics are effective against different species of bacteria, as is explained in ANTIBIOTICS FOR SKIN INFECTIONS. Since no one can anticipate in advance *which* types may infect a wound, it may make good sense to choose a combination product, like the one used on the day-care children described above, rather than a single-ingredient product. These combinations are listed in the chart SAFETY AND EFFECTIVENESS: COMBINATION PRODUCTS at the end of this unit.

Directions for Using First-Aid Antibiotics

Clean the affected area. Apply a small amount of product 1 to 3 times daily. May be covered with a sterile bandage.

WARNING Do not use in the eyes or apply over large areas of the body. In case of puncture wounds, animal bites, or serious burns, consult a doctor. Stop use and consult a doctor if the condition persists or gets worse. Do not use longer than 1 week unless directed by a doctor.

Approved Active Ingredients

Bacitracin   This antibiotic, first isolated in 1943, is produced by a strain of bacteria called *Bacillus subtilis*. It kills gram-positive bacteria by blocking their ability to build cellular walls.

The drug usually is applied to small skin wounds in an ointment, which forms a protective physical cover over the wound. Bacitracin's established value, according to the Panel, is to reduce bacterial growth inside the ointment base itself and at the surface where the wound and ointment meet.

Bacitracin zinc   Formulation of bacitracin as a zinc salt appears to enhance its antibacterial effect, the reviewers say. So bacitracin zinc is judged both safe and effective.

Neomycin   Neomycin is one of a class of potent antibiotics called *aminoglycosides*, which effectively kill bacteria by interfering with their ability to synthesize protein. These antibiotics can injure users' kidneys and damage their hearing when large amounts are ingested. They are unlikely to pose this hazard when small amounts are applied to skin wounds. The FDA says neomycin is safe and effective.

Polymyxin B sulfate   This antibiotic is effective against only a few types of bacteria. But, since these organisms tend to be of the potentially dangerous gram-negative variety, polymyxin is a useful companion with bacitracin or other antibiotics that are more effective against gram-positive organisms. So it is approved as safe and effective only in combination products with other approved antibiotics.

Tetracyclines   Several tetracycline compounds will safely and effectively protect skin wounds against a wide range of bacteria; they include chlortetracycline hydrochloride, oxytetracycline hydrochloride, and tetracycline hydrochloride. These antibiotics interfere with the invading bacteria's ability to synthesize protein; in this manner they inhibit growth of the organisms.

Like all antibiotics, tetracyclines produce adverse effects in a small number of users. But the recommended dose—a dab of tetracycline ointment spread over the wound—is so small that these reactions are quite rare. So the tetracyclines are safe as well as effective.

Conditionally Approved Active Ingredients

Gramicidin   Discovered in the 1930s, this is one of the oldest antibiotics. It has been widely used and has been shown to be mainly effective against gram-positive bacteria. Given the long history of this drug, the Antimicrobial II Panel may have been surprised to discover that there were no clinical studies to demonstrate safety or effectiveness.

Disapproved Active Ingredients

None

Safety and Effectiveness: Active Ingredients in Over-the-Counter Skin Wound Preparations

Active Ingredient	Panel* and FDA's Evaluation as Wound Cleanser†	Panel* and FDA's Evaluation as Wound Protectant
benzalkonium chloride	safe and effective	not proved safe or effective
benzethonium chloride	safe and effective	not proved safe or effective
chloroxylenol (PCMX)	not proved safe or effective	not proved safe or effective
cloflucarban		
in antimicrobial bar soap	not proved safe or effective	not safe or effective
in other formations	not safe	not safe
fluorosalan	not safe	not safe
hexachlorophene	not safe	
hexylresorcinol	safe and effective	safe but not proved effective
iodine complexed with phosphate ester of alkylaryloxy polyethylene glycol	not proved safe or effective	not proved safe or effective
methylbenzethonium chloride	safe and effective	not proved safe or effective
nonylphenoxypoly (ethyleneoxy) ethanoliodine	not proved safe or effective	not proved safe or effective
phenol (over 1.5% in aqueous/alcoholic solution)	not safe	not safe
phenol (under 1.5% in aqueous/alcoholic solution)	not proved effective	not proved effective
poloxamer-iodine	not proved safe or effective	not proved safe or effective
povidone-iodine complex	not proved safe or effective	not proved safe or effective
tincture of iodine	not proved safe	not proved safe
tribromsalan	not safe	not safe
triclocarban		
in antimicrobial bar soap	not proved safe or effective	not safe or effective
in other formulations	not safe	
triclosan	not proved safe or effective	not proved safe or effective
undecoylium chloride-iodine	not proved safe or effective	not proved safe or effective

Safety and Effectiveness: Active Ingredients in Over-the-Counter Skin Wound Preparations (continued)

Antibiotic	Panel† and FDA Evaluation as First-aid Antibiotic
bacitracin	safe and effective (active against gram-positive bacteria)
bacitracin zinc	safe and effective (against gram-positive bacteria)
gramicidin	not proved safe or effective (active against gram-positive bacteria)
neomycin	safe and effective (active against gram-positive and some gram-negative bacteria)
polymyxin B sulfate	safe and effective (active primarily against gram-negative bacteria; approved only in combinations with other antibiotics that are active against gram-positive bacteria)
tetracyclines: chlortetracycline hydrochloride, oxytetracycline hydrochloride, and tetracycline hydrochloride	safe and effective (active against gram-positive and some gram-negative bacteria)

NOTE: The terms gram-positive and gram-negative are explained in the text—especially under CAUSES, EFFECTS, TREATMENTS in ANTIBIOTICS FOR SKIN INFECTION. Any person unsure of what implications this information might have for the usefulness of an OTC product he or she is attempting to select should consult a doctor, pharmacist, or, in some cases, product-information enclosures.

*Evaluated by Antimicrobial Panel I.

†Evaluated by Antimicrobial Panel II. The FDA approved an additional active ingredient: Poloxamer 188.

**Safety and Effectiveness:
Combination Products Sold Over-the-Counter
to Prevent Skin Infections**

Safe and Effective

bacitracin + polymyxin
neomycin + polymyxin + bacitracin
bacitracin + neomycin
any one tetracycline + bacitracin*†
any one tetracycline + polymyxin*

Conditionally Safe and Effective

polymyxin + gramicidin†
any one tetracycline + gramicidin*†

Unsafe and Ineffective

None

NOTE: Determinations made by the Antimicrobial II Panel
and the FDA.
*"Tetracycline" may be *chlortetracycline hydrochloride;
oxytetracycline hydrochloride;* or *tetracycline hydrochloride.*
†These combinations are not yet marketed without prescription in the United States.

First-Aid Preparations: Product Ratings[1]

Skin-Wound Cleansing Products

Product and Distributor	Dosage of Active Ingredients	Rating[2]	Comment
benzalkonium chloride			
Bactine (Miles Labs.)	**spray:** 0.13% **squeeze bottle:** 0.13%	A	
Zephiran (Winthrop)	**tincture:** 1:750 **tincture spray:** 1:750	A	
hexylresorcinol			
S. T. 37 (Beecham Products)	**solution:** 0.1%	A	
povidone-iodine			
Betadine (Purdue-Frederick)	**spray:** liberates approx. 10% free iodine **skin cleanser:** liberates approx. 10% free iodine	B B	not proved safe or effective not proved safe or effective
	skin cleanser, foam: liberates approx. 10% free iodine	B	not proved safe or effective
Polydine (Century)	**solution:** liberates approx. 10% free iodine	B	not proved safe or effective
Povadine (Chaston)	**solution:** liberates approx. 10% free iodine **solution, swabsticks:** liberates approx. 10% free iodine **solution, wipes:** liberates approx. 10% free iodine	B	not proved safe or effective
tincture of iodine			
iodine topical solution (generic)	**solution:** 2% iodine + 2.4% sodium	B	not proved safe; may sting less than

tincture of iodine (generic) — **swabs:** 2% iodine + 2.4% sodium iodide + 50% alcohol — **B** — not proved safe

triclocarban

Coast (Procter & Gamble)	**bar soap:** triclocarban	B	not proved safe or effective
Dial Gold (Armour Dial)	**bar soap:** triclocarban	B	not proved safe or effective
Irish Spring (Colgate-Palmolive)	**bar soap:** triclocarban + triclosan	B	neither ingredient proved safe or effective
Safeguard (Procter & Gamble)	**bar soap:** triclocarban	B	not proved safe or effective

triclosan

Bactal Soap (LaCrosse)	**liquid:** 0.5%	B	not proved safe or effective

Combination Skin-Wound Cleansing Products

Product and Distributor	Dosage	Antimicrobial	Anesthetic	Rating[2]	Comment
Aerocaine (Aeroceuticals)	spray	0.5% benzethonium chloride	13.6% benzocaine	A	
Americaine First Aid (American Critical Care)	spray	0.1% benzethonium chloride	10% benzocaine	A	
Anbesol (Whitehall)	liquid	povidone-iodine yielding 0.04% available iodine + 70% alcohol	6.3% benzocaine	B	povidone-iodine not proved safe and/or not proved effective
Bactine Antiseptic Anesthetic First Aid (Miles)	spray liquid aerosol	0.13% benzalkonium chloride	2.5% lidocaine	A	
Oil-O-Sol (Health Care Industries)	presaturated gauze pads	0.1% hexylresorcinol	6.8% camphor	C	camphor not safe (*see* CAMPHOR: SPECIAL WARNING)
Solarcaine (Plough)	spray	0.18% triclosan	9.4% benzocaine	B	triclosan not proved safe or effective

First-Aid Preparations: Product Ratings[1] (continued)

Skin-Wound Protectant Products

Product and Distributor	Dosage of Active Ingredient	Rating[2]	Comment
benzalkonium chloride			
Bactine (Miles Labs.)	**spray:** 0.13%	**B**	not proved safe or effective
	squeeze bottle: 0.13%	**B**	not proved safe or effective
hexylresorcinol			
S. T. 37 (Beecham Products)	**solution:** 0.1%	**B**	not proved effective
povidone-iodine			
Betadine (Purdue-Frederick)	**spray:** liberates approx. 10% free iodine	**B**	not proved safe or effective
	ointment: liberates approx. 10% free iodine	**B**	not proved safe or effective
Operand (Redi Products)	**spray:** liberates approx. 10% free iodine **ointment:** 1% iodine	**B**	not proved safe or effective
tincture of iodine			
iodine topical solution (generic)	**solution:** 2% iodine + 2.4% sodium iodide in purified water	**B**	not proved safe; may sting less than tincture of iodine
iodine tincture (generic)	**liquid:** 2% iodine + 2.4% sodium iodide	**B**	not proved safe

Combination Skin-Wound Protectant Products

Product and Distributor	Dosage Form	Antimicrobial	Anesthetic	Rating[2]	Comment
Americaine (American Critical Care)	**ointment**	0.1% benzethonium chloride	20% benzocaine	**B**	benzethonium chloride not proved safe or effective
Americane First Aid (American Critical Care)	**spray**	0.1% benzethonium chloride	10% benzocaine	**B**	benzethonium chloride not proved safe or

Product and Distributor		Dosage of Active Ingredients	Rating[2]	Comment
Bactine Antiseptic Anesthetic First Aid (Miles)	spray liquid aerosol	0.13% benzalkonium chloride 2.5% lidocaine	B B C	benzalkonium chloride not proved safe or effective inadequate dosage of benzocaine; triclosan not proved safe or effective
Solarcaine (Plough)	cream	0.2% triclosan 1% benzocaine		
	lotion	0.2% triclosan 0.5% benzocaine	C	inadequate dosage of benzocaine; triclosan not proved safe or effective

Wound-Healer Products

Product and Distributor	Dosage of Active Ingredients	Rating[2]	Comment
allantoin Allantoin (City Chemical)	**powder:** 98%	B	not proved effective
chlorophyll derivatives Chloresium (Rystan)	**ointment:** 0.5% **solution:** 0.2%	B B	not proved effective
cod-liver oil Cod Liver Oil Liquid (Squibb)	**liquid:** 4,250 IU vitamin A + 425 IU vitamin D per teaspoonful	B	not proved effective
cod liver oil, USP (generic)		B	
live yeast-cell derivative Preparation H (Whitehall)	**ointment:** live yeast-cell derivative to provide 2,000 units skin respiratory factor per ounce + 3% shark-liver oil **suppositories:** live yeast-cell derivative to provide 2,000 units skin respiratory factor per ounce + 3% shark-liver oil	B	not proved effective

First-Aid Preparations: Product Ratings[1] (continued)

Wound-Healer Products

Product and Distributor	Dosage of Active Ingredients	Rating[2]	Comment
vitamin A			
Panthoderm (USV)	**lotion** and **cream:** 2% dexpanthenol	B	this drug is a vitamin-A precursor; vitamin A not proved effective as wound-healer

Combination Wound-Healer Products

Product and Distributor	Dosage of Active Ingredients	Rating[2]	Comment
A and D (Schering)	**ointment:** vitamin A + vitamin D	B	not proved effective
Andoin (Ulmer)	**ointment:** vitamin A + vitamin D + 1% allantoin	B	not proved effective
Balmex (Macsil)	**ointment:** vitamin A + vitamin D + Peruvian balsam + zinc oxide + bismuth subnitrate	C	last ingredient not safe or effective (see UNGUENTS AND POWDERS FOR THE SKIN)
Caldesene Medicated (Pharmacraft)	**ointment:** cod-liver oil (vitamin A + vitamin D) + zinc oxide + lanolin + petrolatum + talc	B	not proved effective
Desitin (Leeming)	**ointment:** cod-liver oil (vitamin A + vitamin D) + zinc oxide + petrolatum + lanolin	B	not proved effective
vitamins A and D (generic)	**ointment:** vitamin A + vitamin D	B	not proved effective

1. For rating of products containing antiseptics, see page 77; for ratings of products containing antibiotics, see pages 49 and 351.
2. Author's interpretation of Panel criteria. Based on contents, not claims.

First Aid Antibiotics for Preventing Skin Infections: Product Ratings[1]

Single-Ingredient Products

Product and Distributor	Dosage of Active Ingredients	Rating[2]	Comment
bacitracin			
bacitracin (generic)	**ointment:** 500 units per g	A	active against gram-positive bacteria
Baciguent (Upjohn)		A	active against gram-positive bacteria
chlortetracycline hydrochloride			
Aureomycin (Lederle)	**ointment:** 3%	A	active against gram-positive and some gram-negative bacteria
neomycin sulfate			
neomycin (generic)	**ointment:** 5 mg per g (0.5%)	A	active against gram-positive and some gram-negative bacteria
Myciguent (Upjohn)		A	active against gram-positive and some gram-negative bacteria
tetracycline hydrochloride			
Achromycin (Lederle)	**ointment:** 3%	A	active against gram-positive and some gram-negative bacteria

Combination Products

Product and Distributor	Dosage of Active Ingredients	Rating[2]	Comment
Bacimycin (Merrell-National)	**ointment:** 500 units zinc bacitracin + 3.5 mg neomycin base (as sulfate) per g	A	

First Aid Antibiotics for Preventing Skin Infections: Product Ratings[1] *(continued)*

Combination Products

Product and Distributor	Dosage of Active Ingredients	Rating[2]	Comment
Baximin (Columbia Med.)	**ointment:** 5000 units polymyxin B sulfate + 3.5 mg neomycin base (as sulfate) + 400 units bacitracin per g	A	polymyxin adds protection against gram-negative bacteria
Hysoquen (Tutag)		A	
Neo-Polycin (Dow)		A	
Neosporin (Burroughs-Wellcome)		A	
Epimycin "A" (Delta Drug)	**ointment:** 5000 units polymyxin B sulfate + 3.5 mg neomycin base (as sulfate) + 400 units bacitracin + 10 mg diperodon hydrochloride per g	C	diperodon, a pain reliever, not safe in antibiotic combinations
Spectrocin (Squibb)	**ointment:** 2.5 mg neomycin base (as sulfate) + 0.25 mg gramicidin per g	B	gramicidin not proved safe or effective
Terramycin with Polymyxin B Sulfate (Pfipharmecs)	**ointment:** 30 mg oxytetracycline (as hydrochloride) + 10,000 units polymyxin B sulfate per g	A	
Tri-Salve (Rexall)	**ointment:** 5000 units polymyxin B sulfate + 3.5 mg neomycin base (as sulfate) + 500 units zinc bacitracin per g + 3% benzocaine	C	benzocaine, a pain reliever, not safe in antibiotic combinations

1. For use of these products to *treat* skin infections, once they have arisen, *see* ANTIBIOTICS FOR SKIN INFECTIONS, page 45.
2. Author's interpretation of Panel/FDA criteria. Based on contents, not claims.

Gels for Cavity Prevention

See TOOTHPASTE, RINSES, AND GELS FOR CAVITY PREVENTION

Gum Treatments

Few body tissues weather as much stress and strain as the gums (gingiva). Overlaying our jawbones and ensheathing our teeth, gums are scalded and chilled by food and drink, assaulted by hard and sharp food substances and other objects that are stuck into the mouth, and subjected to extreme pressure when we chew. Finally, infections can arise from bacteria that thrive on food that gets lodged between the gums and teeth and then decays—as well as from bacteria, viruses, and other microorganisms deposited in the gums by body-system infections or even by the air we breathe.

Gum problems are, of course, closely related to teeth. Teething is the first cause of sore gums for most babies. Tooth-straightening braces can be irritating and painful. Later, the buildup of bacteria-laden dental plaque is a principal cause of the persistent gum soreness called gingivitis. False teeth (dentures) often cause gum pain. So, too, do tooth extractions and other dental procedures.

Minor gum sores and irritations soon heal. This natural healing perhaps can be assisted—and the soreness certainly can be relieved—by a variety of drugs that may be applied to the gums. Reviewers caution, however, that many dental products sold for gum care contain ingredients that are useless or even harmful—and some healing claims made for them are extravagant. Also, seriously and persistently painful gums should not be self-treated, says the Panel. A dentist should be consulted.

While the discussion here pertains particularly to the gums, the Panel often speaks more generally of the "oral mucosa." Injuries to and infections of the mucous membranes on the roof, sides, and floor of the mouth, and the nonprescription drugs that may be used to relieve such conditions are described more fully in SORE-THROAT AND MOUTH MEDICINES.

TYPES OF DRUGS THAT CLEAN GUMS

After a lot of deliberation, the Panel identified 5 different types of drugs that may be used to treat the gums.

GUM TREATMENTS is based on the report "Oral Mucosal Injury Drug Products" and on the report "Drug Products for the Relief of Oral Discomfort for OTC Human Use" by the FDA's Advisory Review Panel on OTC Dentifrice and Dental Care Drug Products.

- *Gingival wound cleansers* physically or chemically assist in removing foreign matter from gum wounds.
- *Gingival wound-healing agents* may promote healing of small, superficial wounds.
- *Gingival analgesics* relieve pain.
- *Gingival protectants* are inert (inactive) substances that coat, cover, and protect sore spots on the gum, so that irritation is relieved.
- *Gingival antimicrobial agents* kill or retard the growth of germs and other infectious microorganisms.

In this unit individual active ingredients are sometimes described more than once since some ingredients are claimed to fulfill more than one purpose.

GINGIVITIS

The Panel makes a critical distinction between minor gum disorders and gingivitis. The former refers to inflammation, irritation, and injuries caused principally by "mechanical" forces—such as newly erupting teeth and dentures that fit less than perfectly—and also might include overzealous tooth-picking, burns from hot food or utensils, and other types of injury (trauma). These are conditions that can be successfully self-treated with over-the-counter dental-care products.

The second type of gum inflammation, gingivitis, is the more serious disease. And it is less amenable to self-treatment with nonprescription drugs, or, for that matter, with available prescription drugs. Gingivitis is defined as inflammation in the contact areas where gums and teeth meet. It is caused by bacterial plaque, the sticky, gellike mass of food particles, tissue secretions, and bacteria and their breakdown products that builds up on the teeth, often in spite of brushing. Plaque is the principal cause of dental cavities.

The bacteria in plaque secrete acids and other substances that cause chronic redness, swelling, and soreness of the gum. Besides being extremely irritating, the continued presence of plaque causes the gums to recede from the teeth, which then become loosened in their sockets and eventually fall out or require extraction. For these reasons, the Panel says: "dental plaque and gingivitis represent two of the leading dental-health problems in the country today." Some bacterial plaque can be removed by toothbrushing. But even very diligent brushing may leave significant deposits because tooth alignment and related factors block the bristles' action.

The Panel believes that none of the currently marketed preparations promoted for use against plaque has been demonstrated to be really safe and effective. Such drugs may include cetylpyridinium chloride and domiphen bromide, which have been reported to yield a 30 to 40 percent reduction in plaque when used regularly, as well as more traditional antimicrobial agents like thymol and eucalyptol.

The present Panel, like the Panel on Oral Cavity Drug Products, is particularly worried about antimicrobials in mouthwashes that are recommended for daily use. This routine use may be hazardous (*see* THE WAR ON DENTAL PLAQUE in MOUTHWASH FOR ORAL HYGIENE). Therefore, at least for the moment, reviewers reject as unproved, untrue, or misbranding all claims that antiseptic mouthwashes and gum-care drugs will reduce or prevent plaque or gingivitis. However, they strongly endorse self-treatment with fluoride toothpastes, rinses, and gels for preventing tooth decay (*see* TOOTHPASTES, RINSES, AND GELS FOR CAVITY PREVENTION). The regular use of dental floss to remove food particles between the teeth may help, too. But the most effective method for removing plaque and preventing gingivitis is periodic cleaning and polishing of the teeth by a dentist or oral hygienist, and, when necessary, curettage (scraping under the gumline).

COMBINATION PRODUCTS

A confusing collection of combination products is sold for the relief of sore gums. Evaluators favor single-active-ingredient products and stress that combinations should be used only when one is suffering from both symptoms for which the combined-ingredient product promises relief. To win approval as safe and effective, a combination product must contain safe and effective amounts of 2—but no more than 2—individual safe and effective or active ingredients. The *only* approved combination being marketed is: 1 safe and effective gingival protectant + 1 safe and effective gingival anesthetic.

The present Panel originally planned to include denture adhesives in its findings, and was prepared to give its stamp of approval to all combination products containing a safe and effective gingival anesthetic + a safe and effective denture adhesive. But a change in federal law switched the adhesives from the category of *drugs* to that of *medical devices*—beyond the review process.

GINGIVAL WOUND CLEANSERS

Gingival wound cleansers are widely used. They are swished around in the mouth for a minute or so and then spat out, thus removing foreign matter from small and superficial gum wounds and irritations. These cleansers are not effective against chronically sore gums (gingivitis) or the buildup of bacterial deposits (plaque), which is the principal cause of persistently sore gums.

Many dentists recommend these cleansers to their patients for relieving gum and mucosal injuries and for cleansing the mouth. They usually contain compounds like hydrogen peroxide that rapidly release oxygen when they come in contact with tissue or salivary enzymes. A bubbling, foaming action results. The Panel says that the "wound-cleansing action appears to be a result of this foaming activity, which physically removes debris from the wound." And it adds that evidence for effectiveness comes mostly from clinical impressions rather than scientific study.

CLAIMS FOR WOUND CLEANSERS FOR GUMS

Accurate
for "temporary use in the cleansing of wounds caused by minor oral irritation or injury such as that following minor dental procedures, or from dentures or orthodontic appliances [braces on the teeth]"

for "temporary use in the cleansing of gum irritation due to erupting teeth [teething]"

False or Misleading
"relieves pain"

for "temporary relief of minor congestion and associated pain of surface inflammation"

"apply before a meal for pain relief"

"prevention of minor inflammation"

"an aid to regular oral hygiene"

to "promote firmer and healthier gums"

These cleansers are not indicated for treating bacterial plaque or gingivitis and, similarly, should not be labeled for use in "aphthous ulcers," "canker sores," "periodontal disease," or "pyorrhea"—all of which require dental diagnosis and professional care. Also, no evidence is available to show that massaging the medication onto the area is any more useful than applying it without rubbing.

WARNING These preparations should not be used for more than a week at a time without a dentist's or a physician's supervision.

Approved Active Ingredients

Carbamide peroxide in anhydrous glycerin   In the mouth carbamide peroxide quickly breaks down to about 70 percent urea and 30 percent hydrogen peroxide. The hydrogen peroxide further separates into water and oxygen. The effervescent action of the oxygen bubbles released by the hydrogen peroxide provides the cleansing action—and does so effectively. The glycerin acts as a stabilizing agent.

Currently marketed products that contain 10 percent carbamide peroxide yield about 3 percent hydrogen peroxide—which the Panel says is safe. The glycerin and urea byproducts are also generally considered to be safe, as long as the approved dose—several drops of the preparation—is applied directly to the affected areas of the mouth.

The medication should remain in place at least one minute, then be spit out. It can be used 4 times daily—after meals and before bedtime or as directed by a dentist or physician. Children under 12 should be supervised by their parents in the use of this preparation and it should not be used on babies under age 2, even if they are teething, except with the advice and supervision of a dentist or pediatrician.

Hydrogen peroxide in aqueous solution   The decision that this preparation is safe and effective for temporary use is supported by studies in animals and by considerable medical and dental experience with human patients. Salivary enzymes in the mouth release oxygen bubbles that provide the cleansing action. The assessment of safe and effective is also upheld by manufacturers' marketing data, which show that many, many bottles of the preparation are sold but few complaints are received.

Approved concentrations are 1.5 to 3 percent hydrogen peroxide. Higher levels, particularly if used over a long period of time, can injure the gums and cause a condition that researchers graphically describe as "black hairy tongue." Even at the approved dosages, repeated use may irritate the gums—so hydrogen peroxide should not be used routinely.

The safe and effective dosage for adults and children over 2 is 3 percent hydrogen peroxide. This may be formulated as drops to put onto the affected area of the mouth or as an oral rinse that is to be diluted by half and swished around the teeth and mouth. In either case, the substance should be applied for at least 1 minute, then spit out. Children under 12 should be supervised in their use of this preparation and it should not be used on babies under age 2, even if they are teething, except with the advice and supervision of a dentist or pediatrician.

Conditionally Approved Active Ingredients

None

Disapproved Active Ingredient

Sodium perborate monohydrate   This preparation can release hydrogen peroxide into the mouth, but reviewers have 2 serious complaints about it. One is that it contains the mineral boron, which is toxic. If a 1.2 gram package of sodium perborate monohydrate were used 4 times daily, as the manufacturer suggests, and if the material were swallowed instead of being spit out, as advised by the manufacturer, this would deliver several times the amount of boron that can safely be ingested in a day.

Judging by the preparation's taste when swallowed, this observer believes that users would not go on swallowing sodium perborate monohydrate for very long! But the reviewers reported that in a manufacturer's test on the product, one person in fact did fail to spit out the rinse—and was presumed to have swallowed it. For this reason, the Panel rates the preparation unsafe. Moreover, it adds, when 1.2 grams of the powdered preparation are dissolved in water, as the manufacturer recommends, the rinse that results delivers only 1.3 percent hydrogen peroxide—not the 1.5 percent that experts have set as the minimal effective dose. Conclusion: sodium perborate monohydrate, as presently packaged, is neither safe nor effective.

GINGIVAL WOUND HEALERS

For many years dental products have been marketed with label claims that state or imply that they speed, aid, or enhance the healing of injured or irritated gums. However, there is no convincing evidence that any nonprescription drug ingredient—whether used on the gums or on any other body surface—actually encourages the healing of wounds.

CLAIMS FOR WOUND HEALERS FOR GUMS

Unproved

for "temporary use to aid healing of minor oral soft tissue wounds due to injury"

False or Misleading

"assists nature" (ambiguous and difficult to prove)

references to "oxygenating tissue" (the added oxygen that hydrogen peroxide creates is present only momentarily and oxygen's contribution to healing remains to be proved)

Approved Active Ingredients

None

Conditionally Approved Active Ingredients

Allantoin Although this ingredient has long been promoted and used as a wound-healing agent that the present Panel believes is safe, effectiveness has not been proved.

Carbamide peroxide in anhydrous glycerin This preparation has been marketed in dental products for years, and the Panel judges it to be safe. But studies designed to show that it aids healing—by supplying additional oxygen to the wound—were conducted unscientifically. It is also questionable that the brief, low dosages of oxygen that this preparation provides are useful. The Panel concluded: safe but not proved effective for wound healing.

Chlorophyllins, water-soluble These preparations are derivatives of chlorophyll, the plant material that is responsible for photosynthesis (the process that uses sunlight to convert materials into carbohydrates). On a label, they may be called *potassium-sodium-copper chlorophyllin*.

The chlorophyllins have been used medicinally—both as topical and as systemic drugs—for a variety of medical problems, and have not been reported to have caused toxicity (poisoning). Animal studies also suggest these substances are safe—a judgment in which the present Panel concurs.

Chlorophyllins have been used to control odor and bacteria, and to speed healing of wounds and ulcerated sores. Reports in the medical literature describe cases in which the chorophyll compounds induced healing when all other drugs had failed to do so. The Panel says that more definitive, well-controlled scientific work remains to be done— even though some recent experiments, in tissue culture, indicate that chlorophyllins do act against bacteria found in the mouth. So effectiveness remains in doubt although safety does not.

Hydrogen peroxide in aqueous solution This preparation is safe. But the Panel believes that it remains to be proved whether the small amount of oxygen released in the mouth will increase the oxygenation of gum wounds or speed their healing. Verdict: safe but not proved effective.

Disapproved Active Ingredients

None

GINGIVAL ANALGESICS

Numbing and pain-killing drugs (analgesics) will temporarily relieve sore, irritated gums. A major problem is keeping them in contact with the sore tissue, since saliva, food particles, and other substances in the mouth dilute and neutralize the drug and then it's washed away.

The Oral Cavity Panel notes that when the drugs are formulated into slow-dissolving, candylike lozenges, or troches, they remain in the mouth far longer than liquids. Dental poultices—small, porous sacks which hold drugs that have been formulated in a slow-release base—may be an effective method for self-medicating one's gums and the inside of one's mouth, the Panel says. It adds this caution: be sure to take the poultice out before going to sleep to avoid the possibility of swallowing it and choking on it.

Many of these analgesics have been evaluated by other Panels concerned with use on other parts of the body. In this unit safety and effectiveness will be discussed only in terms of use on the gums.

CLAIMS FOR ANALGESICS FOR GUMS

Accurate

"temporary relief of pain due to minor irritation or injury of soft tissue of the mouth"

"temporary relief of pain due to minor dental procedures"

"temporary relief of pain due to minor irritation of soft tissues caused by dentures [false teeth] or orthodontic appliances [braces]"

for "canker sores when the condition has been previously diagnosed by a dentist"

False or Misleading

for "fast, temporary relief of minor mouth or gum soreness"

"stops baby's tears within seconds"

"subdues the throbbing ache of sore, swollen gums" (vague; this type of suffering may reflect a serious gum infection or other problem requiring professional care).

Approved Active Ingredients

Benzocaine This is a widely used, effective, and very safe analgesic. There is a minor risk that benzocaine will provoke an allergic response.

Pain relief begins within seconds when benzocaine is applied to the gums: this may last for 5 to 10 minutes, perhaps longer. The drug acts only on surface cells, so deep-seated pain will not be relieved.

The best vehicles for benzocaine are polyethylene or propylene glycol water-soluble bases or ointments, or ethyl alcohol (up to 70 percent). The safe and effective dosage for adults, children, and babies over 4 months of age is 5 to 20 percent benzocaine. It should be applied with a swab or small piece of cotton, up to 4 times daily. Children up to age 12 should be supervised when they use benzocaine, and the drug should not be used on infants under 4 months of age without a doctor's supervision.

Parents of infants should note that benzocaine is the only analgesic that the Panel lists as safe and effective for relieving teething distress in children without a doctor's or a dentist's supervision.

The Panel judges the drug safe (despite a minor risk of allergic responses) and effective as a gingival analgesic.

Butacaine sulfate An effective nitrogen-based analgesic, butacaine sulfate has been used by dentists for a long time. The reviewing Panel has recommended that the drug be made available without prescription. Several researchers who studied butacaine sulfate concur that it is very effective in relieving pain after dental work as well as the soreness and discomfort that are caused by braces and dentures.

The trouble with butacaine, as with similar nitrogenous pain relievers, is that it can be highly toxic. It can cause convulsions, coma, slowed heartbeat, heart failure, and death *if* large enough quantities are absorbed through the lining of the mouth and reach the central nervous system or heart. To forestall this hazard, the Panel stipulates that the drug be sold only in tiny, one-use tubes that contain no more than 30 mg of butacaine sulfate. It further warns that only one tube should be used at a time.

Butacaine should not be used for teething infants or for any other reason in children under 12, except under a dentist's or a doctor's supervision.

The safe and effective dose is 30 mg (0.75 gram of a 4 percent ointment) to be taken at no less than 3-hour intervals, up to 3 times daily. Persons allergic to procaine or other *-caine* analgesics should not use this drug.

Phenol and sodium phenolate (under 1.5 percent phenol) These drugs, with their familiar medicinal smell, have been used mainly as germ killers, or antiseptics. The Panel says this analgesic activity stems from their ability to block nerve conduction—a process that has been documented scientifically.

But only very low doses are safe, the Panel stresses. Higher levels can destroy nerve endings in the gums and could help to promote cancer.

The safe and effective dosage of phenol for children over 2 and adults is 0.25 to 1.5 percent phenol, applied up to 4 times daily or as recommended by a dentist or doctor. The total allowable dose in any given day is 300 mg phenol for children and 500 mg phenol for adults, for no more than 7 days. Children under 12 should be supervised when they use phenol preparations, which should not be given to children under 5 except when recommended by a dentist or a doctor.

Conditionally Approved Active Ingredients

Benzyl alcohol Although high concentrations of this alcohol (originally obtained from oil of jasmine) are quite irritating to the gums, the drug has been shown to be safe at low concentrations of up to 3 percent. The Panel admits that benzyl alcohol has some local analgesic properties, but it feels that the results of topical use are uncertain and that the doses needed to relieve pain in soft tissues in the mouth have not been determined. So the Panel's verdict is: benzyl alcohol is safe in concentrations up to 3 percent but has not been proved effective.

Cresol This is a phenollike compound that can be highly irritating to skin and mucous membranes. Dilute solutions are used therapeutically, but the Panel could find no evidence to show that they are safe.

Although studies in humans and animals indicate that cresol does have some local analgesic activity, reviewers found no adequately controlled scientific studies to demonstrate cresol's effectiveness as a pain reliever for the gums. In sum, cresol has not been proved safe or effective.

Thymol preparations: Thymol and thymol iodide These substances are toxic in large doses but apparently safe in the tiny doses for which they may be used to treat sore gums. They are used by dentists to relieve gingival pain, but there is scant scientific documentation of their effectiveness for this purpose. So the thymols are, for now, judged safe but not proved effective.

Disapproved Active Ingredients

Camphor   This is a highly toxic substance, but one that would be unlikely to cause severe problems when applied to the gums in the small amount that a health-product consumer might use. The principal risk—which leads the Panel to brand it unsafe—is that a child might accidentally consume some of the medication and suffer severe symptoms or even death as the result (*see* CAMPHOR).

Camphor is formulated with phenol in a product intended for treating the gums and oral mucosa. The Panel could find little evidence to show that the camphor makes any therapeutic contribution to this combination. (The phenol—at concentrations of 0.25 to 1.5 percent—is safe and effective without the camphor.) After reviewing the matter, the Panel judged camphor to be ineffective as well as unsafe.

Methyl salicylate   The pleasant wintergreen aroma and taste of this aspirinlike drug tend to conceal the fact that it is highly toxic. It is also extremely irritating to the gums. The Panel says it is both unsafe and ineffective.

GINGIVAL PROTECTANTS

A protectant is a pharmacologically inert substance—that is, it is chemically inactive. The way gingival protectants do act is by adhering to the gums and providing a protective coating that insulates a sore area against further irritation. Some protectants form fairly rigid covering layers; others are flexible.

CLAIMS FOR PROTECTANTS FOR GUMS

Accurate
"forms a coating over a wound"
"protects against further irritation"
for "temporary use to protect wounds caused by minor irritations or injury"

Approved Active Ingredients

Benzoin preparations: benzoin tincture and compound benzoin tincture   These are preparations that dentists have used for years to cover and protect small wounds in the gums, lips, and other soft tissues in the mouth. Benzoin is a pine-tree resin with a vanillalike aroma and slightly acrid taste. Benzoin tincture contains 20 percent benzoin in alcohol. Compound benzoin tincture contains 10 percent benzoin, 2 percent aloe, 8 percent storax, 4 percent tolu balsam, and 74 to 80 percent alcohol.

These preparations are relatively toxic, largely because of their high alcohol content. But in the tiny amounts that are required to treat small sores in the mouth, the Panel says they are safe.

No really thorough studies have been conducted to confirm that benzoin preparations are effective when used on the gums. But a host of clinical reports plus the long history of use by dentists convinced reviewers that these compounds are effective for covering and thus easing the pain of chemical or thermal burns, minor injuries, and irritations. They are sometimes applied to canker sores, but the Panel believes they should be used for this purpose only under a doctor's supervision.

Experts urge that these preparations always be used at full strength —*not* diluted—in order to preserve their protectant effectiveness. Before application, the affected tissue must first be dried. Then a few drops of the medicine should be put on with a cotton swab.

For adults and children over 6 months of age, the safe and effective dosage is a few drops used no more often than once every 2 hours. Children under 12 should be supervised when they use such products.

Conditionally Approved Active Ingredient

Myrrh fluid extract This dressing is obtained from a tree resin that the ancient Egyptians used to embalm the dead. The Panel could find no reports of toxicity following the use of small amounts of myrrh on the gums. Neither, however, could it find much data to establish the extract's safety when it's used in this way.

As to effectiveness, evaluators could not find any studies in humans to demonstrate that this preparation is of value as a protectant to injured gums. So both the safety and the effectiveness of this resin remain to be proved.

Disapproved Gingival Protectants

None

ANTIMICROBIALS

Some products sold to relieve sore or irritated gums contain antimicrobial agents, which are claimed to kill or inhibit the bacteria and other microorganisms. The present Panel asked the Panel on Oral Cavity Drug Products—which looked at a wide range of antimicrobials that are used in oral health-care products—to evaluate those ingredients contained in products intended for gum treatments.

Not one antimicrobial was judged both safe and effective for use in the mouth. However, some of these ingredients were judged conditionally safe and effective and it is thought that comparable benefits may be anticipated for sore gums.

CLAIMS FOR ANTIMICROBIALS FOR GUMS

Unproved
for "the temporary relief of minor sore mouth and sore throat by decreasing germs in the mouth"

INACTIVE INGREDIENTS

beeswax
calcium carbonate
cellulose gum
chlorobutanol hydrous
  (chloroform
  derivative)
chloroform
cinnamon oil (cassia
  oil, oil of cassia)
DC red color 11251
distilled water
edetate disodium
  (EDTA)

glycerin
hops
magnesium aluminum
  silicate
nitrogen, compressed
  (propellant)
paraffin wax
petrolatum
pluronic F-127
potassium sulfate
propylene glycol
propylparaben

sassafras root
silica
sodium bicarbonate
sodium chloride
sodium lauryl sulfate
sodium saccharin
sodium sulfate
sorbitol
water

Safety and Effectiveness: Active Ingredients in Over-the-Counter Gum Treatments

Active Ingredient	Panel's Assessment
Gingival Wound Cleansers	
carbamide peroxide in anhydrous glycerin	safe and effective
hydrogen peroxide in aqueous solution	safe and effective
sodium perborate monohydrate	not safe or effective
Gingival Wound Healers	
allantoin	safe but not proved effective
carbamide peroxide in anhydrous glycerin	safe but not proved effective

Safety and Effectiveness: Active Ingredients in Over-the-Counter Gum Treatments *(continued)*

Active Ingredient	*Panel's Assessment*
chlorophyllins, water soluble	safe but not proved effective
hydrogen peroxide in aqueous solution	safe but not proved effective
Gingival Analgesics	
benzocaine	safe and effective
benzyl alcohol	safe but not proved effective
butacaine sulfate	safe and effective
camphor	not safe or effective
cresol	not proved safe or effective
methyl salicylate	not safe or effective
phenol preparations under 1.5% phenol (phenol and sodium phenolate)	safe and effective
thymol	safe but not proved effective
Gingival Protectants	
benzoin preparations: benzoin tincture and compound benzoin tincture	safe and effective
myrrh fluid extract	not proved safe or effective
Gingival Antimicrobials*	
benzoic acid	safe but not proved effective
boric acid	not safe or effective
cetylpyridinium chloride	not proved safe or effective
ethyl alcohol	safe but not proved effective
eucalyptol	safe but not proved effective
menthol	safe but not proved effective
sodium perborate monohydrate	not safe or effective
thymol	safe but not proved effective
thymol iodide	not proved safe or effective

*Antimicrobials were evaluated by the Advisory Review Panel on OTC Oral Cavity Drug Products. (*See* SORE THROAT AND MOUTH MEDICINES).

Safety and Effectiveness: Combination Products Sold Over-the-Counter to Treat Sore Gums

Safe and Effective

all ingredients must be safe and effective
1 gingival protectant + 1 gingival analgesic
1 gingival protectant + 1 oral antiseptic (of which none has been approved)
1 gingival analgesic + 1 oral antiseptic (of which none has been approved)
1 gingival wound cleanser + 1 oral antiseptic (of which none has been approved)
1 gingival wound healer (of which none has been approved) + 1 oral antiseptic (of which none has been approved)

**Safety and Effectiveness: Combination Products
Sold Over-the-Counter to Treat Sore Gums *(continued)***

Conditionally Safe and Effective

any 2 approved or conditionally approved ingredients from the same pharmacological group, acting by different mechanisms, provided both are present within the effective dosage range. (Does not apply to gingival analgesics.)

1 gingival protectant + 1 gingival wound healer

1 gingival analgesic + 1 gingival wound healer

2 toothache relievers acting by different mechanisms

1 toothache reliever + 1 gingival analgesic

1 gingival analgesic + 1 counterirritant

1 gingival protectant + 1 gingival analgesic claimed to have prolonged action (the protectant may hold the analgesic in contact with the affected area for an extended period of time)

1 gingival wound healer + 1 oral antiseptic

1 gingival protectant + 1 oral antiseptic

1 gingival analgesic + 1 oral antiseptic

1 gingival wound cleanser + 1 oral antiseptic

Unsafe or Ineffective

contains any disapproved ingredient

contains any approved ingredient or combination of ingredients in less than the minimum effective dosage

contains any active ingredient that has not been reviewed by an OTC advisory Panel

contains more than 2 active ingredients

contains active ingredients from 2 pharmacological groups but there is no significant population that needs the concurrent therapy

is "irrational"*

contains drugs that are dangerous or neutralize each other when combined

contains 1 gingival protectant + 1 toothache relief agent ("irrational" and dangerous)

contains 1 gingival protectant + 1 counterirritant ("irrationally counterproductive")

contains 1 gingival protectant + 1 tooth desensitizer ("irrational")

contains 1 toothache relief agent + 1 counterirritant ("irrational")

contains 1 toothache relief agent + 1 tooth desensitizer ("irrational")

contains 2 chemically similar gingival analgesics

contains 1 gingival analgesic + 1 tooth desensitizer ("irrational")

contains 2 counterirritants

contains 1 counterirritant + 1 tooth desensitizer

contains 2 tooth desensitizers

contains 1 gingival protectant + 1 gingival wound cleanser ("irrational")

contains 1 toothache relief agent + 1 gingival wound cleanser ("irrational")

contains 1 gingival analgesic + 1 gingival wound cleanser ("irrational")

contains 1 counterirritant + 1 gingival wound cleanser ("irrational")

contains 1 tooth desensitizer + 1 gingival wound cleanser ("irrational")

contains 1 toothache relief agent + 1 gingival wound healer

contains 1 counterirritant + 1 gingival wound healer ("irrational")

**Safety and Effectiveness: Combination Products
Sold Over-the-Counter to Treat Sore Gums** *(continued)*

Unsafe or Ineffective

contains 1 tooth desensitizer + 1 gingival wound healer ("irrational")

contains 1 toothache relief agent + 1 oral antiseptic ("irrational")

contains 1 counterirritant + 1 oral antiseptic ("irrational")

contains 1 tooth desensitizer + 1 oral antiseptic ("irrational")

contains 2 gingival wound healers

contains 1 gingival wound cleanser + 1 tooth desensitizer ("irrational")

contains 1 gingival wound healer + 1 counterirritant ("irrational")

contains 1 gingival wound healer + 1 tooth desensitizer ("irrational")

contains 1 peroxide-containing gingival wound healer + 1 gingival protectant (the peroxide would wash away the protectant)

contains 1 peroxide-containing gingival wound healer + 1 oral analgesic (the peroxide would wash away the analgesic)

contains a gingival wound cleanser formulated as a dentifrice (brushing can aggravate a wound)

contains a gingival wound healer formulated as a dentifrice (brushing can aggravate a wound)

---

*By "irrational" the Panel means a combination that makes no sense because the effects counteract one another, may interfere with specific treatment, could mask a condition so that it becomes worse, or otherwise prove unworkable.

Gum Treatments: Product Ratings

Gingival Wound Cleansers

Product and Distributor	Dosage of Active Ingredients	Rating[1]	Comment
carbamide peroxide in anhydrous glycerin			
Gly-Oxide Liquid (Marion)	**drops:** 10%	**A**	
Periolav (Spectro Med)		**A**	
Proxigel (Reed & Carnrick)	**gel:** 11%	**C**	too much carbamide peroxide
chlorophyllins (water-soluble)			
Chloresium Dental Ointment (Rystan)	**ointment:** 0.5%	**B**	not proved effective
	solution: 0.2%	**B**	not proved effective
hydrogen peroxide			
hydrogen peroxide 3% (generic)	**liquid**	**A**	
PerOxyl Mouthrinse (Hoyt)	**solution:** 1.5%	**A**	

Gum Treatments: Product Ratings *(continued)*

Gingival Wound Cleansers

Product and Distributor	Dosage of Active Ingredients	Rating[1]	Comment
sodium perborate monohydrate			
Amosan (Cooper)	**powder:** 1.2 g per packet	C	not safe or effective

Gingival Anesthetics

Product and Distributor	Dosage of Active Ingredients	Rating[1]	Comment
benzocaine[2]			
Benzodent (Vicks Toiletry Products)	**ointment:** 20%	A	
Orajel (Commerce Drug)	**gel:** 10%	A	
Rid-A-Pain (Abbott)	**gel:** 10%	A	
phenol preparations			
Chloraseptic (Norwich-Eaton)	**gel:** 1.4% phenol as phenol and sodium phenolate	A	

Gingival Protectants

Product and Distributor	Dosage of Active Ingredients	Rating[1]	Comment
benzoin preparations			
benzoin (generic)	**tincture:** 20%	A	
benzoin compound (generic)	**tincture:** 10% benzoin + 2% aloe + 8% storax + 4% tolu balsam + 74–80% alcohol	A	

Combination Products for the Gums

Product and Distributor	Dosage of Active Ingredients	Rating[1]	Comment
Anbesol (Whitehall)	**liquid:** 6.3% benzocaine + 0.5% phenol + 70% alcohol **gel:** 6.3% benzocaine + 0.5% phenol + 70% alcohol	B	2 anesthetics together get only conditional approval; alcohol not proved effective as antiseptic

Gum Treatments: Product Ratings *(continued)*

Combination Products for the Gums

Product and Distributor	Dosage of Active Ingredients	Rating[1]	Comment
Butyn (Abbott)	**ointment:** 4% butacaine + 1% benzyl alcohol	B	contains 2 gingival anesthetics; the butacaine alone would rate an "A"
Kank-a (Blistex)	**liquid:** 0.5% cetylpyridinium chloride + 1% benzocaine + benzoin compound	C	inadequate dosage of benzocaine; the antimicrobial cetylpyridinium is not proved safe or effective
Rid-a-Pain (Pfeiffer)	**gel:** 10% benzocaine + eucalyptol + thymol + menthol + alcohol	C	too many antimicrobial active ingredients, not one of which has been proved effective

1. Author's interpretation of Panel criteria. Based on contents, not claims.
2. For benzocaine lozenges and troches, *see* Product Ratings for Sore Throat and Mouth Medicines, pages 725–726. Benzocaine products rated in this unit are for direct application to the gums.

Hair-Growth Stimulants and Baldness Preventives

If "hair growers" and other products that are purported to prevent or correct baldness actually worked, they would be front-page news, not advertising matter on the inside pages of newspapers, as they now are. The sad fact is that no known drug, whether sold over-the-counter or by prescription, will prevent or reverse baldness. A number of products and ingredients that are now or have been sold for this purpose were assessed by an over-the-counter review panel that declared:

HAIR-GROWTH STIMULANTS AND BALDNESS PREVENTIVES is based on the report "Hair-Grower and Hair-Loss-Prevention Drugs" by the FDA's Advisory Review Panel on OTC Miscellaneous External Drug Products.

"No data are available in the [medical and scientific] literature demonstrating the effectiveness of ingredients reviewed as hair-growers and hair-loss-prevention drug products. . . . All claimed hair-grower and hair-loss-prevention active ingredients reviewed are not effective."

This means that products whose labels promise help against baldness are "misbranded." It also means, if the FDA follows the Panel's recommendations, that all such products will eventually be ordered off the over-the-counter drug market, under penalty of law.

WHY HAIR GROWS AND THEN STOPS GROWING

The commonest type of baldness in men is the receding hairline. The frontal V of balding scalp progresses relentlessly backward until it reaches a second balding area at the crown of the head. Only a horseshoe-shaped remnant of hair is then left, along the side and back of the head. This is called male pattern baldness. It is a hair trait that is inherited from one's forebears—as are hair color, hair texture, and the curl or straightness of one's hair.

Women do not suffer this severe baldness. Their hair may thin out naturally as they grow older, but it does not vanish.

Hair loss over much of the scalp may occur as an aftermath of childbirth, fever, crash dieting, iron deficiency, exposure to X-rays, and hormonal imbalances like hypothyroidism and hyperthyroidism. It also can be caused by drugs, particularly the potent ones used to treat cancer. Smaller and sometimes very unsightly patches of baldness can be caused by fungus infections or by syphilis and other diseases. The hair may regrow normally in these forms of baldness if the hair follicle, where each hair sprouts from the scalp, has not been seriously damaged. Because sudden, excessive hair loss or an unusual pattern of baldness may signal an underlying illness, persons who experience either should consult a doctor.

Under normal circumstances each hair grows for a certain period of time, then enters a transitional stage in which growth slows and stops, and then finally remains in the follicle without growing for a period before it is shed. Then the cycle repeats as the follicle becomes active again and produces a new hair. Under normal circumstances, about 85 percent of the hair on a human scalp is in the growth phase.

A hair grows only in one direction—lengthwise, from the root outward. Above the root, a hair shaft is dead tissue—like a nail. It cannot grow longer or thicker no matter how industriously it is cared for or treated with drugs. Cosmetic substances that cling to the shaft can, of course, make it look and feel thicker.

Many products promoted to prevent baldness claim to strengthen and conserve the hair. Persons tempted to believe these claims may do well to bear in mind the Panel's unequivocal finding that "nothing done to the hair shaft once it emerges from the surface of the scalp will influence the hair growth. Anything that would influence regeneration of the hair would have to work on the hair root. . . . To demonstrate that an ingredient is a hair restorer, it must be proven that the substance gets into the hair root and causes stimulation of hair growth."

To provide this proof a manufacturer, university, or independent researcher would have to demonstrate the following—none of which has been shown to date:

- an increase in the growth rate of the hair
- an increase in the diameter of the hair shaft
- a lengthening of the hair-growth phase
- an increase in the weight of treated hair

Hormones and Hair Growth

One factor that unquestionably does influence hair growth is the level of sex hormones that are circulating in the bloodstream and present in the body. Unfortunately, hormones do not affect hair growth when they are applied directly to the scalp or skin.

Hormones change the growth rate, thickness, and color of the hair on various body surfaces. At puberty, for example, very thin, fine, colorless hair (vellus hair) appears on a boy's chin. Under the influence of the male sex hormone testosterone, this changes to become thick, long, pigmented beard hairs. Around 20 or 30 years later, the changes that produce male pattern baldness essentially reverse this process. The scalp-hair follicles do not simply stop producing hairs; rather, the thick, long, pigmented hair on the scalp is replaced by thin, soft, vellus hairs. The hair-growth phases also become shorter, so that the hairs produced are shorter, too.

The Sebum Theory

Oiliness of the scalp is a condition that *can* be controlled by using shampoos and other drug and cosmetic products. Much of this natural oil—called *sebum*—is produced by glands in the skin called *sebaceous glands*.

One theory states that male baldness may be caused by sebum. If this is true, then so-called sebum hair-loss might be prevented by quickly removing these oily substances from the scalp.

The manufacturer of a hair-preserving regimen submitted studies published some 30 years ago. These reports indicate that when human sebum was appled to rats' skins, their hair fell out. No recent studies and no studies in humans were presented to support this observation or the sebum-hair-loss theory itself, which evaluators say doctors do not accept. On the contrary, a study cited in medical textbooks shows, for example, that sebum secretions are essentially the same on men with bald scalps, on the hairy parts of balding men's scalps, and on the scalps of men with no signs of baldness. The Panel's conclusion: "Balding men did not have abnormally oily scalps, and [there was] no quantitative chemical difference" between the sebum of balding and nonbalding men.

OVER-THE-COUNTER BALDNESS PREPARATIONS

Approved Active Ingredients

None

Conditionally Approved Active Ingredients

None

Disapproved Active Ingredients

Not surprisingly, in view of the information presented earlier in this unit, the Panel discounted the effectiveness of all of the active ingredients it assessed. It dismissed 5 of the ingredients rather summarily, but discussed the female hormone estradiol (a form of estrogen) at length.

Similarly, combination products were also dismissed because all single-entity active ingredients are ineffective.

Ascorbic acid (vitamin C) The manufacturer who submitted a product that contains this substance did not submit, and the Panel could not find, any evidence to show that—by itself or in combination with other ingredients—it has any influence on hair growth. Verdict: not effective.

Benzoic acid The findings and the verdict duplicate those outlined for ascorbic acid (*see* directly above).

Estradiol This substance is a form of the female hormone estrogen. When very potent estradiol compounds are applied to the forehead of normal men, they reduce the production of oil, or sebum. But attempts to inhibit sebum production with estradiol skin creams have been unsuccessful.

Estrogens are readily absorbed through the skin. So there is concern about their use by men, since persistent exposure can cause feminizing changes. For example, male factory workers who handle estrogen develop abnormally large breasts.

To forestall this side effect, estrogenic baldness remedies—like estrogen skin creams that women use for other purposes—are labeled with instructions not to exceed a measured quantity of estrogen. This amount equals 666 International Units (IU) of the hormone per day. Evaluators believe this is a safe amount and they note that in the 30 years that estradiol skin creams have been marketed, only a tiny handful of adverse reactions have been attributed to their use.

The major question, then, is whether estradiol assists hair growth and helps prevent baldness. Since the sebum-hair-loss theory has been scientifically discredited, reviewers had strong doubts about estradiol's effectiveness. The Panel reviewed 4 studies submitted and decided that 3 were "too subjective to be convincing, because they consisted of only favorable testimonials by dermatologists, as well as [by] men and women with hair loss. . . . No descriptions, photographs, or quantitative data on the hair loss of individual patients were given." While evaluators felt the fourth study was well planned, they believed it to be so badly conducted that no significance could be attached to the results.

These studies were based on the manufacturer's recommended regimen: application of a deacidizing scalp conditioner, a scalp cleanser, a shampoo, the hair-growth stimulator, and an antiseptic dressing. The reviewers concluded that while the ingredients in this regimen are safe, neither all of them together nor estradiol alone is effective in preventing hair loss due to sebum or in stimulating hair regrowth. Furthermore, although the Panel specifically says these ingredients are safe, the FDA lists estradiol as unsafe as well as ineffective as a treatment for baldness.

Lanolin   Despite a manufacturer's submission of a product containing this substance, reviewers were not able to locate any evidence that lanolin (alone or in combination) affects hair growth. The verdict: safe but not effective. An FDA summary of the Panel's findings, puzzlingly, lists lanolin as unsafe as well as ineffective for hair growth.

Tetracaine hydrochloride   The manufacturer who submitted a product that contains this ingredient said that it improves circulation, relieves scalp itching, and aids in the development of the hair follicle. But no evidence was submitted or found to show that tetracaine hydrochloride has any effect on hair growth. The Panel concluded that the chemical is safe but not effective.

Wheat-germ oil   This substance—purported to be a source of vitamin E and of thiamine—was included in a baldness remedy submitted for review. But the maker furnished no data to show that wheat germ oil (alone or in combination with other ingredients) has any effect on hair growth, nor could the Panel find any such evidence. Conclusion: topically applied wheat germ oil is safe but not effective in restoring hair or preventing baldness.

Other Ingredients in Baldness Preparations

A variety of drugs are formulated into products promoted for preventing baldness or stimulating hair growth. In sorting them out, reviewers listed the following as inactive ingredients that have no medicinal effect, good or bad, on the scalp or hair.

ammonium lauryl sulfate	polyethylene glycol 400
benzethonium chloride	polysorbate 80
coconut oil	sodium hydroxide
isopropyl alcohol	sulfonated vegetable oil
methyl ethyl ketone	vegetable olive oil
mineral oil	

The Panel came up with a second list of ingredients that it did not classify either as active or inactive, but which it simply disapproved as neither safe nor effective in promoting hair growth or preventing hair loss because no scientific evidence could be found to justify such use. These disapproved ingredients are:

allantoin (5-ureidohydantoin)	lauric diethanolamide
amino acids	olive oil
dichlorophen (dichlorophene)	propylene glycol
essential oils	proteins
eucalyptus oil	tar oil
fatty acids	vegetable oil
hormone constituents	vitamins

Safety and Effectiveness: Active Ingredients in Over-the-Counter Baldness Remedies

Active Ingredient	Panel's Assessment
ascorbic acid (vitamin C)	safe but not effective
benzoic acid	safe but not effective
estradiol	not effective*
lanolin	not effective*
tetracaine hydrochloride	safe but not effective
wheat-germ oil	safe but not effective

*The FDA adds "not safe."

Hair-Growth Stimulant and Baldness Preventives: Product Ratings

The Panel's judgment is that no drug product, over-the-counter or prescription, can safely and effectively stimulate hair growth or prevent baldness. So all products sold for this purpose must be rated "C."

Hangover and Overindulgence Remedies

Almost everyone has had the experience of eating or drinking too much —and then feeling awful. Can anything be done, one despairingly wonders, to calm the stomach and steady the head?

Fortunately, help is close at hand at a drugstore or grocer, if not in the medicine chest. Reviewers who evaluated several familiar products that are sold to relieve these conditions say these preparations can provide significant relief. On the other hand, several drugs that are marketed to *prevent* inebriation and hangover strike the Panel as worthless.

WHAT KINDS OF RELIEF ARE NEEDED?

The over-the-counter drugs assessed by the Panel are intended for the relief of occasional overindulgence or intoxication; they may bring little comfort to chronic alcoholics or inveterate gluttons. As the Panel sees things, 2 somewhat different conditions may require treatment. *Upset stomach* due to overindulgence in food and alcohol results when one eats and drinks too much, together. The key symptoms are heartburn, a sense of fullness, and nausea. *Hangover* results when one simply drinks too much alcohol. The symptoms may include nausea, heartburn, thirst, tremor, unsteadiness, fatigue, aches and pains, headache, and feelings of dullness, depression, or irritability.

HANGOVER AND OVERINDULGENCE REMEDIES is based on the unadopted draft report "OTC Orally Administered Drug Products for Relief of Symptoms Associated with Overindulgence in Alcohol and Food" by the FDA's Advisory Review Panel on OTC Miscellaneous Internal Drug Products.

With this distinction in mind, the Panel divided the products and ingredients it assessed into 3 groups:

- ingredients and drugs intended to relieve overindulgence in food and alcohol
- ingredients and drugs intended to relieve hangover
- ingredients and drugs intended to prevent alcoholic inebriation or speed one's recovery from it

UPSET STOMACH DUE TO OVERINDULGENCE

The Panel decided that the symptoms of overindulgence experienced by people who eat and drink too much are distinct and identifiable. These symptoms are different from hangover alone (which results from alcohol overindulgence) or from overeating alone.

The evaluators' recognition of these symptoms was based mostly on unpublished studies supplied by the manufacturers, in which persons who had overindulged—or who were deliberately overindulged—in rich food and drink were asked to describe their ill feelings. The following symptoms were listed by participants: fullness, heartburn/burning, passing of gas, stomach ache, headache, belching, rumbling stomach, thirsty/dry mouth, sluggishness, taste repeat, nausea, bitter/acid aftertaste. In all the studies, most participants complained of heartburn, fullness, and/or nausea. This led reviewers to identify these as the condition's principal symptoms. According to the Panel, it's the alcohol that is more responsible than the food.

The Panel approached products used to treat upset stomach due to overindulgence with a certain degree of skepticism. One reason is that evaluators could not think of any single active ingredient that will safely and effectively relieve either nausea or fullness, 2 of the 3 main symptoms of overindulgence. The third key symptom, heartburn, can be relieved with a number of safe and effective antacid active ingredients.

COMBINATION PRODUCTS

A fair number of persons with upset stomachs due to overindulgence also suffer headaches and other minor aches and pains. So the experts approve of combining a safe and effective pain reliever—either aspirin or acetaminophen—with safe and effective active ingredients that quell upset stomach; they do not sanction combinations that include 2 different aspirinlike drugs (salicylates). The Panel also approves of one safe and effective stimulant—caffeine—in overindulgence preparations.

One preparation that is marketed for upset stomach due to overindulgence contains aspirin + citric acid + sodium bicarbonate. When this product is immersed in water a chemical reaction occurs: the ingredients are converted into sodium acetylsalicylate (a pain reliever) + sodium citrate (an antacid) + bubbles of carbon dioxide gas. There is some residue of sodium bicarbonate, which also acts as an antacid. Another approved combination consists of acetaminophen + citric acid + caffeine.

CLAIMS FOR OVERINDULGENCE REMEDIES

Accurate
for "the relief of upset stomach due to overindulgence in food and drink"
for "the relief of upset stomach associated with nausea, heartburn and fullness due to overindulgence in food and drink"

False or Misleading
"fast relief" (too vague)
relieves "upset stomach with headache from overindulgence" (the *kinds* of overindulgence aren't specified)

DRUGS FOR UPSET STOMACH DUE TO OVERINDULGENCE

The Panel reviewed 5 ingredients in upset-stomach calmers. Two of them—aspirin and acetaminophen—are pain relievers that have been approved as safe and effective by another Panel; the approved dosages are 325 to 650 mg every 4 hours, except that an initial 975 mg dose is permitted.

A third ingredient—sodium bicarbonate—is judged to be a helper (or adjuvant) to the other active ingredients. Two other drugs are discussed directly below.

Approved Active Ingredients

Bismuth subsalicylate   This bismuth compound has been found safe as a medication to counteract diarrhea at higher dosages than are recommended for the treatment of upset stomach due to overindulgence in food and drink. So the present Panel judges it safe.

The effectiveness of bismuth subsalicylate against upset stomach due to overindulgence was tested in 3 excellently constructed and well-controlled tests. Participants were randomly assigned either to a treatment group or a dummy-medication group; neither the participants nor the investigators knew which people were receiving the bismuth subsalicylate and which the dummy preparation until after the test was over. In one of these tests 132 normal, healthy, nonalcoholic men and women were wined and dined in a dinner-party setting, where they were offered unlimited amounts of champagne, wine, and cordials to drink. Not surprisingly, 91 or them developed gastrointestinal distress during the course of the evening—and they required drug treatment. Roughly half took the bismuth subsalicylate preparation and half the look-alike dummy medication.

When the results were tabulated, it turned out that 9 out of 10 overindulgers who had dosed themselves with bismuth subsalicylate experienced good to excellent relief from their distress—including, particularly, relief from nausea, fullness, and heartburn. Of the overindulgers who took the dummy preparation, only a few more than half experienced good to excellent relief. These are significant findings in favor of the medication's ability to combat both the overall overindulgence syndrome and its 3 principal symptoms.

Evidence from the 2 other studies assessed by the Panel was less convincing, but the general results led reviewers to judge bismuth subsalicylate effective for relieving overindulgers' upset stomach. Appropriate doses are 0.525 grams to be taken no more often than every 30 to 60 minutes, for a total dose of 4.2 grams (or 8 doses) per day.

WARNING If taken with other salicylates, and ringing in the ears occurs, discontinue use. If taking medication for anticoagulation (thinning of the blood), consult a physician before taking this product.

Citric acid As an overindulgence remedy citric acid is very often formulated in tablets or granules, along with sodium bicarbonate and a pain-relieving active ingredient. It fizzes—or effervesces—when put into water. In the resulting reaction, the citric acid is converted to sodium citrate.

Since citric acid has been approved as safe (as well as effective) as an antacid, the present reviewers accept it as safe. The Panel is not persuaded, however, that it effectively relieves gastrointestinal distress due simply to overeating.

Only one scientifically controlled study was submitted to support the claim that citric acid specifically relieves upset stomach associated with overindulgence in rich and spicy foods that are washed down with alcoholic beverages. But statistically significant benefit was recorded only on "the morning after," not during the night.

Although the data on citric acid's effectiveness are less convincing than those for bismuth subsalicylate (*see* above), the Panel decided on the basis of this one study that citric acid is safe and effective in providing general relief of upset stomach due to overindulgence, but that it doesn't act specifically against heartburn, fullness, or nausea. The safe and effective dosage should not exceed approximately 16 grams of sodium citrate for persons under 60 years of age, half that amount for older persons.

WARNING   If you are on a sodium-restricted diet, do not take this product except under the supervision of a physician.

HANGOVER REMEDIES

The Panel defines *hangover* as the "noxious feelings encountered several hours after the occasional ingestion of large amounts of alcohol." The commonest symptoms are nausea, heartburn, thirst, tremor, loss of balance, fatigue, aches and pains, and irritable, dull, or depressed feelings.

Sufferers have long used 3 kinds of drugs to relieve these symptoms: pain relievers like aspirin for the headache, antacids for the gastric distress, and caffeine—a stimulant—for the dullness and fatigue. These are logical choices, reviewers decided, so they approved combinations that include safe and effective doses of these 3 types of ingredients. In essence, the Panel reversed the usual policy of the over-the-counter drug review. That is, it actually recommended that hangover remedies be formulated as combination products rather than as single-entity drugs.

The safe and effective pain relievers are acetaminophen and aspirin. In one preparation, aspirin is mixed with citric acid and sodium bicarbonate in such a way that when the product is put into water before it's swallowed, a chemical reaction occurs. The ingredients are converted into sodium acetylsalicylate (a pain reliever) + sodium citrate (an antacid) + bubbles of carbon dioxide gas + a residue of sodium bicarbonate.

The safe and effective stimulant is caffeine. The safe and effective antacids are aluminum hydroxide, aluminum hydroxide gel, citric acid (sodium citrate), magnesium carbonate, and magnesium trisilicate.

CLAIMS FOR HANGOVER REMEDIES

Accurate

for "the relief of hangover"

if appropriate ingredients are included, symptoms such as "headache," "generalized aches and pains," or "dullness, depression, and/or irritability" may be mentioned

Combination Products

The Panel specifically approves the 4 combination products submitted for its scrutiny.

aspirin + citric acid + sodium bicarbonate (which produces sodium acetyl-salicylate + sodium citrate + carbon dioxide gas + sodium bicarbonate when mixed with water)

acetaminophen + citric acid + sodium bicarbonate (which produces acetaminophen + sodium citrate + carbon dioxide gas + sodium bicarbonate when mixed with water)

aspirin + caffeine + aluminum hydroxide + magnesium carbonate

acetaminophen + aspirin + caffeine + magnesium trisilicate + magnesium carbonate + aluminum hydroxide gel

The Panel notes that the last 2 formulas have too little antacid to meet the FDA's standards for effective antacids. It also notes that persons who use hangover remedies are not attempting to neutralize an excess of stomach acids but rather are trying to protect the stomach—which has been irritated by alcohol—from the burning created by normal acid secretions.

Consumers should choose combination hangover remedies that contain only the ingredients they need to relieve their symptoms. For example, if you are nauseated but have no headache or other aches and pains, then you probably do not require a pain reliever. If you have only a headache, on the other hand, a couple of acetaminophen or aspirin tablets should suffice. The Panel does not approve hangover remedies that contain vitamins.

Approved Active Ingredients

Pain relievers Acetaminophen and aspirin are safe and effective. The approved dosage is 325 to 650 mg every 4 hours, with an initial 975 mg dose permitted.

Stimulants The approved (safe and effective) stimulant is caffeine. It should be taken in doses of 100 to 200 mg.

Antacids Safe and effective antacids are aluminum hydroxide, aluminum hydroxide gel, citric acid (sodium citrate), magnesium carbonate, and magnesium trisilicate.

Conditionally Approved Active Ingredients

None

Disapproved Active Ingredients

None

INEBRIATION AND HANGOVER PREVENTIVES

The best way to prevent hangovers is to drink in moderation. Preparations are marketed with claims about preventing intoxication or minimizing hangover symptoms. Two active ingredients sold for these purposes are activated charcoal, which is claimed to prevent or minimize the symptoms of hangover, and fructose (fruit sugar), which is said to prevent inebriation. (Inactive ingredients in these preparations include dextrose, disaccharide, peat, and xylem.)

The Panel does not believe that either of the 2 active ingredients is effective. So it disapproves both of them.

CLAIMS FOR INEBRIATION PREVENTIVES

False or Misleading
for "the prevention of inebriation"
"to minimize the symptoms of a hangover"
for "the prevention of the symptoms of a hangover"
"an aid in preventing the symptoms of a hangover"

Approved Active Ingredients

None

Conditionally Approved Active Ingredients

None

Disapproved Active Ingredients

Charcoal, activated   This material has a honeycomb structure that allows it to hold and neutralize large amounts of chemical substances. For this reason, it is widely used as an antidote to accidental poisoning, and the Panel judges it safe for use at the lower doses that are recommended for minimizing hangover.

The claim that activated charcoal helps circumvent hangovers is based on the theory that it is the impurities in alcohol—not the alcohol itself—that are largely responsible for unpleasant aftereffects of drinking. According to this theory, vodka, which is largely free of impurities, causes fewer symptoms than an equivalent amount of bourbon, which contains many of these impurities. The problem is that while impurities have been shown to play some role in drunkenness, other studies indicate that it is the *amount* of alcohol consumed—whether as vodka or whiskey—that largely determines drunkenness. Not surprisingly, therefore, another test showed that bourbon produces no worse hangovers than vodka. No direct evidence is available from studies in humans to show that activated charcoal will neutralize impurities or minimize hangover. So the Panel judges activated charcoal safe but not effective when taken for this purpose.

Fructose   Also called *fruit sugar*, or *levulose*, fructose is said to speed up the body's breakdown and neutralization of alcohol. In hospital emergency rooms, fructose is sometimes infused into the bloodstream of grossly intoxicated persons for just this purpose. The rather large doses used in this way appear to be safe, so the Panel believes that taking much smaller amounts of up to 3 grams of fructose (as recommended by the manufacturer) is also safe. Another indication of safety lies in the fact that fructose is a common food substance. It is one of the principal components of honey.

Many studies have been conducted to assess fructose's effectiveness in relieving inebriation. The Panel finds the results inconclusive. The sugar may—or may not—prompt a slight increase in the rate of alcohol metabolism when taken along with, or soon after, the booze. But the reviewers say there is no evidence that it significantly lessens inebriation or the hangover symptoms that follow. So the conclusion is: safe but not effective for preventing inebriation.

**Safety and Effectiveness: Active Ingredients in
Over-the-Counter Remedies to Relieve Upset Stomach
Due to Overindulgence in Food and Drink**

Active Ingredient	Panel's Assessment
acetaminophen	safe and effective
aspirin	safe and effective
bismuth subsalicylate	safe and effective
citric acid	safe and effective
sodium bicarbonate (adjuvant)	safe and effective

**Safety and Effectiveness: Active Ingredients in Over-the-Counter
Remedies for Hangover**

Active Ingredient	Function	Panel's Assessment
acetaminophen	pain reliever	safe and effective
aspirin	pain reliever	safe and effective
aluminum hydroxide	antacid	safe and effective
aluminum hydroxide gel	antacid	safe and effective
caffeine	stimulant	safe and effective
charcoal, activated	preventive	safe but not effective
citric acid (sodium citrate)	antacid	safe and effective
fructose (fruit sugar)	preventive	safe but not effective
magnesium carbonate	antacid	safe and effective
magnesium trisilicate	antacid	safe and effective
sodium bicarbonate	adjuvant	safe and effective

Hangover and Overindulgence Remedies: Product Ratings

Overindulgence Relief Products

Product and Distributor	Dosage of Active Ingredients	Rating[1]	Comment
Alka-Seltzer (Miles)	**effervescent tablets:** 324 mg aspirin + 1.9 g sodium bicarbonate + 1 g citric acid	A	
Bromo Seltzer (Warner-Lambert)	**effervescent granules:** 325 mg acetaminophen + 2.781 g sodium bicarbonate + 2.224 g citric acid per capful measure	A	

Hangover and Overindulgence Remedies: Product Ratings *(continued)*

Overindulgence Relief Products

Product and Distributor	Dosage of Active Ingredients	Rating[1]	Comment
Pepto-Bismol (Norwich-Eaton)	**suspension:** 527 mg bismuth subsalicylate per 2 tablespoonsful dose (30 ml)	A	
	tablets, chewable: 300 mg bismuth subsalicylate	A	

Hangover Relief Products

Product and Distributor	Dosage of Active Ingredients	Rating[1]	Comment
Alka-Seltzer (Miles)	**effervescent tablets:** 324 mg aspirin + 1.9 g sodium bicarbonate + 1 g citric acid	A	
Bromo Seltzer (Warner-Lambert)	**effervescent granules:** 325 mg acetaminophen + 2.781 g sodium bicarbonate + 2.224 g citric acid per capful measure	A	

Products to Prevent Drunkenness or Minimize Hangover

Product and Distributor	Dosage of Active Ingredients	Rating[1]	Comment
Charcocaps (Requa)	**capsules:** 260 mg activated charcoal	C	not effective
Fructose Tablets (Nature's Bounty)	**tablets:** fructose	C	not effective

1. Author's interpretation of Panel criteria. Based on contents, not claims.

Headache Remedies

See PAIN, FEVER, AND ANTI-INFLAMMATORY DRUGS TAKEN INTERNALLY

Hemorrhoid Medication and Other Anorectal Applications

"The U.S. Government has spent over $50 billion to study the backside of the moon, but not one red cent to study the backsides of its citizens."

—LEON BANOV, M.D.

Few self-treatable conditions are as anguishing—physically and emotionally—as hemorrhoids. Reviewers who assessed the ointments and suppositories used to relieve hemorrhoids point to factors that enhance this distress.

- The anorectal region, or anorectum, like the nearby genital area, is richly endowed with sensory nerve receptors—and so hurts and/or itches quite badly when disturbed.
- Among body regions, the anorectum is a "social outcast." Many people, doctors included, are shy about discussing it. This may start with early childhood—when youngsters are encouraged to use euphemisms like "bottom," "fanny," or "behind." Code names are often taught both for defecation itself as well as for the place where this is done—"rest room," "tinkle room," or "potty."

A more frank and forthright acceptance of bowel functions would be beneficial. People could more easily and straightforwardly ask for and receive medical help for anorectal disorders and be spared much immediate suffering.

AN ANATOMIC TOUR OF THE ANORECTUM

Since it is difficult to see one's anus without using a mirror, reviewers offered this brief guided tour. Starting from outside, the perianal area is defined as the 3-inch-wide circle of skin immediately surrounding the anal opening. This skin is moist and is more vulnerable to

HEMORRHOID MEDICATION AND OTHER ANORECTAL APPLICATIONS is based on the report by the FDA's Advisory Review Panel on OTC Hemorrhoidal Drug Products.

pressure, frictional injury, and infection. The perianal area also contains very sensitive pain-receiving nerve endings, which also transmit itching sensations.

The anus is the external opening through which bowel movements pass. The tight, inch-long passage above it is the anal canal. It normally stays tightly closed against leakage and seepage except when one's bowels are moving or gas is being passed. Two sets of muscles open and close the canal. One, which surrounds part of the upper portion of the canal, is the *internal anal sphincter*; it is an involuntary muscle that functions outside our conscious control. Surrounding the terminal portion of the canal is a muscular structure called the *external anal sphincter*, which we "push open" to defecate.

The anal canal is lined with skin and is studded with sensory nerve fibers that convey pain and itching. At its upper end is a demarcation, the anorectal line, where the skin gives way to mucosal surface. There the tight anal canal widens into a 5-inch-long hollow column, the rectum, where feces collect before defecation. Unlike anal skin, the rectal mucosa does not have superficial pain and itch receptors. But its underlying tissues do harbor pressure-sensitive nerves that tell us when to go to the toilet. These nerves also enable us to feel the difference between solid matter and flatus (gas). The anal canal and lower rectum are served by 3 major sets of blood vessels: the inferior (lower), middle, and superior (upper) hemorrhoidal arteries and veins. When affected by swelling they may be a source of considerable discomfort—and, sometimes, more serious disorders.

DISORDERS

Hemorrhoids   The anorectal disease of greatest concern to consumers is hemorrhoids, which sometimes are called *piles*. A hemorrhoid is a swollen or symptom-producing conglomeration of blood vessels, supportive tissue, and overlying mucous membrane or skin. It usually develops along the anal canal or in the lower end of the rectum. Blood may be discharged from the hemorrhoidal blood vessels. But bleeding is by no means the only symptom: hemorrhoids typically cause burning, itching, inflammation, and swelling.

External hemorrhoids, which are those that arise below the anorectal line, constitute a substantial share of the problems for which consumers seek relief with over-the-counter medications. Internal hemorrhoids, which are less common, arise above the anorectal line. When an internal hemorrhoid extends down into the anal canal, or even out through the anus, it is said to be prolapsed.

The sluggish blood-flow through the hemorrhoidal vessels is believed to be a major contributing cause of hemorrhoids. The blood pools up and balloons out the veins and surrounding tissues. Humankind's upright stance may contribute to the problem. Blood in the hemorrhoidal veins must be pumped upward, against gravity, to return to the heart. In most four-legged animals the rectum is higher than the heart. Thus gravity carries the blood back, so it does not collect in vein-stretching pools.

Straining during defecation is another cause of piles because it compresses the hemorrhoidal veins; blood pressure builds up within them, dilating their walls. The increased pressure pregnancy exerts on the pelvis commonly causes hemorrhoids. Another contributing factor may be the accumulation of fecal matter in small pockets (crypts) near the top of the anal canal. An increased intake of roughage may help clean out these pockets.

Perianal abscess   This condition can be defined as an infection and collection of pus due to bacterial penetration of underlying tissues.

Anal fissure   A painful crack or sore in the skin of the anal canal is referred to as an anal fissure.

Anal itchiness   Sufferers experience a persistent and often intense itching in the perianal area. Poor hygiene is a common cause of this complaint, which also may result from the consumption of peppery foods. In children, sudden attacks of intense itching at night often signal pinworm infections (*see* WORM-KILLERS FOR PINWORM). If anal itching does not vanish quickly, a doctor's help should be sought.

A warm sitz bath may resolve the problem. Alternatively, OTC drugs that contain local anesthetics may bring relief. Hydrocortisone preparations may also be particularly helpful.

Polyps   These are benign tumors that arise in, or from just beneath, the mucous membrane of the rectum.

Anorectal cancer   Bleeding and a constant urge to defecate may result from a malignant tumor.

TREATMENT

Uncomplicated hemorrhoids and other minor, noncancerous anorectal disorders can be treated successfully with nonprescription drugs. But if the symptoms do not clear up completely within a week, they require medical attention. Bleeding from the anus, mucus discharge, seepage of fecal matter, and protrusion of a hemorrhoid or of rectal tissue outside the anal canal are all signs of potentially serious medical problems. In these instances, a doctor should always be consulted.

Types of Drugs

A *vasoconstrictor* temporarily shrinks swollen hemorrhoidal blood vessels. A *counterirritant* takes one's mind off pain or itching by producing competing sensations. An *astringent* concentrates and holds (binds) proteins—which may be bacteria, fecal matter, or festering body products—and keeps them away from the skin; it may also produce a bracing sensation. A *skin-peeling agent (keratolytic)* removes dead outer skin. An *anticholinergic* blocks the activity and functions of secretory glands triggered by the nerve-impulse-transmitting substance called acetylcholine. *Anesthetics* deaden pain; *antiseptics* clean wounds; *protectants* provide a protective coating; and *wound-healing agents* assist in the healing process.

For the Panel's comments about hemorrhoid drug ingredients and the symptoms they relieve *see* the DRUGS TO RELIEVE ANORECTAL SYMPTOMS chart.

Drugs to Relieve Anorectal Symptoms

Panel's Expectations for Relief

Symptom or sign	Local Anesthetics	Vasocon-strictors	Protectants	Counter-irritants	Astringents	Wound-healing Agents	Antiseptics	Skin-peeling Agents	Anticho-linergics
itching	yes	yes	yes	yes	yes	maybe	maybe	yes	no
discomfort	yes	maybe	yes	yes	yes	maybe	maybe	no	no
irritation	yes	no	yes	maybe	yes	maybe	maybe	no	no
burning	yes	no	yes	maybe	maybe	maybe	maybe	no	no
swelling	no	yes	no	no	no	maybe	maybe	no	no
pain	yes	maybe	no	yes	yes	maybe	maybe	no	no
inflammation	no	no	maybe	no	no	maybe	maybe	no	no
protrusion	should not be self-treated with over-the-counter products								
seepage	should not be self-treated with over-the-counter products								
bleeding	should not be self-treated with over-the-counter products								

Dosage Forms

Consumers use anorectal drug products to medicate 2 essentially different types of tissues: the perianal area and the rectum (as defined above). These areas respond to drugs in different ways, and different methods are used to treat them. Drugs applied to the perianal area and anal canal are being used *externally*. Drugs slid or pushed through the anal canal into the rectum are being applied *intrarectally*.

Three different delivery systems are used in anorectal products: ointments, suppositories, and foams.

Ointments   These are semisolid preparations that may soften but will not melt into a liquid when they are subjected to normal body temperature of about 98.6°F. Reviewers included creams, gels, jellies, and pastes in their evaluation of anorectal ointments. These substances can be smeared on exposed surfaces and also can be forced upward into the anal canal with the fingertip.

When ointments are used intrarectally, they can be inserted through a tubular applicator sometimes called a *pile pipe*. This is slid past the anal sphincter muscle so that the medication is expelled from the tip and deposited within the rectum. The pile pipe should be flexible and should be well lubricated—perhaps with some of the ointment —so that it slides in easily and does not injure the anal canal or rectal mucosa. Even when they are applying an ointment intrarectally, many people prefer using their fingers—which the Panel says is even safer.

Dosages of anorectal products are hard to standardize. However, evaluators concluded that the average suppository weighs about 2 grams, about 1/14 of an ounce. Studies have shown that patients tend to apply about the same quantity of an anorectal ointment product each time they use it. This amount is enough to provide an effective and protective layer over the perianal area. So the Panel accepts 2 grams —which is the weight of 2 paper clips—as more or less the standard dose for an anorectal product.

Suppositories   Soft, usually slippery, solid formulations, suppositories are oval or bullet-shaped to slide easily through the anal canal and into the rectum. (Reviewers say an hourglass shape would allow the suppository to stay in place longer.) Unlike an ointment, when a suppository is inserted into the rectum little if any of the drug adheres to the anal canal. Suppositories are composed of materials that melt readily at normal body temperature.

This kind of medical treatment has been used at least since biblical times. It continues to be popular, although current reviewers believe the benefit may be more in the mind than in the anorectum and that relief experienced may be dangerously deceptive—that is, one may feel a disorder is being *cured* rather than simply relieved, which could delay a person's seeking appropriate medical attention.

Traditionally, suppositories are made of soap, tallow, candle wax, and, more recently, cocoa butter or glycerin. These substances all relieve constipation and help people move their bowels. The protectant substances in contemporary over-the-counter suppositories may lubricate the anal canal so that stools pass without tearing or irritating the tissue—but consumers are cautioned that the amount of lubricant is not sufficient to act as a laxative. In other words, a suppository will ease but not *induce* a bowel movement. So any claim that such a product facilitates bowel movements is clearly inappropriate, according to the Panel.

The principal use of suppositories as nonprescription anorectal medication is for local treatment of the lower rectum and anal canal, particularly for sufferers of internal hemorrhoids. Since the rectum has no surface receptors for pain and itch, it makes little sense to use such products to treat these symptoms.

A normally functioning sphincter will keep much or all of an anal medication from seeping downward onto itch- and pain-sensitive anal surfaces. Also, caustic fluids normally present higher up in the rectum may quickly break down the active ingredients of these drugs. For these reasons, it may help people who do use suppositories to stand up straight after inserting one. This way the medicine will have a better chance of settling downward into the anal canal.

Foams Use of foams is a new method that has been developed to overcome the shortcomings of suppositories in medicating the anorectum. Active drugs are incorporated into a foam that can be propelled into the anal canal under pressure. However, both the safety and effectiveness of foam products remain to be proved.

Testing of Ingredients

A bewildering array of factors determines how much of an active ingredient reaches a distressed skin surface and how quickly it gets there. For example, fecal matter can hinder drug absorption, so experts recommend using intrarectal drugs after—not before—a bowel movement. Also, ointment may stick to the anal wall and block other drugs' access to it.

In addition, the direction of blood-flow from the rectal vessels plays a role. A drug absorbed from a suppository that has moved to the upper end of the rectum goes to the liver. This may change the composition of many ingredients in the suppository by breaking them down into their components. But if the same suppository—or a dollop of ointment —remains in the lower rectum, the drug is likely to enter the general circulation and be carried, relatively unchanged, throughout the body. For these reasons the Panel found it very difficult to evaluate rectally administered drugs except through studies of finished products. That is, the safety or effectiveness of anorectal drug products cannot always be predicted by individual ingredients.

Choice of Ingredients

The consumer with hemorrhoids or a troublesome itch may be daunted by the discovery that different types of drugs, with dozens of active ingredients, are formulated into a wide variety of combination products that all promise symptomatic relief. The reviewers' sifting and sorting of these drugs—as summarized in the DRUGS TO RELIEVE ANO-RECTAL SYMPTOMS chart, above—should simplify the selective task. This chart allows one to pick the type of drug—local anesthetic, vaso-constrictor, etc.—most likely to relieve one's principal symptoms. Then, in order to choose ingredients that have been approved as safe and effective, one should consult the SAFETY AND EFFECTIVENESS chart at the end of this unit for the type of drug chosen. This chart shows that many protectant ingredients—the bulk of most anorectal products— are safe and effective both for external application to the perianal area and for intrarectal administration in a suppository or with a pile pipe. (Two astringents, calamine and zinc oxide, are also listed as protect-ants.)

Only 2 other drugs from one other group, vasoconstrictors, are safe and effective for intrarectal use. So, a person's choice for safe and effective intrarectal drugs is, in fact, extremely limited.

The range is slightly wider for the consumer interested in choosing a safe and effective preparation for external use. When symptoms re-quire this kind of medication, there are safe and effective agents from 3 other classes—local anesthetics, counterirritants, and skin-peeling agents (keratolytics)—to consider. But even here decision-making is limited by the fact that in all groups other than protectants, there are only 1 to 3 safe and effective ingredients. For 3 pharmacological groups —antiseptics, anticholinergics, and miscellaneous—there are no safe and effective ingredients to consider.

Safety for Women and Children

Only very small amounts of drugs are absorbed into the bloodstream when they are applied externally to the perianal area. So evaluators say women can safely use all approved active ingredients in anorectal preparations. Safe and effective protectant ingredients that have no other pharmacological effect may also be used intrarectally. However, pregnant and nursing women should not use suppositories or intrarectally applied ointments and foams that contain other types of active ingredients.

Hemorrhoids and anorectal complaints are rare in children. When they do occur, the child should be taken to a doctor. The Panel stipulates that nonprofessional diagnosis and treatment of anorectal problems should not be attempted for children under 12. Exceptions can be made in the case of the astringents (calamine, witch hazel, and zinc oxide) and approved protectants that can be used to relieve itching, burning, irritation, discomfort, and pain.

COMBINATION PRODUCTS

Most over-the-counter anorectal products contain a combination of active ingredients to treat 2 or more concurrent symptoms. Evaluators believe that 2 ingredients from 2 different drug groups are usually enough. But as many as 4 of the bland protectant ingredients may be combined if, together, they make up 50 percent or more of a finished product.

Reviewers prefer single-ingredient products and believe a consumer should use a combination product only when he or she suffers all of the symptoms found on the label. Most other Panels maintain that when safe and effective amounts of safe and effective individual ingredients are formulated together the resulting combination *ipso facto* is safe and effective. In a major departure from this practice, the present reviewers say there are so many variables in the formulation of anorectal combination products that each needs to be tested in final formulation to demonstrate safety and effectiveness. The only combinations the Panel accepts without further testing are those that contain protectant ingredients. Two, three or four safe and effective protectants can be assumed to be safe and effective together—without further testing—if they constitute half or more of each suppository or dollop of ointment.

CLAIMS

Accurate
for "the temporary relief of the discomfort associated with hemorrhoids and other anorectal disorders"

for "the temporary relief of anorectal itching"

for "the temporary relief of symptoms of inflammation associated with hemorrhoid tissues"

False or Misleading
The embarrassment that many people feel in talking about anorectal disorders may be one reason why manufacturers use promotional words and phrases that are too general, unclear, or redundant—and so may be misleading. Rejected phrases:

"uncomplicated hemorrhoids"

"simple inflammatory rectal conditions"

"use as a hygienic aid to remove the common cause of local irritation"

"relieves rectal itching" (no sensory nerve endings are in the rectum)

"anal eczema" (too technical)

"recommended by physicians" (misleading)

"provides lubrication and thus facilitates bowel movements" (too weak to act as laxative)

"immediate," "prompt," "fast" relief

DRUG GROUPINGS

The active ingredients in anorectal products were divided by the Panel into 9 groups. To find which group a specific active ingredient belongs in, consult the list that follows. Each group is then described, and a chart showing the safety and effectiveness of all ingredients in each group appears at the end of this unit.

alcloxa	skin-peeling agent
aluminum hydroxide gel	protectant
atropine	anticholinergic
belladonna extract	anticholinergic
benzocaine, polyethylene glycol ointment or gel	local anesthetic
benzyl alcohol	local anesthetic
bismuth oxide	protectant
bismuth subcarbonate	protectant
bismuth subgallate	protectant

bismuth subnitrate	protectant
boric acid	antiseptic
boroglycerin (boric acid glycerite)	antiseptic
calamine (prepared calamine)	protectant and astringent
camphor	counterirritant
cocoa butter (cacao butter)	protectant
cod-liver oil	protectant and wound-healing agent
Collinsonia extract (stone root)	miscellaneous
dibucaine (hydrochloride)	local anesthetic
diperodon	local anesthetic
dyclonine hydrochloride	local anesthetic
E. coli vaccines	miscellaneous
ephedrine sulfate	vasoconstrictor
epinephrine	vasoconstrictor
epinephrine hydrochloride	vasoconstrictor
epinephrine undecylenate	vasoconstrictor
glycerin, aqueous solution	protectant
hydrastis (golden seal)	counterirritant and antiseptic
hydrocortisone	local anesthetic
hydrocortisone acetate	local anesthetic
juniper tar (oil of cade)	counterirritant
kaolin	protectant
lappa extract (burdock root)	miscellaneous
lanolin	protectant
leptandra extract (Culver's root)	miscellaneous
lidocaine	local anesthetic
live yeast-cell derivative (skin respiratory factor)	wound-healing agent
menthol	counterirritant
mineral oil	protectant
mullein	miscellaneous
peruvian balsam	wound-healing agent
petrolatum, white	protectant
phenacaine hydrochloride	local anesthetic
phenol	antiseptic
phenylephrine hydrochloride	vasoconstrictor

pramoxine hydrochloride	local anesthetic
resorcinol	antiseptic and skin-peeling agent
shark-liver oil	protectant and wound-healing agent
sodium salicylic acid phenolate	antiseptic
starch	protectant
sulfur preparations	skin-peeling agents
tannic acid	astringent
tetracaine	local anesthetic
tetracaine hydrochloride	local anesthetic
turpentine oil, rectified	counterirritant
vitamin A	wound-healing agent
vitamin D preparations (ergocalciferol, cholecalciferol)	wound-healing agents
witch-hazel water (Hamamelis water)	astringent
wool alcohols	protectant
zinc oxide	protectant and astringent

ANESTHETICS

The symptoms that may be relieved by local anesthetics—which are also called *topical anesthetics*—include pain, burning, itching, irritation, and discomfort. They are the most important drugs for treating hemorrhoids and other anorectal disorders because they offer relief for a wider variety of symptoms than those of any other group. Such drugs act by temporarily blocking or reducing the activity of sensory nerve receptors in the skin.

Experts disagreed about whether suppositories and other products intended for intrarectal use should contain anesthetics. The majority of the Panel said there is insufficient evidence to show that anesthetics are safe or effective when used intrarectally because drugs may be absorbed into the bloodstream from the rectal mucosa almost as rapidly as if they were injected directly into a vein. Moreover, when they are absorbed from the lower rectum, drugs may immediately enter the general circulation without passing through and being broken down by the liver. This is of concern because some local anesthetics with names ending in the suffix *-caine* can cause serious—even lethal—damage to the heart and nervous system if absorbed into the body in large amounts. The *-caine*-type anesthetic benzocaine is, however, free of this risk. There is another danger in putting anesthetics into the rectum: they may mask the feelings of fullness by which the body normally tells one to sit down on the toilet.

Effectiveness also is at issue. The majority of the Panel said there are no known pain-receiving nerve endings on rectal surfaces. This is clear from the fact that cutting or burning the rectal mucosa during surgical treatments is not painful. It is further supported by 2 studies which show that test subjects could not differentiate between the pain-relieving effects of intrarectal products containing an anesthetic and look-alike dummy drugs.

Reviewers concluded that the usefulness of intrarectal anesthetics has yet to be established—so none was approved. While a minority group disagreed on sensitivity of the rectum itself and also believed that both repeated sales and clinical experience point to safety and effectiveness, the majority opinion prevailed.

CLAIMS FOR ANESTHETICS

Accurate:

for "the temporary relief of pain"

for "the temporary relief of itching"

for "the temporary relief of itching, burning, and pain associated with hemorrhoids or other anorectal disorders"

for "the temporary relief of the discomforts of hemorrhoids [piles]"

Approved Active Ingredients

Only 3 ingredients were granted approval as local anesthetics for the treatment of hemorrhoids and other anorectal disorders. All are approved for external use—not for intrarectal use—for the reasons described above.

For pramoxine hydrochloride cream and pramoxine hydrochloride jelly, approval was specifically limited to 2 brand-name products for which there is ample scientific proof of safety and effectiveness. Acceptance does not extend to other pramoxine hydrochloride formulations until manufacturers can provide satisfactory evidence. This problem arises, reviewers noted, because the action of the active ingredient hinges upon the other compounds in the product and the way they are formulated.

The FDA responded gingerly to the Panel's action, noting that it is a departure from review procedures to approve formulations, and the agency invited comments from doctors, manufacturers, and the public. *Note:* Most of the anesthetics that follow are discussed in greater detail in the unit ITCH AND PAIN REMEDIES. Their application for anorectal problems is described here.

Benzocaine, polyethylene glycol ointment (external use only) While only a few studies have been done on the use of this anesthetic for anorectal distress, evaluators judged them adequate to establish safety and effectiveness. In one study of 39 patients, for example, 20 percent benzocaine in polyethylene glycol ointment relieved anorectal discomfort in all cases; lower concentrations resulted in a lower relief rate. So the Panel approved 5 to 20 percent benzocaine per dosage unit in polythethylene glycol ointment when used up to 6 times in 24 hours.

Hydrocortisone preparations (external use only)   These chemicals and their action as itch-relievers are discussed on pages 457–58. They are very effective, but should be used only externally and are not approved for intrarectal use.

Pramoxine hydrochloride, cream or jelly (external use only) The anesthetic active ingredient in these formulations, pramoxine hydrochloride, may also be called Tronothane hydrochloride. The specific products approved by the present Panel are Tronothane hydrochloride 1 percent topical local anesthetic jelly and Tronothane hydrochloride 1 percent topical anesthetic cream (both from Abbott).

These preparations have been specifically tested in individuals with anorectal complaints. In one study of patients following hemorrhoid surgery, for example, 93 percent reported good to excellent pain relief. In another, 18 of 27 patients had improved enough after 2 weeks' treatment that they did not require surgery. The other 9 reported some symptomatic relief. Patients with anal erosions also felt less pain when they used this drug. The approved dosage, for external use only, is a 2 gram dose of the cream or jelly up to 5 times daily.

Conditionally Approved Ingredients

Benzocaine, polyethylene glycol ointment (internal use only) This drug has been approved for external use (see above). It is safe, but its effectiveness when inserted in the rectum—where the mucosa has no superficial pain receptors—has not been proved.

Benzyl alcohol (external and intrarectal uses)   This anesthetic is unlikely to be absorbed into the bloodstream whether used internally or externally, and so is probably safe for anorectal use. It may also be effective for external use, but the matter requires further study. It seems doubtful that benzyl alcohol relieves itch or pain when used internally in the rectum because of the lack of pain receptors. Thus for both external and intrarectal uses, benzyl alcohol's effectiveness remains to be proved.

Dibucaine and dibucaine hydrochloride (external and intrarectal uses)   When used externally to relieve anorectal disorders, the anesthetic dibucaine may cause allergic responses. But these reactions are not common enough or serious enough to compromise the drug's safety. However, when the drug is used intrarectally, harmful amounts of dibucaine might be absorbed into the systemic circulation—where it has the potential of acting on the heart and central nervous system. So the safety of dibucaine and dibucaine hydrochloride for use inside the rectum remains in doubt.

No studies have been reported on the use of dibucaine in the perianal area, so its effectiveness in relieving external pain and itching must be proved. Two studies of intrarectal use failed to demonstrate that dibucaine is effective, thereby lending support to the Panel majority's view that there are no pain receptors in the rectal mucosa. So the safety and effectiveness of dibucaine preparations when used externally and intrarectally have yet to be established.

Diperodon (intrarectal use only)   Diperodon has been used on many areas of the body since it was first introduced over 40 years ago. Its safety for intrarectal use has not been established. Results of studies are inconclusive, so its effectiveness has not been established. Well-controlled double-blind tests are needed to prove diperodon's safety and effectiveness.

Dyclonine hydrochloride (external and intrarectal uses)   This local anesthetic has been shown to be safe for external use on many parts of the body. While there are no tests on its safety when applied to the rectum, evaluators believe that the recommended low dosage, together with its low toxicity at other sites, vouch for the drug's safety.

A handful of tests have yielded inconclusive data to show that dyclonine hydrochloride works effectively when applied externally—so this claim must be established by further testing. No studies are available on the value of intrarectal use of dyclonine. This, too, must be proved.

Lidocaine (external and intrarectal uses)   This widely employed anesthetic agent has a lower potential for toxic and allergic reactions than many other drugs of its class. Too, published studies on its safe, effective use on many different body sites attest to its safety when it is applied to the perianal area. Because lidocaine is also widely used as an injectable drug and is considered safe in larger doses than those likely to be used in suppositories, evaluators believe it is also safe for intrarectal application.

One study demonstrated that 5 percent lidocaine effectively relieved the pain of anal fissures. But these results were inconclusive since the ointment alone—i.e., the base without the lidocaine—also relieved most patients' pain. So while Panel members are fairly confident that lidocaine is effective in treating perianal itching and pain, they want to see studies that prove this and also prove that lidocaine can relieve pain when it is applied intrarectally in a suppository or ointment.

Pramoxine hydrochloride, cream or jelly (intrarectal use only) These are the 2 formulations the Panel assessed as safe and effective when applied to the perianal area. They also judged them safe intrarectally because no toxic reactions have been reported in studies in which pramoxine hydrochloride was used in the rectum. But the data did not convince the Panel that the drug is effective when applied in this way, so proof is needed.

Tetracaine and tetracaine hydrochloride (external and intrarectal uses) These are relatively potent and also relatively toxic anesthetic agents. Given the relatively small doses that would be used in anorectal preparations, reviewers judged tetracaine and tetracaine hydrochloride safe for external use on perianal surfaces. But the drug is absorbed so readily and so rapidly from mucosal surfaces that evaluators insist that its safety for intrarectal use must be clearly demonstrated.

Tetracaine's effectiveness in relieving anorectal pain has not been studied. Thus, effectiveness must be shown for both external and internal (rectal) application.

Disapproved Active Ingredients

Diperodon (external use only) This anesthetic is conditionally approved for intrarectal use. It probably is safe for external use. But a number of studies have shown that diperodon is of little (if any) benefit when applied to relieve itch and pain due to hemorrhoids and other anorectal disorders. The verdict: not effective.

Phenacaine hydrochloride (external and intrarectal uses) This is one of the most toxic local anesthetics. The Panel says flatly: "this agent cannot be considered a safe local anesthetic for over-the-counter use because the dose required to be effective would produce toxic systemic effects." So it is rejected as unsafe.

VASOCONSTRICTORS

These drugs temporarily constrict small blood vessels. Because hemorrhoids consist in large part of swollen blood vessels, vasoconstrictors can effectively relieve the discomfort of swelling. Vasoconstrictors also seem to offer relief from itching, although *how* is yet to be explained. Also, this itch relief is less than that offered by local anesthetics.

Squeezing an injured blood vessel—whether physically or chemically—is one way to make it stop bleeding. Vasoconstrictors may stop anorectal bleeding in this way. Evaluators warn, however, that blood coming from the anus may originate from a number of sites along the gastrointestinal tract. It could result from any one of several serious diseases—including ulcers and cancer—and so *never* should be self-treated. *If you are bleeding from the anus, see a doctor*.

The major risk of these drugs is that they may be readily absorbed through the hemorrhoidal vessels and carried to the heart, brain, and other central organs. They can raise one's blood pressure, cause irregular or arrhythmic heartbeats, and trigger restlessness, nervousness, sleeplessness, and tremor. Vasoconstrictors may overstimulate the thyroid, adrenal, prostate, and other endocrine glands. Prolonged use can lead to anxiety or even paranoia. Finally, they can profoundly affect the actions of prescription drugs used to treat high blood pressure or mental illness. So reviewers specify that labels contain a warning.

WARNING FOR VASOCONSTRICTORS   Do not use products containing vasoconstrictors if you have heart disease, high blood pressure, hyperthyroidism, diabetes, difficulty in urination, or are taking tranquilizers or nerve pills.

For similar reasons, consumers are warned not to use products containing vasoconstrictors for more than than 7 days. In the nose, where they act as decongestants, and in other regions of the body, vasoconstrictors tend to be effective for only a few days. After that time there is a rebound effect in which the blood vessels relax again, and may become even more dilated than before.

CLAIMS FOR VASOCONSTRICTORS

Claims are made that vasoconstricting products "shrink" hemorrhoids. This may suggest permanent benefit—which nonprescription medication cannot provide. So the word "shrink" must be coupled with the qualifier "temporarily."

Accurate

"temporarily reduces the swelling associated with irritated hemorrhoidal tissue and other anorectal disorders"

"temporarily shrinks hemorrhoidal tissue"

"may temporarily relieve itching"

Approved Active Ingredients

Reviewers decided that 3 compounds provide safe and effective vasoconstrictive results when they are used to treat anorectal vascular swelling. Two were approved for both external use on the perianal area and intrarectal use in suppositories and ointment. One was approved for external use only. However, anyone who plans to use these approved ingredients should note the Panel's warning for vasoconstrictors.

Ephedrine sulfate, aqueous solution (external and intrarectal uses) This is a fine, white, odorless crystal or powder dissolved in water. It is readily absorbed from the rectal mucous membranes, for which reason dosage is restricted to amounts that have been shown to be safe when the drug is injected directly into a vein.

At high doses ephedrine can cause nervousness, insomnia, headache, heart palpitations, and other severe side effects, including anxiety and paranoid feelings. Even at therapeutic doses, death can occur in persons who are also taking certain drugs like phenothiazines (major tranquilizers) or MAO inhibitors, and ephedrine may also trigger cerebral hemorrhage or stroke.

Persons who have heart trouble or thyroid disease, or who are taking digitalis, heart medicine, antidepressants, or other drugs that act on the nervous system should not use ephedrine except under a doctor's care.

For those who do not have these problems, ephedrine sulfate used in the recommended doses is safe for self-treatment of anorectal swelling. However, most studies of effectiveness have been conducted on other body parts—like the nose. Moreover, while an ointment would be the most reasonable base for this drug, reviewers could find no studies of how it works against hemorrhoidal swelling when formulated this way. Nonetheless, because of ephedrine's recognized ability to temporarily constrict superficial vessels and reduce swelling, evaluators said it is effective as well as safe at 2 to 25 mg per dosage unit, up to 4 times daily, not to exceed 100 mg per day.

Epinephrine hydrochloride, aqueous solution (external use only)
This is a short-acting vasoconstrictor. The drug is chemically unstable, so that it degrades rapidly when stored in the medicine chest. Chemically, epinephrine is very similar to ephedrine, described directly above. Thus it carries the same hazards. Note the warning for vasoconstrictors.

Although epinephrine's effectiveness has largely been established on sites other than the anus and rectum, it is still considered safe and effective for relief of anorectal swelling and itching when formulated as a 0.1 percent aqueous solution of which 100 micrograms to 200 micrograms of epinephrine hydrochloride are contained in each dosage unit. It may be used up to 4 times per day. This low dosage limit was set to avoid risk, even though it is unlikely that a toxic amount of the drug can be absorbed into the bloodstream when an ointment is applied externally.

Phenylephrine hydrochloride, aqueous solution (external and intrarectal uses) A potent vasoconstrictor, this drug is related chemically to the hormone epinephrine, but it is safer than epinephrine and the Panel says it is safe. It has little effect on the central nervous system or the rhythmical beats of the heart—although it does increase cardiac output in other ways. Phenylephrine hydrochloride may also be less likely than other vasoconstrictors to cause local irritation.

As with ephedrine and epinephrine, this substance should not be used by persons with hyperthyroidism, hypertension, or cardiovascular disease, or by persons taking MAO inhibitors or other potent psychiatric drugs except under a doctor's direction. Note the warning for vasoconstrictors.

Phenylephrine hydrochloride is very efficient at constricting small blood vessels. So the Panel accepts its effectiveness in relieving hemorrhoidal swelling, itching, and discomfort despite a lack of scientific data on application to the anorectum. The approved dosage—0.5 mg up to 4 times daily—is based on studies of the agent's vasoconstrictive power when used as a nasal decongestant. The drug is approved only in an aqueous solution because there are virtually no data to establish its safety and effectiveness in suppositories or other formulations.

Conditionally Approved Active Ingredients

Epinephrine (external and intrarectal uses) This form of the hormone is pharmacologically quite similar to water-soluble epinephrine hydrochloride even though it is not soluble in water. But both its safety and effectiveness for anorectal symptoms remain to be proved.

Here, too, special caution is advised. Note the warning for vasoconstric-tors.

Epinephrine undecylenate (external use only)   A chemical vari-ant of the epinephrine molecule, this substance is claimed to be a short-acting vasoconstrictor. But data remain to be presented to dem-onstrate safety and effectiveness when the chemical is formulated for use in anorectal products. Again, users are warned. Note the warning for vasoconstrictors.

Phenylephrine hydrochloride suppositories (intrarectal use only)   This stimulant is judged safe when applied intrarectally in a suppository or ointment. But there are too few data to show that it really works when formulated in that manner. Note the warning for vasoconstrictors.

Disapproved Active Ingredients

Evaluators judged 2 vasoconstrictor preparations as not effective when applied into the rectum.

Epinephrine hydrochloride, aqueous solution (intrarectal use only)   Epinephrine is rapidly decomposed in highly alkaline solutions. Since the lower rectum is highly alkaline, reviewers concluded that this preparation is safe but not effective when applied intrarec-tally.

Epinephrine undecylenate (intrarectal use only)   When formu-lated into a suppository or ointment for intrarectal use, epinephrine undecylenate is safe but not effective for the same reason given directly above: it decomposes almost at once.

PROTECTANTS

Most drugs act chemically on the body or on bacteria and other microorganisms. Protectants are different. They are for the most part bland, chemically inert, or inactive substances, and may be formulated as ointments, gels, lotions, creams, or powders. These preparations are intended to provide a physical barrier—that is, they coat and protect the skin or mucous surface where they're applied. In the anorectal area they can offer protection from rough, chemically irritating, bacteria-laden bowel movements. These protectants also prevent loss of mois-ture from anorectal surfaces, which is a major cause of irritation in that area.

Protectants may absorb or bind and hold irritating substances to keep them away from exposed surfaces. Some of these ingredients also soften and lubricate skin tissue.

Few well-controlled scientific studies are available to prove the worth of protectants. Most of the ingredients approved here were judged on the basis of their wide use and few adverse reactions.

Evaluators found no evidence that a combination of 2, 3, or 4 protectants is any more effective than one alone, yet they approved the use of one to 4 such substances provided that they constitute half or more of each dosage unit. Since the standard dose of an anorectal product is about 2 grams, each application will thus provide about 1 gram of active substance(s). Protectants can be applied up to 6 times daily.

CLAIMS FOR PROTECTANTS

Accurate

"form a protective coating over inflamed tissues which can relieve itching"
"temporarily protect irritated areas from irritating materials"
"temporarily help soften and lubricate dry inflamed perianal skin"
"provide lubrication and may help make bowel movements more comfortable"
for "the temporary relief of itching associated with hemorrhoids, inflamed hemorrhoidal tissues, or other anorectal disorders"

Unproved

"[a coating] which may allow healing to occur"

False or Misleading

"promotes wound healing"
"relieves inflammation" (inflammation usually results from an infection or disorder beneath the surface)

Approved Active Ingredients

The Panel reached the safe-and-effective verdict for 13 protectant ingredients. With but one exception (glycerin), all were approved both for external application to the perianal area and for insertion into the rectum. Many of the ingredients discussed below are used as general skin protectants and are described for this use in UNGUENTS AND POWDERS FOR THE SKIN.

Aluminum hydroxide gel (external and intrarectal uses) This white, powdery aluminum compound forms a gel when combined with water. Taken internally, it is widely used as an antacid—which attests its basic safety. This substance, also called *gel of alumina,* has been marketed as a general skin protectant for almost a century.

Aluminum hydroxide gel appears to relieve moist irritations of the anorectal surfaces—but not the irritation related to dry skin. In one study, an aluminum hydroxide gel thickened with kaolin relieved anal itching in 93 of 98 sufferers. This mixture may bind, hold, and neutralize fecal bacteria. It will not work if applied on top of petrolatum or other greasy substances.

Reviewers say that at a concentration of at least 50 percent of the dosage unit, aluminum hydroxide gel—by itself or with other protectants—is safe and effective when applied up to 6 times daily or after each bowel movement.

Calamine (external and intrarectal uses)   This pink mixture consists of at least 98 percent zinc oxide, which is white, and 0.5 percent ferrous oxide, which is red and gives the mixture its pinkish color. Its therapeutic effect is wholly due to the zinc oxide (*see* page 410). Calamine absorbs moisture and chemical irritants, and coats, covers, and protects the skin. The adult dosage is 5 to 25 percent calamine or a combination of calamine and zinc oxide, applied up to 6 times daily or after bowel movements.

Cocoa butter (external and intrarectal uses)   An oily, yellowish-white material, this chocolate-smelling extract of cacao beans has the property of remaining solid until it is warmed to within a few degrees of normal body temperature. Then it melts into a liquid without passing through any appreciable semisoft stage. This quality makes cocoa butter an ideal basic substance for suppositories intended to lubricate the anal canal or soothe abraded and irritated anorectal tissue.

Although cocoa butter has never been studied scientifically as an anorectal drug ingredient, its long use in a variety of other drugs and in cosmetics suggests safety and effectiveness. Cocoa butter is judged to be safe and effective for anorectal use at concentrations of 50 percent or more by itself or with other protectants. It can be used up to 6 times daily or after bowel movements.

Cod-liver oil (external and intrarectal uses)   While scientific studies of the use of this oil are few, the literature reveals no adverse effects when it is used as a skin-softener and protectant. It was judged safe and effective when it comprises at least 50 percent of the dosage unit. Such a product may be applied up to 6 times in 24 hours, or after each bowel movement.

Glycerin, aqueous solution (external use only)   Sometimes called *glycerine* or *glycerol*, this clear, sweetish, syrupy stuff has been used to soothe the skin for some 2 centuries. Tests show glycerin to be safe when applied to rats' tails and the eyes, mucous membranes, and noses of dogs, cats, and rabbits. However, intrarectal application prompts rats and guinea pigs to move their bowels.

When used by itself—that is, as anhydrous glycerin (without water) —this substance has a drying effect on the skin. But certain concentrations in water will hold moisture in the skin and soften it. So glycerin is approved as safe and effective for external use in 20 to 45 percent aqueous solutions when—alone or in combination with other protectants—it constitutes 50 percent or more of the finished product. It can be used up to 6 times daily, or after each bowel movement. But glycerin is *not* approved for intrarectal application because of its laxative potential.

Kaolin (external and intrarectal uses)   Technically a purified and hydrated aluminum silicate, this substance is a powdery, earthy, clayish material. It can absorb large amounts of liquids and can bind, hold, and neutralize noxious substances—including fecal particles and bacteria. Although kaolin is useful for general skin disturbances, its safety in anorectal disorders has never been studied. But because it is inert, and because of its long history of successful use as a skin protectant, reviewers judged it safe. Kaolin is often combined with aluminum hydroxide (*see* above) in products sold to relieve itching due to moisture and irritation of the perianal area. It is ineffective when petrolatum or other greasy substances have been applied before it; so any of those preparations should first be washed away. The safe and effective dose for adults —for both external and intrarectal application—is at least 50 percent concentration per dosage unit, by itself or in combination with other protectants. It may be applied after bowel movements, but daily use should not exceed 6 times.

Lanolin (external and intrarectal uses)   Mixed with water to produce what is called *hydrous wool fat*, lanolin is widely used as a cosmetic or medicinal skin softener (though its effectiveness for this purpose lacks scientific confirmation) and as a base for a variety of other kinds of products.

Lanolin's safety as an anorectal medication has not been determined. Little of it is absorbed through the skin, but it is known to produce localized allergic reactions in a small percentage of users. But evaluators concluded that widespread use in so many preparations and over such an extended period of time suggests effectiveness as a skin-softening protectant. The approved dosage: at least 50 percent by itself or in combination with other protectants. It can be used after bowel movements but should not be applied more often than 6 times a day.

Mineral oil (external and intrarectal uses) This odorless, colorless, transparent oily liquid is refined from crude oil. It is relatively inert, does not turn rancid, and is widely used as a skin softener and as a base for creams and suppositories.

Mineral oil is not absorbed through the skin, so it tends to remain where applied until accidentally or deliberately wiped off. It keeps out air, bacteria, and other irritating substances, holds moisture, and soothes and lubricates the skin. But the Panel could find no specific studies on mineral oil's safety or effectiveness as an ingredient in anorectal products. Approval stems largely from the substance's physical properties and from the fact that it has been safely used on other parts of the body. The dosage should be at least a 50 percent concentration of mineral oil, by itself or with other protectants, and the preparation should be applied no more often than 6 times daily or after each bowel movement.

Petrolatum, white (external and intrarectal uses) A purified petroleum product, white petrolatum can be used to soften, lubricate, and cover the skin. It has been shown in tests to be the most effective ointment for protecting skin surfaces against water. Safety has been demonstrated through almost a century of wide use in pharmaceutical products and cosmetics. Despite the fact that petrolatum has not been specifically studied as an anorectal medication, the Panel considers it effective as a physical barrier. It protects the anorectal area from irritants and may relieve their effects—burning, pain, or itch. The approved dosage is at least 50 percent concentration of white petrolatum in each dosage unit, by itself or in combination with other protectants, applied up to half-a-dozen times daily or after bowel movements.

Shark-liver oil (external and intrarectal uses) This amber-to-brown-colored oily substance soothes and softens irritated skin. No data are available on the use of the oil for anorectal disorders, but experience with its application to other skin surfaces as well as studies of cod-liver oil in diapering products led evaluators to consider shark-liver oil safe and effective for softening and protecting anorectal surfaces and for relieving itching and irritation. The substance must represent 50 percent or more of the dosage unit, by itself or with other protectants. Like so many other remedies noted in this section, it can be applied up to 6 times in 24 hours, or after every bowel movement.

Starch (external and intrarectal uses) Whether manufactured from corn or from rice, starch is an insoluble, chemically inactive substance that, weight for weight, can absorb huge amounts of moisture and noxious substances. It also smoothes the skin and reduces friction. Its safety as a topical dusting powder is well established. Although starch is unstudied as an anorectal medication, the reviewers believe it is safe and effective in concentrations of 50 percent or greater per dosage unit—by itself or in combination with other protectants—when applied up to 6 times daily or after each bowel movement.

Wool alcohols (external and internal uses) These fluids are constituents of lanolin, derived from secretions of sheep's skin. They soften and protect the skin. Some people develop allergy to wool alcohols, but these compounds are otherwise deemed safe and effective for soothing and covering the skin and for relieving itching, burning, and pain. The anorectal dose for adults is 4 to 7 percent wool alcohols per dosage unit, not to exceed 6 applications in 24 hours. Or one may apply the preparation after each bowel movement.

Zinc oxide (external and intrarectal uses) Zinc oxide is applied in a paste or lotion to absorb excess moisture, or it may be sprinkled onto inflamed areas as a powder. It is the principal and the sole *active* ingredient in calamine. For anorectal application, the safe and effective dose is a 5 to 25 percent concentration and the substance can be used up to 6 times daily or after defecating.

Conditionally Approved Active Ingredients

Bismuth oxide (external and intrarectal uses) This compound occurs in nature as the mineral bisemite—a yellow, odorless powder that will not dissolve in water. Although bismuth is toxic, particularly when taken internally, no adverse effects from topical use have been reported in science journals. Evaluators consider it safe when applied in small amounts to the perianal area and rectum. However, there is insufficient evidence to show that it is actually effective.

Bismuth subcarbonate (external and intrarectal uses) This particular bismuth compound has been better studied than the one described directly above. Although bismuth subcarbonate is relatively insoluble, some bismuth, which is toxic, may be absorbed through the skin. But the Panel thinks the risk is so low that the ingredient can be considered safe for short-term use on the anorectal area. However, even though bismuth subcarbonate is listed in one official pharmacological compendium as a skin protectant, evaluators maintain there are no specific reports to substantiate this claim. Verdict: not proven to be effective.

Bismuth subgallate (external and intrarectal uses) The main problem with this compound—as with the other bismuth compounds described directly above—is that little evidence is available to show that it has the various skin-protecting properties claimed for it. So while safety may not be a problem, full approval was not granted because of doubts about its effectiveness.

Disapproved Active Ingredients

Bismuth subnitrate This is the one ingredient used as a skin protectant in anorectal products that evaluators say is dangerous. It is a white powder, which is also called *bismuth oxynitrate*, *Spanish white*, and *bismuth paint*. While there is little data on the toxicity of bismuth subnitrate when it is used to treat anorectal disorders, it has been shown to penetrate and severely damage the oral mucosa when taken orally; purplish lesions appear throughout the digestive tract. A variety of other side effects may occur, some of them serious. While these adverse reactions may be rare, they are common enough and harmful enough for the Panel to decide that bismuth subnitrate is not safe for use in anorectal protectants sold over-the-counter.

COUNTERIRRITANTS

As described earlier, a counterirritant is something that takes one's mind off one's discomfort by creating competing sensations. Drugs, however, are less effective counterirritants than physical methods (such as soaking in a warm bath or using a hot water bottle or ice pack). Since there are apparently no sensory nerve endings in the rectum, counterirritants can work only externally. Claims that they help when applied internally need scientific support. So Panel approval relates only to external use and only for people over the age of 12.

CLAIMS FOR COUNTERIRRITANTS

Accurate
"can help distract from pain or itch"
"temporarily relieves itch or pain in the perianal area"

False or Misleading
"promotes health"

Approved Active Ingredient

Menthol, aqueous solution (external use only)   Menthol is absorbed through the skin, stimulating nerve endings for coolness while it also suppresses those pain sensors responsible for itching. This minty alcohol is the only counterirritant judged to be safe and effective for self-treatment of hemorrhoids and other anorectal complaints. No studies were found of menthol's safety specifically as an anorectal drug, but it has been fairly well studied as a topical treatment on other body sites and appears safe. So the Panel approved menthol as safe and effective for perianal use in concentrations of 0.25 to 1 percent per dosage unit in aqueous solution; application should be limited to 6 times daily.

Conditionally Approved Active Ingredient

Juniper tar (external and intrarectal uses)   This is the only conditionally approved counterirritant active ingredient for anorectal disorders. A dark red oil with a tarlike odor and a bitter taste, it is sometimes called *oil of cade*. Its components include phenol—which is of doubtful safety even when present in small amounts—and other apparently toxic compounds. So juniper tar's safety is in doubt. Also, while the tar has been used for thousands of years to relieve skin conditions, there are no definitive reports on its value for anorectal disorders. Thus, both its safety and effectiveness remain to be proved.

Disapproved Active Ingredients

Camphor (external and intrarectal uses)   This substance produces both warming and cooling sensations. It has a pungent, aromatic taste and a penetrating odor. While camphor has been used for countless years on a variety of skin conditions, the evidence now shows that it may not be safe. In high concentrations it is clearly dangerous, and the Panel was concerned, too, that when camphor is applied to mucosal tissue, like that in the rectum, it is rapidly absorbed into the body. Although it may be effective in the anorectal area (as it is elsewhere on the body) and has been used that way for centuries, evaluators disapproved camphor on the grounds of questionable safety.

Hydrastis (external and intrarectal uses)   Despite the several colorful botanical names that it is known by—including *golden seal*, *yellow root*, *orange root*, *Indian turmeric*, *eye root*, and *eye balm*—this plant extract is neither safe nor effective as a nonprescription anorectal counterirritant ingredient. The Cherokee Indians used it as a pigment and as a medicine for, among other things, stopping internal bleeding.

There is little scientific evidence that hydrastis is effective for this or any of the other conditions—including hemorrhoids and other anorectal distress—for which it has been used. When taken internally, hydrastis can cause convulsions and other serious disorders. So, especially because it is unclear how much, if any, of the substance will be absorbed when it is applied to the anorectal region, reviewers proclaimed it unsafe as well as ineffective.

Menthol, aqueous solution (intrarectal uses only)   This ingredient is safe and effective for external application to the perianal area (*see* MENTHOL, page 412). There seems to be little risk in applying it intrarectally, but because there apparently are no sensory pain receptors in the rectum, menthol was judged ineffective when administered in this way.

Turpentine oil, rectified (external and intrarectal uses)   Distilled from pine-tree gum, this refined oil has the taste and odor of hardware-store turpentine. It can cause headache and other mental and gastrointestinal distress if inhaled, itching and redness if applied to the skin, and death if swallowed. In short: unsafe. There is no evidence that turpentine oil is of any therapeutic value when applied to the anorectum—in fact, it could cause increased tissue damage and make the symptoms worse if applied to inflamed skin.

ASTRINGENTS

The stingy, zesty feeling of witch-hazel lotions and similar astringents is easy to recall but hard to describe in soberly scientific words. An astringent puckers the proteinous outer membranes of skin and mucosal cells, shrinking them. An astringent can also absorb, concentrate, and hold loose proteinous substances on skin and mucosal surfaces —including fecal particles and bacteria—thereby reducing their irritancy. Astringents also have a drying effect.

An astringent will not significantly reduce hemorrhoidal swelling but it may temporarily help relieve symptoms of burning, itching, discomfort, and irritation. Astringent-containing perianal pads and wipes are also useful for cleansing purposes and for relieving itching.

Approved Active Ingredients

The Panel assessed astringents for both external use on the perianal region and intrarectal use—as applied in suppositories and other intrarectal dosage forms.

Calamine (external and intrarectal uses)   This pinkish medication is at least 98 percent zinc oxide, dyed pink with a trace of red iron oxide. The safety and effectiveness of calamine relate directly to that of zinc oxide (*see* below). As an anorectal astringent, it is approved in dosages of 5 to 25 percent for external and intrarectal use when used up to 6 times in 24 hours, or after each bowel movement.

Witch-hazel water (external use only)   This liquid, also called Hamamelis water, is prepared by boiling crushed, dried twigs of the witch-hazel shrub (*Hamamelis virginiana*) for 24 hours. The residue is then distilled and mixed with 15 percent alcohol. It is a clear, colorless liquid that has a pleasant fragrance. The Panel knows of no serious adverse reactions to witch-hazel, although it may be allergenic.

The ingredient's astringency has been attributed to the minute amount of the original plant's volatile oil that is left in the final products. The Panel's guess is that it is the alcohol itself that is the astringent—with the oil accounting only for the drug's appealing aroma. A few studies have shown that witch-hazel water relieves itching, burning, and other discomforts when applied to the anorectal area. The substance is judged safe and effective in concentrations of 10 to 50 percent; it can be applied after each bowel movement up to 6 times daily.

Zinc oxide (external and intrarectal uses)   This substance is widely used to treat skin disorders; it is the essential ingredient of calamine lotion. Zinc oxide's astringent properties are attributed to its ability to gather irritating proteins from the skin or mucosal surface and cover them with a protective film. The chemical appears to be more effective on injured than on unbroken skin. The safe and effective dosage is a 15 to 25 percent concentration of zinc oxide in a suitable base; it can be applied up to 6 times daily or after each bowel movement.

Conditionally Approved Ingredients

None

Disapproved Active Ingredient

Tannic acid (external and intrarectal uses)   Tannic acid was widely used in treating burns and other ailments until it was discovered that it is readily absorbed through the skin and can be lethally toxic. Its medicinal effectiveness has also been challenged—including its use in treating anorectal disorders. Evaluators therefore declared it not safe or effective.

ANTISEPTICS

The anorectal region is, inherently, not very clean—being repeatedly exposed to feces and the bacteria and other microorganisms they carry. When the perianal skin is intact, these noxious substances for the most part remain on its surface. But when the outer skin layer has been broken, they can enter the underlying tissues. This can result in infection, which, of course, complicates healing.

Reducing the number of microorganisms—they can never be wholly removed—can aid healing and relieve some symptoms of anorectal disorders. Antiseptics, which are drugs that act against microorganisms, may help to achieve this aim, but reviewers noted that washing the anorectal area with soap and water is likely to be more effective. Also, putting an antiseptic into the rectum is a futile gesture, due to the huge numbers of bacteria that normally reside there.

Because the bacteria populations of the perianal area are different —and larger—than those on other body surfaces, claims that ingredients can control these bacteria must be proved with studies of the perianal area; they cannot be projected from studies on other body regions.

CLAIMS FOR ANTISEPTICS

Accurate
   "temporarily reduce the number of organisms in the perianal area"
   "reduce the risk of infection"

False or Misleading
   "degerm" or "control infection"
   "form a protective antibacterial film over raw inflamed tissue"

Approved Active Ingredients

   None

Conditionally Approved Active Ingredient

Resorcinol (external use only)   This compound, which also is called *resorcin*, is an alcohol that has long been used in nonprescription itch-relieving products. It is safer—but less effective as an antiseptic—than phenol, which it resembles chemically. The toxic dose of resorcinol is very close to the effective dose, and toxic amounts may be absorbed through unbroken as well as broken skin. The symptoms of mild resorcinol poisoning are ringing in the ears, fast pulse and breathing, and profuse sweating. At higher doses, convulsions and other severe symptoms can occur. Resorcinol also causes allergic reactions.

Despite these problems, reviewers believe that the low doses of resorcinol used in over-the-counter anorectal products are safe—provided consumers heed their warning not to use the substance in open wounds near the anus. But resorcinol's effectiveness remains in doubt. Investigators think it is reasonable to assume that it may limit—but is unlikely to significantly reduce—bacterial populations around the anus. If it does, this ability has not yet been proved.

Disapproved Active Ingredients

Boric acid (external and intrarectal uses)   Although long used as a medicinal standby, boric acid is absorbed through the skin and can cause serious poisoning, even death. Recent reevaluations also cast doubt on boric acid's effectiveness as an antiseptic—and since it has never been studied as an anorectal preparation, the judgment was: not safe and not effective.

Boroglycerin (external and intrarectal uses)   This sticky, yellowish liquid—also called boric acid glycerite—is transformed into boric acid when it becomes wet. So it may be as hazardous as boric acid (*see* directly above). There are no data to show that it is effective in killing germs in the anorectal area, so reviewers disapproved it.

Hydrastis (external and intrarectal uses)   Just as this root derivative was found ineffective as a counterirritant, it was also disapproved as an antiseptic because no data show that it actually kills bacteria. It is not safe.

Phenol (external and intrarectal uses)   This coal-tar derivative readily penetrates the skin, with toxic results. This is thoroughly discussed in the unit PHENOL In short, weak solutions of phenol are of doubtful effectiveness and strong ones are unsafe. The present Panel essentially agrees, and dismisses phenol as neither safe nor effective for nonprescription products intended as antiseptics for anorectal application.

Resorcinol (intrarectal use only)   While probably safe when patted onto the perianal surfaces (*see* RESORCINOL, page 415), resorcinol is rapidly absorbed from the bowel, is toxic, and can be lethal. A safe dose is unlikely to be effective in reducing germ populations, so the ingredient is judged unsafe and ineffective for intrarectal use.

Sodium salicylic acid phenolate (external and internal uses)

This ingredient was listed on the label of a product submitted for evaluation. But neither the Panel members nor the FDA could find it in standard drug compendia. They say, in effect, that they don't know what it is! Neither could any published studies on either its safety or effectiveness be found. The verdict was foreordained: unsafe and ineffective.

WOUND-HEALING AGENTS

This is a murky category of ingredients. On the one hand, claims are made that anorectal ingredients and products "may promote healing," "may help promote tissue repair," or can "temporarily shrink swelling of hemorrhoidal tissue caused by inflammation." On the other hand, it has not been demonstrated—to the satisfaction of this or any other over-the-counter review Panel—that any ingredient in fact actually spurs healing.

It is conceivable that some ingredients in anorectal products do stimulate healing, the reviewers believe. But until this has been demonstrated, all claims for healing and all ingredients for which these claims are made are assessed as only *conditionally* approved. Because these substances are described in detail in the units UNGUENTS AND POWDERS FOR THE SKIN, FIRST-AID PREPARATIONS FOR SKIN WOUNDS, and VITAMINS AND MINERALS, comments here will be confined mainly to discussion of perianal and/or rectal use.

Approved Active Ingredients

None

Conditionally Approved Active Ingredients

Experts classified 6 ingredients as conditionally safe and effective wound-healing agents for anorectal disorders.

Cod-liver oil (external and intrarectal uses) While undoubtedly safe, any active role in healing wounds remains to be proved. It is thought that possibly the protective function simply allows normal healing to go forward unhampered by bacteria or irritants.

Live yeast-cell derivative (external and intrarectal uses) This preparation of baker's yeast is abbreviated LYCD. It's considered safe for use up to a week. The basic notion of action is that applying the yeast to a wound stimulates oxygen uptake, which in turn spurs healing. This correlation is not substantiated—although some studies at least suggest that LYCD might promote healing by helping to build new connective tissue in wounds that have become contaminated by bacteria.

A minority of the Panel's members disagreed. They point out that it would be extremely difficult to do scientifically controlled studies of minor anorectal itching on test subjects recruited at drugstore counters, and they believe that more sophisticated investigations carried out on other anatomical regions (in animals and humans) indicate that LYCD is safe and effective for perianal conditions. But the majority view—that effectiveness needs to be proved—prevailed.

Peruvian balsam (external and intrarectal uses)   Although this balsam may cause an allergic reaction, reviewers believe it is safe to use in treating anorectal disorders. But while a few inadequate reports suggest that the substance stimulates wound healing, there are no studies of its use in the anorectal area. Thus claims of effectiveness need to be established.

Shark-liver oil (external and intrarectal uses)   This substance contains both vitamin A and vitamin D—which are alleged to promote healing. In the low (3 percent) concentration in which shark-liver oil is formulated into nonprescription anorectal products, the danger of causing additional skin disturbances is unlikely, so reviewers consider it safe when used to heal wounds. Whether it is effective is a wholly different matter; convincing evidence is lacking.

Vitamin A (external and intrarectal uses)   In cell cultures, and in tests in animals, this vitamin has been shown to promote the formation of connective tissue. Reviewers say—albeit somewhat hesitantly—that it appears to be safe to apply it to the human skin. However, clinical effectiveness for anorectal use needs to be demonstrated.

Vitamin D preparations: ergocalciferol and cholecalciferol (external and intrarectal uses)   The risks of applying vitamin D preparations to the skin, in the amounts present in over-the-counter rectal products, appear small. Nonetheless, the absence of scientific evidence of effectiveness led the Panel to grant the preparations only conditional approval.

Disapproved Active Ingredients

None

SKIN-PEELING AGENTS (KERATOLYTICS)

A drug that loosens and removes the outer, horny, keratin-containing layer of skin cells is called a *keratolytic*, or skin-peeling, agent. Several types of chemicals—including particularly the phenols—have this ability. They are for the most part used on warts and corns and other conditions where there is an overgrowth of dry, keratin-containing outer skin cells. They reduce itching and may also expose deeper skin layers to medication.

Their value in treating perianal skin disorders—where the skin is usually moist, not dry—remains open to question. The consumer should note that the Panel's approval applies only to *external* application of these drugs to the perianal area, not to intrarectal use. There are no keratin-containing cells in the rectal mucosa.

CLAIMS FOR SKIN-PEELERS

Accurate
"temporary relief of itching"

False or Misleading
"soften" outer skin layers, thus providing "more effective results"

Approved Active Ingredients

Alcloxa (external use only)   This aluminum compound, which is called *aluminum chlorhydroxy allantoinate*, is a form of allantoin, a safe and effective compound that is widely used to soothe irritated skin. A traditional skin remedy, comfrey root, which contains a natural chemical predecessor of allantoin, has been known for several centuries to soften and protect skin.

Like other forms of allantoin, alcloxa has never been shown to harm the skin. Furthermore, it does relieve itching, though how it does so remains unclear. Its skin-peeling capacity appears to be based on its ability to break the bonds of "intercellular cement" in the skin's outer layer. Despite a lack of clarity about how it acts, and a paucity of studies on its activity in the anorectal area, evaluators say alcloxa is safe and effective for adults in concentrations of 0.2 to 2 percent when used up to 6 times in 24 hours.

Resorcinol (external use only)   This phenollike alcohol—whose risks are described on page 415—was judged by the majority of Panel members to be safe for use as an anorectal skin-peeling and skin-softening agent. A minority argued that this has not been proved. However, a number of studies indicate that resorcinol is effective in softening and removing the scales of psoriasis and other conditions in which the perianal skin has become thickened. Also, only relatively weak—1 to 3 percent—preparations were approved. (Another minority objection was that such concentrations have not been shown to be effective.)

Nonetheless, the drug was assessed safe and effective as long as use is confined to adults who do not have open wounds near the anus and as long as one bears in mind the following:

WARNING FOR RESORCINOL   If redness, irritation, swelling, pain, or other symptoms develop or increase, discontinue use and consult a physician.

Conditionally Approved Active Ingredient

Sulfur preparations (external use only)   Few side effects have been reported over the many years sulfur has been used to peel skin —including facial acne lesions. So the Panel believes it is safe. However, no data were submitted to show that sulfur effectively peels thick, dry skin in the perianal area—for which reason the reviewer's verdict is: not proved effective.

Disapproved Active Ingredient

Evaluators found skin-peeling ingredients in—and claims for skin-peeling action on—some products that were also labeled for intrarectal use. They are strongly disapproved. The rectal mucosa contains no keratinized (horny) cells on which this medication might be effective, and this use could be highly risky.

Resorcinol (intrarectal use only)   While this substance can be used for the treatment of thickened, itchy skin in the perianal area, it is unsafe and ineffective when used intrarectally.

Sulfur preparations (intrarectal use only)   These ingredients may damage the rectal mucosa. Their use inside the rectum is neither safe nor effective.

ANTICHOLINERGICS

These drugs act on the tear, salivary, and sweat glands and on the urinary, bladder, and gastrointestinal tracts as well as other glandular tissues, by blocking the action of acetylcholine and thus temporarily blocking or inhibiting the muscles or glands acetylcholine activates. Reviewers concluded that anticholinergics have no place in the self-treatment of anorectal symptoms. No manufacturers offered any good reasons why their companies were formulating anticholinergics into anorectal products—though some do. The Panel says that inclusion of these drugs is quite risky because they are readily absorbed through broken skin or rectal mucosa. This can cause rapid heart rate, urinary retention, dry mouth, visual blurring, and many other distressing and possibly dangerous side effects.

No anticholinergic ingredients are approved or even conditionally approved for anorectal use, and the Panel wants them removed from all such products.

Approved Active Ingredients

None

Conditionally Approved Active Ingredients

None

Disapproved Active Ingredients

Atropine (external and intrarectal uses)   This is a white crystalline substance obtained from the leaves of belladonna, or deadly nightshade. No data are available on its use in anorectal products, but it can be absorbed into the body through broken skin—with the possibility of poisoning the entire body. A potent drug, atropine requires individualized dosage adjustment by a physician in order to prevent toxic side effects. So it was judged unsafe and ineffective for use without prescription.

Belladonna extract (external and intrarectal uses)   Another preparation derived from the leaves of deadly nightshade or related plants, belladonna extract was assessed as being equally dangerous as atropine (*see* directly above) and was hence held unsafe and ineffective.

MISCELLANEOUS INGREDIENTS IN ANORECTAL PREPARATIONS

A half-dozen ingredients that fall outside the standard drug classifications are used in anorectal drugs. Some have been used for decades —or longer. Most are herbal remedies or other traditional remedies that have fallen from favor as more potent and effective agents have come on the market. Despite the continued wide use of at least one of these ingredients, the Panel disapproved them all.

Disapproved Active Ingredients

Collinsonia extract (external and intrarectal uses)   This substance, sometimes called *stone root*, is derived from the dried root of the minty herb called horse balm or citronella (*Collinsonia canadensi*). It was listed in old drug compendia as useful for a variety of ills and in herbal texts is touted for treating snake bite, dumb ague, dropsy, colics, cramps, putrid and malignant fevers, as well as hemorrhoids. But the Panel says that the only evidence of its usefulness for anorectal disorders is limited to a few testimonials for products in which it was used in combination with other ingredients. No report on either the safety or effectiveness of this substance had appeared in the 15 years previous to the review, so evaluators consider it outmoded and neither safe nor effective.

Escherichia coli vaccines (external and intrarectal uses) The *Escherichia coli* bacteria are infectious agents that are normally found in great numbers in the intestinal tract. These materials appear to be the only immunological agents that have been evaluated in the over-the-counter drug review. They pose a puzzle. On one hand, as the Panel noted, *E. coli* vaccines are formulated into a product that has been sold, unchanged, since 1922. Marketing data from a 50-year span show no complaints and no reports of any side effects. On the other hand, there are no reliable data to show that *E. coli* vaccines are actually effective. A vaccine is a biologic substance made from killed or inactivated bacteria or other infectious organisms. It is introduced into the body, usually by injection under the skin. The body's protective, or immunologic, mechanisms respond to the harmless material by making defensive antibodies that will then attack and destroy active forms of the infectious agent if they later enter the body.

The manufacturer said that, for its anorectal preparations, the *E. coli* are grown in laboratory flasks, and then killed—though it did not say how this is done—before they are formulated into products along with a variety of other ingredients. One suppository submitted for review was said to contain conserved breakdown products "and the corpuscular components of approximately 300 million *coli*-bacteria of different types."

The manufacturer claimed these bacterial breakdown products act as local vaccines that prime the body's natural defenses against secondary infections that occur in anorectal diseases. In other words, if a hemorrhoid or anal crack allows gut bacteria to enter the tissue and bloodstream, the presence of the *E. coli* vaccine will stimulate antibody production and other body defense measures to destroy them.

Evaluators were skeptical about these claims, for which there are only 2 studies—both inconclusive and covering fewer than 100 patients. Since normal body defenses become operative in cases of infection, careful investigation would be needed to demonstrate that a locally applied vaccine contributed to this effect. Moreover, anal infections require medical care; they should not be self-treated. Also, if *E. coli* bacteria could be reduced or eliminated from the fecal stream in this way, the result could be bad rather than good: their place might be taken by populations of other bacteria that would not respond to the vaccine. So the conclusion was that *E. coli* vaccines are neither safe nor effective in anorectal medications.

Lappa extract (external and intrarectal uses) This bitter substance is derived from the roots of the burdock (*Arctium lappa* or *A. minus*), which are common thistleweeds. Termed "a relic of old herbal medicine," lappa—formerly taken internally for a variety of ailments—boasts no studies that demonstrate either safety or effectiveness. Nor could dosage be established. Therefore reviewers judged it unsafe and ineffective for anorectal use.

Leptandra extract (external and intrarectal uses) Extracted from the dried rhizomes and roots of Culver's root (*Leptandra virginica*), a North American plant, this substance contains a number of plant chemicals—including alcohol-acid compounds such as cinnamic acid, methaquinones, fatty acids, resins, saponins, tannins, and sugars. It may be safe, but because it has been ignored in the recent medical and pharmacological literatures and no recent data exists to show that it is effective in treating anorectal disease, the ingredient was disapproved.

Mullein (external and intrarectal uses) This is a bland and purportedly soothing substance obtained from mullein dock, great mullein, or verbascum (*V. orientale*), which are common weeds. No evidence was found that mullein is really either safe or effective for relieving discomfort in the anorectal region.

Inactive Ingredients

A variety of inactive ingredients are used in formulating over-the-counter anorectal products—including perfumes, which may cause allergic reactions:

acetone	bismuth oxyiodine	coconut oil (palm
amaranth	carbowaxes	kernel oil)
aromatic oils	cetylpyridinium	eucalpytus oil
beeswax	chloride	mace oil (oil of mace)
benzalkonium chloride	chlorobutanol	methylparaben
benzyl benzoate	chlorothymol	myrrh

perfumes	propylene glycol	sodium lauryl sulfate
phenylmercuric nitrate	secondary	tyloxapol
polyethylene glycol	amyltricresols	white wax
ointment	sodium bisulfite	

While most of these ingredients are likely to be harmless, evaluators questioned the safety not only of perfumes but also of eucalyptus oil, sodium lauryl sulfate, tyloxapol, and benzyl benzoate.

Safety and Effectiveness: Active Ingredients in Over-the-Counter Products for the Treatment of Hemorrhoids and Other Anorectal Conditions

Active Ingredient	Panel's Assessment	
	Applied Externally to Perianal Area	Applied Intrarectally
Local Anesthetics		
benzocaine, polyethylene glycol ointment	safe and effective	safe, but not proved effective
benzyl alcohol	safe, but not proved effective	safe, but not proved effective
dibucaine	not proved safe or effective	not proved safe or effective
dibucaine hydrochloride	not proved safe or effective	not proved safe or effective
diperodon	safe, but not effective	not proved safe or effective
dyclonine hydrochloride	safe, but not proved effective	not proved safe or effective
hydrocortisone and hydrocortisone acetate	safe and effective*	
lidocaine	safe, but not proved effective	safe, but not proved effective
phenacaine hydrochloride	not safe	not safe
pramoxine hydrochloride, cream, 1% (as Tronothane)	safe and effective	safe, but not proved effective
pramoxine hydrochloride, jelly, 1% (as Tronothane)	safe and effective	safe, but not proved effective
pramoxine hydrochloride, 1% (other formulations)	safe, but not proved effective	safe, but not proved effective
tetracaine	safe, but not proved effective	not proved effective
tetracaine hydrochloride	safe, but not proved effective	not proved effective

Safety and Effectiveness: Active Ingredients in Over-the-Counter Products for the Treatment of Hemorrhoids and Other Anorectal Conditions *(continued)*

Active Ingredient	*Panel's Assessment*	
	Applied Externally to Perianal Area	Applied Intrarectally
Vasoconstrictors		
ephedrine sulfate, aqueous solution	safe and effective	safe and effective
epinephrine	not proved safe or effective	not proved safe or effective
epinephrine hydrochloride, aqueous solution	safe and effective	safe, but not effective
epinephrine undecylenate	not proved safe or effective	safe, but not effective
phenylephrine hydrochloride, aqueous solution	safe and effective	safe and effective
phenylephrine hydrochloride suppositories		safe, but not proved effective
Protectants		
aluminum hydroxide gel	safe and effective	safe and effective
bismuth oxide	safe, but not proved effective	safe, but not proved effective
bismuth subcarbonate	safe, but not proved effective	safe, but not proved effective
bismuth subgallate	safe, but not proved effective	safe, but not proved effective
bismuth subnitrate	not safe	not safe
calamine	safe and effective	safe and effective
cocoa butter	safe and effective	safe and effective
cod-liver oil	safe and effective	safe and effective
glycerin, aqueous solution	safe and effective	
kaolin	safe and effective	safe and effective
lanolin	safe and effective	safe and effective

mineral oil	safe and effective	safe and effective
petrolatum, white	safe and effective	safe and effective
shark-liver oil	safe and effective	safe and effective
starch	safe and effective	safe and effective
wool alcohols	safe and effective	safe and effective
zinc oxide	safe and effective	safe and effective
Counterirritants		
camphor	not safe or effective	not safe or effective
hydrastis	not safe or effective	not safe or effective
juniper tar	not proved safe or effective	not proved safe or effective
menthol, aqueous solution	safe and effective	safe, but not proved effective
turpentine oil, rectified	not safe or effective	not safe or effective
Astringents		
calamine	safe and effective	safe and effective
witch-hazel water	safe and effective	safe and effective
tannic acid	not safe or effective	not safe or effective
zinc oxide	safe and effective	safe and effective
Antiseptics		
boric acid	not safe or effective	not safe or effective
boroglycerin	not safe or effective	not safe or effective
hydrastis	not safe or effective	not safe or effective
phenol	not safe or effective	not safe or effective
resorcinol	safe, but not proved effective	not safe or effective
sodium salicylic acid phenolate	not safe or effective	not safe or effective
Wound-Healers		
cod-liver oil	safe, but not proved effective	safe, but not proved effective
live yeast-cell derivative	safe, but not proved effective	safe, but not proved effective

Safety and Effectiveness: Active Ingredients in Over-the-Counter Products for the Treatment of Hemorrhoids and Other Anorectal Conditions *(continued)*

Panel's Assessment

Active Ingredient	Applied Externally to Perianal Area	Applied Intrarectally
Peruvian balsam	safe, but not proved effective	safe, but not proved effective
shark-liver oil	safe, but not proved effective	safe, but not proved effective
vitamin A	safe, but not proved effective	safe, but not proved effective
vitamin D preparations: ergocalciferol and cholecalciferol	safe, but not proved effective	safe, but not proved effective
Skin-Peelers		
alcloxa	safe and effective	not assessed
resorcinol	safe and effective	not safe or effective
sulfur preparations	safe, but not proved effective	not safe or effective
Anticholinergics		
atropine	not safe or effective	not safe or effective
belladonna extract	not safe or effective	not safe or effective
Miscellaneous		
Collinsonia extract (stone root)	not safe or effective	not safe or effective
Escherichia coli vaccines	not safe or effective	not safe or effective
lappa extract	not safe or effective	not safe or effective
leptandra extract	not safe or effective	not safe or effective
mullein	not safe or effective	not safe or effective

*As evaluated by the OTC Panel on Topical Analgesics.

Safety and Effectiveness: Combination Products Sold Over-the-Counter to Treat Hemorrhoids and Other Anorectal Conditions

Safe and Effective

2, 3, or 4 approved protectants, constituting at least 50% of the product

0 to 4 protectants, which if present must constitute 50% of the product + approved amounts of 1, 2, or 3 other approved active ingredients, each from a different 1 of 5 groups (local anesthetics, vasoconstrictors, counterirritants, astringents, skin-peeling agents)—provided that the final formulation has been tested and found to be safe and effective

Conditionally Safe and Effective

0 to 4 protectants, which if present must constitute 50% or more of the product, + approved amounts of 1, 2, or 3 approved active ingredients, each from a different 1 of 5 groups (local anesthetics, vasoconstrictors, counterirritants, astringents, skin-peeling agents)—when the final formulation has *not* been tested and found to be safe and effective

Unsafe or Ineffective

contains any disapproved ingredient or labeling

contains more than 1 ingredient from any group other than protectants

contains 5 or more active ingredients, not counting protectants

contains a counterirritant + a local anesthetic*

---

*This combination makes no sense because the counterirritant acts by stimulating sensory nerve endings that the anesthetic temporarily deadens.

Hemorrhoid Medication and Other Anorectal Applications: Product Ratings

Anesthetic Products

Product and Distributor	Dosage of Active Ingredients	Rating[1] for External Use in Perianal Area	Rating[1] for Use Intrarectally	Comment
benzocaine in polyethylene				
Americaine (American Critical Care)	ointment: 20%	A	B	no pain receptors in rectum, so pain reliever ineffective
dibucaine				
dibucaine hydrochloride (generic)	ointment: 1%	B	B	safety and effectiveness remain unproved
Dibucaine Hydrochloride (Rugby)		B	B	
D-Caine (Century)		B	B	
Nupercainal (Ciba)	cream: 0.5%	B	B	
diperodon				
Diothane (Merrell-Dow)	ointment: 1%	C	B	ineffective externally, and not proved effective or safe for intrarectal use
lidocaine				
Xylocaine (Astra)	ointment: 2.5%	B	B	effectiveness unproved, and considered doubtful when used intrarectally
pramoxine hydrochloride				
Tronothane (Abbott)	cream: 1%	A	B	this brand proved effective for external use; but not proved effective for internal use
	jelly: 1%	A	B	

Product and Distributor	Dosage of Active Ingredients	Rating[1] for External Use in Perianal Area	Rating[1] for Use Intrarectally	Comment
Tronolane (Abbott)	cream: 1%	B	B	newer formulations of pramoxine hydrochloride not assessed by Panel and apparently not proved safe and effective by its criteria
	suppositories: 1%	—	B	
tetracaine Pontocaine (Breon)	ointment: 0.5% tetracaine base + menthol + white petrolatum cream: 1% as hydrochloride	B	B	not proved effective

Steroid Products for Itch, Inflammation, and Swelling

Product and Distributor	Dosage of Active Ingredients	Rating[1] for External Use in Perianal Area	Rating[1] for Use Intrarectally	Comment
hydrocortisone Cortil (Pfipharmecs)	cream: 0.5%	A	—	
Dermolate Anti-Itch (Schering)		A	—	
Hydrocortisone (Fougera)	ointment: 0.5%	A	—	
Hytone (Dermik)		A	—	
Wellcortin (Burroughs-Wellcome)		A	—	

Hemorrhoid Medication and Other Anorectal Applications: Product Ratings (continued)

Steroid Products for Itch, Inflammation, and Swelling

Product and Distributor	Dosage of Active Ingredients	Rating[1] for External Use in Perianal Area	Rating[1] for Use Intrarectally	Comment
hydrocortisone acetate				
CaldeCort (Pharmacraft)	**cream:** 0.5% hydrocortisone equivalent	A	—	
CaldeCort Rectal-Itch (Pharmacraft)	**ointment:** 0.5% hydrocortisone equivalent	A	—	
Cortaid (Upjohn)	**ointment and cream:** 0.5% hydrocortisone equivalent	A	—	
Pharma-Cort (Purepac)	**cream:** 0.5%	A	—	
Resicort (Mentholatum Co.)	**cream:** 0.5%	A	—	

Protectant Products

Product and Distributor	Dosage of Active Ingredients	Rating[1] for External Use in Perianal Area	Rating[1] for Use Intrarectally	Comment
calamine				
calamine (generic)	**lotion:** 8% calamine + 8% zinc oxide + 0.2% glycerin	A	A	
cocoa butter				
cocoa butter (generic)	**cream**	A	A	

Product and Distributor	Dosage of Active Ingredients	Rating[1] for External Use in Perianal Area	Rating[1] for Use Intrarectally	Comment
cod liver oil				
cod liver oil, USP (generic)	**liquid**	**A**	**A**	
Cod Liver Oil Liquid (Squibb)	**liquid**	**A**	**A**	
lanolin				
Lanolin Toilet Creme (Barry Martin)	**cream**	**A**	**A**	
Lanolin Toilet Cream (Squibb)	**cream**	**A**	**A**	
mineral oil				
mineral oil (generic)	**liquid**	**A**	**A**	
petrolatum, white				
Vaseline Pure Petroleum Jelly (Chesebrough-Ponds)	**ointment:** 100%	**A**	**A**	
zinc oxide				
Zincofax (Burroughs-Wellcome)	**cream:** 15% + lanolin	**A**	**A**	
zinc oxide (generic)	**ointment:** 20%	**A**	**A**	
zinc oxide (generic)	**paste:** 25% + 25% starch	**A**	**A**	

Astringents

Product and Distributor	Dosage of Active Ingredients	Rating[1] for External Use in Perianal Area	Rating[1] for Use Intrarectally	Comment
calamine				
See calamine above, under Protectants				
witch hazel water				
witch hazel (generic)	**solution**	**A**	—	

Hemorrhoid Medication and Other Anorectal Applications: Product Ratings *(continued)*

Astringents

Product and Distributor	Dosage of Active Ingredients	Rating[1] for External Use in Perianal Area	Rating[1] for Use Intrarectally	Comment
zinc oxide See zinc oxide above, under Protectants				

Combination Products Containing Pain Relievers

Product and Distributor	Dosage of Active Ingredients	Rating[1] for External Use in Perianal Area	Rating[1] for Use Intrarectally	Comment
A-Caine Rectal (A.V.P.)	**ointment:** 0.25% diperodon hydrochloride + 0.1% pyrilamine maleate + 0.25% phenylephrine hydrochloride + 0.2% bismuth subcarbonate + 5% zinc oxide + cod-liver oil	C	C	diperodon not effective when used externally; pyrilamine maleate not submitted to or assessed by Panel
Emeroid (Delta)		C	C	
Anocaine Hemorrhoidal (Mallard)	**suppositories:** 50 mg benzocaine + 60 mg zinc oxide + 50 mg bismuth subgallate + 20 mg boric acid + bismuth resorcin compound + 20 mg Peruvian balsam		C	boric acid and resorcin not safe or effective for intrarectal use

Product	Formulation			Comments
Anusol (Parke-Davis)	**ointment:** 1% pramoxine hydrochloride + 11% zinc oxide	B	B	pramoxine not proved effective
Epinephricaine Rectal (Upjohn)	**ointment:** 2.5% benzocaine + 0.2% epinephrine + 2% zinc oxide + vitamins A and D	B	B	epinephrine not proved safe or effective for external or intrarectal internal use; vitamins not proved effective as wound healers
Nupercainal (Ciba)	**suppositories:** 2.5 mg dibucaine + zinc oxide + bismuth subgallate + cocoa butter base	—	B	dibucaine not proved safe or effective; bismuth subgallate not proved effective
proctoFoam (Reed & Carrick)	**aerosol foam:** 1% pramoxine hydrochloride (in water miscible, mucoadhesive foam base)	B	B	safety and effectiveness of foams unproved; pramoxine hydrochloride not proved effective
Surfacaine (Lilly)	**suppositories:** 10 mg cyclomethycaine sulfate	—	C	ingredient not assessed by Panel
Tanicaine (Upjohn)	**ointment:** 1.1% phenacaine hydrochloride + 0.05% atropine + 17.3% zinc oxide + 1.3% phenol + 5.3% tannic acid	C	C	phenacaine not safe; atropine and tannic acid not safe or effective
	suppositories: 22 mg phenacaine hydrochloride + 1 mg atropine + 390 mg zinc oxide + 13 mg phenol + 110 mg tannic acid	—	C	

Hemorrhoid Medication and Other Anorectal Applications: Product Ratings (continued)

Combination Products without Pain Relievers

Product and Distributor	Dosage of Active Ingredients	Rating[1] for External Use in Perianal Area	Rating[1] for Use Intrarectally	Comment
Calmol 4 (Leeming)	**suppositories:** cod-liver oil + zinc oxide + bismuth subgallate + cocoa butter	—	B	bismuth subgallate not proved effective; other 3 protectants are safe and effective
Posterisan (Kenwood)	**ointment:** 0.167 ml sterilized Coli vaccine with 330 million Coliform bacteria + 3.3 mg liquefied phenol + 0.16 mg of 2 (ethylmercurithio)-5-benzoxazolcarboxylic acid per g in petrolatum base	C	C	E. coli vaccines and phenol not safe or effective
Preparation H (Whitehall)	**ointment:** Live yeast-cell derivative supplying 2000 units skin respiratory factor per ounce + 3% shark-liver oil	B	B	live yeast-cell derivative not proved effective
	suppositories: live yeast-cell derivative supplying 2000 units skin respiratory factor per ounce + 3% shark-liver oil	—	B	live yeast-cell derivative not proved effective

Wyanoids (Wyeth)

suppositories: 3 mg
ephedrine sulfate + 15 mg
extract belladonna + boric
acid + zinc oxide +
bismuth oxyiodide +
bismuth subcarbonate +
Peruvian balsam + cocoa
butter

belladonna and boric acid not
safe or effective — C

Perianal Hygiene Products

Product and Distributor	Dosage of Active Ingredients	Rating[1] for External Use in Perianal Area	Rating[1] for Use Intrarectally	Comment
Gentz (Philips Roxane)	**wipes:** 1% pramoxine hydrochloride + 0.2% alcloxa + 50% witch hazel	B	—	pramoxine hydrochloride in this combination, and combination itself, not proved effective
Preparation H Cleansing	**pads:** 50% witch hazel + 10% glycerin + octoxynol-9	B	—	less-than-effective amount of glycerin; octoxynol-9 not submitted to or assessed by Panel, but approved as safe and effective for cleansing by Panel on vaginal drug products
Tucks (Parke-Davis)	**pads:** 50% witch hazel + 10% glycerin	B	—	less-than-effective amount of glycerin
	ointment: 50% witch hazel + lanolin + petrolatum	B	—	combination not proved safe and effective
	cream: 50% witch hazel + lanolin + petrolatum	B	—	combination not proved safe and effective

1. Author's interpretation of Panel criteria. Based on contents, not claims.

Hormone Skin Creams and Oils

It is the female hormone estrogen, and to a lesser extent progesterone, that transforms a girl into a woman at puberty. Later, as she grows older and her skin begins to lose its smooth, pliable, youthful feeling and appearance, a woman may be tempted by seductive advertisements to try to rejuvenate her skin by treating it with supplements of these hormones in skin creams, oils, lotions, and other cosmetically appealing preparations.

These products, which contain only low doses of hormones, have been judged safe, but they do not produce visible changes in the skin —so they are not effective.

CLAIMS

All claims are disapproved.

HORMONE PREPARATIONS

The reviewing Panel's assessment of these preparations is summarized in the Safety and Effectiveness chart that concludes this unit. Each one discussed below is disapproved—primarily on grounds of being ineffective.

Approved Active Ingredients

None

Conditionally Approved Active Ingredients

None

Disapproved Active Ingredients

Estrogens: estradiol, estrogen, estrogenic hormones, natural estrogenic homones, natural estrogens, and estrone These hormones are produced naturally by a woman's ovaries and, during pregnancy, by

HORMONE SKIN CREAMS AND OILS is based on the report "Topically Applied Hormone-Containing Drug Products for OTC Human Use" by the FDA's Advisory Review Panel on OTC Miscellaneous External Drug Products.

the placenta. They ready her body for conception and are necessary to sustain pregnancy. Natural and synthetic estrogens are widely used medicinally, principally in oral contraceptives. Estrogens are also formulated into skin creams meant to soften and rejuvenate the skin.

The outer layer of the skin (epidermis) becomes thinner with advancing age. In one study, the use of an estrogen preparation resulted in a doubling of epidermal thickness. However, this increase in number and size of skin cells could be detected only by microscope. Furthermore, other studies have failed to confirm these changes. Some reduction in wrinkling has also been reported from the use of estrogen skin products. But evaluators say wrinkling results from degeneration of the inner skin layer (dermis) and not from the drying out and thinning of the epidermis. So the reviewers strongly doubt that these reports are valid.

It is the Panel's judgment that estrogen in concentrations of up to 10,000 international units (IU) per ounce is safe. Higher concentrations are not. But there is no scientifically acceptable evidence that a product containing up to 10,000 IU estrogen per ounce of cream is any more effective than the same product without it.

In sum: while safe in low doses, estrogen preparations for the skin are not effective. And at higher doses, they are unsafe because, once absorbed through the skin, they may upset the body's natural horomonal balance. The Panel recommends that these products be banned from the over-the-counter drug market.

Progesterones: pregnenolone acetate and progesterone   The reason behind formulating progesterones into skin products is that they are thought to stimulate the sebaceous glands to produce more sebum—a natural skin lubricant—and thus soften the skin. In the concentration in which these hormones are marketed (5 mg progesterone per ounce of cream or oil), the Panel says they seem to be free of side effects.

Progesterone has been shown to increase sebum secretions in female and castrated male rats, but not in women. In one study, progesterone-treated sides of women's faces were compared with untreated sides. Skin samples taken failed to show even microscopic differences. (The male hormone testosterone may stimulate sebum production, but the female hormone progesterone will not, the Panel says.)

Evaluators conclude that 5 mg progesterone per ounce of cream, oil, or lotion is safe but not effective—and recommends such products be barred from availability over-the-counter.

Note: Some progesterone products have been claimed to stimulate breast development. Young women who fear that they are underendowed in this regard may be tempted to try these preparations. The Panel says, in a rough draft report, that progesterone creams are *not effective* as breast developers.

Safety and Effectiveness: Active Ingredients in Over-the-Counter Hormone Skin Treatments*

Active Ingredient	Panel's Assessment
estradiol	not effective
estrogen	not effective
estrogenic hormones	not effective
estrone	not effective
natural estrogenic hormones	not effective
natural estrogens	not effective
pregnenolone acetate	not effective
progesterone	not effective

*Aside from being ineffective, estrogens are unsafe at concentrations of over 10,000 IU estrogen per ounce, and the progesterones are unsafe in concentrations of over 5 mg progesterone per ounce.

Hormone Skin Creams and Oils: Product Ratings

The Panel's judgment is that no hormonal ingredient in a skin cream or oil has discernible benefit to the skin. So all products containing the relatively low concentrations of these hormones that are sold over-the-counter must be rated "C."

Ingrown-Toenail Relievers

An ingrown toenail is like a train that has jumped its track. The nail, which protects the tip of the toe from injury, normally grows slowly outward along tracklike grooves at the edge of the nail bed. But if the nail gets dislocated a bit—when it jumps the track—it digs into the nail bed and groove. This causes pain, inflammation, and swelling. Infections, blood poisoning, and other serious damage may follow.

The Panel that assessed drugs to relieve this condition says that the

INGROWN-TOENAIL RELIEVERS is based on the report "Ingrown Toenail Relief Drug Products for OTC Human Use" by the FDA's Advisory Review Panel on OTC Miscellaneous External Drug Products.

term *ingrown toenail* is a misnomer. The nail does not actually grow into the flesh, but rather becomes embedded in soft tissue.

CLAIMS

Accurate
for "the temporary relief of discomfort from ingrown toenails"

False or Misleading
"fast pain relief" (treatment may require several days)

WARNING Persons with diabetes or other conditions that cause circulatory problems may be insensitive to the pain of an ingrown toenail. Yet they may be especially susceptible to the infection that can result. Such individuals should *not* self-treat ingrown toenails, but should have them treated by a podiatrist or physician.

PEDICURE FOR PREVENTION

Careful and correct cutting will forestall ingrown toenails. The incorrect way to cut is to create a crescentlike curve, as one does with fingernails. This creates tapered corners below the end of the nail groove. These corners may then get pushed up against and embedded in the groove. Toe-pinching shoes, tight hosiery, and too-tight bed clothing can force the side edge of the nail into the softer toe tissue. Even walking may cause poorly pedicured nails to become enclosed in this way.

An alternative—and the best method of preventing this condition —is cutting the toenails straight across. The corners will then be square and they will also be out beyond the ends of the nail grooves. That way there is no chance that a sharp or ragged edge can cut into a groove, nail bed, or other soft tissue. Using this pedicure method should prevent most ingrown toenails, according to the Panel.

DRUGS TO TREAT INGROWN TOENAILS

If caught early enough, there may be merit in self-treatment with nonprescription drugs that can harden the nail groove so it will resist further injury or shrink the soft tissue to provide more space for the nail to resume its normal position—back on track. If self-treatment with drugs does not free the nail, or if the area becomes sore, swollen, or painful, medical help should definitely be sought.

Evaluators assessed the ingredients of 2 products sold to treat ingrown toenails and reviewed several other ingredients that have been used for this purpose in the past. It classified 2 ingredients—isopropyl alcohol and triethanolamine—as inactive. Three others were considered painkillers and referred to another Panel, which judged the ingredients as follows:

benzocaine	safe and effective
chlorobutanol	not proved effective
dibucaine	safe and effective

The present Panel appears to sanction combinations that contain pain-relieving drugs along with ingredients that relieve ingrown toenails. But no product submitted for review contains 2 active ingredients for specific relief of the ingrown nail condition itself.

Approved Active Ingredients

None

Conditionally Approved Active Ingredients

Sodium sulfide   The reason behind the use of this drug is that it softens the keratin (horny material) in the nail and adjacent callused skin. This allegedly relieves the pressure and pain caused by contact between embedded nail and skin.

Tests in rats show that one would have to drink a large amount of a sodium sulfide ingrown-toenail remedy to poison oneself. Other tests in rabbits show that is only slightly irritating to the skin. The Panel judges sodium sulfide to be safe.

The results of a study done with 100 ingrown-toenail patients seem to show that the sodium sulfide produced relief in most subjects within 3 to 7 days while a dummy drug given to some of the patients did not. But in analyzing these findings, the Panel concluded that the test had been conducted in a sloppy manner and stipulated that either this study has to be redone or another one designed and carried out if the manufacturer hopes to show that sodium sulfide really works as an ingrown-toenail-relieving ingredient. In short: effectiveness remains to be proved.

Tannic acid   This compound is believed to harden the skin surrounding the nail and shrink the adjacent soft tissue, making room for the nail to resume its normal position. Another Panel that evaluated tannic acid for treating burns and other skin injuries found that it has little effect—good or bad—on intact skin. This led the present Panel to conclude that it is safe enough for consumers to use (in small amounts) to treat sore toes, but also led it to doubt the compound's effectiveness.

The one published study that the present evaluators reviewed indicates that tannic acid along with a pain-reliever and alcohol proved to be "an excellent aid in helping restore the nail to its proper relationship to the soft tissue of the toe." But it is not clear whether it was the alcohol —which would counteract infection—or the tannic acid that was mainly responsible for these good results.

More recent studies in mice—whose skins were treated with tannic acid and then punctured with needles—support the notion that this substance turns live skin more leathery. But the Panel says a scientifically sound study must be conducted on humans with sore toes from ingrown nails before the substance can be considered effective for relieving this condition.

Disapproved Active Ingredients

Chloroxylenol and Urea   Neither of these two ingredients merits approval because no data were found to show they are safe or effective for self-treatment of ingrown toenails.

Safety and Effectiveness: Active Ingredients in Over-the-Counter Ingrown-Toenail Relievers

Active Ingredient	Panel's Assessment
chloroxylenol	not safe or effective
sodium sulfide	safe, but not proved effective
tannic acid	safe, but not proved effective
urea	not safe or effective

Ingrown-Toenail Relievers: Product Ratings

Product and Distributor	Dosage of Active Ingredients	Rating[1]	Comment
Dr. Scholl's Oxinol (Scholl)	**liquid:** 1% sodium sulfide	B	not proved effective
Nail-A-Cain (Medtech)	**liquid:** 4% tannic acid + 15% benzocaine	B	tannic acid not proved effective
Outgro (Whitehall)	**liquid:** 25% tannic acid + 5% chlorobutanol + isopropyl alcohol 83% by volume	B	tannic acid not proved effective

1. Author's interpretation of Panel criteria. Based on contents, not claims.

Insect Bite and Sting Treatments

For a few individuals who are highly allergic to insects' venom, bee, wasp, or hornet stings can be life-threatening emergencies. For most other persons, such stings and bites are simply a pain in the neck—or wherever else they are struck.

People who are highly sensitive to insect venom may already know their vulnerability. They should be under the care of an allergist, who may be administering desensitizing shots. Susceptible individuals may also have been advised to purchase and carry emergency kits containing hypodermic needles that are preloaded with epinephrine. This substance counteracts anaphylactic shock—a condition that may cause death when highly allergic persons are restung by insects to which they are especially sensitive.

Two approaches are generally available for combating insects. The first is to prevent bites and stings by wearing insect helmets, netting, or other such devices, or by using insect repellents. Most repellents marketed for direct application to the skin are not classified as drugs; one of them, oil of citronella, was judged by the Panel (in a preliminary assessment) to be ineffective. Vitamin B_1, also known as *thiamine hydrochloride*, is marketed as an *internal* insect repellent—to be taken orally. The Panel that reviewed this ingredient assessed it as being ineffective for this purpose.

The second approach to insect stings and bites is to treat them after they occur, with the aim of reducing the swelling and pain and relieving the itching and other discomfort. The idea is to use substances that specifically neutralize the venom. However, the ingredients that manufacturers claimed do have this effect were all assessed as being ineffective.

Therefore, a more fruitful path to relief may be to use the drugs that, generally speaking, are safe and effective for relief of itching and pain on the skin. Many of these ingredients are formulated into products for treating insect bites. They are listed on the next page. Readers who want more information should turn to the unit ITCH AND PAIN REMEDIES APPLIED TO THE SKIN.

INSECT BITE AND STING TREATMENTS is based on the unadopted draft report "OTC Insect Bite Neutralizer Drug Products" by the FDA's Advisory Review Panel on OTC Miscellaneous External Drug Products and the report "Insect Repellent Drug Products for OTC Oral Human Use" by the Advisory Review Panel on OTC Miscellaneous Internal Drug Products.

benzocaine	hydrocortisone	phenolate sodium (0.5
benzyl alcohol	hydrocortisone	to 1.5 percent
butaben picrate	acetate	phenol)
camphor	juniper tar	pramoxine
dibucaine	lidocaine	hydrochloride
dibucaine	lidocaine	resorcinol
hydrochloride	hydrochloride	tetracaine
dimethisoquin	menthol	tetracaine
hydrochloride	methapyrilene	hydrochloride
diphenhydramine	hydrochloride	tripelennamine
hydrochloride	phenol (0.5 to 1.5	hydrochloride
dyclonine	percent)	
hydrochloride		

DRUGS TO NEUTRALIZE INSECT VENOM

Since the reviewers do not believe that any of these ingredients is a safe and effective neutralizer, they were not able to grant full approval to any claim that such products will actually neutralize insect venom.

CLAIMS

Unproved

for "the temporary relief of stings caused by wasps, hornets, bees, mosquitoes, spiders, fleas, chiggers, ticks, and ants"

Approved Active Ingredients

None

Conditionally Approved Active Ingredient

Triethanolamine (trolamine) This chemical penetrates the skin to reach poisons deposited there by insect stings or bites. The amount that would be absorbed into the body from this self-treatment is too small to be dangerous, the Panel says, so it concludes that triethanolamine is safe.

The drug is highly alkaline (pH 10 to 11), which may be why manufacturers formulate it into neutralizing preparations for treating insect stings and bites. The Panel notes that *some* venoms contain acids, but they also contain other, nonacidic irritants. So triethanolamine's effectiveness cannot come solely from its alkalizing capability.

In the one double-blind study submitted for review, triethanolamine was compared with a dummy preparation of salt water. Bee stings were simulated by injecting tiny amounts of bee venom under participants' skin. When the subjects began to feel pain, they were given swabs containing either triethanolamine or the salt water. A full 50 percent of the subjects (13 out of 26) felt relief or elimination of pain within 2 minutes when they used triethanolamine, but only 23 percent (6 of 26) reported comparable relief when they applied the salt-water swabs. Neither the active drug nor the salt water reduced the redness and swelling.

The Panel thinks these findings are interesting, but not persuasive. So it grants conditional approval, pending further testing. Triethanolamine is judged as safe but not proved effective as an insect sting and bite neutralizer.

Disapproved Active Ingredients

Evaluators summarily disapproved of 18 compounds because they could find little or no data on them; *see* the SAFETY AND EFFECTIVENESS chart that concludes this unit. The Panel did receive data on one ingredient: ammonium hydroxide; but it rejected the information on the grounds that alkalization—that is, neutralizing acids—makes little sense in view of the other, nonacid toxins in venom. So ammonium hydroxide, too, is assessed as not effective.

INSECT REPELLENTS, TAKEN ORALLY

Only one oral insect repellent was submitted to the Panel for consideration. Because the Panel ruled it is ineffective, all claims are disapproved.

Approved Active Ingredients

None

Conditionally Approved Active Ingredients

None

Disapproved Active Ingredient

Thiamine hydrochloride (vitamin B₁) This substance is widely used as a vitamin supplement, so the Panel judges it safe. Two studies done in the 1940s and a later one suggest that thiamine supplements reduce the number of bites from mosquitoes and fleas and other insects. The test were not controlled and the Panel took exception to their poorly constructed methodology. Recent double-blind studies showed no advantage for thiamine over dummy medication in reducing the number of insect bites sustained under test conditions. Nor did the drug lessen symptoms. So reviewers conclude that thiamine hydrochloride is safe but not effective as an insect repellent taken orally.

Safety and Effectiveness: Active Ingredients in Over-the-Counter Products for Insect Bites and Stings

Active Ingredient	Panel's Assessment
alcohol	summarily disapproved
ammonium hydroxide	not effective
aqua ammonia	summarily disapproved
benzalkonium chloride	summarily disapproved
bicarbonate of soda*	summarily disapproved
calamine*	summarily disapproved
camphor*	summarily disapproved
ergot fluid extract	summarily disapproved
ethoxylated alkyl alcohol	summarily disapproved
ferric chloride	summarily disapproved
menthol*	summarily disapproved
obtundia surgical dressing	summarily disapproved
oil of turpentine	summarily disapproved
peppermint oil	summarily disapproved
phenol*	summarily disapproved
pyrilamine maleate	summarily disapproved
sodium borate	summarily disapproved
thiamine hydrochloride (vitamin B₁), taken orally	safe but not effective
triethanolamine (trolamine)	safe but not proved effective
zinc oxide*	summarily disapproved
zirconium oxide	summarily disapproved

*Safe and effective as a nonspecific itch and pain reliever or skin protectant.

Insect Bite and Sting Treatments: Product Ratings

Insect Repellents Taken Internally[1]

Product and Distributor	Dosage of Active Ingredients	Rating[2]	Comment
E-Z Mosquito Repellent Tablets (Thompson)	**tablets:** thiamine hydrochloride	C	not effective
E-Z Oral Mosquito Bite Relief Tablets (Cordova Labs.)	**tablets:** thiamine hydrochloride	C	not effective

Neutralizers for Use on Skin

Product and Distributor	Dosage of Active Ingredient	Rating[2]	Comment
After Bite (Tender)	ammonium hydroxide	C	not effective; the manufacturer claims that the Topical Analgesia Panel evaluated ammonium hydroxide safe and effective—warranting an "A" rating here—back in 1974, but then did not include the decision in its report. The present Panel obviously disagrees with that judgment
Aspercreme Cream (Thompson)	**cream:** triethanolamine 10%	C	not effective
Sting-Kill (Milance)	**swabs:** 18.9% benzocaine + 0.9% menthol	C	no data to show that menthol is safe and effective for neutralizing insect venom, but menthol and menthol in combination with benzocaine, may provide non-specific relief for itch and pain

1. For safe and effective itch and pain relievers *see* Itch and Pain Remedies Applied to the Skin: Product Ratings, on page 467.
2. Author's interpretation of Panel criteria. Based on contents, not claims.

Itch and Pain Remedies Applied to the Skin

Some skin irritations are caused by external factors; others are symptoms of diseases originating within the skin itself or even deep in the body. Many remedies have been developed for these complaints, and Panel reviewers found that there is a wide selection of safe and effective active ingredients that will temporarily relieve pain and itching of the skin. A number of these drugs have been sold in over-the-counter preparations for decades. They generally act by directly or indirectly blocking or reducing the activity of sensory nerve receptors in the skin.

On the Panel's recommendation, the FDA has allowed preparations of 2 potent drugs from the class called corticosteroids to be sold without prescription for the first time. They are hydrocortisone and hydrocortisone acetate. Previously all corticosteroids were available only by prescription. But the evaluators judged these preparations safe and effective for self-treatment of minor skin irritations as well as the itching and rashes—*not* the pain—due to eczema, dermatitis, insect bites, poison ivy, poison oak, poison sumac, soaps, detergents, cosmetics, and jewelry, and for itchy genital and anal areas.

Until recently, methapyrilene was the antihistamine most commonly formulated into over-the-counter itch remedies. When it was removed from the market, as a possible cancer-causing agent, manufacturers substituted other antihistamines, including phenyltoloxamine dihydrogen citrate and pyrilamine maleate. The FDA has not yet stated its position on their safety or effectiveness as over-the-counter drugs.

Hydrocortisones and antihistamines may help cure a rash or other skin irritation. But for the most part the drugs described here provide only relief of symptoms. So if the condition does not get better or vanish in a week, it's recommended that it be shown to a doctor.

CLAIMS

Accurate for all products and ingredients except hydrocortisone and hydrocortisone acetate

ITCH AND PAIN REMEDIES APPLIED TO THE SKIN is based on the report on External Analgesic Drug Products, prepared by the FDA's Advisory Review Panel on OTC Topical Analgesic, Antirheumatic, Otic, Burn and Sunburn Prevention and Treatment Drug Products.

for "the temporary relief of pain and itching due to minor burns, sunburn, minor cuts, abrasions, insect bites, and minor skin irritations"

Accurate for hydrocortisone preparations
for "the temporary relief of minor skin irritations, itching, and rashes due to eczema, dermatitis, insect bites, poison ivy, poison oak, poison sumac, soaps, detergents, cosmetics and jewelry, and for itchy genital and anal areas"

False or Misleading
"fast," "swift," "poignant," or "fast cooling" pain relief

WARNING   If condition worsens, or if symptoms persist for more than 7 days, discontinue use of the product and consult a physician.

ITCHING AND SURFACE PAIN

Why We Itch

Feelings of itchiness are close to feelings of pain. They both are produced by the same sensory nerve endings in the skin. Weak stimulation of these nerve fibers causes itching; strong stimulation causes pain. The response, however, is different: we withdraw from a painful stimulus but we attend to an itch by scratching it.

An itch can be produced directly, by an irritative chemical or other foreign substance, or it may result indirectly, from the body's defensive reaction against a certain substance. The latter response is an allergic reaction. The redness and swelling is caused by the release into the skin of histamine, an irritating chemical that is made by the body.

An itch sometimes can be relieved by gently touching the skin with a clean pin about an inch away from the mosquito bite or other source of discomfort; scratching gently at this distance also may help. But scratching *on* the bite—or on poison ivy or other rashes—may release more of the irritative substances into the skin, intensifying the itch and even transforming it to out-and-out pain.

The technical name for an itch is pruritus, so a drug that relieves itch is an antipruritic. Small itchy areas can be self-treated. Large ones —including generalized itching all over the body—require medical care.

Superficial Pain

Pain originating in the skin and tissue layers immediately beneath it differs little from other pain—with the important exception that skin discomfort appears not to be relieved by aspirin or chemically related salicylates. Because of this, there is no merit to product-label claims that aspirin or other salicylates in drugs applied to the skin will relieve the pain of sunburn or shallow cuts and scrapes.

TYPES OF MEDICATIONS

All over-the-counter topical drugs used to relieve itching and pain are characterized by the Panel—somewhat confusingly—as "external analgesics," meaning pain relievers that act on body surfaces.

A drug that acts specifically to block the nerve receptors for pain in the skin is a *topical analgesic*. But since pain and itch travel the same nerve routes, these preparations may also relieve itching. A drug that acts more generally to block all sensation in the skin, causing numbness, is called a *topical anesthetic*. It may block pain and itch sensations as well as feelings of hot, cold, or external pressure.

The medications assessed may act as analgesics by relieving pain, as anesthetics by causing numbness, or as antipruritics by relieving the itch, or they may provide 2 or all 3 of these benefits. Some act only on damaged skin, where they have easy access to the nerve endings. Others penetrate unbroken skin as well.

Benefits of Approved Itch and Pain-Relieving Active Ingredients*

Active Ingredient	Induces Numbness	Stops Pain	Stops Itching	Effective on Damaged Skin	Effective on Intact Skin
benzocaine	yes	yes	yes	yes	yes
benzyl alcohol	yes	yes	yes	yes	yes
butamben picrate	yes	yes	yes	yes	no
camphor	yes	yes	yes	yes	yes
dibucaine	yes	yes	yes	yes	yes
dibucaine hydrochloride	yes	yes	yes	yes	no
dimethisoquin hydrochloride	maybe	yes	yes	yes	maybe
diphenhydramine hydrochloride	feebly	no	yes	yes	no
dyclonine hydrochloride	yes	yes	yes	yes	no
hydrocortisone	no	no	yes	yes	yes
hydrocortisone acetate	no	no	yes	yes	yes
juniper tar	no	unclear	yes	apparently	apparently
lidocaine	yes	yes	yes	yes	yes

Benefits of Approved Itch and Pain-Relieving Active Ingredients* *(continued)*

Active Ingredient	Induces Numbness	Stops Pain	Stops Itching	Effective on Damaged Skin	Effective on Intact Skin
lidocaine hydrochloride	yes	yes	yes	yes	no
menthol	no	yes	yes	yes	yes
phenol	yes	yes	yes	yes	yes
phenolate sodium	yes	yes	yes	yes	yes
pramoxine hydrochloride†	yes	yes	yes	yes	no
resorcinol	no	no	yes	yes	yes
tetracaine	yes	yes	yes	yes	yes
tetracaine hydrochloride	yes	yes	yes	yes	no
tripelennamine hydrochloride	yes	no	yes	yes	unclear

*Author's interpretations, based on Panel's report.
†Pramoxine hydrochloride may relieve pain in unbroken skin, but it does not produce numbness and may not relieve itching unless the deeper layers of skin are exposed.

Pharmacological Class

The Panel attempted to categorize the 3 dozen active ingredients in external analgesics by pharmacological class.

- *Group 1* includes *anesthetics* whose names end in the suffix *-caine* or are amine compounds that resemble them in chemical structure. The *-caines* tend to be stronger and provide faster relief than the amines, but they also are more toxic.
- *Group 2* includes *alcohols* and *ketones* (compounds chemically related to alcohols). They act like the amines, but their therapeutic routes and toxic properties are different.
- *Group 3* are *antihistamines*. They work principally against itching but are also mildly anesthetic.
- *Group 4* are *salicylates*—aspirin-type compounds.
- *Group 5* consists of the *corticosteroids*. They are treated separately because they act against itching but not pain.

General Properties

Taken as a class, the external analgesics tend to be safe as well as effective. Reviewers rejected only one ingredient, chloral hydrate, as unsafe. However, judgments are less well grounded in scientific data than those of most other Panels—largely because the self-limiting nature of these skin problems makes it almost impossible for investigators to conduct meaningful experiments. Thus the evaluators relied to a large extent on less definitive kinds of reports and on manufacturers' data showing that products made with these ingredients have been popular with consumers (effective) and have elicited few complaints of adverse reactions (safe).

Side Effects

The most severe risk posed by external analgesics is also fortunately a rare one: when large amounts of some of the *-caine* preparations are applied to wide areas of bruised or otherwise damaged skin, much of the drug will be absorbed into the body. In some cases reported in the medical literature this has caused life-threatening (and even lethal) toxic reactions. Convulsions and paralysis of the nervous system can occur. The heart may slow down or even stop beating. Reviewers stressed, however, that these complications do not occur when moderate amounts of the drugs are used. Too, it is worth noting that these effects apparently cannot occur with one of the principal *-caine* drugs, benzocaine, because it is insoluble in body fluids. This explains why benzocaine is so widely used and accepted. The more common and less severe side effects of external analgesics are rashes, hives, and other skin eruptions—the very symptoms these products are intended to relieve! The reactions usually abate when use of the drug is discontinued.

The skin is a sensitive organ. So adverse reactions may occur more frequently when analgesic medications are applied to it than they do when the same drugs are taken internally. Persons allergic to a large number of foods and other substances should be especially careful in using these drugs.

The location of a rash or the like—as well as the skin's condition—can influence a drug's action. Some drugs are more readily absorbed through thin than through thick skin. Most are better absorbed, and so are more effective, on mucous membranes like the lips, nostrils, and anus than they are on ordinary skin—but they also may be more toxic when applied to these delicate surfaces.

External analgesics have varying degrees of solubility in water and body fluids. A compound that is insoluble in water may be relatively worthless when placed on unbroken skin, yet may be quite effective when used on cut or broken skin since it then can reach underlying nerve endings. Many external analgesics are soluble in fats and so can reach underlying layers through fatty parts of the skin barrier.

Consumers should keep in mind that newborn babies' skin absorbs drugs very readily. A stable, "adult" absorbency level is reached by about 6 months of age—but to provide an added margin of safety, experts recommend that external analgesics not be used on children under 2 except on the advice of a physician.

Finally, the assessment of the safety and effectiveness of external analgesics is complicated by the fact that most are formulated—as creams, sprays, or lotions—along with inactive ingredients that influence the active drug's ability to reach and remain in contact with the skin. The concentration of the active ingredient also varies from product to product. So consumers may need some trial and error to find those preparations that best meet their own and their families' needs.

COMBINATION PRODUCTS

Many external analgesic products include 2 or more active ingredients. Evaluators took an equivocal stand on combination products. While reviewers maintained that single active ingredients are preferable, they also said that "the Panel is strongly convinced that there is a need for combination products."

A dissenting minority of 2 members of the Panel addressed itself to this contradiction and claimed (1) approval of combination drugs as safe and effective is spurious and unscientific and (2) that consumers should use external analgesics containing a single active ingredient wherever and whenever possible.

Nonetheless, the majority view prevailed, and rules for combining pain and itch relievers are summarized in the SAFETY AND EFFECTIVENESS: COMBINATION PRODUCTS chart at the end of this unit.

TOPICAL ITCH AND PAIN-RELIEVING MEDICATIONS

Reviewers evaluated three-dozen active ingredients that are applied to the skin to relieve pain and itch. The majority were found to be safe and effective (*see* SAFETY AND EFFECTIVENESS chart at the end of unit, which also lists approved concentrations and dosage information).

Approved Active Ingredients

Benzocaine When properly formulated (preferably in propylene glycol) and in adequate concentration (at least 5 percent), this anesthetic is an effective and very safe remedy for pain and itch on the skin. It has been used successfully by tens of millions of people since the turn of the century; over 1.5 million pounds of it are sold in the United States each year.

Benzocaine is relatively insoluble in water; thus very little penetrates beyond the skin to enter the bloodstream. So the serious side effects in the body reported occasionally for other -caine drugs do not occur. For the same reason, benzocaine's beneficial activity occurs almost wholly within the skin and mucous membranes, where it blocks the pain-conducting nerve endings. The drug also provides long-acting relief; a single application may quell pain and itching for 4 to 6 hours.

However, a small percentage of users experience some irritation or sensitivity reactions from benzocaine. While serious side effects have been reported in the medical literature, reviewers believe they are far rarer—and the drug far safer—than sometimes has been suggested. Verdict: safe and effective.

Benzyl alcohol   This substance, which is found naturally in oil of jasmine, is usually synthesized for commercial sale. It has a faint aromatic odor and a sharp, burning taste. It relieves itching, burning, and irritation due to cuts, abrasions, and insect bites—but it is not so effective as benzocaine and its therapeutic action is briefer. When applied to a cut on the lip or other mucous membrane, for example, benzyl alcohol provides relief within 2 minutes—but this effect lasts less than a half-hour.

While benzyl alcohol will kill some bacteria, it is not reliable for this purpose. But it is a very safe drug. For example, the convulsions and heart problems that have been reported with some -caine anesthetics do not occur. Even mild skin sensitization is rare. Conclusion: safe and effective.

Butamben picrate   Insoluble in water, this compound does not readily penetrate the skin's outer layer. So while it relieves pain and itching where the skin has been cut or bruised, it is not very effective on undamaged skin. It works less well than benzocaine (see above) and has the added disadvantage of forming a yellow stain on the skin, on bandages, and on clothing.

Available data indicate that butamben picrate is nontoxic and quite safe to use, although skin sensitization and other allergic responses have been reported. The compound is made in part of picric acid, which has been used as a burn dressing. But because picric acid is no longer considered a wise choice for burn therapy, butamben picrate has no special value for treating burns—although it appears to be safe and effective for pain and itch. Conclusion: safe and effective.

Camphor   This natural extract of the East Asian camphor tree, an evergreen, also is now made synthetically for drug products. In low concentrations, of 0.1 to 2.5 percent, it has a mild warming, numbing effect on the skin. This action relieves itching and burning feelings due to sunburn, insect bites, allergic reactions, and other problems. Camphor's characteristic pinelike aroma is also often associated with healing, which may contribute to its therapeutic value.

Camphor's ability to relieve itch has been widely reported in the medical literature, but this is not confirmed by controlled tests. Long consumer and clinical experience confirm its effectiveness as well as its safety when applied locally in low doses. Higher doses can be harmful (*see* CAMPHOR), and when taken orally can be a deadly poison. Nonetheless, in the recommended dosage, camphor is considered safe and effective for topical use.

Dibucaine   Made synthetically, dibucaine is an extremely potent and long-acting topical anesthetic. It was first introduced a half-century ago. When applied to the skin, dibucaine begins to relieve pain and itch within 15 minutes. If it is formulated in an effective base that keeps it moist and in touch with the skin surface, dibucaine may continue to provide relief for up to 4 hours. When the drug is removed, the noxious sensations return within 15 minutes.

Dibucaine is 15 times stronger than procaine, the reference drug of the *-caine* group; it is a half-dozen times stronger than cocaine. With this degree of potency, very small amounts of dibucaine are required. It should not be used over large areas of the body or applied to badly bruised or cut skin because it is readily absorbed. This could slow the heartbeat and cause convulsions or even death. The drug may also be fatal if swallowed—particularly by children—and it should not be applied in large quantities, especially on raw or blistered surfaces. Nonetheless, this Panel ranked the chemical both safe and effective.

Dibucaine hydrochloride   As one might assume, this drug is similar to dibucaine, described directly above. But it penetrates into skin so slowly that it is not effective unless the skin is cut or damaged. On the other hand, once through the skin, it is more soluble in water than dibucaine—thus it may pose an even greater hazard of generalized poisoning if too much is used. Used judiciously on small areas of unbroken skin, it is safe and effective in approved concentrations and dosages.

Dimethisoquin hydrochloride   Long use indicates that this is a very safe *-caine* topical anesthetic. No serious nerve or heart complications have been reported; it rarely causes skin reactions; and there are few reports of systemic side effects after accidental ingestion. But while studies have demonstrated dimethisoquin hydrochloride's effectiveness in relieving pain and itch on the skin (850 of 1000 patients in one study), it appears to do so less reliably than some other drugs of its class. Investigators are still not clear, for example, if dimethisoquin hydrochloride will penetrate intact skin; it is known to reach and quiet painful nerve endings when the skin is bruised or cut. The Panel's conclusion: safe and effective.

Diphenhydramine hydrochloride This is an antihistamine, whose role as an over-the-counter oral drug for relieving cough-cold symptoms and as a nighttime sleep aid have been controversial. It has been less controversial as an anti-itch medication applied externally to the skin—for which it has been approved.

Evaluators claim that drowsiness and other side effects are rare or nonexistent when diphenhydramine hydrochloride is applied directly to the skin—where it acts protectively by blocking the sites at which the irritating body substance histamine binds to cells in the skin, inducing itching. However, it does not penetrate unbroken skin, and so cannot relieve itching in such a case. (An oral dose—*prescribed by a doctor*—may be helpful under these circumstances.) Also, because diphenhydramine hydrochloride can lose its effectiveness after several days' use, and may eventually cause a skin reaction, experts recommend it be used no longer than a week, except under a doctor's supervision. Evaluation: safe and effective.

Dyclonine hydrochloride This anesthetic is chemically different from the -*caine* drugs with which it is grouped, so it does not produce the convulsions and severe cardiovascular symptoms for which many of these substances are noted. Thus, like benzocaine, it is a very safe drug in its class. Even mild side effects are rare: in one set of trials of 5656 patients, only 2 developed skin sensitivity to this drug.

Dyclonine hydrochloride is particularly effective in relieving pain and itching on mucous membrane and bruised and damaged skin. (It will not pass through undamaged skin.) About half to two-thirds of patients with severe pain and itching find it helpful. It is fast-acting—within 2 or 3 minutes—but affords relief only for about half an hour. Conclusion: safe and effective.

Hydrocortisone and hydrocortisone acetate These drugs are natural extracts of the cortex of the adrenal glands, although they are also made synthetically. They are extremely potent, relieving itching and inflammation—but not pain—due to a variety of causes. Their mode of action is not fully understood.

Hydrocortisone—which also is called cortisol—was introduced as a prescription drug more than 30 years ago. There have been repeated efforts since then to have it approved for nonprescription use, culminating in the present Panel's recommendation that it be sold over-the-counter. The FDA did not object—though it still may do so at some point—and over-the-counter marketing of hydrocortisone preparations began in 1980. A year later, the FDA said it had not seen any problems as a result of this change.

Despite its great potency—which is one reason for the reluctance to permit it to be marketed without prescription—hydrocortisone has been shown to be an extremely safe drug in many scientifically controlled animal and human studies. In fact, aside from aspirin, it may be the best-studied external analgesic ingredient. Hydrocortisone is particularly safe in the relatively weak concentrations for which over-the-counter sale now is authorized. One report reviewed covered 90 different clinical trials on 12,000 human subjects—among whom only 222 adverse reactions were cited. All were mild and, for the most part, were caused by the base in which it was prepared or some contaminant. No case of skin irritation or sensitivity was found.

The hydrocortisone preparations are very effective. The Panel says unequivocally: "Hydrocortisone and hydrocortisone acetate are two of the most potent and effective agents for the treatment of many common skin diseases." In a wide variety of studies on the treatment of contact dermatitis, itchiness of the vulva and anus, eczema, and other skin conditions, the majority of patients experience improvement or total relief of symptoms.

In the low concentrations approved, hydrocortisone and hydrocortisone acetate can be used for the temporary relief of minor skin irritations, itching, and rashes due to eczema, dermatitis, insect bites, poison ivy, poison oak and poison sumac, detergents, cosmetics, and jewelry and for itchy genital and anal areas. They are safe and effective.

Juniper tar   A pungent, oily extract from the wood of the juniper tree, this is a traditional "folk" remedy that has a number of exotic names—including oil of cade, Haarlem oil, bili-drops, Holland balsam and silver balsam. It is dark brown in color, with a smoky aroma and an acrid, slightly aromatic bitter taste.

Although juniper tar can be harmful if accidentally swallowed, localized application is of value in relieving minor skin irritation and itching. Despite scanty scientific data, long use persuades the Panel to judge the ingredient safe and effective for topical use.

Lidocaine   A topical anesthetic of the *-caine* type, lidocaine has been widely used by doctors and first-aiders. It is very safe when applied to small areas of wounded or itchy skin, and irritation and sensitization of the skin are rare. The ingredient is especially effective in treating itchiness, irritation, and pain of the mucous membranes. However, *large* amounts applied to wide areas of bruised or broken skin can cause severe—even fatal—damage to the heart and arteries and the nervous system. Label warnings should caution consumers not to use lidocaine in large quantities—especially over raw or blistered surfaces.

Lidocaine is effective as a topical anesthetic if judiciously used, and, in a suitable base (vehicle), it will penetrate both broken and unbroken skin. It may start to act within minutes and its benefit can continue for several hours if the base keeps the active ingredient in touch with the skin. Verdict: safe and effective.

Lidocaine hydrochloride   This compound is very similar to lidocaine—described directly above—except that it cannot penetrate unbroken skin. So use is not recommended when the skin remains intact, nor should it be used in large quantities over raw or blistered skin. However, when used in the recommended manner, the ingredient is judged safe and effective.

Menthol   A minty-smelling alcohol, menthol is extracted from natural peppermint or manufactured synthetically. At relatively high concentrations of 1.25 to 16 percent it is stimulating and mildly irritating to the skin, and is used as an ingredient in liniments and rubs. When used in low concentrations of 0.1 up to 1 percent, menthol—which is usually combined with camphor or other external analgesic ingredients —is a safe and effective means of relieving itching and pain. Menthol will penetrate unbroken as well as injured skin to reach sensory nerve endings.

Phenol   A coal-tar derivative, phenol is sometimes called carbolic acid. It's the source of what many people have come to think of as *the* "medicinal smell." Phenol easily penetrates the outer layers of the skin and acts somewhat as the *-caine* drugs do, relieving pain and deadening feeling. It also makes itching subside.

The problem with phenol is that in a relatively weak concentration —say 5 percent—it can cause serious skin burns and even internal injury as it is absorbed. Mixed with water, even a 2 percent solution is too irritating to be applied to the skin. However, somewhat stronger concentrations seem to be safe if the substance is dissolved in glycerin.

Despite questions about phenol's capacity to irritate skin and some National Cancer Institute studies that may lead the FDA to ban the substance as a nonprescription ingredient, this Panel says phenol is safe and effective when used as directed and in the proper concentrations (*see* SAFETY AND EFFECTIVENESS chart at the end of this unit). Experts warn that phenol should be applied only to the smallest possible areas of skin, and should *never* be covered with a compress or bandage—which may cause it to burn the skin. *This substance thus should never be used to treat diaper rash in babies.* It also is dangerous if swallowed, and must be kept away from children. Conclusion: safe and effective when used as recommended.

Phenolate sodium   At the name suggests, phenol is the active part of this compound—which may also be called *sodium phenoxide, sodium phenate, sodium carbolate,* or *phenol sodium.* So it has much the same ability to relieve pain and itching as does phenol (described directly above)—but it also shares that substance's risks. In fact, it may be even more risky because the sodium hydroxide in phenolate sodium is also caustic.

Despite these problems, the compound is rated safe on the basis of its wide and apparently safe use. On similar grounds, it is also judged effective in relieving pain and itching. Phenolate sodium rarely is sold as the sole active ingredient in over-the-counter products; but it is usually combined with other active ingredients.

Pramoxine hydrochloride   Also called pramocaine and proxazocain, this topical anesthetic is chemically different from the *-caine*-type drugs and it appears to be essentially free of their systemic side effects. It irritates some mucous membranes and produces a burning sensation in the eyes, but it does not irritate the skin.

Evaluators say there are studies documenting the effectiveness of pramoxine hydrochloride as a nonprescription analgesic for injured skin but not unbroken skin. The assessment: safe and effective.

Resorcinol   This compound, also known as *resorcin,* is a phenol-like alcohol that has the advantage of being less toxic than phenol. In the concentrations that are safe and effective for nonprescription use, it relieves itching but not pain. Resorcinol is readily absorbed through the skin. This enhances its medicinal value but it also means that—to avoid internal poisoning—it must be used only on small areas of skin.

The drug's safety record is difficult to interpret. On one hand, toxic reactions (even death) have been reported when resorcinol has been swallowed—or even applied to the skin of young babies. On the other hand, the Panel reviewed one product that has been marketed for 78 years without any report of substantial toxicity. So approval was granted.

WARNING   Do not apply resorcinol to large areas of the body.

Tetracaine   A potent *-caine*-type anesthetic, tetracaine relieves itching and pain on both damaged and undamaged skin. It is a half-century-old drug, which is also called *amethocaine, pantocaine, decicaine, certacaine* and *anethicaine*. The Panel bases its approval of tetracaine on a few scientific studies and on this ingredient's wide use and clinical acceptance.

Like other *-caine* drugs, tetracaine could interfere with brain and heart function if large amounts were applied to wide areas of injured skin and were absorbed. But this risk is remote if the drug is applied to the relatively small skin areas that a first-aider would treat without a doctor's help. Adverse skin reactions are rare.

Water-based (aqueous) tetracaine solutions lose their potency within months. So products should be replaced if they have been stored for long in the medicine chest.

Tetracaine penetrates both intact and injured skin, relieving itching and pain. When the skin is damaged, it induces numbness, too. The drug provides relatively long-lasting relief.

WARNING   Do not use in large quantities, particularly on raw surfaces or blistered areas.

Tetracaine hydrochloride   This compound has pharmaceutical properties very similar to tetracaine (described directly above). The shelf life is known to be less than one year, so products that have been stored in the medicine cabinet may no longer be effective.

When applied to the mucous membrane, tetracaine hydrochloride is converted to tetracaine and rapidly absorbed. But this conversion does not occur on unbroken skin, which tetracaine hydrochloride penetrates too slowly to be of medicinal value. So it is effective only when the skin is scraped or otherwise broken.

Tetracaine hydrochloride is capable of causing convulsions and slowed heart rate if large amounts are absorbed. Therefore it never should be used over wide areas of damaged skin. However, standard first-aid use of this ingredient has not led to toxicity reports in the medical literature—albeit less serious, allergic reactions have been documented. Verdict: safe and effective.

Tripelennamine hydrochloride   This is an antihistamine that will cause numbness, thus relieving itching in the skin due to allergic and irritative eruptions of poison ivy, bee sting, and similar causes that may be the result of histamine's release in the body.

When taken orally, tripelennamine hydrochloride can result in drowsiness. But too little of the drug is absorbed through the skin from topical ointments and creams to cause this problem. Users eventually may, however, become sensitive to this medication—for which reason it should not be applied longer than a week except under medical supervision. Conclusion: safe and effective.

Conditionally Approved Active Ingredients

Evaluators assessed a number of other anti-itch, antipain agents and could find no solid evidence that they actually work. For camphorated metacresol questions of safety remain.

Aspirin   No one questions the safety and effectiveness of aspirin when taken internally in proper dosages. But applying it (or any of the salicylates) to the skin—while safe enough—appears not to be effective for itch or pain. When aspirin's effect is sought for deeper aches and pains, taking an effective oral dose—of two to three 325 mg tablets—is the way to achieve it. Verdict: not proved effective.

Camphorated metacresol   This ingredient is a combination of camphor and metacresol, which is a form of phenol or carbolic acid. Although it has been marketed for half a century, evaluators could find little data on its safety or its effectiveness in relieving pain and itching. Since phenol can cause skin burns, reviewers expressed deep concern that this preparation, if applied to large areas of damaged skin, might worsen the skin problem. The Panel concluded that the ingredient is not proved either safe or effective.

Chlorobutanol   This is an old drug that has the taste and smell of camphor. On product labels, it may be identified as *acetone chloroform*, *chloretone*, *chlorbutyl*, *methaform*, *acetiform*, or *chlorobutasol*. It does not irritate the skin and is safe for topical application. But the available information does not show that it effectively works on pain or itching of the skin.

Cyclomethycaine sulfate   Although this substance is a potent -*caine*-type anesthetic, there is insufficient evidence that it is effective when used in the relatively low concentrations (around 1 percent) in which it usually is formulated in over-the-counter products. It does not readily pass through intact skin, so any therapeutic value it might possess is limited to scrapes, cuts, and minor burns that have damaged the outer layer of skin. Although it may cause a brief stinging or burning sensation when applied to the skin, serious side effects are extremely rare; the ingredient was assessed as safe, but it is not proved effective.

Eugenol   An aromatic and spicy-tasting substance, eugenol is the main ingredient in oil of clove. It also is extracted from pimiento, cinnamon leaves, sassafras, and canella and can be prepared synthetically from vanillin. Eugenol's safety is attested by its long use in a variety of topical and internal remedies; toxic reactions are rare or nonexistent. But reviewers could find no hard scientific data to substantiate that the substance is effective for use on the skin.

Glycol salicylate   This ingredient is related chemically to aspirin. A label reader may find it listed as *glycol monosalicylate*, *monoglycol salicylate*, *ethylene glycol monosalicylate*, or *2-hydroxyethyl salicylate*. Long use, together with a paucity of reports on adverse effects, indicates that the ingredient is safe. But on the matter of relieving superficial pain or itching when applied to the skin, the Panel noted that no significant topical pain-relieving or numbing activity can be demonstrated. Conclusion: not proved effective.

Hexylresorcinol   Hexylresorcinol is an alcohol-ketone-type ingredient, related to phenol. Long clinical experience—of more than 40 years—indicates that it is less caustic than phenol preparations. Evaluators consider it safe.

When used on the skin, hexylresorcinol has an antimicrobial effect, which is why another Panel found it definitely effective as a skin-wound cleanser and possibly effective as an antiseptic and wound protectant. But, pending further tests, hexylresorcinol rates only conditional approval as being effective for the relief of skin pain and itches.

Salicylamide   When salicylamide is applied, it does not irritate the skin—so evaluators assessed it as safe—even though some of it is absorbed through the skin and can be detected in muscle and in the urine. But its actual effectiveness for topical use remains unestablished.

Thymol   As the name of this volatile oil suggests, thymol is extracted from the field herb thyme. It has a pleasant smell and pungent taste, and evaluators found no real cause for concern about its safety— particularly since little if any of it is absorbed when it is applied to unbroken skin. But thymol's ability to relieve pain and itching—like its ability to relieve any of the dozen other symptoms for which it has been sold over-the-counter—remains to be proved. In short: not proved effective.

Triethanolamine salicylate (trolamine salicylate)   A salicylate, like aspirin, this compound has been used in topical preparations for years. It appears to be harmless—but it also lacks evidence to substantiate how it may work on the skin. Conclusion: not proved effective.

Disapproved Active Ingredient

Chloral hydrate   This chemical is a remarkably effective sedative and sleep inducer when taken orally. It is also an alcohol—which suggests that it will relieve pain when applied topically. But it does not block nerve conduction, so that—after careful evaluation of the scientific literature—evaluators conclude that chloral hydrate is *not* effective against pain or itching when applied to the skin.

Uncategorized Active Ingredients

Phenyltoloxamine dihydrogen citrate   The FDA authorized manufacturers to use this antihistamine in topical preparations in place of methapyrilene, which was withdrawn from the market because it may cause cancer. No assessment of its safety or effectiveness has as yet been published within the context of the OTC Drug Review.

Pyrilamine maleate   The FDA authorized manufacturers to formulate this antihistamine into external analgesic products after methapyrilene was removed from the market because of its cancer-causing risk. The agency has not yet published an assessment of pyrilamine maleate's effectiveness for over-the-counter topical use within the context of the OTC Drug Review.

INACTIVE INGREDIENTS

A wide variety of inactive ingredients is present in topically applied products for the relief of pain and itching. To check the list, *see* INACTIVE INGREDIENTS in LINIMENTS AND POULTICES FOR ACHES AND PAINS.

Safety and Effectiveness: Active Ingredients in Over-the-Counter Itch and Pain Relievers

Active Ingredient*	Pharmacological Group*	Approved Concentration (%)	Maximum Application (Daily)	Panel's Assessment†
aspirin	4			safe, but not proved effective
benzocaine	1	5–20	4	safe and effective
benzyl alcohol	2	10–33	3–4	safe and effective
butamben picrate	1	1	3–4	safe and effective
camphor	2	0.1–2.5	3–4	safe and effective
camphorated metacresol	2			not proved safe or effective
chloral hydrate	2			not safe or effective
chlorobutanol	2			safe, but not proved effective
cyclomethycaine sulfate	1			safe, but not proved effective
dibucaine	1	0.25–1	3–4	safe and effective
dibucaine hydrochloride	1	0.25–1	3–4	safe and effective
dimethisoquin hydrochloride	1	0.3–0.5	4	safe and effective
diphenhydramine hydrochloride	3	1–2	3–4, up to 1 wk	safe and effective
dyclonine hydrochloride	1	0.5–1	4	safe and effective
eugenol	2			safe, but not proved effective
glycol salicylate	4			safe, but not proved effective
hexylresorcinol	2			safe, but not proved effective
hydrocortisone	5	0.25–0.5	3–4	safe and effective
hydrocortisone acetate	5	0.25–0.5	3–4	safe and effective
juniper tar	2	1–5	4	safe and effective
lidocaine	1	0.5–4	3–4	safe and effective
lidocaine hydrochloride	1	0.5–4	3–4	safe and effective
menthol	2	0.1–1	3–4	safe and effective
phenol	2	0.5–1.5	4	safe and effective
phenolate sodium	2	0.5–1.5	4	safe and effective

Safety and Effectiveness: Active Ingredients in Over-the-Counter Itch and Pain Relievers (continued)

Active Ingredient*	Pharmacological Group*	Approved Concentration (%)	Maximum Application (Daily)	Panel's Assessment†
phenyltoloxamine dihydrogen citrate	3			not assessed
pramoxine hydrochloride	1	0.5–1	4	safe and effective
pyrilamine maleate	3			not assessed
resorcinol	2	0.5–3	4	safe and effective
salicylamide	4			safe, but not proved effective
tetracaine	1	1–2	4	safe and effective
tetracaine hydrochloride	1	1–2	4	safe and effective
thymol	2			safe, but not proved effective
triethanolamine salicylate (trolamine salicylate)	4			safe, but not proved effective
tripelennamine hydrochloride	3	0.5–2	4 up to 1 wk	safe and effective

*Group 1, amines and chemically related -caine drugs; group 2, alcohols and ketones; group 3, antihistamines; group 4, salicylates; group 5, hydrocortisone preparations.

†For persons over the age of 2; use on younger children should be supervised by a physician.

Safety and Effectiveness: Combination Products Sold Over-the-Counter to Relieve Itching and Pain

Safe and Effective Combinations

May include a safe and effective combination of these safe and effective ingredients
1 -caine drug and related amines + 1 alcohol and ketone
1 alcohol and ketone + 1 antihistamine
camphor + menthol + any one other alcohol and ketone
1 salicylate + 1 -caine drug and related amines or 1 alcohol and ketone (N.B. no salicylate has as yet been approved as safe and effective.)

Conditionally Safe or Conditionally Effective Combinations

A combination is only conditionally approved if it
contains any conditionally approved active ingredient
any approved ingredient at less than an effective concentration
a safe and effective alcohol and ketone + a safe and effective antihistamine, since these types may not be effective in combination

Disapproved Products are Considered Unsafe or Ineffective If They Contain

any unsafe or ineffective ingredient
a hydrocortisone + any other -caine and related amines, or alcohol and ketone, or antihistamine, or salicylate
any ingredient that has not been evaluated by a panel, or has been found unsafe, ineffective or irrational by another panel
a salicylate + a sunscreen active ingredient (the pain reliever may mask the symptoms of oncoming sunburn)
any active ingredient for relieving itch and pain + any counterirritant active ingredient, since the former depresses and the latter stimulates nerve endings in the skin so that the combination is irrational.

By checking this unit's SAFETY AND EFFECTIVENESS chart, label-readers can determine the pharmacological group to which any single compound belongs. For example, dimethisoquin hydrochloride is a -caine drug; diphenhydramine hydrochloride is an antihistamine, etc. In most cases, the pharmacological group is fairly obvious from the compound's name. For example, benzyl alcohol is an alcohol; tetracaine is a -caine drug; triethanolamine salicylate is a salicylate.

Itch and Pain Remedies Applied to the Skin: Product Ratings

Single-Ingredient Products

Product and Distributor	Dosage of Active Ingredients	Rating[1]	Comment
benzocaine			
Americaine Anesthetic (American Critical Care)	**spray:** 20%	**A**	

Itch and Pain Remedies Applied to the Skin: Product Ratings *(continued)*

Single-Ingredient Products

Product and Distributor	Dosage of Active Ingredients	Rating[1]	Comment
benzocaine topical (generic)	cream: 5% ointment: 5%	A	
butamben picrate Butesin Picrate (Abbott)	ointment: 1%	A	
cyclomethycaine hydrochloride Surfacaine (Lilly)	cream: 0.5% ointment: 1%	B	not proved effective
dibucaine dibucaine hydrochloride (generic)	ointment: 1%	A	
D-Caine (Century)	ointment: 1%	A	
Nupercainal (Ciba)	ointment: 1%	A	
Nupercainal (Ciba)	cream: 0.5%	A	
dimethisoquin hydrochloride Quotane (Menley & James)	ointment: 0.5%	A	
diphenhydramine hydrochloride Benadryl (Parke-Davis)	cream: 2%	A	
dyclonine hydrochloride Resolve Gel (Dow)	gel: 1%	A	
hexylresorcinol S.T. 37 (Beecham Prod.)	solution: 0.1%	B	not proved effective
hydrocortisone Cortil (Pfipharmecs)	cream: 0.5%	A	
Dermolate Anti-Itch (Schering)		A	
Pro-Cort (Barnes-Hind)		A	
Hytone (Dermik)	ointment: 0.5%	A	
Wellcortin (Burroughs-Wellcome)		A	

Itch and Pain Remedies Applied to the Skin: Product Ratings *(continued)*

Single-Ingredient Products

Product and Distributor	Dosage of Active Ingredients	Rating[1]	Comment
hydrocortisone acetate			
CaldeCort Rectal-Itch (Pharmacraft)	ointment: 0.5% hydrocortisone equivalent	A	
Cortaid (Upjohn)		A	
Cortaid (Upjohn)	cream: 0.5% hydrocortisone equivalent	A	
Cortef Feminine Itch (Upjohn)		A	
Rhulicort (Lederle)		A	
Gynecort Feminine Cream Medication (Combe)	cream: 0.5%	A	
Pharma-Cort (Purepac)		A	
lidocaine			
Xylocaine (Astra)	ointment: 2.5%	A	
pramoxine hydrochloride			
Tronothane (Abbott)	cream: 1%	A	
	jelly: 1%	A	
tetracaine			
Pontocaine (Breon)	cream: 1%	A	
	ointment: 0.5%	C	too weak
triethanolamine salicylate (also **trolamine salicylate**)			
Myoflex Creme (Adria)	cream: 10%	B	not proved effective
tripelennamine hydrochloride			
PBZ (Geigy)	cream: 2%	A	

Itch and Pain Remedies Applied to the Skin: Product Ratings *(continued)*

Anesthetic-Based Combination Products—Principally for Pain

Product and Distributor	Dosage of Active Ingredients	Rating[1]	Comment
Americaine (American Critical Care)	**ointment:** 20% benzocaine + 0.1% benzethonium chloride	**B**	benzethonium, an antimicrobial, not prove effective
Burntame (Otis Clapp)	**spray:** 20% benzocaine + 8-hydroxyquinoline	**B**	effectiveness of oxyquinolines questioned by other Panels
Dermoplast (Ayerst)	**spray:** 20% benzocaine + 0.5% menthol	**A**	
Foille (Blistex)	**liquid, spray, and ointment:** 2% benzocaine + 4% benzyl alcohol	**C**	less-than-effective amounts of both ingredients
Solarcaine (Plough)	**cream:** 1% benzocaine + 0.2% triclosan	**C**	less-than-effective amoun of benzocaine; triclosar not proved safe and/or not proved effective as antimicrobial
Unguentine Plus (Norwich-Eaton)	**cream:** 2% lidocaine + 2% chloroxylenol + 0.5% phenol	**B**	chloroxylenol not proved safe or effective as antimicrobial
Vaseline First Aid Carbolated Petroleum Jelly (Chesebrough-Pond's)	**ointment:** 0.2% phenol + 0.5% chloroxylenol + petroleum jelly + lanolin	**C**	too little phenol for pain relief; chloroxylenol not proved safe or effective

Antihistamine-Based Combination Products—Principally for Itchiness

Product and Distributor	Dosage of Active Ingredients	Rating[1]	Comment
Caladryl Cream (Parke-Davis)	**cream:** 1% diphenhydramine hydrochloride + 8% calamine + 0.1% camphor	**A**	
Caladryl Lotion (Parke-Davis)	**lotion:** 1% diphenhydramine hydrochloride + 0.1% camphor + 8% calamine	**A**	

Itch and Pain Remedies Applied to the Skin: Product Ratings *(continued)*

Antihistamine-Based Combination Products—Principally for Itchiness

Product and Distributor	Dosage of Active Ingredients	Rating[1]	Comment
Didelamine (Commerce)	**spray** and **gel:** 1% diphenhydramine hydrochloride + 0.5% tripelennamine hydrochloride + 0.125% benzalkonium chloride	C	2 antihistamines not an approved combination
Histacalma (Rexall)	**lotion:** 1% phenyltoloxamine dihydrogen citrate + 1% benzocaine + 5% calamine	C	antihistamine not assessed by Panel, and as yet not assessed by FDA; too little benzocaine
IVarest (Blistex)	**cream** and **lotion:** 1.5% pyrilamine maleate + 1% benzocaine + 14% calamine	C	antihistamine not assessed by Panel, and as yet not assessed as an over-the-counter topical drug or by FDA; too little benzocaine
Surfadil (Lilly)	**cream:** 1% diphenhydramine hydrochloride + 0.5% cyclomethycaine sulfate	B	cyclomethycaine not proved effective

1. Author's interpretation of Panel/FDA criteria. Based on contents, not claims.

Jock Itch, Athlete's Foot, and Ringworm Cures

Two of the most modern and most effective nonprescription drugs—introduced in the 1960's and 1970's—are topical antifungal agents used to treat jock itch, athlete's foot, and some forms of ringworm. Moreover,

JOCK ITCH, ATHLETE'S FOOT, AND RINGWORM CURES is based on the report "Topical Antifungal Drug Products for OTC Human Use" by the FDA's Advisory Review Panel on OTC Antimicrobial Drug Products (Antimicrobial II Panel).

2 additional potent antifungals may be changed from prescription to nonprescription status at the Panel's recommendation. The Panel describes these drugs' effectiveness succinctly when it says that "unlike other OTC products, [they] treat disease rather than symptoms." That is to say, they are *curative* drugs.

CLAIMS

Accurate
"treats athlete's foot (*tinea pedis*)"

"cures jock itch (*tinea cruris*)"

"clears up athlete's foot, jock itch, and ringworm"

"proven clinically effective in the treatment of ringworm (*tinea corporis*)"

"treats athlete's foot, jock itch, and ringworm"—("jock itch" and "ringworm" may be stated for the drugs haloprogin and tolnaftate only)

"proven to kill dermatophytic fungi and yeast" (causes of athlete's foot)

"prevents," or "helps prevent athlete's foot with daily use," or "guards against athlete's foot with daily use" may be used for the drug tolnaftate against athlete's foot (not jock itch or ringworm)

False or Misleading
"kills most athlete's-foot fungi"

"kills jock-itch fungi on contact"

"proven fungicide for athlete's foot, jock itch, and body ringworm"

for "fast relief of itching and burning of athlete's foot and jock itch"

"kills all known athlete's-foot and jock-itch fungi"

"guards against fungus growth"

WARNING These drugs should not be used on children under 2 except on a doctor's advice, and they should be used by children under 12 only under parental supervision.

WHAT IS FUNGUS?

The funguses that cause human skin diseases are microorganisms that belong to a primitive group of plants which lacks the green pigment chlorophyll. For that reason they must derive their life energy from other plant or animal life rather than from the rays of the sun. The molds that cause jock itch and athlete's foot obtain energy by breaking down keratin, the horny substance that provides strength and structure to hair, nails, and skin. Molds and yeasts are both funguses—and so, of course, are mushrooms. Most of the funguses that cause jock itch, athlete's foot, and ringworm on the body are molds.

The common skin-disease funguses that afflict people normally grow in the soil. But they can also thrive on human bodies—especially in warm, moist areas like the crotch, toewebs, underarms, and in protected and concealed places in the hair or under the nails. They may also cause infection in normal, dry skin.

Fungal Infections

Fungal infections are typically itchy and red. They may become quite painful, particularly if the skin cracks so that bacteria can enter and start secondary infections. The tissue may look and smell decayed or rotten. In some fungal attacks there is a secondary eruption elsewhere on the body, called a *dermatophytid reaction*. It may consist of hard pimples that tend to arise around hair follicles, bruiselike lesions, hives, or ring-shaped red rashes. The cause of these eruptions—which may be accompanied by fever, malaise, and loss of appetite—is unclear. They are not secondary fungal infestations, but rather appear to be defensive overreactions in which the white blood cells attack noninfected skin in much the same way that they attack the moldy skin at the infection site.

More than 200,000 funguses have been discovered and described in the scientific literature. Only very few, fortunately, cause human diseases—although some are grotesquely disfiguring, incurable, and eventually lethal. The funguses that cause jock itch and athlete's foot are much less serious and now are much more successfully treated. Yet anyone who has suffered from these disorders knows they can be tenaciously annoying and frustratingly difficult to cure.

Jock itch and athlete's foot tend to be caused by the same funguses, particularly *Trichophyten rubrum*, *Trichophyten mentagrophytes*, and *Epidermophyton floccosum*. The first is more commonly found on the feet, the last more commonly in the groin. Ringworm of the body is commonly caused by *Microsporum canis*, which, as its name implies, is transmitted by dogs (but also by cats).

A number of different diseases may create itchy, unpleasant-appearing lesions that look a lot like jock itch or athlete's foot. Bacterial infections can cause itchy scaling and redness between the toes. Psoriasis, a scaly disease of unknown cause, creates toeweb and groin-itch patches that look very much like fungus. Allergic responses to shoe material and sock dyes or other footwear components sometimes are mistaken for athlete's foot.

If you are in doubt, or if self-treatment with a nonprescription drug does not quickly relieve the itching and pain and begin to clear up the skin, then seek a dermatologist's help. Simple tests are available to pinpoint the cause of distressing skin complaints in the groin and on the feet.

Athlete's foot   This skin disease is technically called *tinea pedis*, which means foot fungus. Soldiers who suffer severe cases of it in the tropics call it "jungle rot."

Athlete's foot usually originates in the toewebs, the areas between the toes. The rash is itchy, red, and scaling; the toewebs may appear white and soggy. The white scale is particularly common between the fourth and fifth toes. Cracks commonly appear. Blisters and pimples may erupt on the soles of the feet, so that walking becomes painfully difficult at best. These disabling symptoms often occur because the original fungal infection has opened up the skin, providing a way for bacteria to enter and create larger, secondary infections. Sometimes the infectious molds invade and destroy the toenails.

Athlete's foot is more common in men than in women; it occurs most frequently in those between the ages of 15 and 40. It may be picked up at summer camps and resorts, military bases and prisons, and other places where there are many bare or dirty feet. The offending funguses are everywhere, however, so the question of why some people get athlete's foot and others do not has not been satisfactorily answered. The Panel notes that many people who are plagued by recurrent fungal skin diseases also suffer from asthma, hay fever, or atopic eczema—conditions in which the body's protective immune mechanism appears to be somewhat defective.

The standard recommendations for preventing athlete's foot or limiting its spread once it has occurred are to wash the feet once or twice daily with soap and water, keep them dry, and, if possible, cool. One should select absorbent cotton socks and light, ventilated shoes that "breathe" rather than boots or other thick, heavy shoes.

"Curing" athlete's foot, insofar as that means clearing up all symptoms, may not end the problem. Some dermatologists believe the fungus can never be wholly eliminated and that some cells remain hidden in skin cracks and nail beds. Then when conditions are again right for them, they regrow—even many summers afterward.

Since the body *can* build up a protective immunity against these funguses, the question is often asked: Why do these infections recur?

The answer may be that the blood-borne antibodies which can destroy these funguses are unable to reach the outermost layers of the skin (where athlete's foot occurs).

Because of the risk of recurrences, reviewers see some value in using antifungal medication on a *preventive* basis once the original infection has been cleared up. However, only one drug, tolnaftate, is approved as safe and effective for this kind of use.

Jock itch   This fungal infection of the groin is most common in men between the ages of 18 and 40. It is rare in children and uncommon in women. The technical name is *tinea cruris*, but it is more likely to be recognized by the slangier names "crotch rot" and "Dhobie itch." There does not seem to be a generally recognized name for these infections when they occur in women; the Panel suggests that the term *intertrigo*—which has the more general meaning of an inflammation or eruption in a skinfold area—might serve.

Jock itch usually originates in the crease between the inner thigh and the scrotum. It may spread around the groin, down the thigh, and across the scrotum and penis. The rash is red, scaly, and quite itchy, and often has a ringlike curved margin along the thigh and scrotum. This expanding margin may be raised and flaky while the center of the rash, having begun to heal, is stained a light brown color by blood and other breakdown products of inflammation.

No certain way is known to prevent jock itch. But cleanliness and the avoidance of tight, air-tight, or chafing underwear and outerwear undoubtedly help, since fungal infections usually start in warm, moist, damaged skin.

Body ringworm   Itchy ring-shaped eruptions on children's bodies are very likely to be body ringworm, or *tinea corporis*. They commonly are caused by the fungus *Microsporum canis*, carried by pets. The "rings" may be red, scaly, and quite itchy, while the areas inside the rings heal rather quickly. Despite the name *ringworm*, this disorder is a fungus infection. *Ringworm is not caused by or associated with worms of any kind.*

Scalp ringworm and nail ringworm   The technical names for scalp ringworm and nail ringworm are *tinea capitis* and *tinea unguium*: fungal infection of the head and the "claws" (nails), respectively. The ring shape of the lesion is a strong indication that it is caused by a fungus —no worm of any kind is involved.

These fungal infections may be hard to self-diagnose and they are certainly very hard to self-treat since antifungal powders, sprays, and liquids penetrate only poorly to the hair roots and nail beds where the funguses have set up housekeeping. Systemically applied medication prescribed by a doctor will probably be needed.

Evaluators warn that the topical drugs described in this unit are not effective for treating ringworm of the scalp and nails. Persons who think they are suffering such an infection should see their doctor for diagnosis and treatment.

Candidiasis   Not all crotch and toe fungal diseases are caused by molds. Certain yeasts—which are also funguses—can cause horrific itching and other symptoms that may be indistinguishable from those caused by the molds described above.

The best-known—and very likely the least-loved—of these yeasts is a species called *Candida albicans*. The disease it causes is called *candidiasis*, or *monilia*, or *moniliasis*, or, simply yeast.

Like the molds, *C. albicans* thrives in warm, moist body areas like the toewebs and groin. On the feet, it causes redness, toe rot, and cracking between the toes. In the groin it produces bright, red, weepy rashes with many pimplelike bumps along their outer edge. These eruptions are extremely itchy. In men, they often spread to the scrotum and outside of the rectum. In women the pattern may be similar, but the disorder is usually associated with what experts call *extreme* itching of the vulva, as well as with a characteristic white, unpleasant-smelling vaginal discharge. (Women who suspect that they have candidiasis should consult the unit YEAST KILLERS FOR FEMININE ITCHING.)

These eruptions may also occur on other parts of the body. The yeast appears to be everywhere in the human environment, yet most people resist it most of the time. Risk factors include diabetes, pregnancy, obesity, profuse sweating, and the use of certain drugs—particularly birth-control pills, oral corticosteroid drugs, and broad-spectrum antibiotics.

Rapid tests, which can be conducted in a dermatologist's or gynecologist's office, will differentiate yeast infections from the molds that more often are the cause of jock itch, athlete's foot, and ringworm. This diagnostic step is important because most drugs used against molds are not comparably effective against yeast. A few special antifungals, however, will kill both molds and yeast.

Given that the victim of these infections may not be able to tell which organism is causing his or her grief, the Panel feels that there is a therapeutic advantage to be gained by using either a broad-spectrum antifungal or one that acts against molds and against yeast.

The FDA takes a dimmer view of self-treatment of candidal infections. It disapproves the claim, okayed by the Panel, that nonprescription antifungals can be used for the "treatment of superficial skin infections caused by yeast *(Candida),*" and insists, for now, that candidiasis must be diagnosed by a doctor and treated under his or her supervision.

TREATMENT

Though it may seem surprising, since they occur at very different parts of the anatomy, jock itch, athlete's foot, and ringworm of the body respond to the same drugs. This occurs because most cases are caused by very similar species of molds or yeasts.

Many people routinely self-treat jock itch and athlete's foot with medicated powders and sprays. However, as several available drugs will limit fungal growth but will not kill all residual fungus cells, the conditions constantly recur. Sufferers become accustomed to them and come to regard them as an unavoidable annoyance rather than as diseases which can be treated aggressively and very possibly cured.

Fatalistic acceptance of fungal afflictions can have 2 dangerous consequences. At a moment when the body defenses for some reason are suddenly weakened, a minor fungal condition can explode into a serious—even life-threatening—illness. Moreover, continuous use of antifungal drugs, particularly on injured or broken-down skin, can lead to the body's absorbing dangerous amounts of the drugs.

The Panel believes that stand-offs between fungus and hosts are dangerous and should not be allowed to continue. It recommends that sufferers of these conditions use only those drugs that have the potential for eradicating the fungus rather than just holding it in abeyance. The antifungal agents listed as approved have this capacity—although none has been shown to cure every case for which it is used. For this reason, if the condition has not been cleared up after a reasonable period of time—2 weeks for jock itch and feminine itching; a month for athlete's foot and ringworm of the body—it may be wise to switch to a product that contains a different active ingredient or, better yet, visit a doctor.

Infected areas always should be washed with soap and water and dried thoroughly before the medicine is applied. Two applications daily, morning and night, should suffice—unless more frequent treatment is recommended by a doctor.

Comparison of Safe and Effective Antifungal Active Ingredients

Ingredient	Status (7/1/82)	Can Cure Jock Itch, Athlete's Foot, Ringworm of Body	Can Cure Yeast Infections (C. albicans) That Cause Feminine Itching	Proved Safe and Effective for Preventing Athlete's Foot	Safe and Effective in Combination with Hydrocortisone
haloprogin*	Rx	yes	yes	no	yes
iodochlorhydroxyquin	OTC	yes	no	no	yes
miconazole nitrate*	Rx	yes	yes	no	no
tolnaftate	OTC	yes	no	yes	no
undecylenates: undecylenic acid, calcium undecylenate, copper undecylenate, and zinc undecylenate	OTC	yes	no	no	no

*These drugs may become available over-the-counter as the Panel recommends.

Dosage Forms

Antifungal active ingredients are formulated in a variety of bases that includes ointments, creams, powders, liquids, and aerosol sprays. The Panel believes that a soluble form is most effective; these preparations include rapidly evaporating liquids (like alcohol-acetone solutions) and aerosol sprays. These forms dry quickly and leave the antifungal agent in close contact with the skin. It may be much more difficult for the active drug to reach the skin and fungus cells when it is formulated in an ointment, cream, or powder.

Drying Agents

Many antifungal preparations are formulated in a starch, alcohol, or other substance that dries the skin. Drying is useful—but the Panel considers drying agents to be inactive ingredients.

Combination Products

In order for a combination of 2 or 3 antifungals to be approved as safe and effective, each active ingredient must be safe and effective and must be present in the approved dosage. Each must contribute to the product by broadening the range of funguses against which the drug is effective. The FDA says no such combination is currently marketed over-the-counter.

Evaluators also approved several combinations of an antifungal agent with approved active ingredients of other classes. They appear particularly to approve combinations of 0.5 percent hydrocortisone or hydrocortisone acetate with one of the recently developed antifungals. Hydrocortisone acts quickly to relieve inflammation and to reduce itching, burning, and pain. Meanwhile, the antifungal attacks and kills the fungus—which takes a longer time.

Hydrocortisone and the new antifungals seem to act in a complementary fashion. The Panel reports that double-blind clinical studies demonstrate that hydrocortisone with miconazole or with iodochlorhydroxyquin produces a significantly higher rate of cures than either hydrocortisone or one of the antifungals used alone. In one study done in South America with soldiers who had jock itch or athlete's foot, a combination of miconazole (2 percent) and hydrocortisone (1 percent) cured 97 percent of the men in 14 days. This compared with a cure rate of 82 percent for miconazole alone and 6 percent for the hydrocortisone alone. According to the investgator who conducted the tests, these results were particularly impressive because the subjects lived under the "worst conditions of heat, humidity, and poor hygiene."

The Panel also approved combinations of antifungal agents with one other active ingredient that has been approved as safe and effective as an antiperspirant or as a skin-peeling agent. The FDA is less enthusiastic about these combinations, which it says are not proved effective. It will not permit them to be sold over-the-counter. The approved combinations are detailed in the SAFETY AND EFFECTIVENESS: COMBINATION PRODUCTS chart at the end of this unit. Conditional approval was granted to a traditional antifungal preparation called Whitefield's ointment. This is a combination of benzoic and salicylic acids in polyethylene glycol whose effectiveness has never convincingly been demonstrated.

Another widely used combination, called *carbol-fuchsin* solution (sometimes known as *Castellani's paint* or *Magenta paint BPC*), appears to be effective against several types of fungal disease. But most studies concerned with proving the merit of the substance used methods the Panel questioned. Worse, carbol-fuchsin contains carbolic acid (phenol) at dangerously high concentrations (4.5 percent), while the fuchsin, a red dye, is suspected to cause cancer. Given these risks, evaluators assessed carbol-fuchsin as unsafe for over-the-counter sales and self-treatment—although it may be appropriate for use supervised by a doctor.

ANTIFUNGAL DRUGS

Approved Active Ingredients

The Panel identified 6 basic ingredients that it believes are safe and effective for self-treatment of jock itch, athlete's foot, ringworm of the body, or yeast infections caused by *Candida albicans*. Three of them —iodochlorhydroxyquin, tolnaftate, and the undecylenates (undecylenic acid and calcium, copper, and zinc undecylenate)—are already available over-the-counter. Three others are prescription drugs that the evaluators recommended be switched to nonprescription status: haloprogin, miconazole nitrate, and nystatin. All of them have the virtue—absent in the other approved antifungals—of being effective against yeasts, including *C. albicans*. The FDA demurs on switching nystatin to nonprescription status, however; so it is likely to remain a prescription drug.

Haloprogin This prescription drug—which the Panel recommends be switched to nonprescription status—was developed in Japan in 1962. It is already available without prescription in Japan and Canada. It kills the molds responsible for jock itch, athlete's foot, and ringworm of the body and also the yeast (*Candida albicans*) that causes comparable infections at these body sites, as well as intense feminine itching.

Haloprogin was approved for sales by prescription in the United States under the strict regulatory requirements in effect at the FDA during the 1970s. A variety of tests in rabbits, pigs, and other animals (as well as in humans) showed that the drug has a low level of toxicity. The Panel therefore believes it is safe to market over-the-counter.

In clinical tests haloprogin, at a concentration of 1 percent in ointments and solutions, proved to be very effective against jock itch, athlete's foot, and ringworm of the body. When used for 2 to 4 weeks, it cleared up from two-thirds to more than nine-tenths of these infections (as does the standard drug in this group, tolnaftate). Haloprogin also works against yeast infections (tolnaftate does not). It is not, however, very effective against bacterial infections that may occur secondarily to a mold or yeast infection.

The safe and effective dosage is an application of 1 percent haloprogin twice daily for adults and children over 2. Children under 12 should be supervised by adults in the use of this medication.

Iodochlorhydroxyquin   A nonprescription antifungal, this active ingredient effectively combats the molds that cause jock itch, athlete's foot, and ringworm of the body, as well as some bacteria that may be responsible for secondary infections in persons suffering these itch conditions. But iodochlorhydroxyquin is not useful against yeast infections due to *Candida albicans* or its relatives.

This drug was developed in the 1960s and has been carefully tested in animals and people, under stringent drug-approval standards. In the small amounts used on the skin the drug appears to be safe, although very large doses taken internally have been identified as the cause of a severe neurologic disorder called *subacute myelooptic neuropathy*.

Iodochlorhydroxyquin cures between one-half and two-thirds of fungal infections, evaluators report. It seems from the Panel's comments that the drug is a little less likely to work as effectively as tolnaftate or haloprogin.

Iodochlorhydroxyquin is safe and effective when combined with hydrocortisone. This combination provides rapid relief of pain and itching and more gradual elimination of the molds that are their cause. In one study, this combination was found to be dramatically more effective than either the antifungal or the hydrocortisone used alone.

The safe and effective dose of iodochlorhydroxyquin is 3 percent concentration in a cream or other base applied twice daily to the toe-webs, groin, or other body sites of adults and children over 2. Children under 12 should have parental supervision using the drug.

Miconazole nitrate The Panel recommends that this prescription drug be switched to nonprescription status. Miconazole nitrate is a broad-spectrum antifungal that effectively works against the yeast *Candida albicans* as well as the molds that cause jock itch, athlete's foot, and body ringworm.

Miconazole was approved by the FDA in the 1970s under the tight requirements in force at that time for all new drugs. It is one of a very few drugs that is—or may become—over-the-counter, about which an expert body like the present Panel can say: "Adequate, well-controlled animal and human toxicity studies were conducted." It is, in short, safe at manufacturers' recommended dosages.

Careful and well-controlled double-blind clinical tests (tests in which neither the investigator nor the patient knew who was receiving the active medication and who a dummy drug), have shown that miconazole is highly effective—even under difficult conditions. Among patients at an Air Force hospital in Mississippi, for example, 93 percent of the men who received the active drug were cleared of all signs and symptoms of their fungal disease. This compares very favorably with just 19 percent whose conditions cleared up on the dummy medication. No effort was made to induce these servicemen to bathe more often, dress differently, or change their habits in any other way. The miconazole also provided *fast* relief: itching and burning had subsided in three-quarters of the men by the end of the third day.

In another test, in a crowded Florida prison, three-quarters of the inmates treated with the active drug experienced relief of itching within a week—compared with only one-tenth of those who applied the dummy medications to their toewebs, groins, or bodies. There was only one recurrence of fungal infection in the prisoners successfully treated with miconazole nitrate. These results indicate that in most such cases the drug successfully eliminates the causative organisms. Miconazole is also effective against the yeast infection *C. albicans* as well as against several bacterial infections that mimic jock itch and athlete's foot.

The safe and effective dosage is 2 percent miconazole nitrate in cream or another base, applied twice daily, for adults and children over 2. Youngsters under 12 should be overseen by adults when they use this medication.

Nystatin   *See* under DISAPPROVED ACTIVE INGREDIENTS, below.

Tolnaftate   An antifungal introduced in the 1960s, tolnaftate has been shown to be both safe and effective in many studies conducted under the very demanding guidelines then required by the FDA and comparable agencies. In the Panel's view, these studies demonstrate that tolnaftate is safe and effective for treating jock itch, athlete's foot, and ringworm of the body. (Tolnaftate is not effective against bacteria or against *Candida albicans* and other yeasts.)

Tolnaftate is the only nonprescription drug that has been proved safe and effective for *preventing* athlete's foot. But, because the groin is a much more sensitive area than the feet, reviewers do not approve the ongoing use of the drug to prevent jock itch.

In recent years, tolnaftate has become the standard drug against which other topical antifungals are compared. It appears to be best matched by haloprogrin; both drugs give up to 90 percent cure rates in patients with athlete's foot.

The safe and effective dose for the treatment of jock itch, athlete's foot, and ringworm of the body is one percent tolnaftate twice daily in adults and children over 2; children under 12 should be supervised in their use of this drug. One or 2 applications daily are recommended when tolnaftate is used preventively against athlete's foot.

Undecylenic acid and its salts: calcium undecylenate, copper undecylenate, and zinc undecylenate   Although they are only 40 years old, these are the granddaddies among approved antifungal agents. They are less potent than the new agents discussed above, and the cure rates—which in most studies run around 50 percent—are also lower.

The Panel describes a fair number of animal and human tests which indicate that undecylenic acid and its compounds cause little irritation or other toxicity, so safety is not in question. The various undecylenates appear roughly comparable to each other in effectiveness, and they are often combined in products used to treat jock itch, athlete's foot, and ringworm of the body. These compounds do not work against yeast infections caused by *Candida albicans*; neither will they cure bacterial infections.

A concentration of from 10 to 22 percent of one or more undecylenates is safe and effective for adults and children over 2 (children up to 12 should be supervised when they use this medication).

Conditionally Approved Active Ingredients

A wide range of standard over-the-counter drugs—many of them used for a variety of other purposes—are claimed to be beneficial in treating jock itch, athlete's foot, and ringworm of the body. Many are safe in the recommended dosages, according to the Panel. But for most of them, the evidence that allegedly proves that they work is weak or deficient in some way. Since there are several quite effective antifungal drugs that will cure a fair proportion of these infections, the less convincing medications will be described only cursorily.

Aluminum preparations: alcloxa, aluminum sulfate, and potassium alum   These drugs are widely used as astringents and antiperspirants, and are generally regarded as safe. Low doses kill funguses in lab dishes, but higher doses are required to kill them between a person's toes. Tests conducted in an effort to prove effectiveness were questioned on grounds of poor methodology. In short, these aluminum preparations are safe but not proved effective.

Basic fuchsin   This is a red dye that is suspected of causing cancer, so the Panel questions its safety. It does kill bacteria and has been used for years to combat both bacteria and funguses. But there are no studies demonstrating its value against the specific funguses that are known to cause jock itch, athlete's foot, and ringworm of the body. So the Panel says basic fuchsin's safety and effectivenesss remain to be proved.

Benzethonium chloride   This Panel, along with several others, finds that this ingredient, a quaternary ammonium compound, is of doubtful safety—except when used for very brief periods. Furthermore, no data are available showing that it is effective when used alone against fungal infections. Conclusion: both the safety and effectiveness of benzethonium chloride as an antifungal remain to be proved.

Benzoic acid   A widely used over-the-counter medicine that is applied to the skin, benzoic acid is accepted as safe. In one study it was found to be almost as effective as undecylenic acid in treating jock itch and related fungal disorders. But reviewers say this study was flawed, and they want to see a first-rate clinical test done to determine how well benzoic acid actually works. At the moment, the Panel's assessment of benzoic acid is: safe but not proved effective.

Boron compounds: boric acid and sodium borate (borax)   These are common components of athlete's-foot powders. While borates have been used medicinally for over a thousand years, serious doubts have recently been raised concerning both their safety and effectiveness.

In concentrations of under 5 percent, the Panel believes borates are safe—because only very small amounts are absorbed into the bloodstream. However, effectiveness remains much in doubt: only one test has been conducted to assess boric acid as an active ingredient against athlete's foot. Results were not convincing to the evaluators. Wanting better evidence, the Panel says that up to 5 percent boric acid or sodium borate is safe but not proved effective. Concentrations over 5 percent are not safe.

Caprylates: sodium caprylate and zinc caprylate   These compounds are derived from caprylic acid. This fatty acid occurs naturally in human sweat and has been found to inhibit fungal growth. The caprylates may cause some irritation, but clinical studies and long marketing experience—during which few adverse effects have been reported—persuade the Panel that they are safe.

Some old but rather well-conducted studies strongly indicate that these compounds are effective against jock itch, athlete's foot, and ringworm of the body. The Panel believes these compounds can be proved to be effective if rigorous scientific methods are used. Until this is done, however, it assesses them as safe, but not proved effective.

The caprylates have also been used experimentally and clinically against yeast infections caused by *Candida albicans*. The results seem promising, but pending a double-blind controlled study in which caprylates are compared with a dummy medication, the Panel grants them only conditional approval for use against yeast infections.

Chlorothymol   Although chlorothymol is a phenollike drug, it is less toxic dose for dose than phenol (*see* PHENOLATES: PHENOL AND PHENOLATE SODIUM, page 488). However, it is strongly irritating to the skin and mucous membranes and the Panel thinks chlorothymol's safety has yet to be established. As to effectiveness, the substance is strongly active against bacteria and has been shown to possess powerful antifungal properties in lab dishes. But it has not been established clinically whether chlorothymol relieves jock itch, athlete's foot, or ringworm of the body. In short: chlorothymol has not been proved safe or effective.

Chloroxylenol   This Panel concludes that in the low doses (under 3 percent) used in a topical antifungal drug, chloroxylenol is safe. However, while chloroxylenol appears to kill funguses, well-devised double-blind studies that might confirm this supposition have yet to be done. Until they are, the Panel assesses the drug as safe but not proved effective.

Cresols: m-cresol and secondary amyltricresols   These coal-tar derivatives are structurally related to phenol and share its toxic properties. Many cases of cresol toxicity have occurred, and chronic poisoning can result from application of cresols to the skin. The chemicals effectively kill bacteria, and some studies show them to have antifungal properties as well. But only 2 studies—both uncontrolled—have been conducted on cresol's effectiveness against athlete's foot. One was done at an army base, the other in a prison. Neither satisfactorily proved cresols effective. So the Panel decided that cresols are not proved safe or effective against the funguses that cause athlete's foot and related disorders.

Dichlorophen   This substance, commonly called *G-4*, is a phenol-like drug that has been used for flea powders, worm medicines, and other treatments for pets and farm animals. It is not marketed for oral human use in the United States but is in Britain, where it is used against tapeworm. Dichlorophen is chemically related to the antiseptic hexachlorophene, which has been banned for nonprescription use because it is a nerve poison that has killed babies. The Panel is concerned about the risk of its use, and wants its safety carefully studied.

Dichlorophen is a fairly effective antibacterial. It appears to be less effective against funguses, and most studies to prove its effectiveness are poorly documented. Verdict: not proved safe or effective.

Oxyquinolines: benzoxiquine, oxyquinoline, and oxyquinoline sulfate   There is some evidence that these compounds may cause cancer, which concerns the Panel. Studies which purport to show that these substances are effective against fungal diseases were criticized for poor, unscientific design. Wanting better evidence on both counts—that is, safety and effectiveness—the Panel assesses the oxyquinolines as only conditionally approved as antifungal agents.

Parabens: methylparaben and propylparaben   These substances are widely used as drug preservatives at concentrations of 0.4 percent or lower. This is considered too low a level to cure jock itch or athlete's foot. Yet at therapeutic concentrations of 0.5 to 5 percent, the safety of the parabens has not been well established. Neither has their effectiveness been assessed in a systematic and scientific way—although one promising report was published back in 1944 on 5 percent methylparaben as an athlete's-foot medication. Lacking definitive evidence, evaluators concluded: not proved safe or effective.

Phenyl salicylate   Also known as salol, this substance has been around for a century. Despite such a long history of use, manufacturers failed to present the Panel with evidence to prove the substance's safety or effectiveness in treating jock itch or athlete's foot. So, until acceptable data are available, phenyl salicylate is listed as not proved safe or effective.

Povidone-iodine   The povidone in this complex binds iodine and then releases it slowly onto the skin. One fairly good study indicates that povidone-iodine is effective against athlete's foot, but this test was not adequately followed up after treatment ceased. Povidone-iodine was marketed as an athlete's-foot medication only in one year, 1960, and while the Panel finds it to be safe, it is not generally recognized as effective as an antifungal for jock itch, athlete's foot, and similar infections.

Propionic acid and its salts: sodium propionate and zinc propionate   Many studies have demonstrated that these compounds are essentially nontoxic. Also, a number of studies demonstrate the ability of the propionates to quell or prevent athlete's-foot infections. But a carefully controlled, double-blind study on a meaningfully large group of patients has yet to be done. Until it is, the Panel's verdict is: safe but not proved effective.

Salicylic acid   In concentrations of 3 percent or less, salicylic acid applied to the skin is safe. Higher concentrations may be risky, the Panel says. Test data to show that salicylic acid effectively combats athlete's foot and similar fungal infections are inadequate. So pending more definitive results, the judgment is that salicylic acid is safe at concentrations up to 3 percent, but not effective against fungal disorders.

Sulfur   Hippocrates, the Father of Medicine, kept sulfur in his doctor's bag. The chemical has been used for a variety of illnesses since then. Sulfur can irritate the skin, yet its safety when applied to the skin has virtually never been studied! Yet, the Panel hesitantly accepts sulfur as safe because of the drug's almost universal acceptance by dermatologists. However, there are no controlled studies demonstrating that sulfur effectively works against fungal diseases in humans. So the Panel had little choice but to mark it as safe but of unproved effectiveness.

Triacetin   This compound releases glycerin and acetic acid when it is exposed to enzymes produced by some athlete's-foot funguses. Both these breakdown products are noninjurious to the skin; accordingly, the Panel judges that triacetin, too, is noninjurious. The drug appears to be effective against the funguses *Tricophyten mentagrophytes* and *Epidermophyton floccosum,* which produce a soggy-toeweb form of athlete's foot—but supporting studies are still needed. Triacetin does not seem to be effective against *Tricophyten rubrum*, a fungus that produces a drier form of toeweb trouble. Also, its value against jock itch and ringworm of the body remains to be determined. Pending new evidence to show that triacetin works, the drug is judged safe but not proved effective. The Panel notes that the drug should be used only against athlete's foot that takes a soggy, wet form.

Disapproved Active Ingredients

A number of compounds that have been labeled for use against fungal infections of the skin are dismissed by the Panel as unsafe or ineffective.

Camphor   Although there is considerable concern about camphor's safety, the low dosages used in treating athlete's foot are not likely to be hazardous (*see* CAMPHOR). A mixture of camphor and phenol was used for years in the treatment of athlete's foot. While it seems to have been relatively effective, careful and controlled scientific studies were never done. So no evidence of effectiveness was or is available on the antifungal properties of camphor as a single active ingredient. The Panel classifies it as not effective.

Coal tar   This is a blackish-brown distillation product from soft coal. The Panel is worried because coal contains chemicals that may cause cancer, and it is also a skin irritant. On top of that, no adequate studies have shown that the substance is effective against funguses. So the Panel judged coal tar as not safe for treating jock itch or athlete's foot.

Menthol   Can this minty alcohol relieve athlete's foot or other fungal infections? There is no evidence that it can. Its safety has not been established. Verdict: not proved safe and not effective.

Nystatin   This is a prescription drug that the Panel recommended be switched to nonprescription status. It is commonly used for treating feminine itching caused by *Candida albicans* and related yeasts, but has only minimal activity against the molds that cause jock itch, athlete's foot, and ringworm of the body. The FDA did not accept the Panel's recommendation, so nystatin remains a prescription drug.

Phenolates: phenol and phenolate sodium   These coal-tar and benzene derivatives are among the drugs with a characteristically medicinal smell; they have been widely used as antiseptics and disinfectants for over a century. The Antimicrobial I Panel decided that at concentrations above 1.5 percent phenol is dangerous because it is absorbed through both normal and broken skin, and can cause severe internal poisoning, resulting in death (*see* PHENOL). Mild to severe signs of body-system poisoning have been reported following applications of 2 or 3 percent aqueous solutions of phenol to open wounds. So the present Panel concluded there is no rational defense for the continued use of phenol in medications to treat athlete's foot, jock itch, or body ringworm. Also, concentrations of *under* 1.5 percent are likely to be ineffective. The Panel thus rules against the phenolates on grounds both of safety and effectiveness, saying they are not proved safe and are not effective.

Resorcinol   A phenollike compound, resorcinol appears to be more toxic even than phenol (*see* directly above). The one marketed product containing resorcinol that was submitted contains 10 percent of the drug: the Panel considered this level in excess of what might be needed to achieve treatment goals. Worse, evaluators could find no well-conducted clinical studies demonstrating that the drug really works against athlete's foot, jock itch, ringworm of the body, or any other superficial fungus—whether at low dose or high. So the Panel says that resorcinol's effectiveness has not been proved and that lack of safety is a matter of record. Conclusion: not safe.

Tannic acid   Although this substance has been shown to be a potent liver poison, it reacts quickly with surface protein when applied to the skin. So little if any is likely to be absorbed unchanged into the body. The Panel, therefore, regards it as safe. But, because the Panel knows of no studies demonstrating that tannic acid has an antifungal property, it says: not effective.

Thymol   Thymol is irritating to the skin, so the Panel is not convinced of its safety. Does it work? The one controlled study done indicated that thymol is not effective against athlete's foot.

Tolindate   This drug, currently being tested, is somewhat similar to tolnaftate. But no published data are yet available on it, so the Panel lists it as unsafe and ineffective as an over-the-counter drug until such time as formal application is made and supportive evidence is reviewed through the FDA's regular licensing procedures for new drugs.

Inactive Ingredients

The list that follows includes drying agents and other inactive ingredients used in antifungal preparations to provide bulk, or as bases, solvents, dispersants, or preservatives. Some—because of characteristic smell, for example—are included to create product identification in users' minds.

acetone	cetyl alcohol	diethyl sebacate
alcohol	chlorophyll	dioctyl sodium
anhydrous ethanol	cinnamaldehyde	sulfosuccinate
aromatic oils	compound benzoin	essential oils
bentonite	tincture	eucalyptol
benzyl alcohol	corn starch	glycerin
calcium	dehydrated alcohol	hexadecyl alcohol

isopropyl alcohol
magnesium carbonate
magnesium stearate
methyl salicylate
oil of pine
petrolatum
polyethylene glycol
   400
polyethylene glycol
   4000

polyvinylpyrrolidone
propyl alcohol
   (n-propyl alcohol)
propylene glycol
sodium dioctyl-
   sulfosuccinate
starch
talc (talcum)
tincture benzoin
   compound

trimethyloctadec-
   adienylammonium
   chloride
trimethyloctadec-
   enylammonium
   chloride
wormwood oil
   (wormwood)
zinc oxide
zinc stearate

Safety and Effectiveness: Active Ingredients in Over-the-Counter Medications for Treating Athlete's Foot, Jock-Itch and Ringworm

Active Ingredient	Panel's Assessment
alcloxa (see aluminum preparations)	
aluminum preparations: alcloxa, aluminum sulfate, and potassium alum	safe, but not proved effective
aluminum sulfate (see aluminum preparations)	
basic fuchsin	not proved safe or effective
benzethonium chloride	not proved safe or effective
benzoic acid	safe, but not proved effective
benzoxiquine (see oxyquinolines)	
boron compounds: boric acid and sodium borate (borax)	
under 5%	safe, but not proved effective
over 5%	not safe
boric acid (see boron compounds)	
calcium undecylenate (see undecylenic acid and its salts)	
camphor	not effective
caprylates: sodium caprylate and zinc caprylate	safe, but not proved effective
chlorothymol	not proved safe or effective
chloroxylenol	safe, but not proved effective
coal tar	not safe
copper undecylenate (see undecylenic acid and its salts)	
cresols: m-cresol and secondary amyltricresols	not proved safe or effective
dichlorophen	not proved safe or effective
haloprogin (prescription)	safe and effective
iodochlorhydroxyquin	safe and effective
m-cresol (see cresols)	

Safety and Effectiveness: Active Ingredients in Over-the-Counter Medications for Treating Athlete's Foot, Jock-Itch and Ringworm
(continued)

Active Ingredient	*Panel's Assessment*
menthol	not proved safe and not effective
methylparaben (*see* parabens)	
miconazole nitrate *(prescription)*	safe and effective
oxyquinolines: benzoxiquine, oxyquinoline, and oxyquinoline sulfate	not proved safe or effective
oxyquinoline sulfate (*see* oxyquinolines)	
parabens: methylparaben and propylparaben	not proved safe or effective
phenol (*see* phenolates)	
phenolates: phenol and sodium phenolate	
under 1.5%	not proved safe and not effective
over 1.5%	not safe
phenyl salicylate	not proved safe or effective
potassium alum (*see* aluminum preparations)	
povidone-iodine	safe, but not proved effective
propionic acid and its salts: sodium propionate and zinc propionate	safe, but not proved effective
propylparaben (*see* parabens)	
resorcinol	not safe
salicylic acid (up to 3%)	safe, but not proved effective
secondary amyltricresols (*see* cresols)	
sodium borate (*see* boron compounds)	
sodium caprylate (*see* caprylates)	
sodium phenolate (*see* phenolates)	
sodium propionate (*see* propionic acid and its salts)	
sulfur	safe, but not proved effective
tannic acid	safe, but not effective
thymol	not proved safe and not effective
tolindate	not safe or effective
tolnaftate	safe and effective
triacetin	safe, but not proved effective
undecylenic acid and its salts: calcium undecylenate, copper undecylenate, and zinc undecylenate	safe and effective
zinc caprylate (*see* caprylates)	
zinc propionate (*see* propionic acid and its salts)	
zinc undecylenate (*see* undecylenic acid and its salts)	

Safety and Effectiveness: Combination Products Sold Over-the-Counter to Treat Funguses

---

Safe and Effective

2 or 3 approved antifungals, provided that each is present in the approved dosage, and the combination broadens the antifungal preparation (for example, tolnaftate + nystatin) (no such combination has as yet been approved)

1 to 3 approved antifungals + 1 approved antiperspirant*

1 to 3 approved antifungals + 1 approved skin-peeling agent (salicylic acid)*

Conditionally Safe and Effective

includes any conditionally approved ingredient

contains an approved active ingredient at less than the minimal effective dose

includes an antibacterial agent

Whitefield's ointment (benzoic acid 6 percent + salicylic acid 3 percent in polyethylene glycol)

Unsafe or Ineffective

Contains any active ingredient disapproved by the Panel

Contains 4 or more antifungal active ingredients

Contains any local anesthetic, such as benzocaine

carbol-fuchsin

---

*No such combination has as yet been approved.

Jock Itch, Athlete's Foot, and Ringworm Cures: Product Ratings

Single-Ingredient Products

Product and Distributor	Dosage of Active Ingredient	Rating[1]	Comment
aluminum preparations			
Buro-Sol Powder (Doak)	**powder:** 2.36 g packet produces 1 pint of 1:15 Burow's solution (aluminum acetate solution) + benzethonium chloride	**B**	not proved effective; this preparation not specifically assessed by Panel
Burow's solution (generic)	**liquid:** aluminum acetate solution	**B**	not proved effective; this aluminum salt not specifically assessed by Panel

Jock Itch, Athlete's Foot, and Ringworm Cures: Product Ratings *(continued)*

Single-Ingredient Products

Product and Distributor	Dosage of Active Ingredient	Rating[1]	Comment
chloroxylenol (PCMX)			
Metasep (Marion)	**shampoo:** 2%	**B**	not proved effective
nu-FLOW (CooperCare)		**B**	not proved effective
iodochlorhydroxyquin			
iodochlorhydroxyquin (generic)	**cream** and **ointment:** 3%	**A**	
Torofor (Torch)		**A**	
Vioform (Ciba)		**A**	
povidone-iodine			
Betadine (Purdue-Frederick)	**spray** and **solution:** 10% (approx. 1% available iodine)	**B**	not proved safe or effective
tannic acid			
Amertan (Lilly)	**jelly:** 5%	**B**	not proved effective
tolnaftate			
Aftate (Plough)	**gel:** 1% **powder:** 1% **spray:** 1%	**A**	
Aftate for Jock Itch (Plough)	**gel:** 1% **powder:** 1%	**A**	
Tinactin (Schering)	**cream:** 1% **powder:** 1% **solution:** 1%	**A**	
triacetin			
Enzactin (Ayerst)	**cream:** 250 mg per g	**B**	not proved effective
Fungacetin (Blair)	**ointment:** 25%	**B**	not proved effective
undecylenic acid and its salts			
Cruex (Pharmacraft)	**powder:** 10% calcium undecylenate **powder, aerosol:** 10% calcium undecylenate	**A**	
Desenex (Pharmacraft)	**ointment:** 5% undecylenic acid + 20% zinc undecylenate	**A**	

Jock Itch, Athlete's Foot, and Ringworm Cures: Product Ratings *(continued)*

Single-Ingredient Products

Product and Distributor	Dosage of Active Ingredient	Rating[1]	Comment
Medaped (Spencer-Mead)		**A**	
undecylenic compound (generic)		**A**	
Desenex (Pharmacraft)	**powder:** 2% undecylenic acid + 20% zinc undecylenate	**A**	
	solution: 10% undecylenic acid	**A**	
NP-27 (Norwich-Eaton)	**powder, aerosol:** 20% zinc undecylenate	**A**	
Quinsana Plus (Mennen)	**powder:** 2% undecylenic acid + 20% zinc undecylenate	**A**	
Ting Improved (Pharmacraft)		**A**	

Combination Products

Product and Distributor	Dosage of Active Ingredient	Rating[1]	Comment
Blis-To-Sol (Chattem)	**liquid:** 5% undecylenic acid + .9% salicylic acid + thymol	**C**	less-than-effective concentration of undecylenic acid; thymol not effective
Cruex (Pharmacraft)	**cream:** 20% zinc undecylenate + 3% chloroxylenol	**B**	chloroxylenol not proved effective
Deso-Cream (Columbia Med.)	**cream:** 20% zinc undecylenate + 5% caprylic acid + 2% sodium propionate	**B**	latter two ingredients not proved effective
NP-27 (Norwich-Eaton)	**powder:** 1.5% salicylic acid + benzoic acid + boric acid + propylparaben + dichlorophene + zinc undecylenate + thymol + menthol + chlorothymol	**C**	too many antifungal active ingredients, few of which are safe and effective

Jock Itch, Athlete's Foot, and Ringworm Cures: Product Ratings *(continued)*

Combination Products

Product and Distributor	Dosage of Active Ingredient	Rating[1]	Comment
Sopronol (Wyeth)	**ointment:** sodium propionate + sodium caprylate + zinc caprylate	B	not proved effective
Ting (Pharmacraft)	**powder:** 6.5% benzoic acid + 5% boric acid + zinc oxide	B	neither antifungal proved effective
Whitfield's (generic)	**ointment:** 12% benzoic acid + 6% salicylic acid in anhydrous lanolin and petrolatum	C	disapproved combination at these strengths
Whitsphill (Half Strength) (Torch)	**ointment:** 6% benzoic acid + 3% salicylic acid	B	not proved effective

1. Author's interpretation of Panel criteria. Based on contents, not claims.

Kidney and Bladder Drugs: Preliminary Report

Several nonprescription preparations are marketed for the purpose of relieving kidney or bladder irritation and pain, and also for easing the flow of urine. One drug is also marketed for the treatment of benign prostatic hypertrophy (a nonmalignant enlargement of the prostate gland). However, it is unwise to attempt self-treatment of kidney or bladder conditions without asking a doctor for his or her advice.

The over-the-counter drugs sold for the relief of urinary-tract problems were to have been evaluated by the FDA's Advisory Review Panel on Miscellaneous Internal Drug Products. The Panel was terminated before this task was started. At some point, the FDA or a new Panel may

KIDNEY AND BLADDER DRUGS is based on an FDA status report on the OTC drug review.

undertake the review. In the meantime, the active ingredients in these nonprescription drugs intended for kidney and bladder irritation are merely listed below, without comment.

> benzoic acid
> methenamine
> phenazopyridine hydrochloride
> salicylamide
> sodium salicylate

Laxatives

Constipation is defined by *Dorland's Medical Dictionary* simply as "infrequent or difficult evacuation of the feces." Laxatives are drugs used to relieve this condition. This definition is endorsed by the Panel —which comments that constipation is far less common and needs far less treatment than is often believed: "preoccupation with the bowel seems to be the concern of a significant proportion of our population, judging from the inordinately large number of laxative agents available, and by the significant expenditure for over-the-counter laxatives." The July 5, 1982, issue of *Drug Topics* notes that Americans spend more than a third of a billion dollars yearly for laxatives and other elimination aids.

Panel members believe that there is widespread overuse of laxatives and that the pharmaceutical industry has contributed to the false impression that serious and health-endangering consequences will occur if the bowel is not evacuated daily.

NORMAL BOWEL FUNCTION

Many people believe there is a need for one bowel movement a day. This is a myth.

What is normal bowel function? Reviewers found several recent studies that shed light on this question. In one it was shown that on the average test subjects passed stools each 27 hours and 36 minutes, with a range of 9 hours to 57 hours. In another study, researchers found that

LAXATIVES is based on the report of the FDA's Advisory Review Panel on OTC Laxative, Antidiarrheal, Emetic, and Antiemetic Drug Products.

99 percent of adults fall within a range from 3 bowel movements per day down to 3 bowel movements per week. The Panel believes this is the normal range. So unless one is having fewer than 3 bowel movements weekly—or more than 3 each day—experts see no need for medications that either increase or decrease their number.

CONSTIPATION

Most often constipation is caused by poor diet—particularly inadequate intake of dietary fiber or too little water and other fluids. Lack of exercise can also slow the bowels. Traveling, with the need to use unfamiliar toilets, inhibits some people from defecating—and constipation may result.

The cure in these instances is fairly obvious: more roughage in the diet; more water and other beverages; exercise; a prompt response to the urge to defecate when it is first felt.

The use of laxatives should be, at most, a temporary measure. They should not be used on a regular basis, nor should they be used for any extended period of time. Experts say there are few reasons to take laxatives for more than a week, unless one is directed to do so by a physician.

Prolonged use of laxatives can seriously impair normal bowel function: people can become dependent on laxatives. Serious consequences also may follow if laxatives are used when one has a stomach ache, nausea and vomiting, or gastrointestinal symptoms related to conditions other than simple constipation. Any sudden change in bowel habits that persists for 2 weeks should prompt one to consult a doctor—*not* to reach for a laxative. The cause could be the onset of a serious disease.

TYPES OF LAXATIVES

Several words are used to describe drugs that evacuate the bowels. Cathartics and purgatives are strong; they act rapidly to soften the stool or evacuate the bowel and should be used only under a doctor's supervision. Laxatives are supposed to be milder and act less precipitously—though a large dose may have a cathartic effect.

There are several different kinds of laxatives, and they are grouped by drug action.

- *Bulk-forming laxatives* promote evacuation by increasing the stools' bulk volume and water content.

- *Stimulant laxatives* act directly on the intestinal wall to promote peristalsis (waves of muscular contraction that result in defecation).
- *Saline laxatives* draw water into the bowel, promoting movement.
- *Hyperosmotic laxatives* increase the water content of the stool.
- *Stool-softener laxatives* penetrate and soften the stool.
- *Lubricant laxatives* make the intestinal tract and fecal matter more slippery.

The safety and effectiveness chart at the end of this unit indicates which of these categories each laxative active ingredient belongs in and records the Panel's assessment of each ingredient's safety and effectiveness.

Before choosing a laxative, it would be well for the person who believes he is constipated to ask himself if he is trying to achieve an unnecessary regularity in bowel movements. He then should ask himself *what* the problem is—for example, too few bowel movements over a week's time or difficulty in passing a well-formed stool. Then he can select a product which contains an active ingredient that can relieve the specific complaint. The reviewers add one more guide: "The smallest dose of a laxative that is effective is the optimal dose to use."

The Panel found no evidence that any particular type of laxative is particularly advantageous for any set group of people (e.g., older persons, younger ones, men, women). There is one exception: persons whose diets are low in fiber content may benefit from using bulk-forming laxatives.

CLAIMS

Accurate
"laxative [for the] short-term relief of constipation"

The label should also state the product's mode of action. A bulk-forming laxative, for example, should say that it promotes the evacuation of the bowel by increasing bulk volume and water content of the stools.

False or Misleading
"improves well-being" or "promotes good health"
references to "irregularity" (*regularity* is not required for health)
labeling that mentions "natural" or "acts naturally" (a reader might infer that it is a natural thing to do to take these laxatives, an idea evaluators sharply reject)

Combination Products

The fewer active ingredients there are in any over-the-counter medicine, the better. For laxatives, which can waste body fluids and salt and cause cramping and loss of normal bowel function, the least-is-best rule is particularly appropriate.

Reviewers were stymied by a lack of data on the minimal effective doses for most laxative ingredients. In formulating its policy for combination products, the Panel therefore stipulated that each active ingredient be present in an amount *no lower* than the minimal approved dose when the ingredient is used alone. By the same token, there should be *no more* of each ingredient than the maximal approved dose when it is used alone. But these standards would still allow a consumer to take a combined dose that had almost twice the maximal laxative effect of either of 2 ingredients used by itself. To prevent this, the evaluators proposed a formula ensuring that no combination delivers more than 100 percent of a maximal effective dose. This formula is found at the end of the SAFETY AND EFFECTIVENESS: COMBINATION PRODUCTS chart at the end of this unit.

No more than 2 active ingredients are approved in a combination product, and any combination of laxative active ingredients with active ingredients from another drug class also is disapproved. Particularly frowned upon are combinations of laxatives with bismuth subnitrate, capsicum, caroid-papain, ginger, ipecac powder, thiamine, multivitamin preparations, or minerals. Small amounts of nonlaxative ingredients may be present as inactive substances that improve a product's taste or for other pharmacological reasons—but no medicinal claims may be made for them.

BULK-FORMING LAXATIVES

This kind of laxative increases the bulk volume and the water content of stools, which softens them and makes them easier to evacuate. Such preparations are available as a dietary substance, bran, or in medicinal form. Experts view them as one of the safest types of laxative.

Users should always drink an 8-ounce glass of water when taking a bulk-forming laxative. This provides the liquid that the active ingredient needs to soften and expand the stools. The water also guards against the rare possibility that the laxative might become impacted in the digestive tract.

WARNING   Bulk-forming laxatives may interact or combine with other drugs, inhibiting their absorption from the gut. People should not use these laxatives if they are taking aspirin or prescription drugs—particularly if one of them is digitalis or nitrofurantoin.

Approved Active Ingredients

Bran, dietary   Whole-wheat bread, which contains 1 to 2 grams of bran per slice, and bran-rich breakfast cereals, which contain from 2.7 to 6.5 grams per 100 grams of bran flakes, are convenient sources of dietary crude fiber—the beneficial component of bran. This bran is usually obtained from the milling of wheat, though it may come from other grains and plant foods.

Bran acts by attracting water into the stool. It also acts—through mechanisms that remain unclear—directly on the large intestine to prompt it to void its contents.

Reviewers say that 6 to 14 grams of bran—a quarter to half an ounce—each day is safe and effective for laxation. This approval applies to dietary bran, but not to bran tablets (*see* BRAN TABLETS, page 501.)

Cellulose derivatives: methylcellulose and carboxymethylcellulose sodium   These substances are safe and effective in the amounts usually ingested: 4 to 6 grams daily for adults, or 1 to 1.5 grams daily for children over 6. One must drink water when taking this laxative.

The water is absorbed by the cellulose to form a syrupy liquid. When it reaches the colon, some of the fluid is lost, which causes the remaining cellulose and water to form a gel that increases the bulk of the stool and promotes its evacuation.

Karaya (sterculia gum)   A vegetable gum, karaya gum is indigestible, but it does absorb water. It has little effect on the body as a whole, but some people may be allergic to the gum.

The safe and effective dose is 5 to 10 grams daily. Water must be drunk *immediately* after taking karaya in order to avoid the risk of bowel obstruction.

Malt soup extract   This is a powder prepared from partially germinated barley grains. It contains 73 percent maltose, 7 percent protein, and 1.5 percent potassium, plus lesser amounts of calcium and other minerals. The Panel classifies malt soup as a bulk-forming laxative but maintains that it appears to have other laxative actions as well—a matter that merits further study. Malt soup makes the gut acid, but it is not clear how this might promote evacuation. There is no proof that malt soup extract relieves anal itching, as has been claimed.

The safe and effective dosage for adults is 12 to 64 grams daily with water; for infants under 2, it is 6 to 32 grams daily with water.

Polycarbophil Of all the bulk-forming ingredients, polycarbophil absorbs the most liquid: it can bind and absorb 60 times its weight in water. It holds water and other fluids in the stool and in the hollow inside of the colon. In tests, polycarbophil held 120 cubic centimeters of digestive juices per gram of polycarbophil, compared with 36 for methylcellulose, 30 for psyllium preparations, and 14 for agar. Tests in animals indicate that polycarbophil is nontoxic and that it has no undue effects on nutritional status, digestive enzymes, or digestion itself. Tests in humans confirm the substance's safety and effectiveness.

The dose for adults is 4 to 6 grams per day; for children 6 to 12, 1.5 to 3 grams per day; for children 2 through 5, 1 to 1.5 grams per day; and for children under 2, 0.5 to 1 gram per day. One should drink a full glass of water with each dose.

Psyllium preparations: plantago ovata husks, plantago seed, psyllium (hemicellulose), psyllium hydrophilic mucilloid (psyllium hydrocolloid), psyllium seed, psyllium seed (blond), and psyllium seed husks These substances are widely used derivatives of the seeds and husks of plants from the plantain family. An indigestible hemicellulose in these seeds and husks binds and holds water. Some psyllium preparations may cause color changes in the kidney tubules. Other—apparently harmless—biologic changes also have been discovered in humans and in animals dosed with these medications. But evaluators concluded these side effects are minor and that more serious ones—like obstruction of the esophagus or intestines—are too rare to preclude approval.

So psyllium preparations are judged to be both safe and effective in the amounts usually taken orally, with water. Dosage ranges from 2.5 to 30 grams per day for adults and 1.25 to 15 grams per day for children over 6.

Conditionally Approved Active Ingredients

Agar This is a dried, water-absorbing substance obtained from red algae. It is rich in indigestible cellulose and will absorb at least 5 times its weight in water. It probably adds to the bulk of the stool.

Agar is present in many proprietary laxatives. While evaluators judged it safe, its effectiveness—when used alone or with other laxative ingredients—remains to be proved.

Bran tablets While dietary bran is safe and effective as a bulk-forming laxative (*see* BRAN, DIETARY, page 500), there is insufficient evidence to show that pressed and granulated bran tablets are as effective, even though they have been shown to be safe.

Carrageenan, native   Also called *Chondrus crispus* and Irish moss, this is a red seaweed used in ice cream and other foods to stabilize and smoothly bind other ingredients together. It appears to be safe in commonly used laxative dosages—up to 3.5 grams per day—but definitive evidence of its effectiveness is lacking.

Guar gum   This substance is judged to be safe, principally because it is widely used in cheese, salad dressing, and other food products. However, there is no convincing evidence that guar gum effectively promotes defecation in animals or in people.

Disapproved Active Ingredients

None

STIMULANT LAXATIVES

Here the Panel's principal message is: *caution*. These laxatives act directly on the walls of the large intestine, small intestine, or both. They stimulate the slow, wavelike intestinal contractions (peristalsis) that move fecal matter along toward excretion. Some stimulant laxatives may act by irritating the intestinal wall. Others may act by stimulating the nerves that start peristalsis. These pathways of action are as yet not clearly established.

What is clear is that stimulant laxatives can be hard on the user. As the *Handbook of Nonprescription Drugs* (6th ed.) 1979, a guidebook for pharmacists, warns: "All stimulant laxatives produce griping [severe spasmodic bowel pain], increased mucus secretion, and, in some people, excessive evacuation of fluid."

Reviewers warn that stimulant laxatives should be used only on occasion, that they should not be used daily for more than a week (except on the advice of a physician), and that overdosage or persistent use can produce serious side effects. These include a dependence on the laxative that inhibits or blocks a person's ability to move his or her bowels without use of the drug. Body fluids and essential body salts (electrolytes) may also be depleted.

The Panel assessed a number of stimulant laxatives and found many of them safe and effective as long as one keeps in mind the specific limitations cited above.

Approved Active Ingredients

Anthraquinones: aloe, cascara sagrada preparations, danthron, and senna preparations Except for danthron, which is synthetic, these substances where the Panel lists as safe and effective are plant derivatives. The anthraquinones act mainly in the large intestine, but the precise mechanism(s) through which they stimulate bowel movements is not known. They all may discolor the urine, turning acid urine yellowish-brown and alkaline urine reddish-violet—effects that are considered harmless. The senna products are more potent than cascara, according to the authorities, and they may cause greater abdominal discomfort.

Approved Daily Dosage of Laxatives Containing Anthraquinones

Anthraquinone Ingredient	Usual Doses	
	Adults	Children
aloe	120 to 250 mg	under 6: not recommended ages 6–8: 40 to 80 mg ages 8–15: 80 to 120 mg
cascara sagrada preparations aromatic cascara fluid extract	2 to 6 ml	under age 2: 1 to 2 ml ages 2–12: 1 to 3 ml
casanthranol	30 to 90 mg	under age 2: 7 to 22 mg ages 2–12: 15 to 45 mg
cascara sagrada bark	300 mg to 1 gram	under age 2: 75 to 250 mg ages 2–12: 150 to 500 mg
cascara sagrada extract	200 to 400 mg	under age 2: 50 to 100 mg ages 2–12: 100 to 200 mg
cascara sagrada fluid extract	0.5 to 1.5 ml	under age 2: 0.12 to 0.37 ml ages 2–12: 0.25 to 0.75 ml
danthron	75 to 150 mg	under 12: not recommended
senna preparations (single dose) senna fluid extract	2 ml	infants: 250 mg ages 1–5: 500 mg ages 6–12: 1 ml
senna fruit extract	3.4 to 4 grams	infants: 425 to 500 mg ages 1–5: 850 mg to 1 gram ages 6–12: 1.7 to 2 grams

Approved Daily Dosage of Laxatives Containing Anthraquinones *(continued)*

Anthraquinone Ingredient	Usual Doses		
	Adults	Children	
senna leaf powder	500 mg to 2 grams	infants: ages 1–5: ages 6–12:	62 to 250 mg 125 to 500 mg 250 mg to 1 gram
senna pod concentrate (1 to 4 times daily)	600 mg to 1 gram	infants: ages 1–5: ages 6–12:	75 to 250 mg 150 to 250 mg 300 to 500 mg
senna syrup	8 ml	infants: ages 1–5: ages 6–12:	1 ml 2 ml 4 ml
sennosides A and B crystalline	12 to 36 mg	infants: ages 1–5: ages 6–12:	1 to 4 mg 3 to 9 mg 6 to 18 mg

Bisacodyl   This substance—which can be taken orally or inserted intrarectally in a suppository—produces brief but very strong evacuatory movements in the large intestine. When the drug is applied intrarectally, this action occurs within 15 minutes to an hour. Bisacodyl appears to act on the mucous membranes or underlying nerves, but it may also cause water to be secreted into the bowel or be held there.

Although bisacodyl is a very effective laxative, it may be risky to use: excessive use or overdosage can lead to severe diarrhea and the loss of vital body fluids and body salts. Muscle weakness and tremor may result. It can cause abdominal discomfort, faintness, rectal burning, and mild cramps. When given orally, bisacodyl must be swallowed, not chewed, and people who cannot swallow the tablet whole should not take the drug in its oral form. However, the drug was assessed as safe when taken in oral doses of 5 to 15 mg daily for adults or 5 mg for children over 3. Suppository dosage is generally 10 mg for adult use and 5 mg for children under 2. When used judiciously, bisacodyl can be safe as well as effective.

Castor oil   A traditional plant remedy, castor oil more than meets modern standards: one dose of 15 to 60 ml (less for children) will completely clear out the lower bowel. The dose for children is 5 to 15 ml, which is 1 to 3 teaspoonsful of the unpleasant-tasting oil (for infants under 2, it is 1 to 5 ml).

Castor oil's laxative effect comes from ricinoleic acid, a substance that is not produced until the oil reaches the small intestine. There the castor oil is broken down by a pancreatic enzyme called *lipase*. Exactly how the acid product acts to evacuate the bowel remains unclear; what is known is that the colon secretes both water and electrolytes in response to its presence.

While safe and effective in appropriate doses, continued use of castor oil can result in excessive—and dangerous—loss of water and essential body salts. So evaluators warn against overuse.

Dehydrocholic acid   This substance is derived from cholic acid, a natural bile acid. Its presence markedly increases the water content of bile, which is a mixture of digestive juices. How this helps evacuate the stool is not known for sure; the dehydrocholic acid may stimulate the secretion of sodium bicarbonate and water from the colon, or inhibit their absorption by it. Dehydrocholic acid does not relieve "indigestion," "excessive belching," or the "sensation of abdominal fullness," as has been claimed. But tests in animals, as well as in humans, show that it is quite nontoxic. It was judged safe and effective at doses of 750 to 900 mg per day, but it should not be used by children under 12.

Phenolphthalein, white or yellow   These compounds act in the colon, and possibly the small intestine. They apparently prevent water and salt from being reabsorbed from the gut into the body. Yellow phenolphthalein is claimed to be more potent than white. These substances may temporarily turn the urine pink. More seriously, they can lead to excessive laxation and a loss of body salts. So they should be used only occasionally, and should not be given to children under 2.

Nevertheless, the compounds were judged safe and effective when used infrequently by adults and older children, and in the correct amounts. Dosages are 30 to 270 mg per day for adults, 30 to 60 mg for children 6 to 12, and 15 to 20 mg for children 2 through 5.

Conditionally Approved Active Ingredients

Aloin   This microcrystalline powder, derived from the plant aloe, is usually mixed with other ingredients such as phenolphthalein or cascara sagrada. But there are insufficient data to prove that it is either safe or effective.

Bile salts, bile acids, and ox bile   These natural bile acids will stimulate diarrhea when taken in large doses. But because only small amounts are present in laxative products, it remains to be proved that these preparations are effective. Safety, too, needs to be established.

d-Calcium pantothenate   Found naturally in the body, this substance serves a number of important metabolic functions. The Panel says it is safe, but there is virtually no evidence that it works as a laxative.

Frangula   This is the dried bark of the tree *Rhamnus frangula*, which contains a chemical similar to the anthraquinones in aloe, cascara sagrada, and senna. Reviewers could not determine a standard dose, nor could they find studies to show frangula is effective or safe for laxation.

Prune concentrate dehydrate and prune powder   While prunes are a widely accepted home remedy for constipation—although *why* they offer relief is unknown—prune preparations labeled as drugs must prove their worth by meeting certain scientific standards. Such studies are lacking. So while the Panel considers these preparations safe, it says they are not proved effective.

Rhubarb, Chinese   This plant contains chemicals that are related to active laxative ingredients found in aloe, cascara sagrada, and senna. It also contains astringent substances that may pucker the rectal mucosa in much the same way that eating rhubarb puckers the mouth. Whether and how this stimulates bowel movements and whether it does so safely have yet to be proved.

Sodium oleate   This substance is apparently safe. But reviewers could find only one animal study on effectiveness and those results suggest that, in fact, sodium oleate is *not* effective for laxative use. So approval remains conditional.

Disapproved Active Ingredients

Several ingredients—which for the most part no longer are used as laxatives—were assessed as unsafe and/or ineffective. They are:

Calomel (mercurous chloride)   Calomel is unreliable as a laxative. What is worse, it can be unsafe. If it fails to evacuate the bowel promptly, the mercury it contains can build up in the intestine. In the presence of bile and other intestinal substances, this chemical may be converted to a form that is absorbed into the body. In this manner it becomes a toxic substance, and there are reports in the medical literature of people dying of mercury poisoning after chronic use of calomel laxatives. In infants, calomel can cause a severe, feverish disorder called *pink disease*. Verdict: unsafe.

Carrageenan, degraded   This semiprocessed seaweed, which also is known by the botanic names *Chondrus crispus* and *Irish moss*, is much more readily absorbed into the body from the gut than is the native or unprocessed form of carrageenan (*see* CARRAGEENAN, NA-TIVE, page 502). It may remain in the body for a significant period of time, inhibiting normal digestion and also causing a variety of other untoward effects. Thus, evaluators ranked it as unsafe.

Podophyllum resin Also called *podophyllin*, this substance is extremely irritating to skin and mucosal surfaces. It can cause systemic toxicity and may damage an unborn baby if taken by pregnant women. Verdict: not safe.

Other laxative resins: colocynth, elaterin, gamboge, ipomea, and jalap These plant resins, which fortunately are no longer widely used, are profoundly irritating to the intestines and can cause severe spasmodic pain. They may yield watery, blood-tinged stools. Overdosage can lead to severe prostration and other uncomfortable side effects. They have not been well studied as laxative ingredients; the Panel judged all of them to be unsafe.

SALINE LAXATIVES

Saline refers to salt. Saline laxatives—magnesium, phosphate, and tartar salts—were long believed to pull water into the gut by the membrane-penetrating process of osmosis. They may indeed work this way, but investigators believe other, as yet not understood, mechanisms may also be involved. Since serious loss of normal body salts can result from use of saline laxatives, these substances should be taken only occasionally.

Approved Active Ingredients

Magnesium salts: magnesium citrate, magnesium hydroxide (milk of magnesia), and magnesium sulfate These magnesium salts draw water into the gut by osmosis—just as salt water will draw plain water through a semipermeable membrane. But these compounds appear to act through at least one other route as well: they stimulate the release of a hormone called *CCK-PZ* into the gut. This action stimulates motor and secretory activity that may help move stubborn stools along.

(Magnesium hydroxide acts as an antacid. But its ability to neutralize acid in no way contributes to its value as a laxative; acid secretion and constipation are not related.)

The Panel cites no instances of untoward effects in users of these laxatives when taken as recommended and says they are safe and effective. But it indicates that persons with kidney disease should check label warnings, as should persons who need to limit their intake of salt.

Approved Daily Dosages of Laxatives Containing Magnesium

	Daily Dosage*		
Age	Magnesium Citrate	Magnesium Hydroxide	Magnesium Sulfate
Adults	11–18 grams	2.4–4.8 grams	10–30 grams
Children 6–11	5–10 grams	1.2–2.4 grams	5–10 grams
Children 2–5	2.5–5 grams	0.4–1.2 grams	2.5–5 grams

*Daily dosages given should be divided into 2 or 3 individual doses to be taken at different times during the day.

Phosphate salts: disodium phosphate, monosodium phosphate, sodium biphosphate, and sodium phosphate As with the compounds described immediately above, these substances draw water into the gut. They tend to be fast-acting.

Persons with kidney disease should avoid these laxatives, except when use is approved by a doctor. Also, products that contain phosphate salts should not be given orally to children under 6, or in suppositories to children under 2, except on a doctor's orders. Used with these precautions in mind, and taken as recommended, these phosphate-salt laxative ingredients are judged to be safe and effective.

Approved Daily Dosages of Laxatives Containing Phosphate Salts

	Daily Dosage		
Age	Disodium Phosphate	Monosodium Phosphate	Sodium Biphosphate
Adult			
oral	1.9–3.8 grams	8.3–16.6 grams	9.6–19.2 grams
rectal	3.8 grams	16.6 grams	19.2 grams
Children 10–12			
oral	½ adult dose	½ adult dose	½ adult dose
rectal	1.9 grams	8.3 grams	9.6 grams
Children 5–9*			
oral	¼ adult dose	¼ adult dose	¼ adult dose
rectal	1.9 grams	8.3 grams	9.6 grams

*Products containing these phosphates should not be given orally to children under 6 or in suppositories to children under 2, except on a doctor's orders.

Conditionally Approved Active Ingredients

Tartaric acid and tartrate preparations   These compounds are absorbed only slowly into the body, so they tend to attract and hold water in the gut. These substances have not been carefully studied as laxatives and their precise disposition, once swallowed, is not known. Neither the safety nor the effectiveness of using tartaric acid or other tartrate preparations has as yet been established.

Disapproved Active Ingredients

None

HYPEROSMOTIC LAXATIVES

A hyperosmotic laxative attracts water into the stool. It thus acts in much the same way as the saline laxatives—with the clear difference that it is less likely to cause serious imbalances in body salts, and so is likely to be safer. These laxatives are approved for *intrarectal* administration only.

Approved Active Ingredients

Glycerin   This clear, syrupy substance will attract and hold large amounts of water. So it may act by bringing water into the large intestine where it can soften hardened fecal matter. Glycerin also may irritate the rectal mucosa, promoting defecation. A third laxative action also may occur: glycerin's water-absorbing activity may dry the rectal mucosa, which in turn stimulates defecation by a reflex action. For whichever one—or more—of these reasons, a glycerin rectal suppository usually promotes defecation within half an hour in adults and in children. The side effects tend to be minimal, but may include rectal discomfort, burning, and spasmodic bowel pain or stomach cramps. Some rectal bleeding or discharge also may occur.

Glycerin has been administered orally to promote defecation. Evaluators say that the amounts needed to produce this effect could be toxic, so oral usage is disapproved.

When administered intrarectally, however, glycerin is safe and effective for adults and children over 6, in dosages of 3 grams per suppository or 5 to 15 milliliters in an enema. For children under 6, the dosage is 1 to 1.5 grams in suppository form or 2 to 5 ml in an enema.

Sorbitol   An alcohol derived from sugar, sorbitol is effective as a laxative when given either orally or intrarectally. But the Panel says the effective oral dose is too large to be considered a safe medication without prescription, so only rectal use is approved. Administered this way, sorbitol appears to produce similar—but less troublesome—side effects than glycerin. Sorbitol should be used only occasionally. The safe and effective dose for adults is 120 ml as a 25 to 30 percent solution; for children 2 and over, it is 30 to 60 ml in the same percent solution.

Conditionally Approved Active Ingredients

None

Disapproved Active Ingredients

None

STOOL SOFTENERS

The active ingredients characterized by the Panel as stool-softener laxatives may be particularly helpful when the stools are hard and dry, or when hemorrhoids or other anorectal disorders make it difficult to pass a solid stool. Stool softeners should be used only occasionally, and not for longer than a week on a daily basis. This precaution must be observed because these substances can interfere with the absorption of vitamins and other nutrients into the body. If relief is not obtained within a week, experts say, one should consult a physician.

The Panel assessed 4 stool softeners from 2 groups of drugs; 3 were approved.

Approved Active Ingredients

All 3 safe and effective stool-softening agents belong to a single group of drugs, the sulfosuccinates, which were assessed together.

Sulfosuccinate preparations: dioctyl calcium sulfosuccinate, dioctyl potassium sulfosuccinate, and dioctyl sodium sulfosuccinate It is not clear how these compounds soften the stool. It appears that they have a detergent action, according to reviewers. In other words, they lower surface tension at interfaces between oil and water. In that way more oil and more water are absorbed from the gut into the fecal matter—which softens it. One or more of these substances also may stimulate the secretion of water and body salts into the colon. This would also soften the stool. By whichever means they work, these substances are effective, as has been demonstrated by published scientific reports.

Few side effects have been attributed to sulfosuccinate laxatives. They appear to be partially absorbed from the gut into the body—with unknown consequences. This action could enhance the absorption of mineral oil, a common lubricant laxative. Since mineral oil may be quite toxic if it escapes the gut, evaluators warn that it should *never* be used at the same time one is taking a sulfosuccinate. The Panel urges that these laxatives be used only in the smallest possible amounts, and their use limited to brief periods.

Approved Daily Dosages of Laxatives Containing Sulfosuccinates

Age	Dioctyl Calcium Sulfosuccinate oral use only	Dioctyl Potassium Sulfosuccinate rectal use only	Dioctyl Sodium Sulfosuccinate oral use only
Adults	50–360 mg	50–250 mg	50–360 mg
Children 2–11	50–150 mg	100 mg	50 mg
Children under 2	25 mg		20 mg

Conditionally Approved Active Ingredients

Poloxalkol   Also called polykol, this substance is a relatively taste-less surface-acting agent like the sulfosuccinates described immediately above. Evaluators ranked it as safe, but studies demonstrating its effectiveness in relieving simple constipation are inadequate. It also acts slowly, possibly taking several days to soften the stool. So poloxalkol's effectiveness remains to be proved.

Disapproved Active Ingredients

None

LUBRICANT LAXATIVES

The time-honored intestinal lubricant is mineral oil, which may be taken orally or inserted into the rectum. The Panel assessed and approved 2 forms of mineral oil lubricants.

Mineral oil and mineral-oil emulsion   These compounds are widely used to facilitate bowel evacuation, and are safe and effective if properly used. Mineral oil is a clear, tasteless, petroleum byproduct that smoothes the intestinal tract and softens and lubricates fecal material. It is not irritating, is not absorbed from the gut, and is not broken down by gastrointestinal enzymes. So it is quite safe, though it may impair absorption of vitamins and other necessary nutrients. Consequently, mineral oil should be taken orally only at bedtime. Mineral-oil emulsion can be taken upon awakening and at bedtime. Neither form should be used daily for more than a week and mineral oil should never be used if one is taking a sulfosuccinate (*see* above).

When mineral oil is emulsified, magnesium hydroxide or some other compound is added that breaks it into smaller droplets. This appears to enhance the oil's penetration into the fecal mass.

Persistent use of mineral oil can lead to leakage of fecal material between bowel movements and to skin reactions. Except under medical supervision, it should not be taken orally by children under 6, or by pregnant women, or by persons who have difficulty swallowing. These restrictions do not apply to intrarectal use of mineral oil, which is safer in the sense that when taken this way it cannot affect digestion or nutrient uptake. Neither can it get into the lungs and cause trouble as it might when swallowed.

Safe and Effective Dosages of Mineral Oil

Age	Mineral Oil Administered Orally*	Mineral Oil Administered Intrarectally*	Emulsified Mineral Oil Administered Orally†
Adults	15–45 ml	120 ml	15–45 ml
Children over 6	10–15 ml	60 ml	0.25 to 5 ml

*Once daily.
†Twice daily.

MISCELLANEOUS LAXATIVES

The Panel assessed an oral laxative that does not fall under the categories above. Approved as safe and effective, the substance is described immediately below.

The combination of sodium biphosphate anhydrous + sodium acid pyrophosphate + sodium bicarbonate This preparation is formulated as a rectal suppository. When wetted, then inserted into the rectum, the solid ingredients react with the water; this gives off carbon dioxide gas in an amount of about 230 ml. The expanding gas gently increases pressure inside the rectum and the enhanced sense of fullness in turn promotes a bowel movement.

These suppositories are safe and effective when used once daily. They should not be used in children under 12. The approved preparations contain 1.2 to 1.5 grams sodium biphosphate anhydrous, 0.04 to 0.05 gram sodium acid pyrophosphate, and 1 to 1.5 grams sodium bicarbonate. The suppositories should not be lubricated with mineral oil or petrolatum before insertion, as these greasy substances may retard the release of gas.

Safety and Effectiveness: Active Ingredients in Over-the-Counter Laxatives

Active Ingredient	Type of Laxative	Panel's Assessment
agar	bulk-forming	safe, but not proved effective
aloe	stimulant	safe and effective
aloin	stimulant	not proved safe or effective
bile salts and acids	stimulant	not proved safe or effective
bisacodyl	stimulant	safe and effective
bran, dietary	bulk-forming	safe and effective
bran tablets	bulk-forming	safe, but not proved effective
calomel (mercurous chloride)	stimulant	not safe
carboxymethylcellulose sodium	bulk-forming	safe and effective
carrageenan, degraded	stimulant	not safe
carrageenan, native	bulk-forming	safe, but not proved effective
cascara sagrada preparations		
aromatic cascara fluid extract	stimulant	safe and effective
casanthranol	stimulant	safe and effective
cascara sagrada bark	stimulant	safe and effective
cascara sagrada extract	stimulant	safe and effective
cascara sagrada fluid extract	stimulant	safe and effective
castor oil	stimulant	safe and effective
colocynth	stimulant	not safe
danthron	stimulant	safe and effective
d-calcium pantothentate	stimulant	safe, but not proved effective
dehydrocholic acid	stimulant	safe and effective
elaterin	stimulant	not safe
frangula	stimulant	not proved safe or effective
gamboge	stimulant	not safe
glycerin	hyperosmotic	safe and effective
guar gum	bulk-forming	safe, but not proved effective
ipomea	stimulant	not safe
jalap	stimulant	not safe
karaya (sterculia gum)	bulk-forming	safe and effective
magnesium citrate	saline	safe and effective
magnesium hydroxide	saline	safe and effective

Safety and Effectiveness: Active Ingredients in Over-the-Counter Laxatives
(continued)

Active Ingredient	Type of Laxative	Panel's Assessment
magnesium sulfate	saline	safe and effective
malt soup extract	bulk-forming	safe and effective
methylcellulose	bulk-forming	safe and effective
mineral oil	lubricant	safe and effective
mineral-oil, emulsified	lubricant	safe and effective
ox bile	stimulant	not proved safe or effective
phenolphthalein, white	stimulant	safe and effective
phenolphthalein, yellow	stimulant	safe and effective
phosphate preparations		
disodium phosphate	saline	safe and effective
monosodium phosphate	saline	safe and effective
sodium biphosphate	saline	safe and effective
sodium phosphate	saline	safe and effective
plantago ovata husks	bulk-forming	safe and effective
plantago seed	bulk-forming	safe and effective
podophyllum resin	stimulant	not safe
poloxalkol	stool softener	safe, but not proved effective
polycarbophil	bulk-forming	safe and effective
prune concentrate, dehydrate	stimulant	safe, but not proved effective
prune powder	stimulant	safe, but not proved effective
psyllium, hemicellulose	bulk-forming	safe and effective
psyllium, hydrophilic mucilloid (psyllium hydrocolloid)	bulk-forming	safe and effective
psyllium seed	bulk-forming	safe and effective
psyllium seed, blond	bulk-forming	safe and effective
psyllium seed husks	bulk-forming	safe and effective
released carbon dioxide	miscellaneous	safe and effective
rhubarb, Chinese	stimulant	not proved safe or effective
senna preparations		
senna fluid extract	stimulant	safe and effective
senna fruit extract	stimulant	safe and effective
senna leaf powder	stimulant	safe and effective
senna pod concentrate	stimulant	safe and effective
senna syrup	stimulant	safe and effective
sennosides A and B crystalline	stimulant	safe and effective
sodium oleate	stimulant	safe, but not proved effective
sorbitol	hyperosmotic	safe and effective
sulfosuccinate preparations		
dioctyl calcium sulfosuccinate	stool softener	safe and effective
dioctyl potassium sulfosuccinate	stool softener	safe and effective
dioctyl sodium sulfosuccinate	stool softener	safe and effective
tartaric acid	saline	not proved safe or effective

Safety and Effectiveness: Combination Products Sold Over-the-Counter as Laxatives

Safe and Effective Combinations

An approved amount of any of the following 2 ingredients formulated in such a way that the combined effective dosage range does not exceed 100%.*

Oral Dosage Forms
- dioctyl calcium sulfosuccinate + danthron
- dioctyl sodium sulfosuccinate + casanthranol
- dioctyl sodium sulfosuccinate + danthron
- dioctyl sodium sulfosuccinate + phenolphthalein
- cascara sagrada + aloe
- cascara sagrada + magnesium hydroxide
- cascara sagrada + phenolphthalein
- malt soup extract + psyllium seed, blond
- malt soup extract + psyllium seed husks, blond
- mineral oil + casanthranol
- mineral oil + cascara sagrada
- mineral oil + cascara sagrada fluid extract
- mineral oil, emulsified + magnesium hydroxide
- mineral oil, plain + phenolphthalein
- mineral oil, plain + psyllium seed
- plantago ovata husks + methylcellulose
- psyllium (hemicellulose) + senna concentrate
- senna concentrate + dioctyl sodium sulfosuccinate
- carboxymethycellulose sodium + dioctyl sodium sulfosuccinate

Rectal Dosage Forms
- glycerin + dioctyl potassium sulfosuccinate
- sorbitol + dioctyl potassium sulfosuccinate

Conditionally Safe and Effective Combinations

one or both ingredients are present in less than the minimum approved dosage
one or both ingredients are conditionally approved by the Panel as single active
    laxative ingredients

Unsafe or Ineffective Combinations

contains 3 or more active laxative ingredients
dioctyl sodium sulfosuccinate + mineral oil, plain† (The former may enhance the
    latter's absorption into the body).
contains any disapproved active ingredient
contains the maximum dosage set by the panel for 1 ingredient + more than the
    minimum dosage for the second ingredient
the sum of the percentage amounts of each ingredient exceeds 100%*
the combination contains any laxative active ingredient not reviewed by the Panel

Safety and Effectiveness: Combination Products Sold Over-the-Counter as Laxatives *(continued)*

Unsafe or Ineffective Combinations

the combination contains any nonlaxative active ingredient for which a treatment claim is made   *

*To encourage the use of ingredients in amounts at the minimum end of the dosage range (rather than at the maximum end of the range), the Panel devised a formula to express the sum of the percentage amounts of the effective dosage range (EDR) of each ingredient. The EDR of the 2 ingredients must not exceed 100. In this formula *L max d* is the labeled maximum daily dosage listed in the labeling information for the product, *EDR (min)* is the minimum effective dosage range set by the Panel, and *EDR (max)* is the maximum effective dosage range set by the Panel.

$$\frac{L\ max\ d - EDR\ (min)}{EDR\ (max) - EDR\ (min)} \times 100 = \%\ EDR\ of\ each\ ingredient$$

Laxatives: Product Ratings

Single-Ingredient Products:
Bulk-Forming Laxatives

Product and Distributor	Dosage of Active Ingredients	Rating[1]	Comment
cellulose derivatives, semisynthetic			
Cologel (Lilly)	**liquid:** 450 mg methylcellulose per teaspoonful (5 ml)	A	
Hydrolose (Upjohn)	**syrup:** 985 mg methylcellulose per teaspoonful (5 ml)	A	
malt soup extract			
Maltsupex (Wallace)	**tablets:** 750 mg nondiastatic barley malt extract; also in **powder** and **liquid**	A	
polycarbophil			
Mitrolan (A. H. Robins)	**tablets, chewable:** 500 mg (as calcium polycarbophil)	A	
psyllium preparations			
Hydrocil, Plain (Rowell)	**powder:** 50% psyllium hydrophilic mucilloid	A	
Metamucil (Searle)		A	

Laxatives: Product Ratings *(continued)*

Single-Ingredient Products:
Bulk-Forming Laxatives

Product and Distributor	Dosage of Active Ingredients	Rating[1]	Comment
Reguloid (Rugby)		A	
Syllact (Wallace)		A	
Konsyl (Burton, Parsons)	**powder:** 100% psyllium	A	
Metamucil Instant Mix (Searle)	**powder:** 3.6 g psyllium hydrophilic mucilloid per packet	A	
Mucilose (Winthrop)	**flakes** and **granules:** hemicellulose from psyllium seed	A	
Siblin (Parke-Davis)	**granules:** 2.5 g psyllium seed per rounded teaspoonful	A	

Single-Ingredient Products:
Stimulant Laxatives

Anthraquinones

cascara sagrada

cascara sagrada (generic)	**tablets:** 325 mg	A	
cascara sagrada fluid extract (generic)	**liquid**	A	

danthron

danthron (generic)	**tablets:** 75 mg	A	
Dorbane (3M Personal Care)		A	
Modane (Adria)	**liquid:** 37.5 mg per teaspoonful (5 ml)	A	

senna

Black-Draught (Chattem)	**tablets:** 600 mg senna equivalent	A	
	syrup: 20% senna extract	A	
Senexon (Rugby)	**tablets:** 100 mg standardized senna leaf	A	
Senokot (Purdue Frederick)	**tablets:** 187 mg standardized senna concentrate	A	

Laxatives: Product Ratings *(continued)*

Single-Ingredient Products:
Stimulant Laxatives

Product and Distributor	Dosage of Active Ingredients	Rating[1]	Comment
Senokot (Purdue Frederick)	**granules:** 325 mg standardized senna concentrate per teaspoonful	**A**	
Senolax (Schein)	**tablets:** 217 mg senna extract	**A**	
sennosides A and B, calcium salts of			
Glysennid (Dorsey)	**tablets:** 12 mg	**A**	
Nytilax (Leeming)		**A**	
Other Stimulant Laxatives			
bile salts			
Ox Bile Extract Enseals (Lilly)	**capsules:** 325 mg	**B**	not proved safe or effective
bisacodyl			
bisacodyl (generic)	**tablets:** enteric coated: 5 mg	**A**	
Cenalax (Century)		**A**	
Fleet Bisacodyl (Fleet)		**A**	
bisacodyl (generic)	**suppositories:** 10 mg	**A**	
Bisco-Lax (Raway)		**A**	
Dulcolax (Boehringer Ingelheim)		**A**	
castor oil			
castor oil (generic)	**liquid**	**A**	
Kellogg's Castor Oil (Beecham Products)		**A**	
Emulsoil (Paddock)	**emulsion:** castor oil + emulsifying and flavoring agents	**A**	
Neoloid (Lederle)	**emulsion:** 36.4% + emulsifying agents	**A**	
dehydrocholic acid			
Cholan-DH (Pennwalt)	**tablets:** 250 mg	**A**	
Decholin (Dome)		**A**	

Laxatives: Product Ratings *(continued)*

Single-Ingredient Products:
Stimulant Laxatives

Product and Distributor	Dosage of Active Ingredients	Rating[1]	Comment
Other Stimulant Laxatives			
dehydrocholic acid (generic)		A	
phenolphthalein, yellow and white			
Evac-U-Gen (Walker)	**tablets, chewable:** 97.2 mg yellow	A	
Ex-Lax (Ex-Lax Pharm.)	**tablets, chewable:** 90 mg yellow	A	
	pills: 90 mg yellow	A	
Feen-a-Mint (Plough)	**mints:** 97.2 mg yellow	A	
Phenolax (Upjohn)	**wafers:** 64.8 mg	A	
Prulet Liquitab (Mission)	**tablets, chewable:** 60 mg white	A	

Single-Ingredient Products:
Saline Laxatives

Product and Distributor	Dosage of Active Ingredients	Rating[1]	Comment
magnesium salts			
citrate of magnesia (generic)	**liquid**	A	
Citroma (CMC)		A	
magnesium sulfate (generic)	**powder**	A	
milk of magnesia (generic)	**liquid:** magnesium hydroxide	A	
Milk of Magnesia— Concentrated (Philips Roxane)	**liquid:** magnesium hydroxide	A	
phosphate salts			
Phospho-Soda (Fleet)	**solution:** 18 g sodium phosphate + 48 g sodium biphosphate per 100 ml	A	
Sal-Hepatica (Bristol-Myers)	**granules, effervescent:** monosodium phosphate	A	

Laxatives: Product Ratings *(continued)*

Single-Ingredient Products:
Saline Laxatives

Product and Distributor	Dosage of Active Ingredients	Rating[1]	Comment
sodium phosphate (generic)	**powder**	**A**	

Single-Ingredient Products:
Hyperosmotic Laxatives

Product and Distributor	Dosage of Active Ingredients	Rating[1]	Comment
glycerin			
Fleet Babylax (Fleet)	**liquid:** 4 ml per applicator	**A**	
glycerin, USP (generic)	**suppositories**	**A**	
Glycerin (Squibb)		**A**	

Single-Ingredient Products:
Stool-Softeners

Product and Distributor	Dosage of Active Ingredients	Rating[1]	Comment
dioctyl calcium sulfosuccinate (docusate calcium)			
Surfak (Hoechst-Roussel)	**capsules:** 50 mg	**A**	
dioctyl potassium sulfosuccinate (docusate potassium)			
Dialose (Stuart)	**capsules:** 100 mg	**C**	not approved by Panel for oral use
Kasof (Stuart)	**capsules:** 240 mg	**C**	not approved by Panel for oral use
dioctyl sodium sulfosuccinate (docusate sodium, or DSS)			
Colace (Mead Johnson)	**drops:** 50 mg per teaspoonful	**A**	
	syrup: 20 mg per teaspoonful	**A**	

Laxatives: Product Ratings *(continued)*

Single-Ingredient Products:
Stool-Softeners

Product and Distributor	Dosage of Active Ingredients	Rating[1]	Comment
DioMedicone (Medicone)	**tablets:** 50 mg	A	
docusate sodium (generic)	**capsules:** 50 mg	A	
Colace (Mead Johnson)		A	
docusate sodium (generic)	**syrup:** 50 mg per tablespoonful (15 ml)	A	
docusate sodium (generic)	**capsules:** 100 mg	A	
Afko-Lube (American Pharmaceutical)		A	
D-S-S (Parke-Davis)		A	
Laxinate 100 (Mallard)		A	
docusate sodium (generic)	**tablets:** 100 mg	A	
Doctate (Glaxo)		A	
Regutol (Plough)		A	
docusate sodium (generic)	**capsules:** 250 mg	A	
Bu-Lax (Ulmer)		A	
Duosol (Kirkman)		A	

Single-Ingredient Products:
Lubricant Laxatives

Product and Distributor	Dosage of Active Ingredients	Rating[1]	Comment
mineral oil			
Mineral Oil (generic)	**liquid:** liquid petrolatum	A	
Nujol (Plough)	**liquid:** extra-heavy mineral oil	A	
mineral oil, emulsified			
Kondremul Plain (Fisons)	**emulsion:** 55% heavy mineral oil	A	

Laxatives: Product Ratings *(continued)*

Combination Laxative Products

Product and Distributor	Dosage of Active Ingredients	Rating[1]	Comment
Tablets and Capsules			
docusate sodium with casanthranol (generic)	**capsules:** 100 mg DSS + 30 mg casanthranol	A	
Afko-Lube Lax (American Parmaceutical)		A	
D-S-S plus (Parke-Davis)		A	
Dobrantyl (Riker)	**capsules:** 50 mg DSS + 25 mg danthron	A	
Gentlax B (Blair Labs.)	**tablets:** 333 mg guar gum + 108.7 mg standardized senna concentrate	B	guar gum not proved effective
Manalax (Jenkins)	**tablets:** 130 mg phenolphthalein + atropine sulfate + extract of cascara + ox-bile extract	C	too many laxative ingredients
Senokot S (Purdue-Frederick)	**tablets:** 50 mg DSS + 187 mg standardized senna concentrate	A	

Combination Laxative Products

Product and Distributor	Dosage of Active Ingredients	Rating[1]	Comment
Liquids and Syrups			
docusate sodium with casanthranol (generic)	**syrup:** 60 mg DSS + 30 mg casanthranol per tablespoon (15 ml)	A	
Peri-Colace (Mead Johnson)		A	
Haley's M-O (Winthrop)	**emulsion:** 25% mineral oil + 6% magnesium hydroxide	A	
Kondremul with Phenolphthalein (Fisons)	**emulsion:** 55% heavy mineral oil + 147 mg white phenolphthalein per tablespoonful	A	

Laxatives: Product Ratings *(continued)*

Combination Laxative Products

Product and Distributor	Dosage of Active Ingredients	Rating[1]	Comment
Liquids and Syrups			
Petro-Syllium No. 1 (Whitehall)	**emulsion:** 47.5% mineral oil + 0.75% psyllium seed	**A**	
Powders and Granules			
Casyllium (Upjohn)	**granules:** 4.1 g psyllium husk powder + 3 ml cascara fluid extract debittered + 1.2 g prune powder per 6 g packet	**C**	too many active ingredients
Movicol (Norgine)	**granules:** gum karaya + frangula	**B**	frangula not proved safe or effective
Perdiem (Rorer)	**granules:** psyllium + senna	**A**	
Syllamalt (Wallace)	**powder:** 4 g malt soup extract + 3 g powdered psyllium seed husks per rounded teaspoonful	**A**	

Carbon-Dioxide Release

Product and Distributor	Dosage of Active Ingredients	Rating[1]	Comment
Ceo-Two (Beutlich)	**suppositories:** sodium bicarbonate + potassium bitartrate in polyethylene glycol	**A?**	the Panel approves as safe and effective a different combination of ingredients that produce carbon dioxide when moistened, but did not specifically assess sodium bicarbonate + potassium bitartrate, which also release carbon dioxide

1. Author's interpretation of Panel criteria. Based on contents, not claims.

Lice Poisons

In the last decade, lice that suck human blood have been on the rise in the United States—and perhaps elsewhere as well. Officials at the Federal Centers for Disease Control (CDC), in Atlanta, confirm sharp increases of louse infection (pediculosis) in all socioeconomic classes. The reasons for this upsurge of lice are not clearly known. The increase of pubic lice—or *crabs*, as they often are called—has been attributed to less restrained sexual activity. The trend toward transient group living arrangements may favor body lice, which thrive where large groups of people live in close quarters. These changes cannot, however, account for the epidemic rise in head lice, which particularly afflict schoolchildren—since children live now much as they did a few decades ago when lice were only rare classroom visitors. After reviewing nonprescription louse killers (pediculicides), reviewers decided that one combination of 2 ingredients—a poison and a booster, or adjuvant—will effectively control these insects.

CLAIMS

Accurate
"for the treatment of head, pubic (crab), and body lice"

TYPES OF INFESTATION

Three kinds of lice attack humans. All create the same symptom: itchiness. These louse species have different life histories, which must be taken into account in delousing efforts. All, however, are vulnerable to the same insect poisons.

Head lice Technically called *Pediculus humanus capitis*, head lice are 1 to 2 mm long. They rarely are seen because they fade quickly into thick areas of hair, where they escape searching eyes and fingers. What is more likely to be spotted—during what school nurses call *lice inspection*—are the shiny, whitish or silverish egg cases called *nits*. Female lice attach their nits to a hair shaft, within a quarter-inch of the

LICE POISONS is based on report "Pediculicide Drug Products for OTC Human Use" by the FDA's Advisory Review Panel on OTC Miscellaneous External Drug Products.

scalp. One can look for them on the short hairs behind the ears or on the nape of the neck, with a strong light, a magnifying glass, and a fine-toothed comb. Nits may also be found near the base of the combed-out hairs.

The clue to lice is always the itching. Anytime a schoolchild suddenly starts scratching his or her head, lice are suspect. (Boils and other crusty or bloody scalp sores also may occur, as the result of infections caused by the scratching.) Lice feed on human blood. The itching is provoked by their saliva, which they leave in the skin while eating. The bitten area reddens and swells up like a tiny mosquito bite.

Head lice are as common in short hair as in long, so giving children short haircuts will not prevent these lice from occurring. According to recent government data, boys appear less vulnerable than girls, and blacks have a relative immunity to head lice.

School authorities should be informed of head-lice cases since the insects are often transmitted by scarves, hats, coats, and other garments hung together in school cloakrooms. Lice also move from person to person by hiding out in bedding, clothing, or towels.

All suspect clothing and bedding should be disinfected by machine washing in hot water and drying on the dryer's hot cycle for at least 20 minutes. Alternatively, clothing and personal items can be disinfected by dry-cleaning or by sealing them in a plastic bag for at least 2 weeks, until the last louse and last egg die. Brushes and combs and other grooming items should be soaked in hot water (above 130°F) for 5 to 10 minutes. Bedrooms and also all the common rooms of a dwelling should be thoroughly vacuumed.

Pubic lice   Commonly called *crabs*, the technical name for pubic lice is *Phthiris pubis*. The louse has 2 pair of greatly enlarged clawlike legs, so that it looks like a crab when inspected with a magnifying glass or microscrope. It is spread mainly by sexual contact, but it may be picked up from bedding, toilet seats, or shared towels. Crab lice favor the pubic and anal-area hairs, though they sometimes are found elsewhere on the body (especially in eyelashes and eyebrows). Their bites raise pale, bluish-gray blotches on the skin, which may be mildly—or intolerably—itchy. Pubic lice are easier to get rid of than head lice, since they survive only a day when not on a human body. Elaborate disinfecting procedures are not needed.

Body lice   This louse, technically called *Pediculus humanus corporis*, is generally found where many people live together under crowded conditions. It lives in and lays its eggs in clothing seams—so it bites skin areas where clothing rubs along the body (for example, at

the waistline and in the armpits). The bites cause itching, reddish blotches, and hive-like eruptions, as well as raised red bumps like mosquito
bites.

Body lice can survive hungry in clothing for up to 10 days, and their
eggs remain viable for a month. So the disinfectant steps described
above for head lice must be followed—except that heat sterilization or
insecticides should be used on clothing and other personal belongings,
rather than attempts to seal them up in plastic. Body lice can carry
typhus and other illnesses; anyone who has these lice should probably
visit a doctor—particularly if they were picked up in a tropical or
semitropical area outside the United States.

PEDICULICIDES (LICE KILLERS)

Insecticides that kill lice are called *pediculicides*. The Panel assessed a dozen but approves only one regimen, pyrethrins + piperonyl
butoxide. A more effective insecticide, gamma benzene hexachloride
(also called *lindane*) is available by prescription. Because it can be a
systemic poison, it must be used very carefully and once or twice only,
as directed by a doctor.

Approved Active Ingredients

The combination of pyrethrins + piperonyl butoxide   This is a
combination of the insecticide pyrethrins with a booster called piperonyl butoxide. Piperonyl butoxide enhances pyrethrins' effectiveness
because it inhibits the natural detoxification system lice have to combat
these poisons. Pyrethrins ruin the insects' nervous systems. They are
fast-acting, often killing within minutes.

The insecticide and the adjuvant both are poorly absorbed through
intact human skin, so they pose little risk of systemic toxicity. However,
both are slightly irritating, and persons allergic to ragweed may also be
allergic to pyrethrins and should not use them. Generally speaking,
however, the reviewers find this combination safe for the self-treatment
of lice.

A number of studies have demonstrated this preparation's effectiveness against lice. Two or three applications of pyrethrins with
piperonyl butoxide will kill all the lice on most individuals. Itching
usually stops after the initial treatment. While the clinical trials of pyrethrins do not meet the Panel's preferred standards, the panelists were
impressed enough by the available data to declare pyrethrins with

piperonyl butoxide effective as well as safe. However, this mixture does not kill nits, so it must be used a second time—7 to 10 days after the first application—to kill newly hatched lice. The approved dosages are 0.17 to 0.33 percent pyrethrins with 2 to 4 percent piperonyl butoxide.

Conditionally Approved Active Ingredients

None

Disapproved Active Ingredients

As shown in the chart that concludes this unit, one ingredient (described directly below) was rejected as unsafe and ineffective. Eleven of them were summarily disapproved for want of any data about effectiveness or safety.

Isobornyl thiocyanoacetate This chemical has been used in a nonprescription preparation to kill crab, head, and body lice. But virtually no toxicity data were reported to the Panel. In laboratory tests, isobornyl thiocyanoacetate was not quite so effective as pyrethrins with piperonyl butoxide. Furthermore, it appears that no clinical tests were available to the Panel for its assessment. So isobornyl thiocyanoacetate is judged not safe or effective.

WHAT TO DO ABOUT MITES

Intense itching of the skin may result from mites rather than lice. The most common culprit is the bite of *Sarcoptes scabiei,* also known as scabies. This mite burrows under the top layer of skin, causing intense itching and inflammation. Favored spots are the fingerwebs, wrists, penis, buttock, and underarms; unlike the situation with lice, the head and neck are rarely attacked.

Some experts claim cleanliness keeps mites away. Once present, the Panel says—in a rough-draft report—-they can be controlled with use of topical sulfur ointments and lotions containing 5 to 10 percent sulfur.

Safety and Effectiveness: Active Ingredients in Over-the-Counter Louse Killers

Active Ingredient	Panel's Assessment
alkaloids of sabadilla	summarily disapproved
aqueous coconut-oil soap	summarily disapproved

Safety and Effectiveness: Active Ingredients in Over-the-Counter Louse Killers *(continued)*

Active Ingredient	*Panel's Assessment*
benzocaine	summarily disapproved
benzyl alcohol	summarily disapproved
benzyl benzoate	summarily disapproved
DDT (dichlorodiphenyl trichloroethane)	summarily disapproved
dioctyl sodium sulfosuccinate	summarily disapproved
isobornyl thiocyanoacetate	not safe or effective
picrotoxin	summarily disapproved
pyrethrins + piperonyl butoxide	safe and effective
propylene glycol	summarily disapproved
sublimed sulfur	summarily disapproved
thiocyanoacetate	summarily disapproved

Lice Poisons: Product Ratings

Product and Distributor	*Dosage of Active Ingredients*	*Rating[1]*	*Comment*
A-200 Pyrinate (Norcliff Thayer)	**gel:** 0.333% pyrethrins + 4% piperonyl butoxide	A	
Barc (Commerce Drug)	**liquid:** 0.18% pyrethrins + 2.2% piperonyl butoxide	A	principal ingredient not safe or effective
blue (generic)	**gel:** 0.3% pyrethrins + 3% piperonyl butoxide	A	
pyrinyl (generic)	**liquid:** 0.2% pyrethrins + 2% piperonyl butoxide	A	
RID Shampoo (Pfipharmecs)	**liquid:** 0.3% pyrethrins + 3% piperonyl butoxide technical	A	
Vonce (Unipharm)	**shampoo:** 0.165% pyrethrins + 1.65% piperonyl butoxide technical	C	less-than-effective dosage of both ingredients

1. Author's interpretation of Panel criteria. Based on contents, not claims.

Liniments and Poultices for Aches and Pains

When a dentist starts to drill a tooth, many people dig their fingernails into the palms of their hands. The self-inflicted pain, which they control, blocks the drilling pain—which they do not control. Liniments and comparable preparations that are applied to the skin work in roughly the same way; they produce counterirritation, distracting one from more deep-seated pain.

CLAIMS

Accurate

for "the temporary relief of minor aches and pains of muscles and joints, such as simple backache, lumbago, arthritis, neuralgia, strains, bruises, and sprains"

One panelist objected, however, that some of these terms—like "simple backache"—are confusing.

False or Misleading

"penetrates deep into the skin and relieves pain arising from deep down inside"
"penetrating heat relief"
"deep strength"

Including such conditions as "arthritis" and "neuralgia" in labeling is misleading, since consumers should not attempt to self-diagnose and treat these conditions without a doctor's help.

WHAT THEY ARE AND HOW THEY WORK

Counterirritating substances are formulated in different ways:

• A *liniment* is a liquid that is rubbed gently onto the skin.

LINIMENTS AND POULTICES FOR ACHES AND PAINS is based on the report "External Analgesic Drug Products for OTC Human Use" by the Advisory Review Panel on OTC Topical Analgesic, Antirheumatic, Otic, Burn, and Sunburn Prevention and Treatment Drug Products.

- A *rub* may require more vigorous massage.
- A *poultice* is a damp, doughy, or porridgelike mixture that may be spread on a cloth laid over a sore spot.
- A *plaster* is a thicker, self-sticking mixture.
- *Balms* describe those applications concocted of aromatic plant resins and juices, so that they smell sweet.

These preparations mildly stimulate nerve endings in the skin for warmth, coolness, or pain—sometimes all 3 at once—which blocks or distracts one from more bothersome pain deep-seated in muscles, bones, and even viscera (internal organs). To reach the nerve endings, the irritating ingredients in liniments must be absorbed through the protective upper skin layers (the epidermis). Most of this absorption occurs directly through the epidermis—some via hair follicles, which explains why it occurs most readily in hairy areas. Although absorption happens more rapidly if the protective outer layers of skin have been broken or scraped, these preparations should *not* be used in such an instance for fear of damaging underlying tissues.

Oils, water, and other substances are actively absorbed by the skin, which is why counterirritant active ingredients are dissolved in them. Wetting the skin can further enhance absorption, as can heat. Covering the skin with a tight dressing will also markedly increase absorption—but this can increase the risk of damaging the skin after one has applied irritating substances.

Doctors today rarely prescribe or propose the use of these remedies. Nevertheless, they have been a part of traditional medical practice and folk healing for thousands of years. But despite long use of these preparations, relatively few scientific studies have been conducted to demonstrate that they are really effective. So the Panel decided to judge them by less rigorous standards than have been applied to many other classes of drugs in the over-the-counter drug-review process. It took into account popular appeal, as expressed in sales, as one criterion of effectiveness and also noted that complaints have been rare and the problems mild.

WARNING These products should be used only on intact skin surfaces and should not be put onto wounded skin or be covered with bandages or other tight dressings—which can dangerously increase the amount absorbed into the skin and the irritation that results. Even on healthy skin, the margin of safety may be thin. Products must be irritating enough to be felt, but if they are *too* irritating —or are used too often, or incorrectly—they may blister and burn the skin. Use of a liniment or poultice that raises blisters should be discontinued.

All liniments and poultices are for external use only, and should be kept out of children's reach since they may be quite poisonous if swallowed. Because these substances are irritating, they should be kept away from the eyes. They can be used for self-treatment for adults and children over the age of 2, but should be used for younger children only if recommended by a doctor.

Pain and Counterirritation

The deep-lying pains that can be successfully treated with counterirritants tend to be *dull* rather than sharp in feeling. They may originate at the place where they are felt or they may be *referred* pains —which means that a hurt felt in one place may emanate from damaged tissue that is some distance away.

A recent theory may help explain how a poultice applied to the skin can relieve a charley horse deep in the muscle. It was developed to explain how acupuncture—the traditional Chinese therapy in which thin needles are stuck into the body—can relieve pain at other body sites. This gate theory says that stimulating nerve pathways in one place can cause other pathways to close like a gate. This prevents other, more painful impulses from entering these pathways en route to the brain.

The nervous system can be thought of as a railroad, with trunk lines leading to the brain. When irritating—but tolerable—impulses generated by a liniment flow onto the trunk line from a branch line to the skin, the system closes switches (or "gates") that lead on from other branch lines to the muscles and bones. Pain impulses from these areas then cannot enter the trunk—and so are not received or registered by the brain—while the counterirritating impulses continue.

Liniments and rubs are not the only topical remedies for deep-seated pain. Ice packs, heat lamps, hot water bags, and warm or hot baths also act as counterirritants—and heat acts directly to relax painfully tense muscles. The warmth of a hot tub does not penetrate directly more than a fraction of an inch beneath the skin surface. But it warms and relaxes blood vessels in the skin, which enhances the blood-flow through them to deeper tissues. This warming action may also help carry off plasma and other irritating substances that have accumulated in muscle tissues.

Liniments are designed to be rubbed onto the skin. This massage provides part (some experts say *most*) of the benefit of the treatment. Massaging the skin stimulates blood-flow; dexterous fingertips can loosen tight muscles. Massage also is a pleasant-feeling counterirritation —and feeling good, even for a few moments, may break the vicious cycle of pain, tension, and more pain. In the same way, the comforting warmth and agreeably sweet and pungent odors of liniments and balms may contribute to the relief that they bring.

"There is no doubt," the Panel says, "that the action of counterirritants has a psychic component as well as a drug-induced therapeutic component."

When these counterirritants fail to bring relief within a week, a doctor should be consulted. Doctors can provide a variety of more potent prescription medications that may effectively relieve arthritic pain and other nagging, deep-seated discomfort. They also have treatment devices—including diathermy and ultrasound machines—that can beam warming impulses into sore spots deep in the body.

Types of Counterirritants

Reddeners   As their name implies, these substances redden the skin, and also warm it. They tend to be strong counterirritants. This group includes allyl isothiocyanate preparations—in plain language, mustard plasters—and methyl salicylate, turpentine oil, and stronger ammonia water.

Nonreddeners   These are red-pepper preparations that irritate the skin but do not cause it to redden. They are roughly as potent as reddeners.

Coolants   These agents produce a cooling sensation, and yet may stimulate warming and tingling sensations in the skin as well. Counterirritants in this class are camphor, eucalyptus oil, and menthol—all of which stimulate the sense of taste and smell, which may enhance feelings of well-being.

Blood-vessel   expanders   These   agents—technically   called *vasodilators*—widen the capillaries in the skin, which increases blood-flow through them. The 2 used in over-the-counter counterirritants are histamine dihydrochloride and methyl nicotinate.

COMBINATION PRODUCTS

Many counterirritant products are combinations of several active ingredients. Since the Panel interpreted the Drug Regulations on combinations in a liberal way, many liniments can continue to be marketed without proof that each of the several ingredients they contain provides a well-defined therapeutic benefit.

A safe and effective amount of an approved counterirritant from one of the 4 groups discussed above may be combined with a comparably safe and effective amount of an approved ingredient(s) from 1, 2, or 3 other groups. The coolants camphor and menthol *both* can be used, so that approved products may have as many as 5 active ingredients. No ingredient is allowable if it diminishes the effectiveness or the safety of any other.

A combination that contains less than an effective concentration of any other ingredient, or one that contains eucalyptus oil, rates only conditional approval. A combination that contains an active ingredient that had not been assessed by one of the review Panels would be disapproved—as would one that contains chloral hydrate.

Safe and effective counterirritants can also be combined with safe and effective ingredients in other drug groups. But combining a counterirritant with a skin anesthetic, which deadens feeling in the skin, makes no sense, since the 2 drug actions are working against each other. Similarly, a counterirritant should not be combined with a skin protectant, since they have opposing purposes.

Two Panel members raised strenuous objections to the majority's proposals. They objected to the combining of 2 or more counterirritants because the potential hazards of blending them have not been carefully studied. The only justification for such a combination would be if it provided some well-defined therapeutic advantage that was not present when one ingredient alone was used. They felt this has not been established: "The minority of the Panel is not impressed by statements appearing in manufacturers' submissions, such as 'marketing experience has been favorable,' or 'no complaints have been reported.'"

COUNTERIRRITANT INGREDIENTS

As noted earlier, standards for the approval of these products were less scientifically rigorous than those used by some other review Panels. In particular, they are less exacting than the standards used by reviewers who evaluated aspirin and other drugs taken internally to relieve aches and pains similar to those for which liniments and poultices are applied externally (*see* PAIN, FEVER, AND ANTI-INFLAMMATORY DRUGS TAKEN INTERNALLY).

Approved Active Ingredients

Allyl isothiocyanate (mustard oil)   This volatile oil is a powerful irritant and stimulates nerve endings in the skin. It is the active ingredient in mustard plasters (considered poultices), which consist of powdered mustard seed and flour fixed to a cloth or paper backing that can be dampened and pressed to the skin. Body heat releases the allyl isothiocyanate from the powdered mustard. It produces a decided warmth and reddening of the skin within 5 minutes.

In one test of 9 reddening counterirritants, allyl isothiocyanate was one of the few that both reddened *and* warmed the skin.

Blistering of the skin may occur in some instances. But manufacturers' data show that in an 11-year period—1962 through 1972—during which 15 *million* package units were sold, only 43 complaints, all minor, were received. This translates into a ratio of one complaint per 350,000 packages. On the basis of these data, the Panel says allyl isothiocyanate—in 0.5 to 5 percent concentrations and applied no more than 4 times daily—is a safe and effective counterirritant ingredient for the self-treatment of aches and pains in adults and children over 2.

Ammonia water, stronger This peculiarly named colorless solution is, in fact, stronger than ordinary household ammonia. But it is diluted for use in liniments and is safe when formulated in 1 to 2.5 percent concentrations.

Ammonia irritates the skin because it is strongly corrosive. But stronger-ammonia-water liniments—which are formulated as soaps by combining them with oleic acid and sesame oil—have caused few adverse reactions, according to marketing data. Without citing any scientific study on effectiveness, the Panel concluded that stronger ammonia water is effective as well as safe for use on adults and children over 2 as long as it is not applied more than 4 times daily.

Camphor At low dosage levels, camphor has a cooling, numbing effect on skin receptors, and is used to relieve pain and itching. But, paradoxically, in somewhat higher concentrations it produces a warming sensation that helps to block and relieve aches and pains. Camphor's persistent, pungent odor may well contribute to the sense of relief people experience.

Taken orally, camphor can be a deadly poison. It is absorbed through both intact and injured skin—and the Panel on Miscellaneous External Drugs has declared it unsafe in concentrations over 2.5 percent. This Panel disagrees, saying it is unaware of any poisonings attributable to applying camphor to the skin and believes such application is safe.

Camphor usually is mixed with other irritating substances in liniments and related products. Although the report cites no published scientific data, camphor—in concentrations of 3 to 11 percent, used no more than 4 times a day by adults and children over 2—was judged by this Panel to be safe and effective for use as a counterirritant. However, the FDA ruled that camphor formulated in water-base preparations is possibly effective and safe only in concentrations up to 2.5 percent.

Capsicum preparations: capsaicin, capsicum, and capsicum oleoresin These counterirritant ingredients are derived from a variety of peppers. Paradoxically (in view of the word "red"), red-pepper preparations create a warm—even burning—feeling on the skin without reddening it. They do not raise skin temperature or dilate superficial blood vessels to enhance blood-flow. Neither do they cause blistering, although they may feel intolerably hot.

The way capsicum preparations do work and their therapeutic effectiveness have not been adequately studied. Yet the sense of warmth they produce is highly accepted by users, and they do not appear dangerous. Two companies that were selling more than 4 million product units annually in the early 1970s reported only 16 customer complaints in one of those years—all of them minor.

In most of these products red-pepper extract is mixed with other counterirritant ingredients. Insofar as the pepper is concerned, the safe and effective concentration is 0.025 to 0.25 percent capsaicin. Also approved is its equivalent in less refined form, such as capsicum, which is the whole ground dried red pepper, or capsicum oleoresin, which is obtained by percolating the whole pepper in volatile solvents. These preparations are approved as safe and effective for use up to 4 times daily on adults and children over 2.

Histamine dihydrochloride Histamine is naturally present, in a bound and inactive form, in most body cells. When released, it stimulates smooth muscle; increases the heart rate, blood-flow, and metabolic rate; and causes a generalized flushing and feeling of warmth around the head and neck. In the same way, when histamine is vigorously massaged into intact skin or simply *applied* to broken skin, it penetrates to the underlying layers. There it dilates small blood vessels and increases the blood-flow through them. A warming effect results. At the low doses in which histamine dihydrochloride is used in nonprescription medications there have been few—and minor—side effects reported. The Panel cites no published studies to show that histamine is therapeutically effective at these low levels. Yet it says it is effective, as well as safe, at concentrations of 0.025 to 0.25 percent when applied no more often than 3 to 4 times daily to the skin of adults and children over 2.

Menthol This aromatic substance is sometimes called *peppermint camphor*. When rubbed vigorously onto the skin, relatively high concentrations of menthol produce an intense feeling of coolness even though the skin temperature in the treated area is likely to be warmer than the surrounding skin. The chemical seems to stimulate the nerves for cold perception. The cool feeling is then often followed by a sense of warmth. Menthol also depresses the activity of nerve receptors for pain, so it can be effectively used in low doses to treat pain and itching. (*See* MENTHOL, page 459.)

Menthol penetrates both unbroken and broken skin. But there are few reports of toxicity when it is rubbed onto the skin, nor do the sharply aromatic menthol vapors appear to harm the lungs. Some 32 million dosage units of mentholated counterirritant products are sold each year, and manufacturers report no more than one to 3 complaints per million dosage units—none of them serious.

The Panel concludes that menthol is safe and effective as a counterirritant alone or in combination products when the concentrations are 1.25 to 16 percent, the preparation is applied no more than 3 or 4 times daily, and use is confined to adults and children over 2.

Methyl nicotinate   Judging by the Panel's assessment, this derivative of the vitamin niacin is both widely used and poorly studied as a reddening counterirritant. Approval was based on a handful of scientific studies and on marketing reports that show, for example, that in one recent year 3 companies which sold 2.7 million product units received only 16 customer complaints—all about minor problems.

Methyl nicotinate rapidly penetrates the skin's protective barrier and stimulates underlying sense receptors. These receptors in turn trigger return impulses from the brain that expand small blood vessels in the skin, which increases blood-flow. This warms and reddens the skin. In doses of 0.25 to 1 percent, applied no more than 4 times daily, methyl nicotinate was evaluated as a safe and effective counterirritant for self-treatment by adults and children over 2.

Methyl salicylate   This sweet- and pungent-smelling chemical member of the aspirin family is one of the most widely used counterirritant active ingredients—it is also one of the better studied. It is sometimes still called *wintergreen oil*.

If eaten, methyl salicylate is quite poisonous and it now must be sold in childproof containers. Even so, products that contain it should be kept out of reach of children.

Despite its toxic risk, however, a 3-year search of records of the National Clearinghouse for Poison Control Centers in Bethesda, Maryland, showed no fatal cases and only a few serious ones resulting from accidental ingestion of methyl salicylate in the forms used as counterirritants for aches, pains, and bruises. Ten manufacturers who sold 35 million packages of these products in 1972 also reported no serious customer complaints, and only about one minor complaint for each half-million packages sold.

Methyl salicylate's effectiveness has been tested by controlled scientific studies. They show subjectively experienced pain relief and objectively measured reduction in muscle tension after treatment with lotions that contained the active ingredient.

When applied to the skin of adults and children over 2, no more than 4 times daily, methyl salicylate is safe and effective in concentrations of 10 to 60 percent.

Turpentine oil   Medicinal-grade turpentine oil, the Panel says, is of better quality than hardware-store turpentine sold as paint thinner —even though it shares its pungent odor and irritant properties. Turpentine's use for aches and pains has become a part of American folklore. It appears to be safe as well as effective. One company that sold 40 million bottles of a turpentine-oil liniment for 80 years claimed it had received no reports of customer problems; another manufacturer, who sold 9 million ounces of it in 1972, reported only 2 minor problems.

Turpentine is a potent skin irritant. It also causes allergic reactions in 5 to 10 percent of its users.

While no scientifically controlled studies have been conducted, wide acceptance by consumers and doctors led the evaluators to declare turpentine oil safe and effective when applied up to 4 times a day on adults and children over 2 and in concentrations of 6 to 50 percent.

Conditionally Approved Active Ingredients

Eucalyptus oil   This distillate of Australian and Malaysian eucalyptus-tree leaves is so widely used in drug and health products that many people consider its pungent odor to be *the* medicinal smell. Eucalyptus oil (or eucalyptol) is used as a fragrance and flavoring in a variety of products—including counterirritants—and is considered to be safe. But evaluators could find no convincing evidence that it actually irritates the skin. Thus, eucalyptus cannot be considered an accepted counterirritant and its effectiveness has yet to be proved.

Triethanolamine salicylate (trolamine salicylate)   This is a salicylate, like aspirin, long used in topical preparations to relieve deep-seated aches and pains. Its long usage, without problems, convinces the Panel that the substance is safe. Although it is absorbed through the skin, experts could find no evidence that it acts on underlying tissues to relieve muscle ache or other painful symptoms. Conclusion: effectiveness remains to be proved.

Disapproved Active Ingredient

Chloral hydrate   This bitter-tasting, acrid-smelling chemical has been used for a long time as a sleeping aid—and it is considered to be very safe and very effective for that purpose. Since it is potent, toxic in high doses, and can be habit-forming, it is a prescription drug.

Chloral hydrate has been used as an active ingredient in counterirritants. While it is considered safe for topical application, it has been suggested that it may be too irritating for this purpose. Our Panel says it is not as stable as or as effective as other counterirritants and judges it safe but not effective for this purpose. So the Panel elected to disapprove chloral hydrate's use in counterirritants.

Safety and Effectiveness: Active Ingredients in Over-the-Counter Liniments and Poultices

Active Ingredient	Mode of Action	Panel's Assessment
allyl isothiocyanate (mustard oil)	reddener	safe and effective
ammonia water stronger	reddener	safe and effective
camphor	coolant	safe and effective
capsicum preparations (capsaicin, capsicum, capsicum oleoresin)	nonreddeners	safe and effective
chloral hydrate	reddener(?)	safe, but not effective
eucalyptus oil	coolant	safe, but not proved effective
histamine dihydrochloride	blood-vessel expander	safe and effective
menthol	coolant	safe and effective
methyl nicotinate	blood-vessel expander	safe and effective
methyl salicylate	reddener	safe and effective
triethanolamine salicylate (trolamine salicylate)	not categorized by Panel or FDA	safe, but not proved effective
turpentine oil	reddener	safe and effective

Liniments and Poultices for Aches and Pains: Product Ratings

Single-Ingredient Products

Product and Distributor	Dosage of Active Ingredients	Rating[1]	Comment
methyl salicylate			
Gordogesic Cream (Gordon)	cream: 10%	A	
triethanolamine salicylate (trolamine salicylate)			
Aspercreme (Thompson)	cream and lotion: 10%	B	not proved effective

Combination Products

Product and Distributor	Dosage of Active Ingredients	Rating[1]	Comment
Gels, Creams, and Ointments			
Analgesic Balm (Lilly)	15.2% methyl salicylate + 15% menthol	A	
Ben Gay Original Ointment (Leeming)	18.3% methyl salicylate + 16% menthol	A	
Exocaine Plus Rub (Commerce Drug)	30% methyl salicylate + 5% benzocaine	C	it makes no sense to combine counterirritant with skin anesthetic
InfaRUB Cream (Whitehall)	0.1% histamine dihydrochloride + 0.4% capsicum oleoresin	A	
Men-Balm (Jenkins)	15% methyl salicylate + 2% menthol + 3% eucalyptus oil	B	eucalyptus oil not proved effective
Minut-Rub (Bristol-Myers)	10% methyl salicylate + 4.4% camphor + 3.5% menthol	C	the Panel approves this dosage of camphor, but the Misc. External Drugs Panel says this dosage is unsafe
Musterole Extra Strength Ointment (Plough)	0.6% methyl salicylate + 2.8% mustard oil + 5.7% camphor + 1.9% menthol + 1.9% glycol monosalicylate	C	too much camphor (*see* comment on Minut-Rub, above)
Lotions and Liniments			
Ben Gay Lotion (Leeming)	15% methyl salicylate + 7% menthol	A	

Liniments and Poultices for Aches and Pains: Product Ratings (continued)

Combination Products

Product and Distributor	Dosage of Active Ingredients	Rating[1]	Comment
Lotions and Liniments			
Heet Spray (Whitehall)	25% methyl salicylate + 3% camphor + 1% methyl nicotinate + 3% menthol	C	the Misc. External Drugs Panel says 3% camphor unsafe
Heet Liniment (Whitehall)	15% methyl salicylate + 3.6% camphor + 0.025 capsicum oleoresin	C	unsafe level of camphor
Panalgesic Rub (Poythress)	55.78% methyl salicylate + 5.32% aspirin + 2% camphor + 0.95% menthol	B	aspirin not proved effective when used on the skin; too little menthol
Sloan's Liniment (Warner-Lambert)	2.66% methyl salicylate + 3.35% oil of camphor + 0.62% capsicum oleoresin + 46.76% oil of turpentine + 6.74% oil of pine	C	unsafe dosage of camphor; too little methyl salicylate; oil of pine not assessed by Panel
Thru Penetrating Analgesic, Cooling Liquid (Rexall)	5% salicylamide + 1% benzocaine + 48% isopropyl alcohol	C	too little benzocaine; salicylamide not proved effective
Thru Penetrating Analgesic, Warming Liquid (Rexall)	7.95% methyl salicylate + 5% salicylamide + 5% menthol + 2.5% camphor + 1.86% benzocaine + 66% isopropyl alcohol	C	benzocaine should not be combined with counterirritant like methyl salicylate, as they counteract each other

1. Author's interpretation of Panel criteria. Based on contents, not claims.

Menstrual-Distress Preparations

Many women experience bloating and other unpleasant symptoms in the week before their menstrual periods. Many, too, experience cramp-

MENSTRUAL-DISTRESS PREPARATIONS is based on the unadopted draft report "OTC Orally Administered Menstrual Drug Products" by the FDA's Advisory Review Panel on OTC Miscellaneous Internal Drug Products.

ing and other discomfort once they start to bleed. No single cause has been identified for either of these situations but, fortunately, a few nonprescription and prescription drugs have been developed that will effectively relieve them.

Reviewers say that the nonprescription drugs should be used only for the *mildest* symptoms of premenstrual distress or painful menstruation (technically called *dysmenorrhea*). Severely disturbing or disabling pain and other serious symptoms should lead a woman to visit her gynecologist or family physician. Recent discoveries have opened new ways of successfully treating menstrual distress with prescription drugs.

WHY SOME WOMEN SUFFER MONTHLY

The Panel tried to differentiate between 2 conditions: premenstrual syndrome (occurring in the week before menstruation) and dysmenorrhea (which occurs during menstruation). But their several symptoms—including weight-gain, pain, and jangled nerves—may occur during one or both. So evaluators found it difficult to draw sharp lines between these 2 conditions.

The principal symptoms of premenstrual syndrome are water retention (edema), weight-gain, abdominal bloating and pain, tender breasts, headache, fatigue, and feelings of depression, irritability, tension, and anxiety.

The symptoms of dysmenorrhea consist primarily of sharp, cramping pelvic pain, which may radiate to other parts of the body. Related symptoms include nausea, vomiting, diarrhea, headache, dizziness, and fatigue.

Many theories have been advanced to explain these syndromes. Two facts stand out in the reviewers' report:

- The key premenstrual symptom for many women is water retention. Relieving this condition allows the pain, irritability, and other symptoms to subside. One may suceed in doing this simply by decreasing fluid load in the week before menstruation—without recourse to drugs. In addition to drinking less fluid, a woman should avoid salt- and sodium-rich foods like potato chips, pickles, sodas, and table salt on the 3 or 4 preperiod days, since salt and sodium hold water in the body tissues.
- Women who suffer premenstrual distress and painful periods tend to have high levels of body chemicals called *prostaglandins* when they menstruate. When these women are treated for a few days each

month with prescription drugs called *prostaglandin inhibitors*, many experience a remarkable symptomatic relief.

DRUGS FOR RELIEF

Most nonprescription menstrual-relief products contain one or more of the following ingredients:

- *Pain relievers*: These drugs, also called analgesics, act on the nervous system to block sensations of pain and discomfort.
- *Antihistamines*: These drugs block the activity of irritating substances called histamines, which the body may produce in excess during menstruation. Antihistamines also have a mild pain-relieving effect, and they may counteract anxiety, tension, and irritability. (Their exact contribution is not clearly spelled out by the Panel.)
- *Diuretics*: These drugs act on the kidney or other organs to eliminate excess water that has accumulated in the body.
- *Smooth-muscle relaxants*: These drugs may relieve cramping by relaxing the muscles of the uterus, where the pain appears to originate, but their effectiveness has not been proved.
- *Botanical or vegetable compounds*: Extracts from plants have been formulated into menstrual drugs for more than a century, but appear to lack real medicinal value. (It may be the alcohol in which they are formulated that provides some relief.)
- *Vitamins*: The value of these essential nutritional ingredients in treating menstrual distress remains to be proved.

The Panel viewed many of the active ingredients in menstrual products according to the categories described above, so this unit follows that grouping. Many other ingredients were not categorized or assessed for want of meaningful data; they are simply listed as "summarily disapproved" in the first of the 2 SAFETY AND EFFECTIVENESS charts that conclude this unit. In this welter of ingredients, only the following compounds in products submitted to the Panel are graded safe and effective:

- *Pain relievers:* acetaminophen and aspirin
- *Antihistamines:* pyrilamine maleate
- *Diuretics:* ammonium chloride, caffeine, and pamabrom.

Combination Products

Since premenstrual syndrome and dysmenorrhea cause a variety of symptoms, it made sense to the Panel—as it has to manufacturers and to women who use these products—that the symptoms be treated concurrently, with combination products. The Panel suggests that for premenstrual relief one should choose a diuretic, supplemented perhaps by an antihistamine and/or pain-reliever. Once bleeding—and cramping—have started, a pain-reliever is likely to be the best drug, supplemented perhaps by a smooth-muscle relaxant.

Naturally, the claims that can legitimately be made for menstrual-relief products depend on their specific ingredients. For example, a claim for the relief of bloatedness or other signs of fluid retention can be made only if a diuretic is included. Pain-relief claims require that aspirin or another safe and effective pain reliever be present.

PAIN RELIEVERS

Drugs that relieve pain are principal ingredients in many combination products sold for the self-treatment of premenstrual and menstrual symptoms. The two most widely used safe and effective pain relievers —aspirin and acetaminophen—can, of course, be purchased as single-entity drugs that are far cheaper than combination products labeled for menstrual distress. An aspirin and a cup of coffee provide essentially the same relief as the aspirin and caffeine in a tablet sold for menstrual pain.

CLAIMS FOR PAIN RELIEVERS

Accurate

for "relief of pain of the premenstrual period"
for "relief of pain of the cramping of the premenstrual period"
for "relief of pain of the menstrual period"
for "relief of pain of menstrual cramps"
for "relief of pain of dysmennorrhea"

Approved Active Ingredients

This Panel accepts the findings of the Advisory Review Panel on OTC Internal Analgesic and Antirheumatic Drug Products on the safety and effectiveness of over-the-counter pain relievers. Thus it approves the ingredients noted immediately below. These ingredients, as well as those conditionally approved or disapproved as pain relievers, are discussed more fully in the unit PAIN, FEVER, AND ANTI-INFLAMMA-TORY DRUGS TAKEN INTERNALLY.

Acetaminophen   This ingredient is safe and effective in doses of 325 to 650 mg every 4 hours, up to 4000 mg in 24 hours.

Aspirin   This ingredient is safe and effective in doses of 325 to 650 mg every 4 hours, up to 4000 mg in 24 hours.

Calcium carbaspirin   This ingredient is safe and effective in doses of 414 to 828 mg every 4 hours, up to 4000 mg in 24 hours.

Choline salicylate   This ingredient is safe and effective in doses of 435 to 870 mg every 4 hours, up to 5220 mg in 24 hours.

Magnesium salicylate   This ingredient is safe and effective in doses of 325 to 650 mg every 4 hours, up to 4000 mg in 24 hours.

Sodium salicylate   This ingredient is safe and effective in doses of 325 to 650 mg every 4 hours, up to 4000 mg in 24 hours.

Conditionally Approved Active Ingredients

One helper drug (or adjuvant) and one pain reliever are granted only tentative aproval by the Panel.

Caffeine   Manufacturers allege that caffeine relieves pain or enhances the effectiveness of pain relievers like aspirin. The Panel dismisses the notion that caffeine is itself a pain reliever, but says it may enhance the effect of aspirin or acetaminophen. So it gives caffeine conditional approval for this purpose—that is, the ingredient is safe but not proved effective.

Salicylamide   This drug is promoted as a pain reliever, but neither its safety nor its effectiveness has been established. Therefore it merits only conditional approval.

Disapproved Active Ingredients

Two compounds that have been formulated into drugs sold for relief of premenstrual syndrome and dysmenorrhea are specifically disapproved by the evaluators.

Codeine   In the low doses in which it is formulated into nonprescription products, codeine is not effective. In higher doses that *are* effective, it is not safe—and for the most part is not sold over-the-counter.

Phenacetin   This drug is a kidney poison, and so is unsafe.

ANTIHISTAMINES

Data are available on the one antihistamine that is used in menstrual remedies. The drug is discussed below.

CLAIMS FOR ANTIHISTAMINES

Accurate

"an aid in relieving symptoms of premenstrual tension such as nervous irritability"

for "premenstrual tension"

"relieves premenstrual tension"

for relief of premenstrual "anxiety, irritability, and tension"

Approved Active Ingredient

Pyrilamine maleate Because of wide use over many years, this drug is judged safe even though it may make the user drowsy (*see* PYRILAMINE MALEATE, page 131).

The question of *how* pyrilamine maleate helps relieve premenstrual syndrome remains, in the Panel's word, "uncertain." A manufacturer claims that initial discomfort is caused in part by the release of the body substance histamine, which is blocked by the drug—a theory that authorities say is highly conjectural. Pyrilamine maleate, like other antihistamines, does have mild anesthetic (numbing) and analgesic (pain-killing) properties, and a sedative effect that may not be related to its effects on histamine.

In 2 recent controlled studies, pyrilamine maleate was shown to be significantly more effective than a dummy medication in relieving irritability, depression, and premenstrual tension. It also acted to reduce water retention. Basing its decision on these studies, reviewers judged pyrilamine maleate to be safe and effective in doses of 25 mg every 3 to 4 hours, or 60 mg every 12 hours, not to exceed 200 mg in any 24-hour period.

Conditionally Approved Active Ingredients

None

Disapproved Active Ingredients

None

DIURETICS

A diuretic—sometimes called a *water pill*—stimulates the kidneys or acts in other ways to remove excess water that has accumulated in body tissues. This fluid excess is called edema; why it occurs on premenstrual days is not known. Water is believed to be largely responsible for the bloated feeling that many women experience before their menstrual periods, and much of the other pain and discomfort that go with it. Removing water therefore relieves many of these symptoms.

Only very weak diuretics are formulated into over-the-counter preparations. Water pills do alter key physiologic functions that are intimately tied to water levels, which explains why almost all diuretics are prescription drugs, for use only under medical supervision.

Premenstrual syndrome is the *only* approved use for nonprescription diuretics. If you are using over-the-counter water pills for any other purpose, you should stop using them and see a doctor. Nonprescription diuretics are safe for treating premenstrual syndrome, the Panel says, "because [it] is self-diagnosable, limited in duration, occurs intermittently, disappears abruptly at the onset of the menstrual flow—and is not a sign of a potentially serious underlying disorder."

CLAIMS FOR DIURETICS

Accurate

"a clinically tested diuretic that gives relief of premenstrual water-weight gain"

"proven effective in helping avoid bloatedness, weight-gain, and swelling associated with menstruation"

"an aid in relieving the symptoms of premenstrual tension such as nervous irritability, sleeplessness, painful breasts, and a bloated, full feeling"

"a diuretic which helps to control temporary weight-gain during the menstrual period"

WARNING   Do not use diuretics if you have kidney disease, liver disease, or pulmonary insufficiency.

Approved Active Ingredients

Ammonium chloride   This ingredient has seen many years of use as a diuretic, as a means of acidifying urine, and as an expectorant—for which purpose it has been found safe. The present Panel accepts the other reviewers' finding that the drug is safe in the low dosages used for premenstrual relief. (In higher doses of 8 or more grams daily, ammonium chloride frequently causes nausea, vomiting, and stomach ache.)

After the diuretic dose is swallowed and absorbed into the bloodstream, the ammonium and the chloride are separated from each other in the liver. The chloride combines with sodium—from sodium bicarbonate in the body—to form sodium chloride (salt). Loss of the sodium bicarbonate decreases the tissues' ability to bind water, so both water and salt are freed for elimination from the body. This reaction can be maintained by fresh doses of ammonium chloride only for a couple of days, after which the body blocks it—so there is no point in taking the drug for long periods of time.

Only one controlled study was available concerning ammonium chloride's use in the treatment of premenstrual edema. The drug was combined with caffeine, which also is a diuretic, so that results were confounded. Nevertheless, on the basis of this study and wide clinical use, the Panel deems ammonium chloride effective (as well as safe) in a dosage of 1 gram 3 times daily for up to 6 days for the relief of premenstrual syndrome.

Caffeine The stimulant that is found in coffee, tea, chocolate, and many soft drinks, caffeine increases the rate at which the kidneys remove water from the blood and excrete it. The present reviewers accept the findings of another Panel that in customarily used doses the drug is safe.

Caffeine is a mild diuretic, the effectiveness of which is well established. The Panel approves it as effective for the relief of premenstrual and menstrual bloating at a dosage of 100 to 200 mg every 3 or 4 hours. (The same effect can be obtained by drinking a cup of coffee.)

Pamabrom (2-amino-1-methyl-1-propanol-8-bromotheophyllinate) The safety of this compound by itself—and in combination with pyrilamine maleate or pyrilamine maleate and pain relievers—was certified by the FDA in the 1950s when it licensed pamabrom as a new drug. Since then, no evidence of significant toxicity or adverse reactions has been reported—so the present Panel finds pamabrom safe.

When given to healthy women when they are not accumulating fluid before menstruation, pamabrom doubles urinary output for at least one hour. When tested in the premenstrual week, however, the results are less persuasive. In one study of 194 subjects over several menstrual periods, the drug significantly lessened the women's pain, cramps, tension, irritability, and feelings of depression. But it did not significantly reduce the excess fluid. Because of these equivocal results, the Panel approves pamabrom as safe and effective for relieving the symptoms of premenstrual tension—but *not* edema specifically. Dosage is set at 50 mg per dose, not to exceed 200 mg daily.

Conditionally Approved Active Ingredients

Theobromine This compound, which is a diuretic, is formulated into some premenstrual-distress products. The Panel feels its safety and effectiveness have yet to be proved.

Theophylline While relatively potent as a diuretic in the same class as caffeine and theobromine, theophylline is also occasionally toxic. The Panel is not persuaded that the drug is safe. Reviewers decided at their very last meeting—which was also the last meeting of any Panel —that theophylline's safety and effectiveness for premenstrual syndrome remain to be established.

Disapproved Active Ingredients

Theobromine sodium salicylate This is a caffeinelike compound that stimulates the kidneys to produce urine. Although it is safe, the drug is an especially weak diuretic and the Panel could find no evidence to show that it effectively relieves edema or other premenstrual symptoms. Conclusion: safe but not effective.

SMOOTH-MUSCLE RELAXANTS

The crampy pain of dysmenorrhea is attributed by many experts to spasmodic contractions of the smooth muscles that make up the wall of the uterus. So there may be merit in using a drug that will relax smooth muscle once bleeding has started, if not beforehand. Unfortunately, of the 2 relaxants formulated into these products, the Panel could grant only conditional approval to one; it disapproved of the other.

CLAIMS FOR MUSCLE RELAXANTS

If an active ingredient were approved, the following claims would be allowed:
    for "relief of menstrual pain"
    "relieves painful menstrual cramps"
    "relieves menstrual cramps"
    for "the treatment of dysmenorrhea"

Approved Active Ingredients

None

Conditionally Approved Active Ingredient

Cinnamedrine hydrochloride   The safety of this compound as a single ingredient has not been studied. But in lab tests in mice in which it was combined with other ingredients, it appeared to be relatively nontoxic. Moreover, in the 35 years cinnamedrine has been marketed in nonprescription menstrual products, only 23 instances of side effects have been attributed to its use. This leads the Panel to judge it safe.

But evaluators could not find any clinical material that establishes cinnamedrine hydrochloride's effectiveness—by itself—in treating cramps. One study shows that cinnamedrine combined with other ingredients works better than other combinations. This suggests some promising potential, but for the time being the Panel assesses cinnamedrine hydrochloride safe but not proved effective.

Disapproved Active Ingredients

Homatropine methylbromide   This is a belladonna derivative, sometimes used as a digestive aid. This Panel judged it safe for that purpose. Because even lower doses are used in menstrual products, the Panel judges the drug safe for such preparations. The problem is that these doses are probably too low to be effective. Worse, no evidence at all was available to demonstrate that homatropine methylbromide relieves menstrual cramps. If fact, one authority on this class of drugs states that the substance has very little effect on the uterus. So the verdict is: safe but not effective.

BOTANICAL OR VEGETABLE COMPOUNDS

Plant extracts, usually formulated in alcohol, were widely marketed in the last century for use when women were in what was then called "a delicate condition." Some of these products survive, if somewhat changed.

One preparation, sold both as an elixir and in tablet form, was submitted to the Panel. Reviewers judged that 2 of its ingredients—a bitter extract of the herb *Gentiana lutea* and licorice root *Glycrrhiza glabra*—are simply flavoring and not active drugs. The Panel evaluated the 5 other plant substances in these products. Since it could not find any one of them that merited the "safe and effective" designation, it rejected as scientifically untenable or misleading all claims that the substances really combat the pain or distress of menstruation.

CLAIMS FOR PLANT EXTRACTS

False or Misleading
"relieve cramps and other distress of monthly periods" (menstruation)
"acts as a uterine sedative"

Approved Active Ingredients
None

Conditionally Approved Active Ingredients
None

Disapproved Active Ingredients

Asclepias tuberosa (pleurisy root) Drug reference books indicate that this compound has been used medicinally for a variety of purposes, for almost a century. But records are nonexistent concerning its use for dysmenorrhea. No scientific studies of *Asclepias'* safety for humans were submitted to the Panel—although women have taken the drug, apparently without hazard, for many decades. And no evidence indicates that this root extract effectively relieves cramps or other menstrual symptoms. The Panel judges *Asclepias* safe but ineffective.

Cimcifuga racemosa (black cohosh) Here we have a folk remedy that has been used for many purposes, one of which is inducing menstruation. The Panel is somewhat reassured about safety because of a 150-year history of the drug's use. But it notes that *Cimcifuga* has been shown to be fairly toxic in animal tests, and its safety for human use has not been scientifically established. No studies have been done on its effectiveness in relieving menstrual discomfort. Animal tests conducted a half-century ago indicate that the substance is therapeutically worthless. So evaluators conclude that *Cimcifuga* is neither safe nor effective.

Piscidia erythrina (Jamaica dogwood) This tree is also called the *fish-poison tree* because when its crushed bark, twigs, and leaves are dragged through water, fish become stupefied and float to the surface. Extracts of the bark have been promoted as a pain reliever for menstrual cramps. Although no safety studies have been conducted on humans, the Panel says that long use and studies on rats and mice indicate that *Piscidia* is safe. Some tests in animals show that the bark extract depresses uterine muscle tone; other tests do not. No studies have been done to specifically assess *Piscidia erythrina*'s effect on menstrual cramps. Conclusion: safe but not effective.

Senecio aureus (life root)   The manufacturer of the product that contains this material conceded back in 1975 that the drug's safety is questionable and said that the preparation would be quickly reformulated. But as of April 1981, this had not been done. The Panel takes the manufacturer at his word that *Senecio aureus* is unsafe. Furthermore, no data were submitted to show that the ingredient has medicinal value in treating menstrual distress. So the verdict is: not safe and not effective.

Taraxacum officinale (dandelion root)   This bitter plant root has a lengthy history of medicinal use in stimulating the gastrointestinal tract and for its laxative properties. More recently it has been found to also act as a diuretic. Long use and a handful of animal tests persuaded the Panel that *Taraxacum officinale* is safe. But no scientific evidence was submitted that suggests a role for it in treating dysmenorrhea. The Panel concluded that the substance is safe but not effective.

VITAMINS

A smattering of data is available to suggest that one vitamin might be of value in relieving premenstrual and menstrual distress. *How* it might do so remains wholly unclear.

Approved Active Ingredients

None

Conditionally Approved Active Ingredient

Pyridoxine hydrochloride (vitamin B₆)   One of the B vitamins, this compound has been found to be safe and effective when given as a supplement to people who are deficient in it. One researcher has suggested that pyridoxine hydrochloride has an antispasmodic effect, which would relieve cramps. But the few studies cited to bolster this viewpoint cover only a few women and are not well constructed for scientific validity. One double-blind study failed to show that the B vitamin is any better at relieving menstrual symptoms than a dummy preparation. In view of all this, the Panel judges pyridoxine hydrochloride to be safe but not proved effective when used to relieve menstrual symptoms.

Disapproved Active Ingredients

None

Safety and Effectiveness: Active Ingredients in Over-the-Counter Menstrual-Distress Preparations

Active Ingredient	Function	Panel's Assessment
acetaminophen	pain reliever	safe and effective
alfalfa leaves	not categorized	summarily disapproved
aloes	not categorized	summarily disapproved
ammonium chloride	diuretic	safe and effective
Asclepias tuberosa (pleurisy root)	uncertain	safe, but not effective
asparagus	not categorized	summarily disapproved
aspirin	pain reliever	safe and effective
barosma	not categorized	summarily disapproved
caffeine	as pain reliever	safe, but not proved effective
	as diuretic	safe and effective
calcium carbaspirin	pain reliever	safe and effective
calcium lactate	not categorized	summarily disapproved
calcium pantothenate	not categorized	summarily disapproved
choline salicylate	pain reliever	safe and effective
chlorprophenpyridamine maleate	not categorized	summarily disapproved
Cimcifuga racemosa (black cohosh)	uncertain	summarily disapproved
cinnamedrine hydrochloride	smooth-muscle relaxant	safe, but not proved effective
Cnicus benedictus (blessed thistle)	not categorized	summarily disapproved
codeine	pain reliever	not safe (high dose); not effective (low dose)
corn silk	not categorized	summarily disapproved
couch grass	not categorized	summarily disapproved
dog-grass extract	not categorized	summarily disapproved
essence pepsin	not categorized	summarily disapproved
ethyl nitrite	not categorized	summarily disapproved
extract buchu	not categorized	summarily disapproved
extract hydrangea	not categorized	summarily disapproved
extract stone root	not categorized	summarily disapproved
extract uva-ursi	not categorized	summarily disapproved
extract of bearberry (cascada sagrada)	not categorized	summarily disapproved

Safety and Effectiveness: Active Ingredients in Over-the-Counter Menstrual-Distress Preparations *(continued)*

Active Ingredient	Function	Panel's Assessment
extract of cascara	not categorized	summarily disapproved
ferric chloride	not categorized	summarily disapproved
homatropine methylbromide	smooth-muscle relaxant	safe, but not effective
Hydrastis canadensis (golden seal)	not categorized	summarily disapproved
hyoscyamine sulfate	not categorized	summarily disapproved
magnesium salicylate	pain reliever	safe and effective
magnesium sulfate	not categorized	summarily disapproved
methapyrilene hydrochloride	not categorized	summarily disapproved
methenamine	not categorized	summarily disapproved
methylene blue	not categorized	summarily disapproved
natural estrogenic hormone	not categorized	summarily disapproved
niacinamide	not categorized	summarily disapproved
oil of erigeron	not categorized	summarily disapproved
oil of juniper	not categorized	summarily disapproved
oil of nutmeg	not categorized	summarily disapproved
oleoresin capsicum	not categorized	not safe or effective
pamabrom (2-amino-1-methyl-1-propanol-8-bromotheophyllinate)	diuretic	safe and effective
parsley	not categorized	summarily disapproved
phenacetin	pain reliever	not safe
phenindamine tartrate	not categorized	summarily disapproved
phenyl salicylate (salol)	not categorized	summarily disapproved
pipsissewa	not categorized	summarily disapproved
Piscidia erythrina (Jamaica dogwood)	uncertain	safe, but not effective
potassium acetate	not categorized	summarily disapproved
potassium nitrate	not categorized	summarily disapproved
pyridoxine hydrochloride (vitamin B_6)	not categorized	not proved effective
pyrilamine maleate	antihistamine	safe and effective
riboflavin	not categorized	summarily disapproved
salicylamide	pain-reliever	not proved safe or effective
saw palmetto	not categorized	summarily disapproved
Senecio aureus (life root)	uncertain	summarily disapproved
sodium benzoate	not categorized	summarily disapproved
sodium salicylate	pain reliever	safe and effective
spirit of peppermint	not categorized	summarily disapproved
sucrose	not categorized	summarily disapproved

**Safety and Effectiveness: Active Ingredients in Over-the-Counter
Menstrual-Distress Preparations (continued)**

Active Ingredient	Function	Panel's Assessment
sulfurated oils of turpentine	not categorized	
Taraxacum officinale (dandelion root)	uncertain	safe, but not effective
theobromine	diuretic	not proved safe or effective
theobromine sodium salicylate	diuretic	safe, but not effective
theophylline	diuretic	not proved safe or effective
thiamine hydrochloride	not categorized	summarily disapproved
triticum	not categorized	summarily disapproved
urea	not categorized	summarily disapproved
venice turpentine	not categorized	summarily disapproved

**Safety and Effectiveness: Combination Products Sold Over-the-Counter
to Relieve Premenstrual and Menstrual Distress**

Safe and Effective

caffeine + ammonium chloride
pamabrom + pyrilamine maleate
pamabrom + pyrilamine maleate + acetaminophen

Conditionally Safe and Effective

aspirin + cinnamedrine hydrochloride + caffeine

Unsafe and/or Ineffective Combinations

Piscidia erythrina + Asclepias tuberosa + Cimcifuga racemosa + Taraxacum officinale + Senecio aureus
Cimcifuga racemosa + Senecio aureus + Taraxacum officinale + ferrous sulfate

Menstrual-Distress Preparations: Product Ratings[1]

Single-Ingredient Products

Product and Distributor	Dosage of Active Ingredients	Rating[2]	Comment
ammonium chloride (diuretic)			
Ammonium Chloride (Bowman)	**tablets:** 325 mg	**A**	approved for brief, monthly use only
ammonium chloride (generic)	**tablets:** 500 mg	**A**	approved for brief, monthly use only
	tablets, enteric coated: 500 mg	**A**	approved for brief, monthly use only
Ammonium Chloride (Lilly)	**tablets, enteric coated:** 1 g	**A**	approved for brief, monthly use only

Combination Products

Product and Distributor	Pain Reliever	Diuretic	Antihistamine	Caffeine	Other	Rating[2]	Comment
Aqua Ban (Thompson)		325 mg ammonium chloride		100 mg		**A**	
Cardui (Chattem)	325 mg acetaminophen	25 mg pamabrom	12.5 mg pyrilamine maleate			**A**	
Femcaps (Otis Clapp)	324.4 mg acetaminophen			32.4 mg	8.04 mg ephedrine sulfate + 0.0325 mg atropine sulfate	**C**	"other" ingredients not submitted to or assessed by Panel

Menstrual-Distress Preparations: Product Ratings[1] (continued)

Combination Products

Product and Distributor	Pain Reliever	Diuretic	Antihistamine	Caffeine	Other	Rating[2]	Comment
Fluidex (O'Connor)		65 mg powdered buchu extract + 65 mg powdered couch grass extract + 65 mg powdered corn silk extract + 32.5 mg powdered hydrangea extract				C	none of these ingredients is safe and/or effective
Lydia Pinkham Vegetable Compound Liquid (Cooper)					extract of Jamaica dogwood + pleurisy root + licorice + alcohol	C	disapproved combination; the first two ingredients not effective
Midol (Glenbrook)	454 mg aspirin			32.4 mg	14.9 mg cinnamedrine hydrochloride	B	cinnamedrine not proved effective
Trendar (Whitehall)	325 mg acetaminophen	25 mg pamabrom				A	

1. For ratings of pain relievers, see page 602; for ratings of caffeine products, see pages 606–608.
2. Author's interpretation of Panel criteria. Based on contents, not claims.

Minerals

See VITAMINS AND MINERALS ·

Motion-Sickness Medicines

"Severe nausea, and the realization that one is about to vomit, is one of the more dreadful conditions suffered by man!"

—THE PANEL

Motion sickness occurs when our sense of what we are seeing with our eyes is out of sync with our sense of balance, which is maintained by sensitive organs of the inner ear. Trouble is particularly likely to arise as the head rotates and one becomes dizzy. While some people are less susceptible than others—including astronauts, ballet dancers, and others who are specially trained to overcome these effects—no one is wholly immune to this distress.

Fortunately, several nonprescription drugs are available that can be taken before departure or during a trip to quell the discomforting symptoms of airsickness, carsickness, seasickness, and other forms of motion sickness. While motion sickness is by no means the only cause of nausea or vomiting, discussion in this unit will center around over-the-counter remedies for nausea and vomiting as they relate to it.

CLAIMS

Accurate
for "the prevention and treatment of nausea and vomiting associated with motion sickness"

MOTION-SICKNESS MEDICINES is based on the report of the FDA's Advisory Review Panel on OTC Laxative, Antidiarrheal, Emetic, and Antiemetic Drug Products, and on the FDA's "Temporary Final Monograph on Antiemetic Drug Products for OTC Human Use."

PRODUCTS TO TREAT MOTION SICKNESS

Emesis is the Greek term for vomiting. An antiemetic, of course, blocks this action. Many effective antiemetics require a doctor's prescription. Others are available over-the-counter, but both the Panel and the FDA believe that these preparations should be used only to quell the nausea and vomiting associated with motion sickness.

Authorities also disapprove the formulation of antiemetics into combination products; they say such combinations are unsafe, ineffective, or both.

Approved Active Ingredients

Benzhydryl piperazines: meclizine hydrochloride and cyclizine hydrochloride   The antihistamines meclizine hydrochloride and cyclizine hydrochloride are both evaluated as safe and effective for the prevention and treatment of motion sickness—especially when they are taken a half-hour *before* one sets out on a journey. There is no explanation of exactly why or how these antihistamines work, although they are thought to reduce the excitability of balance centers within the inner ear.

Meclizine hydrochloride is a well-studied and widely used drug that has been available by prescription for more than a quarter of a century. The evaluators' decision that it is also safe and effective in over-the-counter products allowed manufacturers to begin marketing it in this way for the first time. Cyclizine hydrochloride, which is chemically similar, appears to have been used and studied less extensively.

Fears were raised in the 1960s that these drugs could cause birth defects if used by pregnant women. However, a study of more than 1000 women who used meclizine hydrochloride during their first trimester indicates that this is not true. So the FDA is withdrawing its presently required label warning which suggests that these drugs not be used during pregnancy unless urgently needed. But neither of these drugs, it should be emphasized, is approved—or regarded as safe—for treating the nausea and vomiting associated with morning sickness of early pregnancy.

Both meclizine and cyclizine cause drowsiness in some users and should not be taken by persons driving a car or piloting a boat, plane, or other vehicle, or operating heavy machinery. Nor should they be taken when one is drinking; alcohol and antihistamines have an additive, sleep-inducing effect.

Meclizine hydrochloride has the advantage that a single 25 to 50 mg dose remains effective up to 24 hours.

The adult dosage for cyclizine hydrochloride is 50 mg every 4 to 6 hours, up to 4 times in 24 hours. For children 6 to 12, it is 25 mg per dose, up to 3 times in 24 hours.

Dimenhydrinate This is a form of the antihistamine diphenhydramine. Its safety and effectiveness against seasickness and airsickness has been shown repeatedly in the 30 years since it was introduced, evaluators noted. It is relatively free of side effects in the recommended doses, although some users do become drowsy. So passengers can use it—but not drivers, pilots, or nautical captains. Drinking liquor may make one drowsier still, which some seasickish passengers may find welcome!

Antihistamines have a drying effect on some glands and tissues. So dimenhydrinate should not be used by sufferers of asthma, glaucoma, or enlarged prostate (disorders already marked by glandular problems) except under a doctor's supervision.

The dosage of dimenhydrinate required to prevent or relieve motion sickness in adults is 50 to 100 mg every 4 to 6 hours, not to exceed 400 mg in 24 hours. For children 6 to 12, it is 25 to 50 mg every 6 to 8 hours, not to exceed 150 mg in 24 hours. For youngsters 2 to 6, the dosage is 12.5 to 25 mg every 6 to 8 hours, not to exceed 75 mg in 24 hours. Dimenhydrinate is the only antiemetic approved for young children.

Meclizine hydrochloride See BENZHYDRYL PIPERAZINES, above.

Conditionally Approved Active Ingredients

Bismuth subsalicylate This substance has been used for a long time in widely marketed over-the-counter products labeled for antidiarrheal symptoms and other forms of gastrointestinal distress. Both the Panel and the FDA say it is safe. Bismuth subsalicylate has not been claimed to relieve motion sickness, but proof of its worth for this purpose would be required if manufacturers now wished to advance this claim. Products containing bismuth subsalicylate have been said to coat and protect the stomach and relieve "nausea" and "upset stomach." Experimental data show that this substance does in fact inhibit experimentally induced vomiting in dogs. But in humans, 1 ounce of a liquid preparation of bismuth subsalicylate was no more effective than 1 ounce of water in preventing vomiting induced by a tablespoonful of ipecac syrup. So claims that bismuth subsalicylate controls the nausea of motion sickness remain to be proved.

Diphenhydramine hydrochloride For many years this antihistamine has been available by prescription for nausea and vomiting. It was not submitted to the reviewers but the FDA agreed to give it an in-house review after the Panel had completed its report. The agency notes that diphenhydramine is both the chemical base and apparent source of the antiemetic properties of dimenhydrinate, which is approved for nonprescription antiemetics (*see* DIMENHYDRINATE, above).

But the FDA has a lingering concern about all nonprescription uses of diphenhydramine hydrochloride because the drug induces drowsiness in a third of all users—a side effect that the agency concedes is not necessarily unpleasant or unwelcome to a seasick passenger, although hazardous for a captain. So the FDA says on the one hand that diphenhydramine hydrochloride is safe enough for over-the-counter marketing as a motion-sickness medication, but on the other hand it recommends that manufacturers compare its incidence of drowsiness to that of dimenhydrinate. If the 2 are about equal, the agency suggests, it would approve diphenhydramine hydrochloride for nonprescription use against motion sickness. But the FDA indicates that if the drug is significantly more sleep-inducing, it might withhold this approval on grounds that dimenhydrinate provides comparable benefit with less risk.

Diphenhydramine hydrochloride was categorized as not proved safe but effective. It is still not available over-the-counter as an antiemetic.

Phosphorated carbohydrate   This preparation is a sweet mixture of grape sugar, fruit sugar, and phosphoric acid that also is called *levulose-dextrose-orthophosphoric acid*. The manufacturer recommends a dosage of 1 to 2 tablespoonsful every 15 minutes—up to 5 doses—until the distress subsides. This means swallowing a lot of sugar, which could be risky for diabetics or persons intolerant of fruit sugar (fructose).

This mixture slows the emptying of stomach contents into the small intestine. But neither the reviewers nor the federal agency is persuaded that this action will reduce nausea or vomiting: no convincing studies support the claim that it does. So while phosphorated carbohydrate is rated safe, when sold with appropriate warnings about sugar intake, proof is still lacking that it is effective in relieving motion sickness.

Scopolamine hydrobromide   This is an anticholinergic—a material that blocks receptor sites for the nerve-impulse transmitting substance called acetylcholine; it is a potent but also relatively toxic drug. Claims have been made that it acts on the body's balance control center in the inner ear, thus decreasing sensitivity to imbalance and preventing dizziness and nausea. Scopolamine hydrobromide was not submitted for review as a motion-sickness remedy, but because it has long been sold over-the-counter for that purpose, the FDA agreed to a special review.

The special evaluators concluded that at higher prescription doses, scopolamine hydrobromide *is* effective against motion sickness. But because of the high incidence of side effects—which include dry mouth, blurred vision, drowsiness, forgetfulness, cardiac irregularities, and reduced brain function—these prescription doses of 0.6 mg and above are not safe for use without prescription. However, used at the lower amount (0.25 mg per dose) contained in nonprescription products, scopolamine hydrobromide appears safe when taken up to 4 times daily. But because existing data do not clearly establish that these doses will really prevent or curtail motion sickness, effectiveness remains to be proved.

Disapproved Active Ingredients

Aminoacetic acid   Also called *glycine* or *glycocol*, this amino acid is safe and effective when used as an antacid. So it is judged to be safe by the Panel and the FDA. But stomach acid does not cause nausea or vomiting, so there is no clear rationale to support the use of an antacid like aminoacetic acid to prevent or treat these symptoms. Verdict: not effective.

Phenyl salicylate   This substance, which also is called salol, is judged to be safe. But no evidence could be found to show that it is effective against the nausea or vomiting of motion sickness.

Zinc phenosulfonate   Zinc phenosulfonate was assessed as safe in the amounts usually present in over-the-counter products. But neither the Panel nor the FDA could find evidence to support claims that the substance is an effective antidote for the symptoms of motion sickness.

Safety and Effectiveness: Active Ingredients in Over-the-Counter Motion-Sickness Medicines

Active Ingredient	Panel's and FDA's† Assessment
aminoacetic acid	not effective
bismuth subsalicylate	not proved effective
cyclizine hydrochloride	safe and effective
dimenhydrinate	safe and effective
diphenhydramine hydrochloride*	not proved safe
meclizine hydrochloride	safe and effective
phenyl salicylate	not effective

Safety and Effectiveness: Active Ingredients in
Over-the-Counter Motion-Sickness Medicines *(continued)*

Active Ingredient	Panel's and FDA's† Assessment
phosphorated carbohydrate	not proved effective
scopolamine hydrobromide	not proved effective
zinc phenolsulfonate	not proved effective

*Not sold over-the-counter as an antiemetic in the United States as of 1982.
†Judgments reaffirmed or modified by the FDA, or originated by it.

Motion-Sickness Medicines: Product Ratings

Product and Distributor	Dosage of Active Ingredients	Rating[1]	Comment
bismuth subsalicylate			
Pepto-Bismol (Norwich-Eaton)	**suspension:** 527 mg per 2 tablespoonsful **tablets, chewable:** 300 mg	**B**	not proved effective
cyclizine hydrochloride			
Marezine (Burroughs-Wellcome)	**tablets:** 50 mg	**A**	
dimenhydrinate			
dimenhydrinate (generic)	**tablets:** 50 mg	**A**	
dimentabs (generic)		**A**	
Dramamine (Searle)		**A**	
dimenhydrinate (generic)	**liquid:** 12.5 mg per 4 ml	**A**	
Dramamine Junior Syrup (Searle)		**A**	for children
meclizine hydrochloride			
meclizine hydrochloride (generic)	**tablets:** 12.5 mg	**A**	
meclizine hydrochloride (generic)	**tablets:** 25 mg	**A**	
Wehvert (Hauck)		**A**	
meclizine hydrochloride (generic)	**tablets, chewable:** 25 mg	**A**	
Bonine (Pfipharmecs)		**A**	
Motion Cure (Wisconsin Pharm.)	**capsules, chewable:** 25 mg	**A**	

Motion-Sickness Medicines: Product Ratings *(continued)*

Product and Distributor	Dosage of Active Ingredients	Rating[1]	Comment
phosphorated carbohydrate solution			
Controflex (Bowman)	**syrup:** sucrose + orthophosphoric acid + peppermint	B	not proved effective
Emetrol (Rorer)	**solution:** levulose (fructose) + dextrose (glucose) + orthophosphoric acid	B	not proved effective
scopolamine hydrobromide			
Scopodex (CMC)	**pellets:** 0.5 mg	B	not proved effective
Triptone (Commerce Drug)	**capsules:** 0.25 mg	B	not proved effective

1. Author's interpretation of Panel criteria. Based on contents, not claims.

Mouth Medicines

See SORE THROAT AND MOUTH MEDICINES

Mouthwash for Oral Hygiene

Bad breath *is* unpleasant. But, if one goes by mouthwash commercials, it is the ultimate social sin. So it is no wonder that Americans spend a million dollars a day on mouthwashes, gargles, and other breath fresheners.

These products are promoted to encourage daily use by persons with no symptoms or evidence of disease. However, manufacturers claim these products prevent dental decay and gum and mouth diseases, which, of course, are medicinal claims. Many mouthwashes con-

MOUTHWASH FOR ORAL HYGIENE is based on the unapproved draft report of the FDA's Advisory Review Panel on OTC Oral-Cavity Drug Products.

tain pharmacologically active ingredients—principally antimicrobials (germicides), which kill or inhibit the growth of bacteria, viruses, funguses, and other microorganisms. Both the medicinal claims and the pharmacological ingredients define these products legally as drugs as opposed to cosmetics, and, therefore, they were assessed as part of the Drug Review.

The Panel takes a dim view of medicated mouthwashes. It rates many of the claims made for them as sheer hogwash. Aside from questionable benefits, there seems to be a significant risk in the daily use of antimicrobials by healthy people—a cautionary view shared by the FDA and the National Academy of Sciences. "The absurd notion that antimicrobial agents in gargles, mouthwashes, and mouth rinses are necessary for daily cleansing of the mouth and throat is based on tradition, promotional appeal by manufacturers, and misunderstandings concerning their effectiveness and safety, rather than on well-documented facts," the evaluators charge. "There are few, if any, indications justifying the use of [these products] for self-medication or for oral health care by lay consumers."

None of the germicides used in these products has been demonstrated to be safe and effective for routine use by healthy people. However, some of these preparations are also marketed for brief use in treating sore throat, sore mouth, and other minor oral-cavity irritation (*see* SORE THROAT AND MOUTH MEDICINES).

CLAIMS

False or Misleading
"inhibits odor-forming bacteria"
"deodorizing mouthwash and gargle"
"oral antiseptic cleanser"
"for oral hygiene, bad breath"
"management of mouth odors, bad breath"
"an aid to daily care of the mouth"
"for causing the mouth to feel clean"

THE HEALTHY MOUTH

Millions of microorganisms enter our nose and mouth each day in the air we breathe, the food we eat, and the water we drink. Many come to rest in the gastrointestinal tract or respiratory system. These "germs" normally do not cause disease because the body has a potent defense system to kill or remove them.

A third of a liter of saliva is secreted into the mouth each day. It cleans the inside of the mouth and the teeth and also inhibits bacterial growth. The body's immunologic defense mechanisms are constantly at work in the mouth. Bacteria that are normally present in the mouth also appear to help resist colonization by their invading, disease-producing relatives.

These defense mechanisms sometimes fail, and infections and other disorders may result. But a healthy mouth requires no ongoing help in the form of medicated mouthwash to stay fresh and clean. And there is no evidence, the Panel says, that using these products will prevent infections and diseases.

THE WAR ON DENTAL PLAQUE

One of the major dental-health needs in the United States is the development of effective over-the-counter drugs to combat dental plaque. This is the buildup of acid-forming bacteria, body secretions, and food debris on the teeth and gums. It is said to be the main cause of inflamed gums (gingivitis) and dental cavities.

Manufacturers claim that antiseptic mouthwashes kill the bacteria that form dental plaque, thereby preventing gingivitis and cavities. Specifically, cetylpyridinium chloride and domiphen bromide (quaternary ammonium compounds) have been reported to reduce plaque by 30 to 40 percent. Other antimicrobials that are potentially effective for this action include thymol and eucalyptol, the Panel says.

However, these benefits are still uncertain. After carefully weighing the available reports on antiplaque ingredients and the theories advanced to explain their protective action, reviewers concluded that the matter is too controversial to allow approval. The Panel decided that all claims about prevention and control of plaque are untrue, unproved, or misbranding—and it recommended that manufacturers be required to go through the FDA's formal drug-approval procedures if they hope to market such a product for daily use.

ORAL MALODOR

Whether it is called *bad breath*, *halitosis*, *foul breath*, or, as the Panel prefers, *oral malodor*, the problem is age-old. Remedies employed against it have ranged from the chewing of pleasant-smelling berries like teaberry to taking enemas, tongue scraping, the use of perfumes, and the smoking of flavored cigarettes. Today, the principal remedy is scented mouthwashes. These are cleansing and freshening preparations—that is, cosmetics—unless they contain an antimicrobial or other drug or carry medicinal claims on their labels—as many do. Any substance that is promoted as a germ killer is being promoted as a drug.

Some diseases cause unusual—and in some instances quite unpleasant—odors on the breath, but the Panel says that most oral malodor is not associated with sore throat, sore mouth, or any particular systemic or local oral-cavity disease. Bad breath, the Panel says, is not a disease.

Oddly, bad breath usually is not detected by the person who has it. Putting into more delicate language the script of many a mouthwash commercial, the Panel declares: "Unless a social contact informs an individual that he or she has malodor, the individual may be unaware of its presence."

Of course, bad breath can sometimes be associated with certain medical conditions. Diabetes, for example, creates a sweetish smell on the breath. Persons whose kidneys are failing and who no longer can get rid of body wastes in their urine may have a urinelike smell on their breath. Upper-respiratory infections, not surprisingly, can produce a purulent smell. These malodors, of course, do not occur in healthy people.

Having studied the medical literature, the Panel concludes that only about 10 percent of all oral malodors are due to outside causes like food and drink, or disease. The rest represent local oral conditions in people who are healthy.

Researchers long quarreled about what *kind* of chemicals produce bad breath. In recent years, an analytic method called *gas chromatography*—which can detect airborne molecules in parts-per-billon concentrations—has demonstrated that a halitosis-affected mouth has minute traces of sulfur compounds. These volatile and foul-smelling gases include hydrogen sulfide, methyl mercaptan, and, to a lesser extent dimethylsufides.

These sulfurous gases cannot be made by cells of the human body. But they can be—and are—made by bacteria that are normally present in the mouth. Two species, fusobacterium and peptostreptococcus, are principal culprits. These microbes thrive in places where there is little or no oxygen. This means they are principally found in crevices in the gums, between the teeth, in small folds in the tonsils, and in tiny intercellular spaces in the tongue. (This last has long been believed to be one of their principal places of concealment.)

Neither the volatile sulfurs nor the bacteria that produce them appear to be dangerous.

Eating candy and other sweets does not lead to bad breath—contrary to what some parents tell their children. Rather, according to the experts, the offensive bacteria consume sulfur-containing proteins and amino acids that are most abundant in meat, fish, and dairy products.

Methods for Eliminating Bad Breath

The Panel has several suggestions for eliminating bad breath. These suggestions refer specifically to malodor that arises from within the throat and mouth—*not* to "garlic breath" and other such situations that can be avoided simply by not eating or drinking the offending substance before a date or other social function.

Purging   It is often possible to temporarily rid oneself of bad breath by rinsing out one's mouth with water, brushing one's teeth, using dental floss, or eating a meal. These methods sometimes work and sometimes do not. The improvement results from the physical removal or dilution of volatile sulfur compounds, the bacteria that produce them, and the food debris they consume. This dilution is part of the beneficial effect of most liquid preparations and products sold to relieve mouth odor—but water will serve as well.

Masking   Bad odors sometimes can be covered up with good odors. Many mouthwashes contain anise oil, cinnamon oil, peppermint, spearmint, or sage oil to provide this coverup. These masking agents are effective only until the saliva dilutes them and carries them away—usually about 15 to 20 minutes.

Chemical neutralization   Some substances react chemically with bad-smelling airborne compounds to form nonodorous substances, usually nonvolatile sulfides. The effect they produce depends on how long the neutralizing agent remains in the mouth and how much of the malodorous compounds needs to be neutralized. This method provides longer-lasting protection than purging or masking substances. Unfortunately, the Panel failed to identify what these neutralizing substances are.

Bacterial inhibition   An antimicrobial that kills or slows the growth and reproduction of the bacteria that cause mouth malodor will freshen the breath for longer periods than purging or masking methods. But after a meal or during sleep, the Panel says, the bacteria will usually return to their original numbers, bringing back the odor.

Theoretically, the best results should be obtained by using germicides that specifically and selectively attack the relatively few bacteria that appear to be responsible for bad breath. But the Panel says it does not know whether antimicrobials really work this way. What is known is that the bacteria rarely if ever are completely destroyed, and they will quickly repopulate the mouth once the antimicrobial is gone.

Evaluators estimate that to obtain long-lasting protection the antimicrobial dose would have to be repeated every 3 or 4 hours, as long as the malodor persists. This heavy use of antimicrobials—which can upset the normal, healthy balance of microorganisms in the mouth—cannot be justified. So the Panel stresses its objection to the routine, self-prescribed use of medicated oral-health preparations—particularly those with antimicrobial agents.

This hard stance against over-the-counter sales and self-treatment with antimicrobial mouthwashes does not mean that the reviewers wholly oppose efforts to use drugs to eliminate odor-forming bacteria in the mouth. Rather, they feel that drug-research progress—which has produced far more effective germ-killing agents than the ones found in over-the-counter preparations—makes it necessary that such treatment be supervised by a doctor or dentist. The professional may be able to identify the responsible microorganisms and then prescribe a potent prescription antimicrobial prescription that will fairly specifically and selectively reduce or eliminate them. These drugs for the most part are administered systemically, not topically in mouthwashes.

ACTIVE INGREDIENTS IN OVER-THE-COUNTER MOUTHWASH

A glance at mouthwash labels in any drugstore will reveal that most contain antimicrobials. A few also contain astringents, anesthetics, or other types of drugs. The Panel assessed all ingredients in the preparations submitted for its evaluation, and automatically disapproved any that were not submitted for review. (For the Panel's assessment of all active ingredients in oral-health-care products, *see* SORE THROAT AND MOUTH MEDICINES.)

Among the astringents that may be found in mouthwashes, alum and zinc chloride are safe and effective, but tincture of myrrh is neither safe nor effective. Among the many antimicrobials that are the principal medicinal ingredients in these washes, the Panel could not find even one that it felt was safe and effective for self-treatment under any circumstances. Brief use of some of these antimicrobials to relieve specific symptoms of sore throat and mouth *may* be safe and effective—though this has not been clearly established. But the evidence to establish their safety when used daily or for extended periods in healthy mouths simply does not exist.

The compound cetylpyridinium chloride, to take one example, is an antimicrobial active ingredient in mouthwash. The Panel notes that there are no data on its cumulative effects, metabolism, or excretion from the body during long-term use. Neither is there evidence about whether it might cause cancer or birth defects in users or their descendants.

While all of these safety questions remain unresolved, the Panel finds no reason to support routine, long-term use when no symptoms exist and no benefits can be shown. Because the Panel—like the FDA —believes there is little if any valid reason to put antimicrobials into nonprescription mouthwashes, it did not specifically evaluate safety and effectiveness for this use. Rather—as noted in the Assessment of Antimicrobial Active Ingredients chart at the end of this unit—evaluators, in many instances, simply declared an ingredient "not recommended."

Some of these antimicrobials were evaluated for brief use in treating sore-throat and sore-mouth symptoms. It makes sense that a drug the reviewers found not safe even for this brief use is certainly not safe for long-term, routine use.

Assessment of Antimicrobial Active Ingredients in Over-the-Counter Mouthwash Products

Active Ingredient	Panel's Assessment
benzalkonium chloride	not recommended
benzethonium chloride	not recommended
benzoic acid	not recommended
borax	not safe or effective
boric acid	not safe or effective
boroglycerin glycerite	not safe or effective
camphor	not safe or effective
carbamide peroxide in anhydrous glycerin	not recommended
cetalkonium chloride	not recommended
cetylpyridinium chloride	not recommended
chlorophyll	not recommended
cresol	not safe
dequalinium chloride	not recommended
domiphen bromide	not recommended
ethyl alcohol	not recommended
eucalyptol	not recommended
ferric chloride	not safe
gentian violet	not recommended
hydrogen peroxide	not recommended
iodine	not recommended

Assessment of Antimicrobial Active Ingredients in Over-the-Counter Mouthwash Products
(continued)

Active Ingredient	Panel's Assessment
menthol	not recommended
meralein sodium	not safe or effective
methyl salicylate	not recommended
nitromersol	not safe or effective
oxyquinoline sulfate	not recommended
phenol	not recommended
phenolate sodium	not recommended
potassium chlorate	not safe or effective
povidone-iodine	not recommended
secondary amyltricresols	not recommended
sodium bichromate	not safe
sodium borate	not safe or effective
sodium caprylate	not recommended
sodium dichromate	not safe
thymol	not recommended
thymol iodide	not recommended
tolu balsam	not recommended

Mouthwash for Oral Hygiene: Product Ratings[1]

Product and Distributor	Dosage of Active Ingredients	Rating[2]	Comment
Cēpacol (Merrell-National)	**mouthwash:** 1:2,000 cetylpyridinium chloride + alcohol	**C**	both ingredients not recommended
Cēpastat (Merrell-National)	**mouthwash:** 1.4% phenol	**C**	not recommended
Chloraseptic (Norwich-Eaton)	**mouthwash** and **spray:** 1.4% phenol as phenol and sodium phenolate	**C**	not recommended
dalidyne (Dalin)	**spray:** lidocaine + cetalkonium chloride + ethyl alcohol	**C**	cetalkonium chloride and alcohol not recommended

Mouthwash for Oral Hygiene: Product Ratings[1] *(continued)*

Product and Distributor	Dosage of Active Ingredients	Rating[2]	Comment
aryglan (Ayerst)	**spray:** 0.3% antipyrine + 0.05% pyrilamine maleate + 0.5% sodium caprylate + menthol + gentian violet + methyl salicylate + peppermint oil + spearmint oil + anise oil + cinnamon oil + isobornyl acetate + 0.05% benzyl alcohol + 1% ethyl alcohol	C	several ingredients are not recommended

The Panel does not approve regular daily use of any mouthwash product that contains active medicinal ingredients.
Author's interpretation of Panel criteria. Based on contents, not claims.

Nail-Biting and Thumb-Sucking Deterrents

Drugs used to discourage children from biting their fingernails or sucking their thumbs rely on a very basic drug-making principle: make things taste bad enough and people will not put them in their mouth!

This approach may work, according to the Panel that assessed the 2 active ingredients used in these deterrent products. And these bitter drugs are considered safe. But reviewers say the evidence of their value in breaking bad biting and sucking habits remains inconclusive—and it suggests caution in using such preparations.

A common error of parents is to worry too much and too early about thumb-sucking. It's a natural act that may continue normally until about age 4. To forestall parental efforts to stop it prematurely, the reviewers stipulate that these drugs should not be used on children under 4.

NAIL-BITING AND THUMB-SUCKING DETERRENTS is based on the report on nail-biting and thumb-sucking deterrent drug products by the FDA's Advisory Review Panel on OTC Miscellaneous External Drug Products.

FINGERNAILS AND THEIR BITERS

Nail-biters are quite numerous. One recent study reports that 43 percent of children bite their nails, as do 25 percent of college students and 10 percent of other adults.

Hard-bitten nails, surprisingly, grow back faster than nails that are not bitten. The normal growth rate for fingernails is about 0.1 mm per day—which means 36 mm (just under an 1½ inches) per year. Nail-biters can expect almost 3 inches of annual growth.

The horny keratin (hard material) of the nail is produced continuously by the matrix, that white, half-moon-shaped material visible at the base of the exposed part of the nail, which extends back under the skin.

Nail-biting goes by the technical name *onychophagia*. People who do it may nip and pull the ends off the nails until they are past the normal attachment point of nail and bed. The bed then may bulge upward where the nail should be. The sharp and rough edges left by biting can cause inflammation, and excessive biting can cause open wounds that are apt to become infected.

Why people bite their nails is not fully known. Biting is sometimes thought to express discontent, stress, or emotional maladjustment. In most cases, it is an unconscious habit that seems to provide oral gratification. The consequences can nevertheless be quite distressing not only to parents and friends but also to nail-biters themselves, who often try the nail-biting drug products available in hopes of breaking the habit.

Less distasteful approaches may, however, be more effective. Reviewers cite one study of a behavioral modification method called The Habit Reversal procedure. Children are reminded by their parents and therapist that they are biting their nails; then they are helped to understand why this is a bad habit; finally they are offered alternative self-gratifying behavioral choices. In a study of 13 chronic nail-biters, all stopped biting their nails after a month of treatment. Pediatricians, dentists, psychologists, and psychiatrists may be able to provide this type of therapy.

The drugs used to discourage nail-biting are the same ones used to deter thumb-sucking, and will be described later in this unit.

THUMB-SUCKERS

Many children suck their thumbs: studies indicate that between 16 and 40 percent of kids of various ages do. Thumb-sucking is so natural that it starts before birth—as has been shown in X-rays of unborn babies.

It usually stops at about age 4. Why it continues longer in some children than others is not known, but the Panel says the current professional belief is that thumb-sucking in older children is an "empty or simple habit, a result of [previously] learned behavior" and does not signify that a child is emotionally disturbed.

Thumb-sucking may, however, be damaging—more so to the mouth that sucks them than to the thumbs that are sucked. Sucking may delay or disrupt the eruption of a child's incisor teeth. It can distort the development of muscles in the lips, affecting a child's ability to swallow. The dental arch and palate of the mouth may become deformed, causing difficulties in breathing, chewing, and speaking.

DETERRENT DRUGS

The active ingredients in drugs intended to keep fingers out of mouths taste extremely bitter. They are meant to be painted onto the fingertips or nails. They are *not* to be swallowed. Neither of the 2 active ingredients has been demonstrated to be effective, so no drug was granted full approval (nor was any totally disapproved). But if one should be fully approved, the only claim that can be made for it is the one that follows.

for "use as a nail-biting and thumb-sucking deterrent in persons aged 4 years and older"

Approved Active Ingredients

None

Conditionally Approved Active Ingredients

The Panel approved 2 individual ingredients—and a combination of the 2 of them—as safe and as possibly effective for deterring nail-biting and thumb-sucking.

Denatonium benzoate This substance has such an extremely bitter taste that it is added to poisonous industrial alcohol to discourage alcoholics from drinking it. It is also added to lead-base paint to discourage children from chewing paint chips. There have been a few studies that have established the drug's safety. In most of these experiments, which have been conducted in rats, varying doses of denatonium benzoate were introduced into the animals' stomachs through tubes—since no right-minded rat would choose to eat it. Enormous doses had to be administered to kill the rats.

In one test in humans, 90 volunteers painted their fingernails with a product containing 0.15 percent denatonium benzoate and 6 percent sucrose octaacetate (*see* immediately below). Then they licked their nails at 4-hour intervals. The subjects' nails, tongues, and mouths were checked daily for signs of irritation. None was found. The test continued for 30 days.

The effectiveness of this combination product was tested in 19 inveterate nail-biters out of the 90 volunteers. The researchers reported good nail regrowth in 12 of the 19, fair regrowth in 3, and little or no regrowth in the remaining 4. In another study of denatonium benzoate (0.35 percent) by itself, two-thirds of the test subjects reported good results while the other third said the product was only partially effective or ineffective. The manufacturer concluded that this study proved that the product is effective, but evaluators were not convinced—citing the absence of proper controls. While judging denatonium benzoate to be safe, the Panel says its effectiveness still needs to be demonstrated in a carefully controlled scientific study.

Sucrose octaacetate   This ingredient is so bitter that wildlife biologists have tried to use it to keep nuisance species of wild birds from eating food crops. In one test concerning safety, a researcher was unable to feed or force-feed animals enough of the chemical to kill them. He could not detect toxic changes after dosing animals with sucrose octaacetate for 90 days. Two other researchers believe that stomach irritation or vomiting would occur long before a dangerous dose could be ingested.

On the basis of such findings, evaluators concluded that sucrose octaacetate is safe. But they believe there is insufficient data from controlled scientific studies to adequately judge how well it works. In fact, the only study of this substance in humans that the Panel cited is the one involving combination with denatonium benzoate (*see* above). Verdict: safe but not proved effective.

The combination of denatonium benzoate + sucrose octaacetate One marketed product contains a combination of 0.15 percent denatonium benzoate and 6 percent sucrose octaacetate. Based on the fact that peoples' perceptions of tastes—even very bad tastes—may differ, the Panel recognizes the possible value of such a combination.

Disapproved Active Ingredients

None

Safety and Effectiveness: Active Ingredients in Over-the-Counter Nail-Biting and Thumb-Sucking Remedies

Active Ingredient	Panel's Assessment
denatonium benzoate	safe, but not proved effective
sucrose octaacetate	safe, but not proved effective

Nail-Biting Deterrents: Product Ratings

Product and Distributor	Dosage of Active Ingredients	Rating[1]	Comment
Stop 'n Grow (Mentholatum)	denatonium benzoate 0.15% + sucrose octaacetate 6%	B	not proved effective
Thum (Num)	**Liquid:** cayenne pepper extract 16.6% + citric acid	C	ingredients not submitted to or assessed in over-the-counter drug review

1. Author's interpretation of Panel criteria. Based on contents, not claims.
Note: Other nail-biting and thumb-sucking deterrent products are available; however, they are not included here as manufacturers have declined to provide ingredient listings.

Pain, Fever, and Anti-Inflammatory Drugs Taken Internally

Pain is the most common problem for which people use medicines, and pain relief is the most common reason why people take nonprescription

PAIN, FEVER AND ANTI-INFLAMMATORY DRUGS TAKEN INTERNALLY is based on the report of the FDA's Advisory Review Panel on OTC Internal Analgesic and Antirheumatic Drug Products and the FDA Notice on Proposal to Withdraw Approval of New Drug Applications for Phenacetin.

drugs. The pain relievers that work externally and that are applied to the skin are described elsewhere in the book. This unit is concerned with pain relievers taken internally.

Many internal analgesic drugs also relieve fever—that is, they have an antipyretic (antifever) effect. Many, too, soothe the inflammatory distress of arthritis and so are said to have an antirheumatic effect. All 3 factors—pain, fever, and inflammation—are treated together by the Panel because most safe and effective drugs in the group are advertised and used for 2 or even all 3 effects. So, for convenience, drugs that provide these several benefits are referred to collectively as *pain-relievers* or *analgesics*.

Drugs that thus far have been proved to be safe and effective include aspirin and several chemically related salicylates, and acetaminophen (although the latter is not effective against inflammation). Evaluations of effectiveness were based on published and unpublished studies that the Panel believed to be scientifically valid. Criteria for judging safety included the incidence and risk of adverse reactions and significant side effects when the drug is used correctly, the potential for misuse or abuse when easily available without prescription, and the benefit-to-risk ratio.

More money is spent advertising internal analgesics than any other category of nonprescription drugs. Ad campaigns have reached a new level of sophistication, with advertisers' referring to wholly new—and medically unrecognized—ailments like "file-cabinet backache" and "camper-noise tension." The Panel says that more effective government regulation of such promotions—particularly on TV commercials that are seen by children—is needed.

CLAIMS

Labeling "Musts"
amount of each active ingredient (in milligrams or grams and in grains)
conditions for which the drug is useful
clear and brief directions for use

Accurate
for "the temporary relief of occasional minor aches, pains, and headache, and for the reduction of fever"

False or Misleading
product is especially effective against certain types of pain—e.g., "postpartum pain," "pain due to cancer," "tooth extraction pain" (If one label lists a

particular pain that the product is supposed to relieve but the label of another product does not list it, a consumer can be led to believe—erroneously—that the first product will help his or her problem, while the second will not.)

confusing terms like "jumpy nerves," "fretfulness," "nighttime pain and its tension," and "under the weather"

"fast pain relief," "special pain-relieving formula," "so strong and and so gentle," "so gentle can be taken on an empty stomach," "acts 5 times faster than aspirin," "reaches peak action 12 times faster than aspirin," "long-lasting pain reliever," "enhanced relief of pain"

references to "depression" and "nervous tension" (over-the-counter pain relievers are clearly ineffective against them)

"arthritis strength" or "arthritis pain formula" (arthritis symptoms should not be treated with nonprescription drugs except as directed by a doctor)

PAIN

It is usually best to have a doctor determine the cause of pain. On the other hand, minor pain—of mild to moderate intensity—can often be successfully treated by over-the-counter drugs used at home. Minor pain is sometimes referred to as *self-limited pain*. That means it can be expected to go away by itself, without a docotor's diagnosis or treatment.

Persons who must work or maintain other normal daily activities in the face of such pain may find over-the-counter analgesics particularly useful. The several active ingredients and many products that are safe and effective work predominantly by blocking the transmission of pain impulses to the brain.

These nonprescription drugs should not be taken for more than 10 days by adults, or more than 5 days by children. And, if pain persists, one should see a doctor.

Headache

In the Panel's view, headache is in a class by itself because it is so common—almost everyone suffers one from time to time—and also because nonprescription analgesics are widely used and vigorously promoted to treat it. While self-medication is most often both appropriate and successful, experts caution that headaches vary greatly in intensity, feeling, persistence, and cause—as well as in the part of the head where pain is felt. So in some instances prescription medication or medical supervision is needed, as outlined below.

Vascular headache This pain usually occurs when blood vessels inside the brain and adjacent areas dilate or distend, so that their walls do not adapt well to blood-pressure changes. As a result, pressure variations are more keenly felt by sensory receptors in the blood-vessel walls. These sensations are experienced as pain.

One common vascular headache, hypertensive headache, is caused by a sudden rise in blood pressure. It is a dull, generalized pain, usually in the forehead, that characteristically is worse in the morning, then lessens as the day progresses.

Migraine headache, a recurrent, throbbing headache often on one side of the head, is another common form of vascular headache. Millions of people are afflicted by migraine.

Authorities say that *neither hypertensive nor migraine headache should be treated with nonprescription analgesics. Both require medical diagnosis and, usually, prescription drugs*. However, the same authorities note that headaches from fever, hangover, and caffeine withdrawal (all of which involve the vascular system) can be successfully treated with nonprescription drugs.

Psychogenic headache This malady is an extremely common plight that accounts for up to 9 out of 10 headache complaints for which sufferers see doctors. Causes include apprehension, anxiety, depression, and other emotional states. Job, social, or marital stress can also induce these headaches. Psychogenic headaches are more common after age 30. The pain usually is diffuse and difficult to describe; it is rarely confined to one side of the head. Some people experience these emotionally induced headaches as "pressure" rather than pain; this sensation may be accompanied by persistent contractions of the head, neck, and facial muscles.

Because investigators found that over-the-counter pain relievers provide little if any relief for these headaches, the Panel concurs with experts who maintain that it is advisable to get medical help. Prescription drugs are available that will provide temporary but effective relief.

Traction and inflammatory headaches Much rarer than the 2 types described above, these headaches are caused by organic disease. For example, inflammation of the sinuses (sinusitis, or allergic rhinitis) may cause a deep, dull, nonpulsating pain in the front of the head. Such headaches may also result from pressure (or traction), from brain tumors, or from inflammation of the membranes surrounding the brain. Clearly, medical care is required.

FEVER

Normal body temperature is about 98.6°F (37°C). There is slight variation in baseline temperatures among individuals and most peoples' temperatures rise and fall slightly throughout the day. Fever is defined medically as temperature above 98.6°F.

The body's balance between heat production and heat loss is controlled by the hypothalamic nuclei—tiny areas in the brain stem. In fever, this "thermostat" is set too high. Fever-lowering drugs, it is believed, act to reset this regulator so that the temperature falls back toward normal. The hypothalamus accomplishes this by increasing blood flow to vessels near the body surface and by inducing sweating —both of which serve to carry off heat.

Fever is a signal that something is wrong in the body. Current medical practice focuses on finding and treating what has caused the rise in temperature; treating the fever itself is of secondary importance. Antibiotics can be used, with good result, to treat many infections that cause fever. So, in general, fever is a less common and less persistent problem than it once was. But many pain relievers—such as acetaminophen, aspirin, and some other salicylates—do relieve fever, and they can be safely used for this purpose. Since high or persistent fever may indicate a serious illness, a doctor should be called or seen whenever an individual's temperature goes above 103°F (39.5°C) or fever persists for more than 3 days (72 hours).

ARTHRITIS

A major use of aspirin and other nonprescription analgesics is to combat the pain and inflammation of red, swollen, sore joints that are the hallmark of osteoarthritis, rheumatoid arthritis, gout, and other rheumatic disorders. Between 20 and 50 million Americans are estimated to suffer from these conditions—which together are called *arthritis*. Arthritis usually comes on with age, so that most people will have some arthritic aches and pains by the time they are 65. Yet some forms of arthritis strike very young children—so no age group is exempt.

Aspirin and related salicylates are effective ingredients for relieving this distress; acetaminophen is not. The exact way in which salicylates relieve arthritic tenderness and swelling is still not known, even though these medications have been widely used for this purpose for many decades. One current theory is that aspirin and similar drugs inhibit the body's production of substances called *prostaglandins*, which are believed to contribute to the inflammatory process.

Despite the wide use of salicylates to relieve rheumatic symptoms and related muscular discomfort, the Panel urged the FDA not to let nonprescription drugs be labeled for this purpose. It recommends that claims such as "for temporary relief of minor arthritic and rheumatic aches and pains" be forbidden because salicylates act on 2 levels, depending on dosage. Lower doses—up to 4000 mg (4 grams) of aspirin daily—can be taken safely as self-medication for temporary relief of pain and perhaps with some limited effect on the inflammation and underlying symptoms. But the larger doses—5300 mg (5.3 grams) daily —that actually appear to stop the underlying disease process may be toxic for some people. So these amounts should be taken only on prescription and under close medical supervision.

Reviewers also saw danger in the fact that self-medication at the safer, lower dosage level may relieve the immediate pain but allow the underlying disease to smolder on. So individuals who self-treat an arthritic condition with nonprescription pain relievers and do not get medical help may do irreversible damage to their joints and other tissues.

DOSAGE

Aspirin is the most widely used and widely studied of the effective over-the-counter pain relievers, so it is used as the baseline for dosage recommendations that also apply to sodium salicylate and to acetaminophen. The Panel believes they are roughly equivalent in potency. Acetaminophen has somewhat different side effects than the salicylates, and it is not effective against inflammation and other arthritic symptoms. It also has been used and studied far less than aspirin; so until there are more data, dosages for acetaminophen should not exceed those for aspirin.

The standard dosage unit for these drugs—that is, the amount that should be contained in a standard tablet, pill, or capsule—is 325 mg. This amount, 325 mg, is also considered the minimum effective dose.

Equivalent doses

Dosage for over-the-counter pain relievers are sometimes given in grains (an apothecary measure), instead of in milligrams or grams, measurements that reflect the now-preferred metric system. A 325 mg tablet contains 5 grains. Here are some common equivalences:

    1 grain—65 mg
    1.25 grains—81 mg (standard child's dosage unit)
    5 grains—325 mg (standard adult dosage unit)
    10 grains—650 mg (standard adult dosage)
    61.54 grains—4000 mg (maximum 24 hours dosage for adults)

Of the other approved over-the-counter pain relievers, magnesium salicylate, while less well studied than aspirin, is believed to be equally potent. Thus its minimum effective dose is also 325 mg. The other 2 approved salicylates are weaker. The minimum effective dose of calcium carbaspirin is 414 mg; that of choline salicylate is 435 mg.

These drugs would be far safer and easier to use if they were sold only in the standard 325 mg dosage unit (or the equivalent for the weaker ones), as the Panel recommends. But at present products are sold in nonstandard units that may deliver as little as 590 mg of aspirin when one takes 2 tablets. This amount is less than the 650 mg dose usually recommended for an adult. Or a product might provide as much as 1300 mg, which is dangerously high (more than should be taken as self-medication). This means that nonprescription-product users should never take 2 double-strength (650 mg) tablets of a pain reliever at one time, except on a doctor's advice.

If the simplification of standardizing to 325 mg dosage units cannot be achieved, evaluators recommend that dosage units be labeled as "standard" or "nonstandard," with both the standard and actual content of the tablets listed on the label.

Dosage for Adults

Two tablets every 4 hours is the most common dosage recommendation for nonprescription pain relievers for adults. This amount is the standard and correct dosage for aspirin, sodium salicylate, and acetaminophen—provided that tablets or other dosage units each contain 325 mg (5 grains) of one of these active ingredients. Translated into total quantities, this dosage means 650 mg (10 grains) of an active ingredient every 4 hours.

An initial dose of 975 mg—or 3 tablets—provides increased benefit for some people. But only *one* such dose is safe; a repeat could cause bad reactions. In light of this 975 mg safety limit, it is clear that single 1300 mg (20 grain) aspirin tablets are not safe for self-medication.

Just as there is a standard adult dose for these drugs, there also is a maximum daily amount—except for arthritics under a doctor's supervision. No one should take over 4000 mg of aspirin, sodium salicylate, or acetaminophen (or their equivalents in other nonprescription pain relievers) in 24 hours. This limit comes to about 167 mg per hour. What this means is that no more than 12 standard tables or capsules of acetaminophen, aspirin, or sodium salicylate should be taken during a 24-hour period. Beyond these limits, there is a dramatic, rapidly rising risk of toxic side effects—with little, if any, added pain relief.

Recommended Adult Dosage Schedule for Aspirin, Acetaminophen, and Sodium Salicylate

Dosage Unit	First Dose*	Subsequent Doses	24-hour Maximum Dosage
Standard dosage			
325 mg	2 tablets (650 mg)	2 after 4 hours	12 tablets (3900 mg)
Nonstandard Dosages			
325 mg	2 to 3 tablets (650 to 975 mg)	2 after 4 hours	12 tablets (3900 mg)
400 mg	1 to 2 tablets (400 to 800 mg)	1 after 3 hours	9 tablets (3600 mg)
421 mg	1 to 2 tablets (421 to 842 mg)	1 after 3 hours	9 tablets (3790 mg)
485 mg	1 to 2 tablets (485 to 970 mg)	1 after 4 hours or 2 after 6 hours	8 tablets (3880 mg)
500 mg	1 to 2 tablets (500 to 1000 mg)	1 after 3 hours or 2 after 6 hours	8 tablets (4000 mg)
650 mg	1 tablet (650 mg)	1 after 4 hours	6 tablets (3900 mg)

*A *tablet* may be a capsule, packet of powder, or measure of liquid containing the same amount of the drug.

Dosage for Children

The standard dosage unit for children is 81 mg (about 1.23 grains) of aspirin or acetaminophen. Children under age 2 should not be medicated with these drugs except when recommended by a doctor, who should determine the dose. For older children, the dose rises with age from 160 mg (2 tablets) for 2-to 4-year-olds, up to 480 mg (6 tablets) for 11-to 12-year-olds. Older children can use adult doses in the recommended schedule of one dose every 4 hours.

Recommended Children's Dosage Schedule for Aspirin or Acetaminophen

Age in Years	Dose and Frequency (Standard Dosage: 81 mg, or about 1.23 Grains)*	24-hour Maximum Dosage
Under 2	No recommended dosage except with advice and supervision of doctor	
2 to under 4	2 tablets every 4 hours (or a total of 160 mg)	800 mg
4 to under 6	3 tablets every 4 hours (or a total of 240 mg)	1200 mg
6 to under 9	4 tablets every 4 hours (or a total of 320 mg)	1600 mg
9 to under 11	5 tablets every 4 hours (or a total of 400 mg)	2000 mg
11 to under 12	6 tablets every 4 hours (or a total of 480 mg)	2400 mg
Over 12	See Recommended Adult Dosage Schedule	

*Dosage units are listed here as tablets but may be capsules, syrups, or other products containing the same amount of drug.

If children's-strength products are unavailable, the second column can be used to reckon appropriate amounts of standard, 325 mg aspirin or acetaminophen tablets. Examples: for a 2-year-old, 160 mg recommended dosage is ½ of a standard 325 mg adult aspirin tablet; for an 11-year old, 480 mg is 1½ the standard 325 mg adult tablet.

PAIN RELIEVERS

Approved Active Ingredients

Six drugs are approved as active ingredients for nonprescription pain relievers: acetaminophen, aspirin, calcium carbaspirin, choline salicylate, magnesium salicylate, and sodium salicylate. They are safe and effective for allaying mild to moderate pain.

Acetaminophen Acetaminophen is a safe, effective over-the-counter pain reliever when taken in the recommended dosage of 325 to 650 mg (5 to 10 grains) every 4 hours with limits of 4000 mg per 24-hour period and use of no longer than 10 days. (If pain persists after that period, one should seek a doctor's help.)

Acetaminophen was introduced before aspirin, in 1893. Milligram for milligram, it has been shown to be about as effective as aspirin— except against inflammatory conditions like arthritis, for which it is not effective.

Numerous clinical studies have shown that in recommended doses, the drug is relatively free of adverse effects in most age groups—even in persons suffering a variety of illnesses. Unlike aspirin, for example, it does not cause gastrointestinal bleeding and it does not interfere with drugs used to treat gout. However, it may minimally affect blood-clotting, and some people are allergic to it (and so should not use it).

Some advertising claims that acetaminophen is safer and less toxic than aspirin. Actually, the drug is metabolized by the liver, and overdoses can cause severe liver damage, even death. Alcoholics and other persons whose livers are damaged or diseased may be more vulnerable to acetaminophen toxicity—even at lower doses—than normal people with healthy livers.

CLAIMS FOR ACETAMINOPHEN

Accurate

for "the temporary relief of occasional minor aches, pains, and headache"

False or Misleading

for "nervous tension headache," "cold symptoms," "simple exertion," "simple pain of teething," "simple pain of immunization," "simple pain of tonsillectomy," "toothache," "fretfulness," "pain of neuralgia," "pain of neuritis," "pain of flu," "pain following dental procedures," "sinusitis," "overexertion," "bursitis," "sprains"

Aspirin   When taken in the recommended dosage of 325 to 650 mg (5 to 10 grains) every 4 hours, aspirin is a safe and effective nonprescription pain reliever. Self-medication with aspirin should not go beyond 10 days (after which one should consult a doctor if the pain persists), nor should one take more than 4000 mg in a 24-hour period.

Aspirin's technical name is *acetylsalicylic acid*; it is one of a group of compounds that are called *salicylates*. It is by far the most widely used over-the-counter drug in the United States; over 20 billion dosage units are sold each year. This works out to about 100 aspirin tablets per annum for every American man, woman, and child.

Aspirin is effective against mild to moderate pain that is localized or widespread, including some cancer pain. But it is not effective against severe pain. The lowest effective dose of aspirin is a little over 300 mg; increments of around 200 to 300 mg—up to somewhat over 900 mg—produce noticeable increases in pain relief. But different people respond differently to any pain reliever—so a dose of aspirin that quells one person's pain may not help another's. However, interestingly enough, 2 standard-dose aspirin tablets (a total of 650 mg) have been found to be more effective than the standard (60 mg) dose of the narcotic pain killer codeine in calming the pain of some types of advanced cancer.

Because aspirin has been widely used for such a long time and has produced comparatively few serious side effects, its safety has been well established for the majority of people; the risk-benefit ratio is low. But in some cases aspirin does have adverse effects:

- *Effects on Blood*: Aspirin interferes with blood-clotting (coagulation). So persons who have blood-coagulation defects, who are receiving anticoagulant drugs, or who suffer severe anemia should avoid it. Constant use may also cause persistent iron-deficiency anemia.
- *Effects on gastrointestinal tract*: Aspirin can trigger or aggravate peptic ulcer, and may cause stomach upset or heartburn. It can cause imperceptible bleeding from the stomach lining, and in some individuals can trigger massive bleeding into the stomach.
- *Allergic effects*: Aspirin produces allergic reactions in an estimated 2 persons per 1000 who are hypersensitive to the drug, and, more commonly, in some asthma sufferers. These reactions range from rash, hives, and swelling to asthmatic attacks that may be life-threatening.
- *Effects in pregnancy*: Aspirin interferes with blood-clotting in both mother and fetus; it can lengthen pregnancy and the process of delivery. It produces birth defects in animals and increases the incidence of stillbirths and deaths of newborn babies. It should not be taken in the last 3 months of pregnancy except under the advice and supervision of a physician.
- *Effects on central nervous system*: Aspirin overdoses may stimulate the brain and spinal cord, producing ringing in the ears (tinnitus)—a warning sign. Subsequently there is a depression in central-nervous-system functioning that may appear as respiratory failure, circulatory collapse, coma, then death.
- *Effect on kidneys*: In rare instances, aspirin can make a severe existing kidney disorder worse.

- *Effect on the liver*: High doses of aspirin may interfere with liver function. When the drug is stopped, function returns.
- *Effects of taking aspirin with other drugs*: Aspirin interferes with the action of some anticlotting and antidiabetic drugs, as well as some drugs used to treat gout. It may also enhance the ulcer-producing risk of medications taken for arthritis.

Ringing in the ears (tinnitus) is the most common and reliable sign that one is taking too much aspirin or too much of another salicylate. Hearing loss is also a fairly common early warning sign. If either occurs, the drug must be discontinued or the dose drastically reduced. These symptoms will vanish—one's hearing will return to normal—within hours to days, and at most a month after the medication is stopped.

Other early signs of aspirin toxicity include headache, dizziness, vomiting, rapid breathing, extreme irritability, and even bizarre behavior. The danger signs of aspirin toxicity in children may be different from those in adults. For example, nausea or rapid breathing may occur before ringing in the ears does.

As noted in the list of adverse reactions, aspirin interferes with the blood's ability to clot. So persons who are scheduled for surgery or dental work should tell their doctors ahead of time if they are taking aspirin.

A new risk for children has been reported. In 1982 the FDA was in the process of preparing a new mandatory label warning against using aspirin to treat youngsters who have chicken pox, flu, or late-winter flulike symptoms. The danger is this: a very high percentage of children who suffer or who die from a rare liver disorder called Reye's syndrome turn out to have been treated with aspirin to relieve chicken pox or flu symptoms. Whether—and if so, how—aspirin enhances their risk is not known. Treatment with acetaminophen appears *not* to carry this risk.

CLAIMS FOR ASPIRIN

Accurate

for "the temporary relief of occasional minor aches, pains, and headache"

False or Misleading

for "comforting relief of aches," "pains caused by: colds and flu, inoculations, minor ailments, tonsillectomy," "pains caused by teething," "under the weather," "pains of neuralgia," "pains of neuritis," "gargle for sore throat," "sinusitis," "pains of mild migraine," "tooth extraction," "pains of minor injuries," "pains of dysmenorrhea," "discomfort of ordinary colds," "pains of sciatica," "swollen tissues," "jumpy nerves," "minor sore-throat irritation," "sleeplessness caused by minor painful distress," "normal menstrual distress," "premenstrual tension," "functional menstrual pains and cramps," "the blues," "nervous tension headache," "feeling of depression," "minor pain of arthritis," "minor pain of rheumatism," "sore, stiff aching muscles," "muscular fatigue," "muscle tension," "low back pain," "bursitis," "lumbago," "low body ache due to fatigue," "body aches," "fever of colds and flu," "reduc[ing] fever in simple headaches, minor muscular aches, neuritis, neuralgia"

Aspirin, far more than any other approved pain reliever, has been formulated into a wide variety of special products intended to enhance effectiveness, safety, and appeal. Some of these formulations—chewable aspirin for children and buffered aspirin, to name just 2—make the medication easier to take for persons who tolerate the ordinary tablets poorly.

Some of these special formulations have been demonstrated to be safe and effective. A few have not. In some cases, while the product itself is judged to be okay, the manufacturer's claims are exaggerated or unproved. These are the principal special aspirin formulations:

• *Buffered aspirin*: Buffering agents, principally antacid compounds—that is, they are *alkaline* as opposed to *acid*—are added to aspirin to make it dissolve faster in the stomach. This is supposed to make the active ingredient act faster to relieve pain. Buffering is also intended to reduce gastric irritation. The stomach is naturally acidic. When its contents are neutralized by the alkaline buffer, acidic aspirin can supposedly dissolve and be absorbed more rapidly.

There is more alkaline in highly buffered *effervescent powders*—which must be mixed with water before being swallowed—than there is in the buffered tablets. Both kinds of preparations—which usually are identified as such in the product name or on the label—*may* speed up the absorption of aspirin from the stomach. Also, some highly buffered aspirins have been shown to significantly decrease mild, unnoticed bleeding in the stomach. Because they facilitate absorption, highly buffered preparations are an ideal way to take aspirin. There is, however, little scientifically meaningful difference in the absorption rates between many buffered and nonbuffered aspirin products. Moreover, there are no data satisfactorily demonstrating that buffered aspirin provides pain relief with a more rapid onset, a greater peak intensity, or prolonged duration.

Buffered and highly buffered aspirins may diminish the stomach distress that a relatively small number of people experience when they take aspirin. But they do not necessarily reduce the rare-but-real risk of massive gastrointestinal bleeding—so they cannot be considered safer in that regard. Some buffering ingredients are more effective than others, and some poorly formulated preparations may dissolve no more rapidly than ordinary aspirin. Also, some unbuffered calcium salts of aspirin dissolve more rapidly than buffered aspirin.

- *Chewable aspirin tablets:* Flavored, chewable tablets are convenient for children or for grown-ups who cannot or will not swallow whole tablets; they are an acceptable way to formulate aspirin. Children should be told to drink water after they take chewable aspirin.
- *Enteric-coated tablets:* Aspirin tablets can be given special coatings to keep them from dissolving in the stomach, as a way to prevent gastric irritation and possible bleeding. The aim is to delay dissolving until they leave the stomach and can be absorbed from the small intestine instead. But there are problems: the tablets may take several hours to reach the intestine, so that pain relief may be delayed, and some tablets may fail to dissolve at all. For these reasons, enteric-coated preparations are only conditionally approved, pending tests to prove they will produce reliable and adequate levels of aspirin in the blood.
- *Time-release aspirin:* These products are designed to dissolve more slowly than ordinary aspirin, and over a longer period of time. But effective time-release products have been difficult to produce because of technical deficiencies. Too, it is debatable whether a 1300 mg sustained-release aspirin tablet is as effective as two 650 mg doses of ordinary aspirin given 4 hours apart. So these products were given only a qualified approval from the Panel, which wants the manufacturers to prove that such preparations provide comparable relief and no more side effects than ordinary aspirin.
- *Micronized aspirin:* There is no convincing scientific evidence that formulating aspirin in tinier-than-ordinary particles improves it in any way.
- *Aspirin capsules:* Some people find smooth-sided capsules easier to swallow than tablets. These products are otherwise comparable to ordinary aspirins.
- *Aspirin powders:* While not commonly used, aspirin powders are absorbed and reach effective blood levels faster than tablets. They may be easier to give to children than tablets or capsules are, once the powder is dissolved in a full glass of water.

- *Chewing-gum aspirin:* Aspirin in a gum base is effective—but it may not be safe if a person has sore gums or a sore mouth.
- *Rectal suppositories:* Aspirin-impregnated rectal suppositories are a good way of giving the drug to people who are vomiting, unconscious, or otherwise unable to take it by mouth. But absorption is slow and the suppositories can slip out—thus their value as nonprescription medications remains to be proved outside of use in these special circumstances.

Calcium carbaspirin   This is a safe and effective nonprescription pain reliever when one takes the recommended dosage of 414 to 828 mg every 4 hours, no more than 4970 mg during 24 hours, and for no longer than 10 days. (After that length of time, a doctor should be seen if the pain persists.)

Calcium carbaspirin—frequently called *soluble calcium aspirin*—is similar to aspirin but it contains calcium and urea (which aspirin does not). It is only four-fifths as strong on a milligram-for-milligram basis, so *more* must be taken to get the same result as aspirin might afford.

The standard dosage unit of calcium carbaspirin is 414 mg (roughly one and a quarter times the 325-mg standard dose for aspirin), so the standard adult dose is 828 mg. (For children, multiply the dosages in the RECOMMENDED CHILDREN'S DOSAGE SCHEDULE on page 583 by 1.24 to obtain the right equivalences.)

Calcium carbaspirin dissolves in the stomach more rapidly than ordinary aspirin, but one team of researchers found that it offers no significant advantage over aspirin in the rate at which it gives relief from pain. It may produce slightly less gastrointestinal bleeding than aspirin, but this has not been scientifically demonstrated. Beyond the possibility that calcium carbaspirin might be slightly less irrritating to the stomach and intestines, the drug's effectiveness and safety are quite like aspirin's—given the difference in dosage requirements.

CLAIMS FOR CALCIUM CARBASPIRIN

Accurate
for "the temporary relief of occasional minor aches, pains, and headache"

False or Misleading
for "pains due to sinusitis," "minor aches and pains of arthritis," "minor aches and pains of rheumatism"

Choline salicylate   Choline salicylate is a safe and effective nonprescription product for relief of pain as long as it is taken as recommended: 435 to 870 mg every 4 hours with no more than 5220 mg in a 24-hour period. If pain persists after 10 days, medical care should be sought.

Choline salicylate is similar to aspirin, but unlike aspirin it is highly soluble. Because of this, it may be sold and stored as a stable, palatable liquid. One of its particular advantages is that it is the *only* aspirinlike drug available over-the-counter in liquid form.

Choline salicylate is absorbed from the stomach rapidly, which may forestall the stomach aches and cramps that sometimes follow ingestion of ordinary aspirin. But there is no evidence that this faster absorption brings quicker relief of pain; one investigator noted that even if this were so, it would be absurd to claim advantages for any compound that may hasten relief by no more than a few minutes.

Milligram for milligram, choline salicylate is weaker than aspirin, so that a larger dose is needed to produce the equivalent pain relief. The standard dosage unit of the drug, 435 mg, is 1.3 times greater than the standard dosage of aspirin. The choline salicylate standard dosage for adults is 870 mg (the equivalent of 650 mg of aspirin) every 4 hours. For children, multiply by 1.3 the aspirin doses in the RECOMMENDED CHILDREN'S DOSAGE SCHEDULE on page 583.

Choline salicylate is less well studied than aspirin, but the comparisons that have been made suggest that its actions and risks appear comparable to those of aspirin.

CLAIMS FOR CHOLINE SALICYLATE

Accurate
for "the temporary relief of occasional minor aches, pains, and headache"

False or Misleading
for "menstruation," "menstrual cramps," "neuralgia," "pains of arthritis," "pains of rheumatism"

Magnesium salicylate   This magnesium-aspirin compound is a safe and effective nonprescription analgesic when taken as recommended. It is equal in potency to aspirin: 650 mg every 4 hours, no more than 4000 mg in 24 hours, and use no longer than 10 days without consulting a doctor.

Magnesium salicylate has been studied far less extensively than ordinary aspirin, but it seems essentially equivalent. Claims that it may be the drug to use when aspirin is not tolerated remain to be proved —although thus far it appears that it does *not* cause asthmatic attacks in susceptible persons, which can happen with aspirin and some other salicylates. Thus the compound may be particularly useful for the few asthmatic individuals who are sensitive to aspirin.

CLAIMS FOR MAGNESIUM SALICYLATE

Accurate
for "the temporary relief of occasional minor aches, pains, and headaches"

False or Misleading
for "pain of menstrual period," "pains of sciatica," "dental pains," "overexertion," "fatigue," "minor aches and pains of rheumatism," "minor aches and pains of arthritis," "minor muscle aches," "aches and pains due to fatigue"

Sodium salicylate   When used in the recommended dosage—325 to 650 mg every 4 hours, no more than 4000 mg in a 24-hour period, and for no longer than 10 days without a doctor's consultation—this compound is safe and effective.

Originally, aspirin was introduced to the market because it was believed to be more palatable and cause less stomach distress than sodium salicylate. But the 2 ingredients are essentially similar in these and all other matters of safety—save that sodium salicylate appears not to provoke asthmatic attacks in susceptible persons, as ordinary aspirin does. However, persons who are on sodium-restricted diets because of high blood pressure or other disorders would be wise to use other over-the-counter pain relievers that do not contain sodium.

CLAIMS FOR SODIUM SALICYLATE

Accurate
for "the temporary relief of occasional minor aches, pains, and headache"

False or Misleading
for "minor muscle pains and aches," "arthritis," "rheumatism"

Conditionally Approved Active Ingredients

There are several pain-relieving nonprescription drugs for which there still is too little evidence for evaluators to decide about safety and effectiveness.

Aluminum aspirin   This salicylate, very similar to ordinary aspirin, is safe. But it may not be wholly effective in the recommended dosage of 365 to 730 mg every 4 hours. No more than 4380 mg should be taken in a 24-hour period; if pain continues beyond 10 days, a doctor should be consulted.

The problem with aluminum aspirin is not its safety, which appears to be comparable to aspirin's, but its efficacy, since it dissolves very slowly in the stomach and may be absorbed far less rapidly than ordinary aspirin. There are some indications in unpublished reports that this slow dissolution and absorption may prolong the pain relief it provides. However, this claim remains to be proved.

Antipyrine   While widely used in Europe, antipyrine has seen limited use in the United States. It is in a wholly different class of drugs from aspirin and acetaminophen. In terms of safety, it is said not to interfere with blood-clotting, as aspirin does, nor is it believed to damage the liver—even when taken in large doses—as acetaminophen does. But more studies are needed to confirm these tentative findings. The major block to full approval is that a small number of persons, apparently many of them blacks, are highly allergic to antipyrine. Before 1950, 394 poisoning cases and 23 deaths were reported; since 1950 there have been no reported fatalities. Severe skin eruptions are one of the principal allergic reactions; anyone who notices a rash while taking antipyrine should stop using the drug and see a doctor.

Antipyrine has a long-lasting effect against pain—a single dose of 975 mg provides relief for 24 hours. So the majority of Panel members believe it should be carefully studied, as it has not yet been, to see if antipyrine can be recommended for persons who cannot tolerate other analgesics. But a minority of the evaluators—in an unusual division of opinion—feel that the drug's side effects can be so severe in the small percentage of people who appear to be highly allergic to it, that it is too dangerous to study in human subjects. These members argued that antipyrine should be banned at once as a nonprescription drug.

Antipyrine is *not* recommended for children under 12.

Salicylamide   Chemically less closely related to aspirin than its name would suggest, salicylamide became widely used in the last 30 years in combination products: that is, in pain relievers combined with cold preparations in quantities between 100 and 400 mg per dosage unit. There are too little data to determine whether it is either safe or effective in these doses.

Much larger amounts—up to 1000 mg or even 2000 mg every 4 to 6 hours—appear to be effective, but studies that would establish the safety of these larger quantities have not been completed as yet. Reviewers' skepticism about the lower doses that are currently used reflects the finding that small amounts of salicylamide are almost completely broken down—extremely quickly—in the body. Most of the substance is gone before it ever gets into the bloodstream, where it could be carried throughout the body to relieve pain. It appears that the only way to get an effective amount of this drug into the bloodstream is to give a dose of 1000 mg or more—enough to overwhelm the enzyme system that controls its breakdown. On the other hand, in doses under 600 mg, salicylamide has been shown to provide no more pain relief than dummy medication. Salicylamide also lacks aspirin's anti-inflammatory property, so it is far less effective against arthritic symptoms.

The drug's safety has been inadequately studied. It does not cause the gastrointestinal irritation and bleeding that aspirin can, and ought to be safer in this respect—although large doses can produce stomach aches. Very large doses have also produced toxic effects in other organs —particularly in children, for whom it is not recommended for use without prescription.

Salsalate   Also called *salicylsalicylic acid*, this drug has not been shown to be safe or effective in the recommended dosage of 500 to 1000 mg every 4 hours. Little research has been done on the substance. It is known to dissolve rather slowly, so it might be expected to be absorbed slowly or incompletely. Because of the slow absorption, salsalate is at best only two-thirds as potent as aspirin—despite claims that it may approach aspirin in its ability to relieve pain and fever.

Because salsalate is composed of 2 molecules of salicylic acid, the active ingredient in ordinary aspirin, it has been assumed that its safety is like aspirin's. This simplistic view is not justified and studies to establish the agent's safety remain to be done. Claims that it is safer than aspirin particularly need to be proved. In the meantime, the drug seems comparable to aspirin in the severity and incidence of its side effects—so that warnings applicable to aspirin are appropriate for salsalate too.

CLAIMS FOR SALSALATE

Accurate

for "the temporary relief of occasional minor aches, pains, and headache"

False or Misleading

for "minor pains, swelling, stiffness of arthritis," "minor pains, swelling, stiffness of fibrositis," "minor pains, swelling, stiffness of osteoarthritis" "aspirin—for relief of arthritis"

Disapproved Active Ingredients

Many over-the-counter pain relievers still marketed contain active ingredients that are ineffective, unsafe, or mislabeled. The Panel has recommended that they be banned from nonprescription products sold in the United States.

Acetanilid Though marketed for many years for the relief of pain and fever, this drug is currently not readily found in over-the-counter products because the effective dose is very close to the toxic dose. There are many reports of poisoning; a number of these incidents resulted in death. The toxic compound is the breakdown product aniline, which has no beneficial effect. The pain-relieving property of acetanilid comes from another breakdown product, acetaminophen, which does *not* have aniline's poisonous properties. But acetaminophen is available as such (*see* ACETAMINOPHEN, page 583), so it makes no sense to take acetanilid to obtain acetaminophen's benefits.

Codeine This narcotic agent, derived from opium, is a very effective pain killer in the dosages used in prescription drugs. But in the small amounts—from 10 to 20 mg codeine per dose—that the federal government now allows in nonprescription products, it is ineffective against pain. Moreover, because it is a narcotic, codeine has the potential for abuse; it may cause narcotic dependence when taken in large amounts over a period of time.

Because of its addictive properties codeine is not sold over-the-counter as a single-ingredient product in the United States. It is available in combination products for treating coughs—for which it is recognized as safe and very effective (*see* CODEINE in COLD, COUGH, AND ALLERGY DRUGS).

Iodopyrine There is no scientific evidence to show that this compound—more widely used in Europe than in the United States—is actually effective. As for safety, it liberates free iodide in the body. This can cause iodine poisoning, so the risks outweigh any possible benefits from its use.

Phenacetin   This is the "P" in popular, once widely sold APC tablets that are used for pain relief and fever. Phenacetin has been used for 80 years, usually in combination with other ingredients. It is an effective drug against pain and fever, although not against rheumatic complaints. But it is less effective than aspirin or acetaminophen, and since the latter—a breakdown product of phenacetin—is available on its own there is no reason to take phenacetin to get the benefits of the acetaminophen.

But aside from the question of effectiveness, the main problem with phenacetin is its safety—or lack of it. Short-term use at recommended doses has not posed a major hazard, but potentially fatal blood disorders can be triggered in unborn babies when their mothers take only 1 or 2 usual doses. Long-term use is especially hazardous. Excessive use of phenacetin over a long period of time can cause life-threatening diseases of the kidneys and lower urinary tract, including kidney and bladder cancer.

Because of the risk of kidney failure and cancer, phenacetin already is banned or restricted as a nonprescription ingredient in Canada and in England, Sweden, and Denmark. Most of the reported cases of phenacetin-related kidney disease have thus far been from Europe. If American doctors had been on the lookout for this type of poisoning—and they appear not to have been—they might have found it to be a major health problem in the United States as well.

Adding to phenacetin's danger is the fact that its effects stimulate feelings of euphoria (an exaggerated sense of well-being). Many users —a large proportion of whom studies show to be anxious, middle-aged women—do not take phenacetin to relieve pain, strictly speaking. Rather, they take it because the drug appears to act as a mood elevator. Phenacetin is also abused by factory workers, who sometimes take it to increase their work output. But after prolonged use it causes headache, fatigue, and apathy—mood depression. These central-nervous symptoms diminish or vanish when use of the drug is discontinued.

The potential for abuse inherent in phenacetin does not appear to persist in its breakdown product acetaminophen—which the panel says is a safe and effective pain-relieving drug (*see* ACETAMINOPHEN, page 583), nor have phenacetin's other serious risks been shown to afflict acetaminophen users.

Because of its high potential for abuse and its high potential for serious harm, phenacetin is not safe for use as an analgesic in over-the-counter pain relievers. It has been banned by the FDA from over-the-counter products as of August, 1983.

Quinine The ground-up bark of the cinchona tree has long been known to relieve fever. It also relieves pain. Lately it has been particularly recommended for relief of nighttime leg cramps. However, reviewers concluded that the high dosage required for this kind of relief should be prescribed by a doctor.

Quinine is quite toxic, causing ringing in the ears, headache, nausea, visual disturbances, and other symptoms. The drug is poisonous to the cardiovascular system, and can cause death. Such risks heavily outweigh any value that it might have as an over-the-counter drug.

Other Ingredients

A number of substances besides active ingredients are put into over-the-counter pain relievers. Some are believed by manufacturers to be active ingredients, contrary to the Panel's judgment. Others are included for different reasons, and reviewers classify them as described below.

Adjuvants In the amounts used, adjuvants, or "helpers," have no significant pain-relieving ability—but they may *contribute* (directly or indirectly) to the effectiveness of an active ingredient. Some adjuvants enhance a drug's response by increasing its effect at the site(s) where it acts in the body. Others act elsewhere to modify the drug's absorption, breakdown, distribution, or excretion from the body.

• *Caffeine* This substance is one of the best known of those believed to act as an adjuvant. Caffeine is the "C" in the popular, once widely marketed APC tablets. People who cannot tolerate caffeine should, clearly, avoid APCs. It is safe in amounts up to 65 mg per dose.
Caffeine is mildly habit-forming and mildly toxic. More important, while it has been said to have pain-relieving properties in its own right, this has not been demonstrated scientifically—so caffeine cannot be claimed to be an active ingredient in over-the-counter pain medication. However, there is some evidence that relatively small amounts—65 mg per dosage unit or less—may enhance the effects of active pain-relieving drugs with which it is combined. In these circumstances the caffeine may be acting as a mood elevator. Another possibility is that caffeine helps to relieve headaches by tightening up the distended blood vessels that are causing the pain. But exactly how this ingredient works remains to be established.

- *Antihistamines*: Small amounts of antihistamines are sometimes added to over-the-counter pain relievers.
  While these substances are useful for other purposes (described elsewhere in several units of this book), they are not effective against pain. They *may* have adjuvant value in boosting the pain relief provided by aspirin and other active ingredients, but this has not been proved. They are safe for this purpose. Compounds in this category include pheniramine maleate, phenyltoloxamine, and pyrilamine maleate.
- *Salicylamide*: Despite some questions regarding safety, this compound, discussed as an active ingredient on page 592, is known to be effective in doses of 1000 mg every 4 hours. But because it is so rapidly broken down before it reaches the general circulation, lower doses are unlikely to have any direct pain-killing activity. Yet salicylamide is marketed in a variety of over-the-counter pain-killing combination products—usually with aspirin or acetaminophen—in amounts of about 200 mg per dose. There is some evidence that in these lower doses it enhances the analgesic effect of the other compounds. But this remains to be demonstrated conclusively, and, if true, knowledge of how it actually works and what doses are appropriate must be more clearly defined.
- *Benzoic acid compounds*: Some over-the-counter antirheumatic medications contain benzoic acid and related compounds. They include aminobenzoic acid, which is also called para-aminobenzoic acid (or PABA), and sodium para-aminobenzoate. These compounds have not been proved effective, and they are not safe.

Correctives (side-effect reducers) These ingredients are intended to reduce one or more undesirable side effects of an active agent. Their principal role in over-the-counter analgesics is to act as antacid and buffering agents—for example, speeding aspirin's dissolution and buffering the stomach lining against its acidity. These compounds include:

aminoacetic acid (glycine, glycocol)	dihydroxyaluminum sodium
calcium carbonate	carbonate
calcium phosphate dibasic	dried aluminum hydroxide gel
(monocalcium phosphate)	magnesium carbonate
citric acid (sodium citrate)	magnesium hydroxide
dihydroxyaluminum aminoacetate	sodium bicarbonate
(aluminum glycinate)	sodium carbonate

Descriptions and Panel evaluations can be found in the unit ANTA-CIDS.

COMBINATION PRODUCTS

The nonprescription pain-relieving active ingredients are formulated into a large number of combination products. The medicinal advantage of buffering ingredients has been established. But the advantage of most other combined products—which consumer sources say may be much more expensive than single-ingredient products—has not been established. In general, the Panel ruled that an over-the-counter product with fewer ingredients provides greater safety. The standards of the Panel for combination pain-relieving products are summarized below.

Combinations of Two Pain Relievers

Under the Panel's standards, no product should contain more than 2 active pain-relieving ingredients. Combinations of 2 safe and effective pain relievers are approved—*provided* that each tablet or dosage unit contains at least the minimally effective dose but no more than the maximum recommended amount of each ingredient.

The minimum effective dose of both aspirin and acetaminophen is 325 mg. So, for example, a product containing 400 mg of aspirin and 250 mg of acetaminophen per tablet would not meet this standard of approval because it contains too little of the latter ingredient. This would rate only conditional approval.

No combination product is specifically approved for the relief of arthritic pain or other rheumatic symptoms. Evaluators believe that arthritis medication should be purchased and used only under medical supervision.

Combination products that contain conditionally approved or disapproved active ingredients are categorized as conditionally approved or disapproved by the applicable standards. For example, a combination containing salicylamide plus 325 mg of aspirin would be conditionally approved. One that contained phenacetin (a disapproved ingredient) plus 325 mg aspirin would be disapproved.

Combinations of Pain Relievers + Other Active Ingredients

One or 2 safe and effective pain relievers, in effective amounts, may be combined with other approved active ingredients intended to achieve a different purpose. But *all* active ingredients must help relieve at least one of the symptoms for which the combination is intended. Further, the whole must be as safe and as effective as any of its parts.

Mixes that the Panel approved as reasonable are those with one or more safe and effective pain relievers combined with one or more safe and effective antitussive agents, expectorants, nasal decongestants, or antihistamines.

Nonsalicylates may be combined with antacids. Aspirin and other salicylates are combined with small amounts of antacids that act to buffer acidity. But such a product cannot be promoted for the treatment of heartburn, sour stomach, and/or acid indigestion, because aspirin can *cause* heartburn and stomach distress. Authorities say that people who need antacids for their stomach should not take them in combination with aspirin. If they want to treat their stomachs and relieve pain at the same time, they would do better to select a combination of an antacid plus acetaminophen—which is less irritating.

Combinations of aspirin plus a bronchodilator (bronchial muscle relaxer) are unsafe because a small percentage of asthmatic persons who may have urgent need for bronchodilators are also fatally allergic to aspirin. Another disapproved combination is analgesics that are mixed with laxatives or vitamins; despite wide availability, their use makes no sense because the need for the amount of each ingredient should be determined individually. Premixed combinations may not meet these individual needs.

All combinations that contain caffeine are only conditionally approved. Caffeine is not in itself an effective pain reliever and it remains to be determined whether relatively small amounts of it will boost the pain relief provided by other ingredients.

Safety and Effectiveness: Active Ingredients in Over-the-Counter Drugs for Pain, Fever, and Rheumatic Symptoms

Active Ingredient	Pain Relief†	Fever	Rheumatic (Arthritic) Symptoms‡
acetaminophen	safe and effective	safe and effective	safe, but not effective
acetanilid	not safe	not safe	not safe or effective
aluminum aspirin*	safe, but not proved effective	safe, but not proved effective	safe, but not proved effective
antipyrine	not proved safe or effective	not proved safe or effective	not proved safe or effective
aspirin (acetylsalicylic acid)*	safe and effective	safe and effective	safe and effective
calcium carbaspirin*	safe and effective	safe and effective	safe and effective
choline salicylate*	safe and effective	safe and effective	safe and effective
codeine	not safe or effective	not safe or effective	not safe or effective
iodopyrine	not safe	not safe	not safe
magnesium salicylate*	safe and effective	safe and effective	safe and effective
phenacetin	not safe	not safe	not safe or effective
quinine	not safe	not safe	not safe or effective
salicylamide	not proved safe or effective	not proved safe or effective	not effective
salsalate*	not proved safe or effective	not proved safe or effective	not proved safe or effective
sodium salicylate*	safe and effective	safe and effective	safe and effective

*These ingredients belong to aspirin family (salicylates).
†Pain-relief listing includes simple headache.
‡OTC drugs should not be taken for rheumatic symptoms except when prescribed by a doctor.

Safety and Effectiveness: Adjuvant ("Helper") Ingredients in Over-the-Counter Drugs for Pain, Fever, and Rheumatic Symptoms

Adjuvant	Evaluation
aminobenzoic acid (PABA)	not safe
sodium para-aminobenzoate	not safe
caffeine	safe, but not proved effective
pheniramine maleate	safe, but not proved effective
phenyltoloxamine	safe, but not proved effective
pyrilamine maleate	safe, but not proved effective
salicylamide	not proved safe or effective

Pain, Fever, and Anti-Inflammatory Drugs Taken Internally: Product Ratings

Single-Ingredient Products

Product and Distributor	Dosage of Active Ingredients	Rating[1]	Comment
acetaminophen[2]			
acetaminophen or APAP (generic)	tablets: 325 mg	A	adult dosage
Datril (Bristol-Myers)		A	
Febrinol (Vitarine)		A	
SK-APAP (SKF)		A	
Tylenol Regular Strength (McNeil)		A	
acetaminophen (generic)	tablets: 500 mg	C	nonstandard dosage
Datril 500 (Bristol-Myers)		C	nonstandard dosage
Acetaminophen (Philips Roxane)	tablets: 650 mg	A	
acetaminophen or APAP (generic)	elixir: 120 mg per teaspoonful (5 ml)	C	nonstandard dosage
Pedric (Vale)		C	nonstandard dosage
Tenol (Vortech)		C	nonstandard dosage
Acetaminophen Uniserts (Usher-Smith)	suppositories: 120 mg	C	this dosage form not assessed by Panel
	325 mg		
Dolanex (Lannett)	elixir: 325 mg per teaspoonful (5 ml)	A	
Phenaphen (Robins)	capsules: 325 mg	A	
Tylenol (McNeil)	tablets, chewable: 80 mg	A	children's dosage
Tylenol Extra Strength (McNeil)	liquid: 165 mg per teaspoonful (5 ml)	A	2 teaspoonful is the approved minimally effective adult dosage
	capsules: 500 mg	C	nonstandard dosage
aspirin (acetylsalicylic acid)			
A.S.A. (Lilly)	tablets: 325 mg	A	standard adult dosage unit
aspirin (generic)		A	
Bayer Aspirin (Glenbrook)			

Drug (manufacturer)	Dosage form	Rating	Notes
Empirin Analgesic (Burroughs-Wellcome)		A	
A.S.A. Enseals (Lilly)	tablets, enteric coated: 325 mg	B	this form not proved effective
aspirin (generic)		B	this form not proved effective
A.S.A. (Lilly)	capsules: 325 mg	A	nonstandard dosage
Aspirin (Bowman)	tablets: 500 mg	C	nonstandard dosage
aspirin (generic)	tablets: 650 mg	A	
aspirin (generic)	suppositories: 65 mg through 1.2 g	B	not proved safe or effective for self-treatment outside of emergency situations
Aspergum (Plough)	chewable gum tablets: 210 mg	C	nonstandard dosage
Bayer Timed-Release Aspirin (Glenbrook)	tablets, timed release: 650 mg	B	timed-release aspirin not proved safe or effective
Measurin (Breon)		B	timed-release aspirin not proved safe or effective
children's aspirin (generic)	tablets: 65 mg	C	nonstandard dosage
children's aspirin (generic)	tablets: 81 mg	A	children's dosage unit
Bayer Children's Aspirin (Glenbrook)		A	children's dosage unit
aspirin, buffered			
Aluprin (Lemmon)	tablets: 300 mg + magnesium hydroxide + aluminum hydroxide	C	nonstandard dosage
Antalgesic (Spencer-Mead)	tablets: 325 mg + 97.5 mg magnesium carbonate and aluminum glycinate	A	
Arthritis Pain Formula (Whitehall)	tablets: 487.5 mg + 60 mg magnesium hydroxide + 20 mg dried aluminum hydroxide	C	nonstandard dosage
Ascriptin (Rorer)	tablets: 325 mg + 150 mg aluminum magnesium hydroxide	A	
buffered aspirin (generic)	tablets: 325 mg + buffers	A	

Pain, Fever, and Anti-Inflammatory Drugs Taken Internally: Product Ratings *(continued)*

Single-Ingredient Products

Product and Distributor	Dosage of Active Ingredients	Rating[1]	Comment
Bufferin (Bristol-Myers)	**tablets:** 324 mg + 97.2 mg magnesium carbonate + 48.6 mg aluminum glycinate	A	
Bufferin, Arthritis Strength (Bristol-Myers)	**tablets:** 486 mg + 145.8 mg magnesium carbonate + 72.9 mg dried aluminum glycinate	C	nonstandard dosage
Bufferin Extra Strength (Bristol-Myers)	**capsules:** 500 mg + magnesium oxide + magnesium carbonate + calcium carbonate	C	nonstandard dosage; too much aspirin
Cama Inlay-Tabs (Dorsey)	**tablets:** 600 mg + 150 mg magnesium hydroxide + 150 mg aluminum hydroxide	C	nonstandard dosage
choline salicylate			
Arthropan (Purdue-Frederick)	**liquid:** 870 mg per teaspoonful (5 ml)	A	
magnesium salicylate			
Doan's Pills (Jeffrey Martin)	**tablets:** 325 mg	A	
quinine sulfate			
Quinine Sulfate (Lilly)	**tablets:** 325 mg	C	not safe
	capsules: 325 mg, 200 mg, 130 mg	C	not safe
salicylamide			
salicylamide (generic)	**tablets:** 325 mg	B	not proved safe or effective; not effective against inflammation
	650 mg	B	
Uromide (Edwards)	**tablets:** 667 mg	B	not proved safe or effective; not

sodium salicylate

Product and Distributor	Dosage	Rating¹	Comment
sodium salicylate (generic)	**tablets:** 325 mg	A	
	650 mg	A	
sodium salicylate (generic)	**tablets, enteric-coated:** 325 mg	B	enteric-coated tablets not proved effective
	650 mg	B	
Uracel 5 (North American)	**tablets, enteric-coated:** 324 mg	B	enteric-coated tablets not proved effective

Effervescent Products

Product and Distributor	Dosage of Active Ingredients	Rating¹	Comment
Alka-Seltzer (Miles)	**effervescent tablets:** 324 mg aspirin + 1.9 g sodium bicarbonate + 1 g citric acid	A	
Bromo Seltzer (Warner-Lambert)	**effervescent granules:** 325 mg acetaminophen + 2.781 g sodium bicarbonate + 2.224 g citric acid per capful measure	A	

Narcotic Liquid Combination Products³

Product and Distributor	Narcotic	Acetaminophen	Rating¹	Comment
acetaminophen with codeine elixir (generic)	12 mg codeine phosphate	120 mg per teaspoonful	C	codeine not safe or effective
Bayapap with Codeine Elixir (Bay)			C	
Tylenol with Codeine Elixir (McNeil)			C	

Pain, Fever, and Anti-Inflammatory Drugs Taken Internally: Product Ratings *(continued)*

Non-Narcotic Combination Products

Product and Distributor	Aspirin	Acetaminophen	Other Analgesic	Other	Rating[1]	Comment
Anacin Tablets (Whitehall)	400 mg			32 mg caffeine	C	nonstandard dosage; caffeine not proved effective
Anacin-3 (Aspirin-Free) Tablets (Whitehall)		500 mg		32 mg caffeine	C	nonstandard dosage
A.P.C. Buffered Tablets (Bowman)	162.5 mg		162.5 mg phenacetin	16.25 mg caffeine + glycine	C	phenacetin not safe
A.P.C. capsules or tablets (generic) P-A-C Compound Tablets (Upjohn)	227.5 mg		162.5 mg phenacetin	32.5 mg caffeine	C	phenacetin not safe
BC Powder (Block)	650 mg			195 mg salicylamide + 32 mg caffeine	B	salicylamide and caffeine not proved effective
BC Tablets (Block)	325 mg			95 mg salicylamide + 16 mg caffeine	B	salicylamide and caffeine not proved effective
Cope (Glenbrook)	421 mg			32 mg caffeine + 50 mg magnesium hydroxide + 25 mg aluminum hydroxide magnesium hydroxide	C	nonstandard dosage of aspirin; caffeine not proved effective
Duragesic Tablets (Glaxo)	325 mg		162 mg salsalate		B	salsalate not proved effective

Product					Rating	Comment
Excedrin Capsules (Bristol-Myers)	250 mg	250 mg		65 mg caffeine	C	nonstandard dosage; caffeine not proved effective
Excedrin Tablets (Bristol-Myers)	250 mg	250 mg		65 mg caffeine	C	nonstandard dosage of active ingredients; caffeine not proved effective
Gaysal-S Tablets (Geriatric)	180 mg		300 mg sodium salicylate	60 mg aluminum hydroxide	C	less-than-effective dosage of both pain relievers
Gemnisyn Tablets (Rorer)	325 mg	325 mg			A	
Momentum Tablets (Whitehall)	162.5 mg (microfined)		325 mg salsalate	12.5 mg phenyltoloxamine citrate	B	salsalate and antihistamine not proved effective
Persistin Tablets (Fisons)	162.5 mg		487.5 mg salsalate		B	salsalate not proved effective
Presalin Tablets (Mallard)	260 mg	120 mg		120 mg salicylamide + 100 mg aluminum hydroxide	B	less-than-effective dosage of pain relievers; adjuvant not proved effective
Pirin-C (Scrip)			450 mg salicylamide	30 mg vitamin C	C	pain killer + vitamin combination makes no sense
Rid-A-Pain Compound Capsules (Pfeiffer)	226.8 mg		97.2 mg salicylamide	32.4 mg caffeine	C	less-than-effective dosage of acetaminophen; other ingredients not proved effective

Pain, Fever, and Anti-Inflammatory Drugs Taken Internally: Product Ratings (continued)

Non-Narcotic Combination Products

Product and Distributor	Aspirin	Acetaminophen	Other Analgesic	Other	Rating[1]	Comment
Salatin Capsules (Ferndale)	259.2 mg	129.6 mg		16.2 mg caffeine	C	less-than-effective dosage of pain relievers
Vanquish Caplets (Glenbrook)	227 mg	194 mg		33 mg caffeine + 50 mg magnesium hydroxide + 25 mg aluminum hydroxide	C	less-than-effective dosage of pain relievers; caffeine not proved effective

1. Author's interpretation of Panel criteria. Based on contents, not claims.
2. The acetaminophen ratings are for pain and fever relief. Acetaminophen is not effective, and so is rated "C" for use against *inflammation* due to arthritis and other conditions and injuries.
3. Not available in all states, and if available may not be displayed on open shelves.

Pain: Liniments and Poultices
See LINIMENTS AND POULTICES FOR ACHES AND PAINS

Pain Remedies for the Skin
See ITCH AND PAIN REMEDIES APPLIED TO THE SKIN

Pancreatic Enzyme Supplements

The pancreas—a fish-shaped organ between the stomach and kidneys—produces digestive enzymes which play an important role in breaking down food so that it can be absorbed from the intestinal tract and used by the body for energy. When these enzymes are unavailable because the pancreas is diseased, or had to be removed surgically because of illness or injury, digestion may be seriously impaired. Foodstuffs, and particularly fats, may pass through the gut and be excreted basically unchanged. As a result, diarrhea and malnutrition may occur.

The lack of pancreatic enzymes can be made up for by replacements sold to fulfill this purpose. The approved supplements come from hog pancreases. However, the Panel cautions that the need for these preparations cannot be self-diagnosed and the serious illnesses which cause them cannot be self-treated. So while some of these products are available over-the-counter, both the diagnosis and the treatment of pancreatic insufficiency must be supervised by a doctor.

The normal human pancreas has the capacity to produce far greater amounts of these enzymes than the body actually needs. Some 90 percent of the organ—and thus, its enzymes—must be gone before digestive function is threatened. Short of serious pancreatic insufficiency, therefore, these supplements are not needed.

PANCREATIC ENZYME SUPPLEMENTS is based on the report "Exocrine Pancreatic Insufficiency Drug Products" by the FDA's Advisory Review Panel on Miscellaneous Internal Drug Products.

CLAIMS

Accurate
for "the treatment of exocrine pancreatic insufficiency when conducted under the care of the physician"

False or Misleading
references to "enteritis," "postgastrectomy syndrome," "chronic hepatitis," "gall-bladder disease," and postsurgical conditions (all require medical treatment)

THE PANCREAS AND ITS ENZYMES

Normally the pancreas produces 3 digestive enzymes, each with a different function:

- *Lipase* digests fat.
- *Protease* digests protein.
- *Amylase* digests starch.

Supplements of these enzymes together are called *pancreatin*. A similar prescription drug, which contains a higher proportion of lipase, is called *pancrelipase*. Since both preparations are obtained from hogs, persons allergic to pork should not use them.

The Panel stipulates that all nonprescription pancreatic supplements contain all 3 enzymes—lipase, protease, and amylase—in a single dosage form. Reviewers consider pancreatin and pancrelipase to be single-entity drugs, not combinations. In fact, no combinations were submitted for review; if they had been, evaluators say, such products probably would not have met the over-the-counter drug-review standards.

PANCREATIC ENZYME SUPPLEMENTS

Approved Active Ingredients

The Panel assessed 2 pancreatic supplements together, as it finds that they are essentially alike.

Pancreatin and pancrelipase Both of these substances are obtained from hog pancreases. Both contain lipase, protease, and amylase. Pancrelipase—as its name implies—contains relatively more lipase. It is presently available only on prescription. The Panel recommended that it be switched to nonprescription status, but at least two manufacturers of these preparations have told the FDA that they do not want this switch to be made since the treatment of pancreatic insufficiency should be directed by a doctor.

Basing its decision on a long record of medical use, the Panel judged these preparations to be safe. However, in high doses, they may cause nausea, vomiting, and diarrhea. For this reason the approved daily dosage—up to 14 grams triple-strength pancreatin or its equivalent—should be divided and taken with each of the day's meals. Dosage should be determined by a doctor.

Medical records also indicate that the substances are effective, so full approval was granted—providing use is under a doctor's supervision and pancrelipase continues to be available only by prescription.

Conditionally Approved Active Ingredients

None

Disapproved Active Ingredient

Hemicellulase This enzyme, obtained from molds, helps digest cellulose plant fibers in food. It has no relationship to pancreatic enzymes. Therefore, while it generally is recognized as safe, the Panel says it has no value in supplementing missing pancreatic enzymes. So the evaluators disapproved hemicellulase because it is not effective.

Safety and Effectiveness: Active Ingredients in Over-the-Counter Pancreatic Supplements

Active Ingredient	Panel's Assessment
hemicellulase	safe but not effective
pancreatin	safe and effective†
pancrelipase*	safe and effective†

*Not yet available over-the-counter.
†When used under a doctor's supervision.

Pancreatic Enzyme Supplements: Product Ratings

Product and Distributor	Dosage of Active Ingredients	Rating[1]
Elzyme 303 (Elder)	**tablets, enteric-coated:** 300 mg pancreatin USP (7500 units amylase + 600 units lipase + 7500 units protease)	A

Pancreatic Enzyme Supplements: Product Ratings *(continued)*

Product and Distributor	*Dosage of Active Ingredients*	*Rating[1]*
Pancreatin (Lilly)	**tablets:** 325 mg pancreatin USP (8125 units amylase + 650 units lipase + 8125 units protease)	**A**
Pancreatin Enseals (Lilly)	**tablets, enteric-coated:** 1000 mg pancreatin USP (25,000 units amylase + 2000 units lipase + 25,000 units protease)	**A**

1. Author's interpretation of Panel criteria. Based on contents, not claims.

Phenol: Special Warning

The phenol story is one of the classics in pharmacology. This drug—of lowly origins, coming as it does from coal tar—rose quickly to world fame a century ago. Then it was pushed from center stage by new and better performers, and also by the growing awareness of its inherently destructive nature. Phenol's popular appeal remains strong to this day. Nevertheless, as signaled by the over-the-counter drug review, its use as a drug may be diminishing.

Phenol is an alcohol. It was discovered in 1834, as a constituent of coal tar, which is why it also is called *carbolic acid*. Later it was discovered that phenol can also be distilled from hardwoods and can be made synthetically from benzene. In 1867, phenol became important to the practice of medicine when the English surgeon Joseph Lister showed that the high death toll from postoperative infections could be greatly reduced by spraying phenol in the operating room, cleansing a patient's skin with it before surgery, and applying phenol-soaked dressings to the surgical wound afterward. The drug quickly gained wide acceptance among doctors and lay people as a disinfectant for sanitary, medical, and surgical purposes. There is no denying its ability to kill or inhibit

PHENOL is based on the report "OTC Topical Antimicrobial Products" by the FDA's Advisory Review Panel on OTC Topical Antimicrobial Drug Products for Repeated Daily Human Use (Antimicrobial I Panel); the FDA's Tentative Final Monograph on OTC Topical Antimicrobial Products; and reports by other OTC Review Panels.

disease-causing bacteria and other microorganisms, and its characteristic, easily recognized pungent odor conveys the notion of "medicine."

Even today, in medical facilities, phenol continues to be widely used as a disinfectant—that is, a chemical used to cleanse and degerm objects, floors, and other surfaces. People continue to think of phenol as the germ-killing solution with the "medicinal smell."

For many years phenol was the principal odoriferous ingredient in a popular soap that was widely and successfully promoted for its ability to kill bacteria that suppposedly cause body odor. It is a clear sign of phenol's decline that—in the United States at least—this soap no longer contains phenol or its engaging smell.

It was discovered through the years that phenol has useful pharmacological properties other than killing germs. It can, for example, penetrate the sensory nerve endings in the skin and temporarily inactivate them, providing an anesthetic or numbing effect. So phenol has been widely used in topical drugs for relieving pain and itching. The drug is also used as an acne remedy, an antifungal against athlete's foot, and for many other purposes. It is one of the most widely represented active ingredients in over-the-counter drugs and has been assessed, for different purposes, by 7 of the 17 review Panels.

THE DANGERS OF USE

The fates changed for phenol early in this century, when more effective germicide and anesthetic drugs began to come on the market. Meanwhile phenol was found to be extremely toxic. It can be—and is —dangerous, whether swallowed, applied to the skin or mucous membranes, or even when it's inhaled from the air.

When taken orally, just a half-ounce of concentrated phenol is lethal; death occurs within minutes. Smaller amounts or weaker concentrations produce nausea, vomiting, physical collapse, pallor, cold sweats, and a feeble pulse rate. The victim may sink into a stupor. For these reasons, it is not safe to keep phenol around the house, particularly if there are children in the family.

When phenol is applied to the skin, concentrations of over 2 percent in water are irritating and may cause the skin to peel and die. The drug is readily absorbed through both normal and injured skin or mucous membranes, so that systemic poisoning can result from its use on body surfaces.

It is particularly dangerous to use phenol to treat diaper rash—a practice that may still continue. The drug is more readily absorbed through a rash than it would be through normal skin, and a large area of the baby's body is involved. Putting a fresh diaper on over the phenol retards its evaporation and increases its absorption. Worst of all, an infant's ability to break down and neutralize the drug may not be fully developed, so toxic amounts accumulate quickly in the liver and other organs.

Many chemical injuries in people of all age groups have now been attributed to phenol's use. Recent studies suggest the drug also may cause cancer.

Similar risks are being found or are suspected for a number of other compounds that are related to phenol. They include:

> chlorothymol
> chloroxylenol
> cresols (including *m*-cresol and secondary amyltricresols)
> dichlorophen
> phenolate sodium (also called sodium phenolate)
> resorcinol

Few of these drugs were assessed as safe and effective—except when they are used on very tiny body areas (such as the gums) or in extremely weak solutions.

After a careful study of phenol drugs (phenolates), the Antimicrobial I Panel proposed a formulation standard for phenol that was then endorsed by the FDA. This standard is now being applied to most nonprescription uses of these drugs.

WARNING Do not use for diaper rash, or over large areas of the body, or cover the treated area with a bandage or dressings.

SPECIFIC PHENOL CONCENTRATIONS

Phenol 1.5 percent or greater in aqueous or alcoholic solutions
Concentrations above 1.5 percent are too dangerous for use without prescription, according to the Antimicrobial I Panel and the FDA. The FDA plans to ban their use unless manufacturers present satisfactory evidence on safety and effectiveness.

Phenol 5 percent or less in glycerin or oil bases Phenol is released onto and absorbed into the skin less rapidly when it is formulated with glycerin—or in an oil-base preparation with camphor. So it appears that the FDA has for the moment set a 5 percent upper limit for safety on these formulations. However, preparations that contain over 2.5 percent *camphor* are dangerous and may be removed from the market (*see* CAMPHOR).

Phenol 1.5 percent or less in aqueous or alcoholic solutions Low concentrations of 1.5 percent phenol or less in aqueous or alcoholic solutions do not present a known hazard to the consumer. But they may be too weak to be effective. Whether manufacturers will try to prove that weak phenol preparations are effective remains to be seen. At present, however, only 2 uses are approved as both safe and effective by OTC review panels.

• Phenol is judged to be safe and effective for relieving itching and pain on the skin at concentrations of 0.5 to 1.5 percent.
• Phenol is judged to be safe and effective at concentrations of 0.5 to 1.5 percent for the relief of soreness and irritation of the gums and mucous membranes of the mouth and throat.

Conditional approval—pending proof of safety, effectiveness, or both—has been granted to phenol by a number of Panels for a variety of other uses. Phenol is used in many products. (To locate where these products are discussed consult the index.) However, to prevent serious mishaps, the FDA will require the following notice to appear on all drug products that contain phenol in concentrations of 0.5 to 1.5 percent.

Do not use for diaper rash, or over large areas of the body, or cover the treated area with a bandage or dressings.

Phenol under 0.5 percent as an inactive ingredient At very low concentrations—under 0.5 percent, or one-half of 1 percent—phenol is safe, the FDA says, and may continue to be used as "an inactive ingredient for its aromatic characteristics." In other words, the FDA is willing to allow manufacturers to practice a small deception on over-the-counter drug users, since the "medicinal smell" will come from an ingredient that no longer is present in concentrations high enough to be of medicinal value.

Safety and Effectiveness: The Phenolates

Active Ingredient	Assessment*
phenol over 1.5% in aqueous or alcoholic solutions	not safe
phenol over 5% in anhydrous glycerin, or formulated in oily preparation with camphor	not safe

Safety and Effectiveness: The Phenolates *(continued)*

Active Ingredient	Assessment*
phenol 0.5 to 1.5% in aqueous or alcoholic solutions	safe, or may be safe— but may not be effective
phenol under 5%	safe, or may be safe—
in anhydrous glycerin	but may not be effective
in oily preparations with camphor over 2.5%	not safe
in oily preparations with camphor under 2.5%	safe, or may be safe— but may not be effective
phenol under 0.5%	safe but inactive as a drug

*Made by Antimicrobial I Panel and FDA.

Phenol: Product Ratings—Rated for Safety Only[1,2]

Product and Distributor	Phenol Dosage	Rating	Comment
Anbesol (Whitehall)	0.5%	A	
Campho-Phenique (Winthrop)	4.7%	C	not safe because contains 10.8% camphor
Cēpastat Mouthwash (Merrell-National)	1.4%	A or B	depends on usage
Chloraseptic Mouthwash and Spray (Norwich-Eaton)	1.4%	A or B	depends on usage
Schamberg's Lotion (C & M Pharm.)	1%	A or B	depends on usage
Unguentine Plus (Norwich-Eaton)	0.5%	A	

1. Author's interpretation of Panel/FDA criteria. Based on contents, not claims.
2. Based on F&C and industry sources.

Pinworm Medications

See WORM-KILLERS FOR PINWORM

Poisoning Antidotes

Most poisonings occur in children and are accidental. Adults must be prepared to provide first aid, with the help—if available—of poison experts. Teen-agers and adults who overdose on licit or illicit drugs, or who have taken poison deliberately are a different matter; they are likely to be uncooperative—police help should be sought.

STEPS TO TAKE RIGHT NOW

Find the phone number of 2 nearby poison-control centers. Ask your telephone information operator, local or state health department, family doctor, hospital, police or fire department, or call the National Poison Center Network at (412) 647-5600. It is best to have 2 poison-center numbers because one may be closed at the time you need it, or may not answer for some other reason. Write the phone numbers of these centers, and the other phone numbers indicated, in the spaces below:

Poison Control Center #1 _____
Poison Control Center #2 _____
Dr. _____
Police _____
Emergency Room _____

Purchase over-the-counter antidotes from your druggist. Buy syrup of ipecac. (*Do* not *buy ipecac fluid extract; if you have some in the house, discard it—it's dangerous*.) Also buy activated charcoal. These ingredients are available in kits that contain several premeasured doses of each antidote, plus instructions. Keep kit where it is in clear sight—in a bathroom, kitchen, or bedroom—and from time to time remind all adults in the house where it is.

POISONING ANTIDOTES is based on the report of the FDA's Advisory Review Panel on OTC Laxative, Antidiarrheal, Emetic, and Antiemetic Drug Products; the FDA's Tentative Final Order on Emetic Drug Products for OTC Human Use; the report "Drug Products for OTC Use for the Treatment of Acute Toxic Ingestion" by the Advisory Review Panel on OTC Miscellaneous Internal Drugs; and material on first aid provided by the director of the National Poison Center Network.

STEPS TO TAKE IN CASE OF POISONING

In case of poisoning or suspected poisoning, follow these steps in order. Do not panic.

General First Aid

1. Call poison control center, doctor, or emergency room *immediately*. If possible, begin first-aid treatment at once while another person does the phoning.
2. Loosen tight clothing—be sure airway is clear. You may have to remove or reposition false teeth in older persons.
3. Apply artificial ventilation—mouth-to-mouth resuscitation—if breathing has stopped. Keep airway open if victim is unconscious.
4. Keep victim warm (not hot) with blankets.
5. Do not give liquor, soft drinks, or drugs in any form.

Treating the Poisoning

Take these steps next. Stay calm.

1. If you can, tell the poison control center or other medical authority, the victim's condition, type of poison, and the amount taken. Decide with the medical authority whether to bring the victim to an emergency room, wait for an ambulance, or begin additional treatment on the spot.
2. If the victim is transported for help, take along the poison container—or if the victim has vomited, a sample of vomited matter.
3. If a petroleum distillate product has been swallowed—for example, *furniture polish*, *gasoline*, *lighter fluid*, or *kerosene*—first-aid instruction must come from the poison center, your physician, or hospital emergency room. You may be able to smell a petroleum distillate on the victim's breath if no container can be found.
4. Do *not* induce vomiting if victim
     - is unconscious
     - is having convulsions
     - complains of pain or burning sensation in mouth or throat and
     - has swallowed a *corrosive acid* or *corrosive alkali*
         - Corrosive acids include
             toilet-bowl cleaner (sodium acid sulfate)
             sulfuric, nitric, oxalic, hydrochloric, and phosphoric acids

caustic or styptic pencils (silver nitrate)
chlorine bleach (calcium hypochlorite)
•Corrosive alkalis include
lye or drain cleaner (sodium or potassium hydroxide)
washing soda (sodium carbonate)
ammonia water
bleaching powder (sodium perborate)
dishwashing detergent

A. If the victim of corrosive poisoning is conscious, alert, and can swallow, give him water or milk.
For babies up to age 5, 1 to 2 cups of fluid.
For older persons, 2 to 3 cups of fluid.
B. Do *not* give activated charcoal and—repeat—do *not* induce vomiting.

5. If the poison is not a corrosive substance, first give 1 to 2 cups of *water*—not soda, milk, or any other fluid—to dilute the poison in the stomach.

6. Induce vomiting if directed to do so by medical authority—or take the responsibility yourself if no emergency medical source can be reached.

A. You can usually induce vomiting by irritating the back of the victim's throat with back end of a spoon or with your finger. This stimulates the gag reflex. When retching and vomiting begins, help victim stand or sit, leaning forward, with head lower than hips. This prevents poisoned vomitus from being sucked into the lungs—which could cause further damage.
B. If this mechanical method does not work—and it often does not —attempt to induce vomiting with *syrup of ipecac*. (Don't use ipecac fluid extract.) For infants under 1, 1 to 2 teaspoonsful (5 to 10 ml), followed by ½ to 1 glass of water. For older persons, 1 to 2 tablespoonsful (15 to 30 ml), followed by 1 to 2 glasses of water.
C. If vomiting has not occurred within 20 minutes, repeat ipecac dose and water.
D. If vomiting *still* has not occurred, seek emergency medical help.
E. After vomiting has occurred—*not before*—give activated charcoal. This is an adsorbent which will grab onto, bind, and so neutralize many poisons. If you know how much of the toxic substance was swallowed, give 8 to 10 times that amount of

activated charcoal. Otherwise, give at least 6 tablespoonsful (30 grams). Each 6-tablespoon dose should be mixed in ½ glassful of water (4 ounces) to facilitate swallowing.

7. Bring the victim to a medical facility as quickly as possible.

UNDERSTANDING THE POISONING PROBLEM

The need to know about and be able to deliver first-aid treatment for poisoning is clear from the statistics: about a million poisonings occur in the United States each year. The National Safety Council says 5000 of these episodes are fatal.

Most accidental poisonings occur in youngsters under 5. According to one estimate, these children account for 70 percent of accidental poisonings. Between 100 and 200 of these victims die—as do an additional 100 young people between the ages of 5 and 14.

Many of these poisonings could be prevented by what some parents call "child-proofing" the house as soon as an infant is able to crawl.

- *In the kitchen:* Put household chemicals and cleaners in a locked cabinet or on high shelves out of reach. A bicycle padlock with a long hasp can be used to secure kitchen cabinet-door handles.
- *In the bathroom:* Lock the medicine cabinet if possible, and keep all drugs and medicines on a high shelf. Don't trust safety caps. Get "Mr. Yuck" stickers from your poison control center or druggist for all medicine bottles.
- *In the bedroom:* Take perfumes and other cosmetics and medicines off the nightstand or dresser and store them in a secure place children can't reach.
- *In the basement and garage:* Don't put paint-thinner, solvents, fuels, or other toxic substances in milk or soft-drink bottles that children can find. Store weed killers and pesticides as manufacturers recommend: out of children's reach. Be sure that laundry detergents are out of reach, too.

DRUGS USED TO COUNTERACT POISONING

A number of chemicals and mixtures have been used as antidotes. Most are ineffective—and hence dangerous. Contrary to what some people believe, there is no universal antidote. Preparations recommended for this purpose in the past have consisted of activated charcoal, tannic acid, and magnesium oxide. While activated charcoal can be helpful, tannic acid and magnesium oxide are worthless and may interfere with the activated charcoal's action.

The only 2 useful antidotes to keep in the house are syrup of ipecac and activated charcoal.

CLAIMS

Accurate for Syrup of Ipecac
"to cause vomiting [emesis] in case of poisoning"

Accurate for Activated Charcoal
for "the treatment of acute poisoning"

WARNING Before using, call a physician, poison control center, or emergency room for advice. Do not use on a semiconscious or unconscious person.

Approved Antidotes

Ipecac syrup This is the *first* antidote to use (*see* above, under STEPS TO TAKE IN CASE OF POISONING). Ipecac is prepared from a powder obtained from the plant *Cephaelis ipecacuanha*, where it gets its unusual name. Its only recommended use is as an antidote in poisoning, and it has been shown to be safe and effective for this purpose.

The recommended dose for children under 1 is 1 to 2 teaspoonsful of ipecac syrup (5 to 10 ml), followed by ½ to 1 glass of water (4 to 8 ounces). If vomiting does not occur within 20 minutes, repeat dosage *once*. Do not repeat a second time—seek emergency medical help.

For older children and for adults, the FDA recommends a dose of 1 tablespoonful (15 ml), followed by 1 to 2 glasses of water (8 to 16 ounces). The director of the National Poison Control Center suggests an initial dose of 1 tablespoonful (15 ml) for children, and 2 tablespoonsful (30 ml) for adults, followed by at least one glass of water. If vomiting does not occur within 20 minutes, the initial dose can be repeated *once*. Do not repeat a second time—seek emergency help.

Charcoal, activated This substance should be taken *after* ipecac has been given and *after* vomiting has occurred. Otherwise it will interfere with the ipecac's ability to stimulate vomiting. Strictly speaking, activated charcoal is not an antidote—that is, it does not act specifically against any poison or group of poisons. Rather, it acts by binding to, holding, and thus neutralizing many toxic substances—a pharmacological and chemical property called adsorption.

Activated charcoal's enormous adsorptive capacity comes in large part from its highly porous, honeycomblike internal structure. It is here that poisonous particles become stuck and entrapped. Unbelievable as it may seem, the internal surface area of a standard 1 ounce (30 gram) dose of activated charcoal is 300,000 square feet—the equivalent of a square that is 500 feet on a side.

Many tests in animals and long clinical use in humans have demonstrated that activated charcoal is safe. Its binding and neutralizing functions have been demonstrated in the laboratory, in emergency rooms and hopitals, and through the follow-up of poisoning victims who were treated at home. It will not adsorb all poisons, however, and should be used as advised by your poison control center or other health-care professionals.

While activated charcoal should not be given in advance of ipecac syrup, it works best when it is given within the first half-hour after poisoning—before the poison leaves the stomach and enters the small intestine. Luckily the charcoal *can* catch up with the poisons, and so it can be given later if necessary.

Activated charcoal is a black powder and is unpleasant to take. The Panel recommends that drug makers find an inactive base like carboxymethylcellulose that will make it more palatable. Meanwhile, each 6 tablespoon (30 gram) dose should be mixed in a half glassful of water (4 ounces). This is the usual dose, but the more that the victim can be made to take, the better.

Conditionally Approved Antidotes

None

Disapproved Antidotes

The Panel lists, without comment, several substances that have been used to treat poisoning but that the reviewers summarily disapproved because data to prove safety and effectiveness are lacking. They are:

> alcohol
> magnesium hydroxide
> potassium arsenite
> tannic acid
> toast, burnt

Safety and Effectiveness: Active Ingredients in Over-the-Counter Antidotes for Poisons

Active Ingredient	Assessments*
alcohol	summarily disapproved
charcoal, activated	safe and effective
ipecac syrup	safe and effective
magnesium hydroxide	summarily disapproved
potassium arsenite	summarily disapproved
tannic acid	summarily disapproved
toast, burnt	summarily disapproved

*By the FDA and two Panels.

Poisoning Antidotes: Product Ratings

Single-Ingredient Products

Product and Distributor	Dosage of Active Ingredients	Rating[1]	Comment
ipecac syrup			
ipecac (generic)	**syrup:** 15 ml and 30 ml	**A**	
charcoal, activated			
Activated Charcoal Liquid (Bowman)	**liquid:** 12.5 g in propylene glycol per 60 ml bottle	**C**	this may be the "palatable" formulation the Panel asks,
	liquid: 25 g in propylene glycol per 120 ml bottle	**C**	but the unit dosage is too low
charcoal, activated (generic)	**powder:** 15, 30, 120, 240g, and 1 lb.	**A**	
Charcodote (Panray)	**powder:** 15 g	**A**	

Combination Products

Product and Distributor	Dosage of Active Ingredients	Rating[1]	Comment
Res-Q (Boyle)	**powder:** activated charcoal + magnesium hydroxide + tannic acid in 15 g packets	**C**	magnesium hydroxide and tannic acid not safe or effective; combination not effective

Poisoning Antidotes: Product Ratings *(continued)*

Emergency Antidote Kits

Product and Distributor	Dosage of Active Ingredients	Rating[1]	Comment
Poison Antidote Kit (Bowman)	**package includes:** 2 bottles syrup of ipecac (15 ml) + 4 bottles charcoal suspension (45 ml)	C	Panel favors kits, and suspension of charcoal in palatable medium. But safety and effectiveness of this particular kit not specifically assessed by Panel and, apparently not by FDA either; ipecac dosage adequate for adult by Over-the-Counter Drug Review criteria, but not by National Poison Control Center criteria, which specify up to 2 doses of 30 ml
Poison Safeguard Kit (Marshall Electronics)	**package includes:** 2 bottles syrup of ipecac (15 ml) + 1 bottle activated charcoal (25 g)	C	charcoal dose too small; kit does not contain enough activated charcoal to provide second dose; ipecac dosage adequate for adult by Over-the-Counter Drug Review criteria, but not by National Poison Control Center criteria, which specify up to 2 doses of 30 ml

1. Author's interpretation of Panel/FDA criteria. Based on contents, not claims.

Poison-Ivy Preventives and Palliatives

The plant poisons—poison ivy, oak, and sumac—are the scourge of many a fishing trip, golf game, and gardening day. It would be nice if there were preventive medicines that could be swallowed or rubbed onto the skin before exposure; but no drug is available that fulfills this need. It would be nice, too, if there were effective drugs that could be used after exposure to prevent the rashes from erupting on the skin— but there are none.

Once the rash has erupted, more can be done about it: safe and effective drugs are available to relieve the itching and pain. Some are marketed specifically for plant poisoning, others as general remedies for skin rashes.

PREVENTIVE MEASURES

The best way to avoid poison ivy is to learn to recognize these poisonous plants and stay away from them. One should remember, too, that direct contact with the plant is not required. For example, a dog that runs through patches of the plant, or a boat or other equipment that is dragged through them, will pick up enough toxin to cause a serious rash if one pets the dog or handles the equipment. Even air-borne material from the plants can be poisonous to highly sensitive persons, particularly when the plants are burned in brush-clearing efforts.

Persons seriously afflicted with poison ivy should discuss their problem with an allergist. Some helpful medical measures are available, including oral desensitizing doses of ivy toxin.

PREVENTIVE DRUGS

At least one nonprescription oral drug is marketed with the claim that it prevents plant poisoning. The Panel concerned with miscella-

POISON-IVY PREVENTIVES AND PALLIATIVES is based on the unadopted draft report "OTC Poison-Ivy, -Oak, and -Sumac Prevention Drug Products" by the FDA's Advisory Review Panel on OTC Miscellaneous External Drug Products.

neous internal drugs was supposed to assess such compounds but it was disbanded before it could do so.

Several preparations are currently available with *claims* that they help prevent ivy poisoning when applied to the skin. No data were submitted—or were otherwise available—on 2 of the 3 active ingredients. The third, an experimental drug, was conditionally approved, but the manufacturer's New Drug Application is no longer active—so the preparation is not marketed in the United States. (A New Drug Application is submitted to the FDA when manufacturers wish to introduce a drug into the public marketplace.)

Approved Active Ingredients

None

Conditionally Approved Active Ingredient

The combination of cation + anion exchange resins, buffered Not sold in the United States, this preparation contains resins that are said to pick up both acid and base plant proteins (antigens) that provoke reactions to plant poisons. The resins are then washed off, carrying the toxins away.

A few safety tests were submitted for review. They indicate that the mixture produces little skin irritation during the first 2 weeks of use, but later it can provoke severe sores in the skin and underlying tissues. So the mixture was judged safe when used briefly.

Evaluators were not impressed by the evidence about how well the drug works. In an uncontrolled study, 13 doctors reported on 32 instances in which they used the resin. All claimed it was effective. Another doctor said the rashes dried up quickly in the 40 patients he treated with the resins. But in a controlled study of 20 men who were sensitive to poison ivy, the mixture was not clearly superior to dummy medication. The Panel concluded that, while safe, a buffered mixture of anion and cation exchange resins has not been proved effective.

Disapproved Active Ingredients

The Panel tried to evaluate 2 active ingredients in products marketed for the prevention of poison-ivy rashes, but it could find no data on either of them and so summarily disapproved both *ferric chloride* and *zirconium oxide*.

DRUGS TO RELIEVE POISON IVY

Many products are available to treat bumps, blisters, rashes, and other eruptions from poison ivy and related plant poisons. Because of fiscal and governmental policy constraints, the present Panel was disbanded by the FDA before it could specifically evaluate active ingredients in these preparations—except for approving a wet astringent dressing of aluminum acetate solution, called Burow's solution, which it says is safe and effective for treating poison ivy (see ALUMINUM ACE-TATE, page 735).

However, reviewers did note that many of these ingredients had already been evaluated, in more general terms, as skin protectants and as itch and pain relievers. Unfortunately, some others were not evaluated in this way, including the antihistamines chlorpheniramine maleate, phenyltoloxamine citrate, and pyrilamine maleate. Since histamine is a principal irritant in ivy poisoning, and since one antihistamine (diphenhydramine hydrochloride) is safe and effective, it would be helpful to know if these other antihistamines are, too.

The ingredients hydrocortisone and hydrocortisone acetate, which were both assessed by The Topical Analgesics Panel as safe and effective anti-itch medications, were not in any of the poison-ivy preparations reviewed by this Panel because they were only recently approved for use without prescription. Many doctors believe these drugs are highly effective for treating poison ivy, oak, and sumac and the Topical Analgesics Panel says these hydrocortisone preparations are safe and effective for treating these conditions. In fact, it approves the following claim.

for "the temporary relief of . . . poison ivy, poison oak, poison sumac."

All available judgments on active ingredients in poison-ivy relievers are summarized in the SAFETY AND EFFECTIVENESS chart at the end of this unit. For more information on the pain relievers, see ITCH AND PAIN REMEDIES APPLIED TO THE SKIN; for more on skin protectants, see UNGUENTS AND POWDERS FOR THE SKIN.

Safety and Effectiveness: Active Ingredients in Over-the-Counter Medications Used to Treat Poison Ivy, Oak, and Sumac

Active Ingredient	Function	Panel's Assessment*
alcohol		inactive ingredient
allantoin	skin protectant	safe and effective
	wound healer	not proved effective

**Safety and Effectiveness: Active Ingredients in Over-the-Counter Medications
Used to Treat Poison Ivy, Oak, and Sumac** *(continued)*

Active Ingredient	Function	Panel's Assessment*
aluminum acetate solution (Burow's solution)	astringent	safe and effective†
benzethonium chloride	skin protectant (antiseptic)	not proved effective‡
benzocaine	itch-pain reliever	safe and effective
benzyl alcohol	itch-pain reliever	safe and effective
bithionol		not assessed
buffered mixture of cation and anion exchange resins	preventive	safe, but not proved effective†
Burow's solution, *See* aluminum acetate solution		
calamine	skin protectant	safe and effective
camphor	itch-pain reliever	safe and effective
cetalkonium chloride		not assessed
chloral hydrate	itch-pain reliever	safe, but not effective
chlorpheniramine maleate	antihistamine	not assessed
creosote (beechwood)		not assessed
diperodon hydrochloride		not assessed
diphenhydramine hydrochloride	antihistamine	safe and effective
endothermic hectorite		not assessed
eucalyptus oil	counterirritant	unclear§
ferric chloride	preventive	summarily disapproved†
glycerin	skin protectant	safe and effective
hydrocortisone preparations (hydrocortisone, hydrocortisone acetate)**	itch relievers	safe and effective
hydrogen peroxide		not assessed
iron oxide		not assessed
isopropyl alcohol		inactive ingredient††
lanolin	skin protectant	safe and effective
lead acetate		not assessed
lidocaine	itch-pain reliever	safe and effective
menthol (0.1 to 1%)	itch-pain reliever	safe and effective†
merbromin (Mercurochrome)	antiseptic	not effective†
mercuric chloride	antiseptic	not safe or effective†
oil of turpentine	counterirritant	unclear§
panthenol		not assessed
parethoxycaine hydrochloride		not assessed

**Safety and Effectiveness: Active Ingredients in Over-the-Counter Medications
Used to Treat Poison Ivy, Oak, and Sumac *(continued)***

Active Ingredient	Function	Panel's Assessment*
phenol (0.5 to 1.5%, in aqueous or alcoholic solution)	itch-pain reliever	safe and effective
phenyltoloxamine citrate	antihistamine	not assessed
polyvinylpyrrolidone		not assessed
pyrilamine maleate	antihistamine	not assessed
salicylic acid		inactive ingredient
simethicone		not assessed
sodium bicarbonate	skin protectant	safe and effective
tannic acid	skin protectant	not safe or effective
tincture of impatiens bi-flora		not assessed
tripelennamine hydrochloride	antihistamine	safe and effective
triethanolamine salicylate (trolamine)		not assessed
zinc acetate	skin protectant	safe and effective
zirconium oxide	symptomatic relief	not assessed
zyloxin	antiseptic	not safe or effective†

*These conclusions apply to itching and skin pain, generally speaking, not specifically to the effects of plant poisons. Judgments were made by the Topical Analgesic Panel unless otherwise noted.
†Assessed by the FDA's Miscellaneous External Drug Panel.
‡Assessed by the FDA's Advisory Review Panel on OTC Antimicrobial Drug Products for Repeated Daily Human Use and by FDA.
§Assessed by the External Analgesic Panel as safe and effective as a counterirritant against deep-seated pain; it is not approved for relieving superficial itching and pain in the skin.
**Not contained in poison-ivy products submitted to the Miscellaneous External Drug Panel because it was not approved for use without prescription at that time. However, the Panel on External Analgesic Drug Products specifically approves it for such use.
††In concentrations of 60 to 91.3%, isopropyl alcohol is listed by the Miscellaneous External Drug Panel as a safe and effective antiseptic active ingredient. It is not recommended for poison ivy or similar plant poisons.

Poison-Ivy Preventives and Palliatives: Product Ratings

Single-Ingredient Products[1]

Product and Distributor	Dosage of Active Ingredients	Rating[2]	Comment
aluminum acetate solution (Burow's solution)			
Burow's solution (generic)	**liquid:** aluminum acetate solution	A	

Poison-Ivy Preventives and Palliatives: Product Ratings *(continued)*

Single-Ingredient Products[1]

Product and Distributor	Dosage of Active Ingredients	Rating[2]	Comment
Buro-Sol Powder (Doak)	**powder:** 2.36 g packet produces 1 pint 1:15 Burow's solution + 4.4% benzethonium chloride	B	benzethonium chloride not proved effective
calamine calamine (generic)	**lotion:** 8% calamine + 8% zinc oxide	A	
diphenhydramine hydrochloride Benadryl (Parke-Davis)	**cream:** 2%	A	
sodium bicarbonate Arm & Hammer Baking Soda (Church & Dwight)	**powder**	A	
sodium bicarbonate (generic)		A	
tripelennamine hydrochloride PBZ (Geigy)	**cream:** 2%	A	this antihistamine not submitted as poison-ivy remedy, but judged safe and effective for that purpose by Topical Analgesic Panel

Combination Products

Product and Distributor	Dosage of Active Ingredients	Rating[2]	Comment
Ablitox (Pfeiffer)	**lotion:** 3% benzocaine + 0.136% benzalkonium chloride	C	less-than-effective concentration of benzocaine
	spray: 3% benzocaine + 0.5% chloroxylenol	C	less-than-effective concentration of benzocaine

Poison-Ivy Preventives and Palliatives: Product Ratings *(continued)*

Combination Products

Product and Distributor	Dosage of Active Ingredients	Rating[2]	Comment
Americaine First Aid Spray (Arnar-Stone)	**spray:** 10% benzocaine + 0.1% benzethonium chloride	B	benzethonium chloride not proved effective; *but* this is only combination product listed here with effective dosage of benzocaine
Caladryl (Parke-Davis)	**cream:** 1% diphenhydramine hydrochloride + calamine	A	
	lotion: 1% diphenhydramine hydrochloride + calamine + 1% camphor	A	
Calamatum (Blair)	**lotion:** calamine + zinc oxide + phenol + camphor + 3% benzocaine	C	ineffective dosage of benzocaine; maker does not indicate concentrations of other ingredients
Ivy-Chex (Bowman)	**spray:** polyvinylpyrrolidone-vinylacetate copolymers + methyl salicylate + benzalkonium chloride	C	initial ingredient as yet unassessed in Over-the-Counter Drug Review
phenolated calamine (generic)	**lotion:** 8% calamine + 8% zinc oxide (plus 0.1% phenol)	A	not a medically active amount of phenol
Rhulicream (Lederle)	**cream:** 1% zirconium oxide + 1% benzocaine + 0.7% menthol + 0.3% camphor	B	ineffectively low dose of benzocaine
Rhulihist (Lederle)	**lotion:** 1% tripelennamine hydrochloride + 1% zirconium oxide + 1% benzocaine + 3% calamine + 0.1% camphor + 0.1% menthol	B	ineffectively low dose of benzocaine

Poison-Ivy Preventives and Palliatives: Product Ratings *(continued)*

Single-Ingredient Products[1]

Product and Distributor	Dosage of Active Ingredients	Rating[2]	Comment
Surfadil (Lilly)	**cream:** 1% diphenhydramine hydrochloride + 0.5% cyclomethycaine sulfate	B	latter ingredient not proved effective
	lotion: 1% diphenhydramine hydrochloride + 2% cyclomethycaine sulfate + 0.5% benzyl alcohol	B	cyclomethycaine not proved effective
Ziradryl (Parke-Davis)	**lotion:** 2% diphenhydramine hydrochloride + 2% zinc oxide	A	

1. For benzocaine product ratings and for hydrocortisone product ratings, *see* pages 467–469.
2. Author's interpretation of Panel criteria. Based on contents, not claims.

Poultices for Aches and Pains

See LINIMENTS AND POULTICES FOR ACHES AND PAINS

Powders for the Skin

See UNGUENTS AND POWDERS FOR THE SKIN

Premature Ejaculation Retardants

Many men reach sexual climax too soon—when the penis first enters the vagina, or even before. This is embarrassing for the man and frustrating for his partner.

Premature ejaculation is caused by a variety of problems, some of which require medical or psychiatric correction. But the Panel that evaluated self-treatment products believes that their use can be beneficial to many men. These preparations may carry labels that describe them as "cream for relief of premature ejaculation," "desensitizing lubricant for men," "world-famous delay spray for men," or "climax-control spray for men." The active ingredients are topical anesthetics, which act by temporarily diminishing penile sensations. Although some claims made for these products are judged misleading or inappropriate, the Panel decided that the drugs themselves are safe and effective.

CLAIMS

Accurate

for "temporary male genital desensitization helping to slow the onset of ejaculation"

aids in temporarily "retarding the onset of ejaculation," or "slowing the onset of ejaculation," or "prolonging time until ejaculation"

for "reducing oversensitivity in the male in advance of intercourse"

"as an aid in the prevention of premature ejaculation"

False or Misleading

aids in "temporarily retarding rapidity of ejaculation" or "slowing the speed of ejaculation" (the preparation can *delay* ejaculation but not slow it once it has started)

"to strengthen sexual confidence"

"original and unchallenged throughout the world for quality, effectiveness, and satisfaction"

WARNING Premature ejaculation may be due to a condition requiring medical supervision. If a product, used as directed, does not provide relief, stop

PREMATURE EJACULATION RETARDANTS is based on the unadopted draft report "OTC Male Genital Desensitizing Drug Products" by the FDA's Advisory Review Panel on OTC Miscellaneous External Drug Products.

using it and consult a doctor. If the skin to which you apply a product becomes irritated, stop using it and consult a doctor. The effect of these products on sperm and fertility has not been determined.

In about 75 percent of men, orgasm occurs about 2 minutes after entry of the penis into the vagina. But in what the Panel says is a "considerable number" of others, climax is reached in under a minute —or even within 10 or 20 seconds or less. The Panel got these statistics from a urological specialist who pointed out that the condition can usually be attributed to 1 of 3 basic causes.

- A penis may be so highly sensitive to sexual stimulation that it starts the ejaculatory response before it is welcome.
- Inflammation of the urethral tissues can serve as an ejaculatory trigger mechanism.
- Psychoneurotic problems can interfere with the individual's sex life.

The same report notes that a man's orgasm may occur within a normal span of time but that his partner may require a much longer time to reach climax if his partner does so at all. Pondering this problem, the urologist hit on the idea of delaying the male partner's ejaculation by temporarily desensitizing the penis by using a numbing (anesthetic) drug. He tried this method with his patients and reported (in 1963) that anesthetic preparations in fact raised the level of resistance to sexual excitation, thereby delaying a man's orgasm.

In a study of 13 men—aged 22 to 39—who complained that they ejaculated prior to or upon insertion of the penis into the vagina, the researcher found that treating the head and shaft of the penis with 3 percent benzocaine cream corrected premature ejaculation in all 13. The average time from insertion to orgasm lengthened to a minute and a half. Other studies, described below, have confirmed this initial finding. According to inconclusive evidence related by the Panel in its report, the anesthetic drug does not desensitize the clitoris or diminish the woman's pleasure.

DRUGS USED TO TREAT PREMATURE EJACULATION

Products marketed to retard ejaculation all contain an anesthetic. None contains more than one active ingredient. But they also may contain benzyl alcohol, ephedrine hydrochloride or passion fruit— which the Panel lists as inactive ingredients.

Approved Active Ingredients

Benzocaine   This is a widely used topical anesthetic. Because of its excellent safety record, reviewers assess it as safe for use as a penile anesthetic. Benzocaine's effectiveness was initially suggested by the study described above. In a larger study with 120 men who had premature-ejaculation problems, another investigator reported that 108 benefited: they were able to maintain control over the ejaculatory reflex for 2 minutes or longer when they used a 7.5 percent benzocaine ointment before intercourse; 72 were able to delay orgasm for 3 minutes or more. Only 8 of the 120 benefited from using a dummy preparation.

Use of the active drug was reported to please their partners, too; 72 percent of them achieved orgasm when the man used the active drug, compared with only 2.5 percent when the man used an ointment without the benzocaine.

The Panel concludes that benzocaine is safe and effective in concentrations of 3 to 7.5 percent when applied in small amounts to the head and shaft of the penis before intercourse. It should be washed off afterward.

Lidocaine   Another widely used local anesthetic, lidocaine has a good safety record when used in small amounts. The Panel says it is safe for use on the penis. The studies submitted to demonstrate lidocaine's effectiveness as a penile anesthetic showed that the drug significantly prolonged the time required for men to masturbate to orgasm. Another study showed that it reduced the penis's sensitivity to a variety of stimuli—including pressure, pain, warmth, cold, and mechanical vibrations. The Panel says it considers these results show lidocaine's ability to retard the onset of ejaculation, and assesses it safe and effective for that purpose. The approved concentration is 9.6 percent lidocaine in an aerosol spray dispensed from a dose-metered container that delivers measured amounts of the lidocaine. The Panel says that a nonmetered spray container is unsafe because the amount of anesthetic applied is not measured.

Conditionally Approved Active Ingredients

None

Disapproved Active Ingredients

None

**Safety and Effectiveness: Active Ingredients
in Over-the-Counter Premature Ejaculation
Relievers**

Active Ingredient	Panel's Assessment
benzocaine	safe and effective
lidocaine	safe and effective

Premature Ejaculation Retardants: Product Ratings

Product and Distributor	Dosage of Active Ingredients	Rating[1]
benzocaine topical (generic)	**cream:** 5%	**A**
	ointment: 5%	**A**
Detane (Commerce Drug)	**gel:** benzocaine 7.5%	**A**
Stud 100 (Pound)	**spray:** lidocaine 9.6%	**A**

1. Author's interpretation of Panel criteria. Based on contents, not claims.

Psoriasis Lotions

Sufferers of psoriasis usually are well aware of their problem *and* its name. This intensely itchy and often unsightly skin disorder may wax and wane, but once present it usually remains for a lifetime.

Severe psoriasis is a demoralizing, occasionally life-threatening ailment that requires medical management. Mild cases may fall more into the nuisance category. It's this latter group that may be appropriate for self-treatment with nonprescription drugs. The Panel that evaluated nonprescription products used for psoriasis finds that 2 types of drugs —coal-tar preparations and salicylic acid—are safe and effective for relieving the itching, inflammation, and scaling that occur in these mild cases.

PSORIASIS LOTIONS is based on the unadopted draft report "Dandruff, Seborrheic Dermatitis, Psoriasis Control Drug Products," by the FDA's Advisory Review Panel on OTC Miscellaneous External Drug Products.

CLAIMS

Accurate
"relieves the itching, redness, and scaling associated with psoriasis on the body and/or scalp"

WARNING   If psoriasis covers a large area of the body, one should consult a doctor before attempting self-treatment. If the condition worsens or fails to improve after several days, a physician should be seen. These drugs should not be used on children under 2 except as directed by a doctor.

PINK PATCHES AND SILVERY SCALES

Psoriasis is a chronic inflammatory disease that afflicts several million Americans. The cause is unknown. The disease is characterized by sharply demarcated pink or dull red splotches on the skin that are covered with tiny silvery scales. These lesions may come and go or they may be continually present.

In persons with psoriasis, the outer layer of the skin (the epidermis) turns over extremely rapidly. Skin cells may take only 3 or 4 days to grow, mature, and die. This turnover rate is 10 to 20 times faster than normal, which is 25 to 30 days.

The plaques of psoriasis may appear on the scalp or on virtually any other body surface; common sites are the elbows and knees. These plaques are particularly likely to develop at the site of a cut, burn, sunburn, or preexisting rash. Emotional stress can also bring on eruptions. Pregnancy, on the other hand, may bring dramatic remissions. So, too, might the onset of hot summer weather.

DRUGS USED FOR PSORIASIS

The drugs formulated into body lotions, shampoos, and other over-the-counter preparations for treating psoriasis fall into several classes. They may be *cytostatic agents*, which retard skin-cell growth; *keratolytic agents*, which loosen and dissolve scales; *tar preparations*, whose mode of action is uncertain; *hydrocortisone preparations*, which reduce itching and inflammation; *anti-itch preparations*; or *antimicrobials* (*see* more about these different kinds of drugs in DANDRUFF AND SEBORRHEIC SCALE SHAMPOOS).

Combination Products

Many over-the-counter preparations that are claimed to relieve psoriasis contain more than one active ingredient. No combination has been shown to be safe and effective. Many inactive ingredients are also formulated into lotions, shampoos, and over-the-counter products for treating psoriasis (*see* INACTIVE INGREDIENTS in DANDRUFF AND SE-BORRHEIC SCALE SHAMPOOS, page 217.)

The Panel assessed about a dozen active ingredients that are marketed over-the-counter for treating mild psoriasis.

Approved Active Ingredients

Coal-tar shampoos These tar preparations, derived from coal and petroleum products, are assessed as safe when formulated as shampoos for twice-weekly application to the scalp. Tars have been used for a long time to treat psoriasis and other skin conditions. But there have been no double-blind studies in which coal tar by itself was tested against the base in which it was formulated. This is the kind of testing the Panel preferred.

But in one study, 7.5 percent coal-tar solution with 1.5 percent menthol proved to be superior to shampoo alone after a month of regular shampooing. The redness, itching, and scaling were measurably reduced in participants who used the medicated product. Basing their judgment on this and other studies, reviewers list coal-tar shampoos as safe and effective for twice-weekly use to relieve scalp psoriasis.

The approved dosages are:

coal tar extract	2 to 8 percent
coal tar USP	0.5 to 5 percent
coal tar solution	2.5 to 5 percent
coal tar distillate	4 percent

The Panel's approval of coal-tar shampoos does *not* extend to coal-tar lotions and other formulations that are intended to remain on the skin, rather than quickly be washed off as shampoos are.

The Panel warns that coal-tar products may make the skin hypersensitive to sunlight. So any user should try to stay out of bright, direct sun for a day following application.

Salicylic acid This is a keratolytic (skin-peeling) agent that is widely used to treat skin disorders. The Panel has assessed it as safe. Evaluators were not presented with results from any scientifically controlled, double-blind study of salicylic acid used by itself as a psoriasis treatment. (It may have seen—but does not describe any—studies in which the drug was used in combination with other ingredients to treat this condition.) Nevertheless, salicylic acid in concentrations of 1.8 to 3 percent was judged safe and effective for controlling psoriasis of the body and scalp.

Conditionally Approved Active Ingredients

Allantoin   A safe skin-peeling active ingredient, allantoin's effectiveness has not been clearly established. Material submitted failed to demonstrate the substance's therapeutic effect. So allantoin is classified as safe but not proved effective against psoriasis.

Coal-tar body lotions   These tar lotions are intended to be applied to the body—once or twice daily—to relieve itching and other distress of psoriasis. The Panel approved coal-tar drugs as safe and effective against psoriasis of the scalp because shampoos come into only brief contact with the skin and are then washed off.

While several fairly convincing scientific studies suggest that these lotions effectively relieve psoriatic itching and inflammation, there is a lingering fear among Panel members that continued use of coal-tar products may eventually lead to skin cancer. The evaluators say the weight of evidence available is that the preparations are safe. But until the matter is resolved, the Panel chooses to assess coal tar effective but not proved safe for use against psoriasis on the body.

Hydrocortisone preparations: hydrocortisone acetate and hydrocortisone alcohol   Potent anti-inflammatory agents, these drugs have excellent safety records. But their safety and effectiveness in treating dandruff and seborrheic dermatitis have not been demonstrated, and the Panel says the same holds true for their proposed use as self-treatment psoriasis balms. Pending further data, reviewers list hydrocortisone preparations as not proved safe or effective in relieving psoriasis.

Juniper tar   This tar preparation is widely used to treat skin disease. The Panel labels it safe, but could find no study that demonstrates the effectiveness of juniper tar (used by itself) for relieving psoriasis. Conclusion: safe but not proved effective.

Menthol   An antimicrobial agent that also relieves itching, menthol is judged safe. But reviewers appear to have received virtually no evidence to show how menthol works against psoriasis. The Panel has little to say on the matter except that the ingredient is safe but not proved effective for psoriasis relief.

Phenol preparations: phenol and phenolate sodium   These germicides also have a numbing and anti-itching effect on the skin. The Panel says they are safe in concentrations of 0.5 to 1.5 percent (*see* PHENOL). The evidence on whether phenol and phenolate sodium are helpful in relieving psoriasis symptoms is conflicting and inconclusive. So the Panel judges these ingredients safe but not proved effective.

Pine-tar preparations: pine tar and rectified pine tar   Traditional skin remedies, these substances were granted the "safe" label because of a long historical record and Panel members' own clinical experience using pine-tar preparations to treat their own patients. But since no firm scientific evidence is available to confirm effectiveness, the verdict is: safe but not proved effective.

Disapproved Active Ingredients

Benzocaine   No evidence was submitted to show that this anesthetic is effective in relieving symptoms of psoriasis. Since there is also a small but real risk of side effects from benzocaine's use, the Panel decided that the drug is not safe or effective.

Colloidal oatmeal   The Panel could think of no way that oatmeal could be dangerous. But no data were submitted—nor was the Panel aware of any—to show that oats suspended in lotion might be effective in relieving psoriasis. Conclusion: safe but not effective.
Note: An FDA summary document indicates that this ingredient will be listed as safe and effective in the Panel's final published report.

Cresol, saponated   This is cresol formulated in soap. Cresol is a phenollike coal-tar derivative, with many of phenol's anti-itch and antimicrobial properties. It is put up into soaps because it is more soluble in fats than it is in water. In the low doses of under 2 percent in which it is formulated in antipsoriasis products, cresol is judged safe; this decision is based on an assessment by the Panel concerned with over-the-counter topical analgesics, sunburn preventers, and other drugs.

The problem is that while one cresol soap carries a label saying it is "for removing the crusts and scales and relieving other discomforts of psoriasis," the Panel could not find any evidence—and none was submitted by the manufacturer—to demonstrate that the product lives up to this claim. Verdict: cresol is not effective.

Mercury oleate   A mercury preparation, this drug could be dangerous if large amounts were absorbed through the skin (mercury is a systemic poison). The Panel appears to feel, however—and its draft report is not altogether clear on the matter—that too little of this substance would be absorbed through the skin to do much harm. The greater problem, it says, is that no acceptable test results were submitted or found to show that mercury oleate effectively relieves psoriasis. Therefore the drug is assessed as safe but not effective.

Resorcinol   This antimicrobial is widely used in treating skin conditions—in part because it also has skin-peeling and itch-relieving properties. It is a phenollike compound, which can be irritating to the skin, and it may also occasionally stimulate an allergic reaction. If absorbed, resorcinol can cause internal poisoning. The Panel thinks this absorption is unlikely to occur, and it decided that the drug is safe for use on the scalp. But lacking evidence that resorcinol actually combats psoriasis, the Panel calls it safe but not effective.

Safety and Effectiveness: Active Ingredients in Over-the-Counter Psoriasis Drugs

Active Ingredient	Panel's Assessment
allantoin	safe, but not proved effective
benzocaine	not safe or effective
coal-tar shampoos	safe and effective
coal-tar body lotions	not proved safe
colloidal oatmeal	safe, but not effective*
cresol, saponated	safe, but not effective
hydrocortisone preparations: hydrocortisone acetate and hydrocortisone alcohol	not proved safe or effective
juniper tar	safe, but not proved effective
menthol	safe, but not proved effective
mercury oleate	safe, but not effective
phenol preparations: phenol and phenolate sodium	safe, but not proved effective
pine-tar preparations: pine tar and rectified pine tar	safe, but not proved effective
resorcinol	safe, but not effective
salicylic acid	safe and effective

*An FDA summary document indicates that this ingredient will be upgraded to safe and effective in the Panel's published report.

Safety and Effectiveness: Combination Products Sold Over-the-Counter for Relieving Psoriasis

Safe and Effective

None

**Safety and Effectiveness: Combination
Products Sold Over-the-Counter for
Relieving Psoriasis** *(continued)*

Conditionally Safe and Effective

allantoin + phenol
coal-tar extract + allantoin
coal-tar extract + hydrocortisone alcohol
coal-tar extract + menthol
coal-tar solution + menthol
coal tar + pine tar + juniper tar
coal tar + salicylic acid

Not Safe or Effective

Contains any active ingredient not
  approved for use against psoriasis

Psoriasis Lotions: Product Ratings[1]

Product and Distributor	Dosage of Active Ingredients	Rating[2]	Comment
ammoniated mercury			
Ammoniated Mercury (Lilly)	**ointment:** 5%	**C**	not submitted to or assessed by Panel
coal-tar shampoos			
DHS Tar (Person & Covey)	**shampoo:** 0.5% coal-tar USP equivalent	**A**	
Pentrax Tar (Cooper)	**shampoo:** 4.3% crude coal tar	**A**	
Tersa-Tar (Doak)	**shampoo:** 3% tar distillate	**A**	
coal-tar body lotions and bath preparations			
Alphosyl (Reed & Carnrick)	**lotion** and **cream:** 5% crude coal-tar extract + 1.7% allantoin	**B**	tar not proved safe; allantoin not proved effective
Balnetar (Westwood)	**bath additive:** 2.5% coal tar	**B**	not proved safe
coal tar or Carbonis Detergens (generic)	**solution:** 20% coal tar	**B**	not proved safe
Polytar Bath (Stiefel)	**bath additive:** 25% polytar (coal-tar solution + crude coal tar + pine tar + juniper tar)	**B**	some ingredients not proved safe or effective

Psoriasis Lotions: Product Ratings[1] *(continued)*

Product and Distributor	Dosage of Active Ingredients	Rating[2]	Comment
Pragmatar (Menley & James)	**ointment:** 4% cetyl alcohol–coal-tar distillate + 3% precipitated sulfur + 3% salicylic acid	C	sulfur not approved for use against psoriasis
Tar Doak (Doak)	**lotion:** 5% tar distillate	B	not proved safe
Tarlene (Medeco Labs.)	**lotion:** 2% refined crude coal tar + 2.5% salicylic acid	B	conditionally approved combination
icthammol			
Ichthyol (Stiefel)	**ointment:** 10%	C	ingredient not submitted to or assessed by Panel as psoriasis reliever
pine-tar preparations			
Packer's Pine Tar (Cooper)	**soap:** 0.82% pine tar	B	not proved effective
salicylic acid			
Salicylic Acid (Stiefel)	**soap:** 3.5%	A	

1. For hydrocortisone preparations, *see* ratings pages 468–469.
2. Author's interpretation of Panel criteria. Based on contents, not claims.

Reducing Aids

The 17 Review Panels made tens of thousands of decisions about the safety and effectiveness of ingredients in a quarter-million brands of over-the-counter drugs sold in the United States. But if one had to decide which was the most controversial of all these decisions, the choice would be easy: the vote to list the drug phenylpropanolamine hydrochloride (PPA) as safe and effective as a reducing aid.

REDUCING AIDS is based on the report "Weight-Control Drug Products for OTC Human Use" by the FDA's Advisory Review Panel on OTC Miscellaneous Internal Drug Products.

This endorsement of PPA triggered a major marketing effort that helped boost sales sharply to close to a quarter billion dollars a year, according to industry sources. The Panel's approval also set off a sharp backlash among medical colleagues and other health authorities, who charge that PPA is a fad and a fraud—and dangerous to boot.

Officials at the FDA were disquieted by the Panel's decision on PPA. The agency has demanded further safety testing and has already cut back the Panel's recommended dosages.

The reasons for the Panel's approval of PPA are not altogether clear. Members perhaps felt that the wide public constituency for aids to combat overweight was entitled to some help in the over-the-counter marketplace. But the reviewers conceded that the studies upon which they based their approval were flawed—and they were also unpublished. It certainly seems reasonable to want far better evidence to support a drug that is taken for weeks at a time by millions of people —many of them women of childbearing age.

CLAIMS

Accurate

for "appetite control to aid weight reduction"
"helps curb appetite"
"appetite depressant in the treatment of obesity"
"an aid in the control of appetite"
for "use as an adjunct to diet control"

Unproved

"provides bulk to add to low caloric intake and helps to satisy the feeling of hunger caused by emptiness"
"contains one of the most powerful diet aids available without prescription"
"Easy-to-follow reducing plan built around food you love to eat. You will eat well but less and lose weight without going hungry."
"the modern aid to appetite control"
"Now enjoy a slim, trim figure. Lose pounds. Reduce inches."
"Lose weight starting today. . . . Look your best, feel your best"
"the delightful aid to appetite control"
"delightfully delicious, scientifically formulated to help you control your appetite quickly, pleasantly"
"trim pounds and inches without crash diets or strenuous exercise"
"get rid of unsightly bulges"

WARNING These products should not be used for longer than 3 months. They should not be given to children under 12, since there is no evidence to show they are safe and effective for youngsters.

APPETITE SUPPRESSANTS

Many Americans *are* fat and many others *fear* that they are. And we all face a world in which thinness is prized. Little wonder then that there is tremendous demand for new and better ways to lose weight— a miracle drug that has yet to be developed!

The Panel says that over-the-counter reducing aids (anorexiants) have a real—if brief—therapeutic role to play in helping people lose weight. These drugs can help one eat less and may contribute to the development of a long-standing self-commitment to staying in negative caloric balance—that is, to burn more calories than one consumes. However, the experts stress that these preparations must be used only temporarily, and never longer than 3 months—which may be time enough to develop new, sparer eating habits.

An enormous range of drugs and other substances claimed by manufacturers to have medicinal benefit have been formulated into weight-loss products. Some have no pharmacological activity at all, and many others are dismissed out-of-hand by the Panel for want of any shred of evidence that suggests they may be helpful. Of the multitude, reviewers winnowed out a dozen drugs that have at least promise of benefit. They further decided that 2 of them—PPA and benzocaine (plus one combination)—are safe and effective.

COMBINATION PRODUCTS

The Panel approves as safe and effective the combination of PPA and 100 to 200 mg of caffeine or caffeine citrate. This is about the amount of caffeine in a cup of coffee. The Panel says one unpublished study showed a statistically significant weight loss with these ingredients—but not with a dummy medication. No really well-controlled study has shown that PPA with caffeine is any more effective than the PPA alone. Nevertheless, the combination makes sense because caffeine can relieve the fatigue that accompanies weight-reduction efforts.

To indicate that the caffeine does not directly help take off pounds, the Panel stipulated that this combination be labeled as an "anoretic/- stimulant."

The evaluators took a far dimmer view of combination diet products that contain vitamins and minerals—an addition said to serve no useful purpose. These combinations are disapproved.

A Stiff Word About Starch Blockers

As the PPA fad peaked in the early 1980s, manufacturers produced another "revolutionary new" weight-loss method: starch blockers, also known as amylase inhibitors and alpha amylase blockers. The active ingredient in these products is the enzyme alpha amylase, which is derived from a variety of kidney beans.

Manufacturers say these products block the breakdown of starch, an important source of calories—and thus of body weight—so that the starch passes through the intestinal tract undigested. One manufacturer claims that a single tablet of his product blocks the digestion and absorption of 150 grams of starch, which represents 600 starch calories.

The problem with this theory is that there are little data to support it, and little or no data to show that starch blockers are safe. The manufacturers claim these products are "food," since they are derived from beans. But the FDA disagrees, citing a clause in the Food, Drug & Cosmetic Act which says that any substance that "may affect the body's normal metabolic functions" is a drug and therefore must be proved safe and effective. This has not been done, the FDA says, and in fact many consumers have complained to the FDA of nausea, vomiting, diarrhea, headache, and other symptoms when taking these products. The FDA has banned starch blockers from the market—an action that the manufacturers were fighting as this guide went to press. The FDA's conclusion: starch blockers are unproved and misbranded drugs. They are not safe and not effective.

Approved Active Ingredients

Benzocaine   This is a widely used anesthetic with an excellent safety record. The Panel lists it as safe. We eat partly because we like the taste of our food. Benzocaine acts as an appetite suppressant by temporarily deadening the taste receptors in the mouth, dulling our pleasure. It particularly interferes with our ability to detect varying degrees of sweetness. The Panel reviewed several studies which suggest that benzocaine can help one lose weight, but did not indicate if the studies were controlled or not controlled, nor how they were conducted. The Panel also neglects to say whether appetite returns when the benzocaine wears off. Nevertheless, in a conclusion based on this seemingly meager record, the Panel says 3 to 15 mg of benzocaine in chewing gum or candy used just before eating is safe and effective for weight control.

Phenylpropanolamine hydrochloride (PPA) This is a weak anticholinergic agent, like ephedrine—which means it can block certain nerve impulses, affecting glandular secretions. Its therapeutic activity is similar to that of the amphetamines, a class of prescription drugs that have long been used as dieting aids, but which have a high potential for abuse and dependence because of the "highs" they produce. PPA may be free of this addictive risk. However, the Panel does say that low doses of PPA can be expected to tighten blood vessels and speed up the heart rate—which will elevate one's blood pressure. Large doses may cause anxiety, excitement, sleeplessness, headache, heartbeat irregularities, convulsions, and circulatory distress.

Despite these hazards, the Panel says that in manufacturers' recommended doses of 25 to 50 mg before meals, PPA has low toxicity and can be safely used without professional supervision. Of course, because of PPA's stimulating effect on the body, persons with high blood pressure, heart disease, diabetes, or thyroid disease should ask their doctor's advice before they use the drug.

The question of how PPA acts to reduce appetite remains unanswered. But work it does, the Panel says, at least temporarily. The Panel cites double-blind, dummy-medication controlled investigations that show the drug's effectiveness, but concedes that the studies were flawed, and may be criticized for improper study design that has resulted in "confusing or contradictory findings." Some studies are inconclusive. Nonetheless, the evaluators say that the studies adequately establish PPA's ability to facilitate weight loss over short periods, of 4 to 6 weeks. One study shows that the active drug is better than dummy medication for up to 16 weeks. So the Panel considered the available data adequate to establish PPA's effectiveness for periods of up to 12 weeks, in dosages up to 150 mg daily, divided into 25 to 50 mg doses before meals.

The reviewers did not say how many people were studied, what percentage lost weight, or how much was lost. All these questions seem highly relevant when one considers the virtually simultaneous assessment by the American Medical Association's Department of Drugs. That group maintains that products containing PPA—with or without caffeine—"are only minimally effective" (*AMA Drug Evaluations*, 4th ed., 1980).

The Panel's approval of PPA proved to be a fast-acting stimulant to the diet-aid business. The leading United States manufacturer—Thompson Medical Company—promised druggists $21 million in advertising in 1980 to launch what it called a "gigantic growth in diet-aid sales" that aimed at exceeding $300 million dollars per year. As sales rose, so did adverse-reaction reports. Particularly worrisome to the FDA was a report from Australia, published in *The Lancet* (January 12, 1980), about tests in which a single 85 mg dose of PPA was given to normal, healthy medical students in their twenties. The capsule pushed the blood pressure up in one-third of them; 3 of the 37 subjects required antihypertensive medication. The Australian investigators concluded that the high-dose PPA capsules are potentially hazardous.

The FDA reacted by noting that, based on the Panel's recommendations, United States drug companies were selling higher-dosage units of PPA than it had formally approved. The agency said the maximum dosage it would sanction is 75 mg daily—not the 150 mg that the Panel had recommended. It set a limit of 37.5 mg for ordinary, immediate-release tablets or capsules and 75 mg for sustained-release PPA capsules.

Reporter Joseph Carey meanwhile searched out the studies upon which the Panel based its approval of PPA. He noted in New York's *Daily News* (February 2, 1981) that one study, conducted by a Philadelphia internist, was funded by Thompson Medical. In the test, 35 subjects were given PPA plus caffeine, and 35 were given dummy drugs. Of the participants who took the active drug, 50 percent lost 6 or more pounds; only 22 percent of those who took the dummy drug lost this much. Of those who took the active drug, 35 percent lost 8 or more pounds while only 9 percent of those on the dummy drug achieved this result.

But after considering all the published evidence on PPA, a number of medical authorities came to conclusions quite at odds with the Panel's. The well-regarded *Medical Letter on Drugs and Therapeutics* (vol. 21, no. 16) declared: "There is no good evidence that PPA . . . can help obese patients achieve long-term weight reduction." An editorial in the *Journal of the American Medical Association* (vol. 245, no. 13) said: "Clearly, the use of PPA poses a danger to the public."

When the FDA published the Panel's report, approving PPA, it expressed strong doubts about the drug's safety, but did not override the Panel's decision that it is safe and effective. The agency did insist, however, that "further studies" be conducted "to resolve the safety questions," and promised to monitor dieters' use of the drug with the eye to "immediate . . . regulatory action" if new evidence of risk were to warrant it. The agency noted, too, that sustained-released capsules and tablets that contain more PPA than immediate-action ones will have to be proved safe and effective under the stringent guidelines that apply to all new drugs.

WARNING FOR PHENYLPROPANOLAMINE HYDROCHLORIDE (PPA)

Do not exceed the recommended dosage. If nervousness, dizziness, or sleeplessness occur, stop the medication and consult your physician. If you are being treated for high blood pressure or depression, or have heart disease, diabetes, or thyroid disease, do not take this product except under the supervision of a physician.

Conditionally Approved Active Ingredients

Alginic acid   This foam-making ingredient is used in some antacid preparations, and the present Panel concurs that it is safe. When taken along with sodium bicarbonate and water, alginic acid creates a bulk-producing foam in the stomach. This supposedly creates a full feeling, discouraging further eating. Four double-blind, dummy-drug controlled studies were submitted for review and one of them suggests that alginic acid combined with sodium bicarbonate and carboxymethylcellulose sodium may be beneficial. But the Panel believes this still remains to be proved. In sum: alginic acid is not proved effective as a diet aid in combination with sodium bicarbonate.

Carboxymethylcellulose sodium   This is a derivative of plant cellulose, which has been assessed as safe and effective as a bulk-forming laxative. The present Panel says the medical record demonstrates that the drug is safe. However, because it binds digitalis, nitrofurantoin, and salicylates, it should not be used by persons taking these drugs unless a doctor approves.

When swallowed with a full glass of water, a dose of carboxymethylcellulose sodium forms a soft wad in the belly. This creates a feeling of fullness, which is supposed to reduce one's appetite. But the substance leaves the stomach within 30 minutes. Its passage is marked by strong rumblings, which may signal a rapid return of appetite. In one large study, significant reduction in hunger was reported by participants who took the carboxymethylcellulose as compared with subjects who took dummy medication. But after 2 weeks, there was no difference in weight loss between the 2 groups. So, while safe, carboxymethylcellulose sodium's effectiveness remains to be proved.

Carrageenan   This derivative of seaweed is widely used as a thickener and stabilizer in ice cream and other foods, and so the Panel judges it safe. Like carboxymethlcellulose sodium, described directly above, it absorbs water, and will produce a soft, bulky wad in the stomach. It may therefore have value for weight reduction—but this remains to be proved.

Chondrus   This seaweed material is used in foods, and is safe, but has not been proved effective as a diet aid.

Guar gum   This substance, used as a food additive, has been found safe for use as a bulk laxative by the Advisory Review Panel on OTC Laxative, Antidiarrheal, Emetic and Antiemetic Drug Products. Like carboxymethylcellulose sodium, described above, it absorbs water and so may be effective as a diet-aid active ingredient—although this remains to be proved.

Karya gum   This substance is very similar to guar gum, described immediately above, and like it, it is safe. But the gum has not been proved effective as a reducing aid.

Methylcellulose   A bulking agent, this material is very similar to carboxymethylcellulose sodium, described above, and the same conclusions apply.

Psyllium   This seed material is assessed as safe and effective as a bulk-forming laxative. So the Panel says it would be safe for use as a diet-aid ingredient. It acts in the same way as carboxymethylcellulose sodium, described above, and may have a similar beneficial action in creating a full feeling in the pit of the stomach. But this remains to be proved. The Panel's assessment: not proved effective.

Sea kelp   This seaweed is used as a food additive, and so is safe. It absorbs water, and could create a filling wad in the stomach, yielding a full feeling. But it is not proved effective as an appetite suppressant.

The combination of sodium bicarbonate + alginic acid   The only role for this household remedy as a diet aid comes from its reaction with alginic acid (*see* ALGINIC ACID, above). This combination is safe but it has not been proved effective.

Xanthan gum   This substance is an approved food additive, so the Panel accepts it as safe for use as an over-the-counter weight-loss drug. Xanthan combines easily with water to form a gelatinous mass, which is thought to create a full feeling that discourages eating. The gum passes through the gut unchanged—although it may produce soft stools. The data submitted to the Panel did not demonstrate that xanthan gum works any better than a dummy medication. So, while safe, its effectiveness remains to be proved.

Disapproved Active Ingredients

Many ingredients are formulated into products that allegedly help one lose weight. The Panel summarily dismissed *several dozen* of these ingredients owing to lack of data about safety and effectiveness. These substances will not be described here, but each of them is listed as summarily disapproved in the SAFETY AND EFFECTIVENESS chart below.

Safety and Effectiveness: Ingredients in Over-the-Counter Reducing Aids

Active Ingredient	Panel's Assessment
alcohol	summarily disapproved
alfalfa	summarily disapproved
alginic acid	safe, but not proved effective
alpha amylase blockers	not safe and not effective*
amylase inhibitors	not safe and not effective*
anise oil	summarily disapproved
arginine	summarily disapproved
benzocaine	safe and effective
biotin	summarily disapproved
bone marrow-red-glycerin extract	summarily disapproved
buchu	summarily disapproved
buchu, potassium extract	summarily disapproved
calcium	summarily disapproved
calcium carbonate	summarily disapproved
calcium caseinate	summarily disapproved
calcium lactate	summarily disapproved
calcium pantothenate	summarily disapproved
carrageenan	safe, but not proved effective
carboxymethylcellulose sodium	safe, but not proved effective
choline	summarily disapproved
chondrus	safe, but not proved effective
citric acid	summarily disapproved
Cnicus benedictus	summarily disapproved
copper	summarily disapproved
copper gluconate	summarily disapproved
corn oil	summarily disapproved
corn silk, potassium extract	summarily disapproved
corn syrup	summarily disapproved
cupric sulfate	summarily disapproved
cystine	summarily disapproved
dextrose	summarily disapproved
dioctyl sodium sulfosuccinate	summarily disapproved
ferric ammonium citrate	summarily disapproved
ferric pyrophosphate	summarily disapproved
ferrous fumarate	summarily disapproved

**Safety and Effectiveness: Ingredients in
Over-the-Counter Reducing Aids** *(continued)*

Active Ingredient	*Panel's Assessment*
ferrous gluconate	summarily disapproved
ferrous sulfate	summarily disapproved
flax seed	summarily disapproved
folic acid	summarily disapproved
fructose	summarily disapproved
glycerides	summarily disapproved
guar gum	safe, but not proved effective
histidine	summarily disapproved
Hydrastis canadensis	summarily disapproved
inositol	summarily disapproved
iodine	summarily disapproved
isoleucine	summarily disapproved
juniper, potassium extract	summarily disapproved
karaya gum	safe, but not proved effective
lactose	summarily disapproved
lecithin	summarily disapproved
leucine	summarily disapproved
liver concentrate	summarily disapproved
L-lysine	summarily disapproved
L-lysine monohydrochloride	summarily disapproved
magnesium	summarily disapproved
magnesium oxide	summarily disapproved
malt	summarily disapproved
maltodextrin	summarily disapproved
manganese citrate	summarily disapproved
mannitol	summarily disapproved
methionine	summarily disapproved
methylcellulose	safe, but not proved effective
niacinamide	summarily disapproved
organic vegetables	summarily disapproved
pancreatin enzymes	summarily disapproved
pantothenic acid	summarily disapproved
papain	summarily disapproved
papaya enzymes	summarily disapproved
pepsin	summarily disapproved
phenacetin	summarily disapproved
phenylalanine	summarily disapproved
phenylpropanolamine hydrochloride (PPA)	safe and effective
phosphorus	summarily disapproved
phytolacca berry juice	summarily disapproved
pineapple enzymes	summarily disapproved
potassium citrate	summarily disapproved
PPA (*see* phenylpropanolamine hydrochloride)	

Safety and Effectiveness: Ingredients in
Over-the-Counter Reducing Aids *(continued)*

Active Ingredient	Panel's Assessment
psyllium	safe, but not proved effective
riboflavin	summarily disapproved
rice polishings	summarily disapproved
saccharin	summarily disapproved
sea kelp	safe, but not proved effective
sea minerals	summarily disapproved
sesame seed	summarily disapproved
sodium	summarily disapproved
sodium bicarbonate + alginic acid	safe, but not proved effective
sodium caseinate	summarily disapproved
sodium chloride	summarily disapproved
soybean protein	summarily disapproved
soy meal	summarily disapproved
starch blockers	not safe and not effective
sucrose	summarily disapproved
threonine	summarily disapproved
tricalcium phosphate	summarily disapproved
tryptophan	summarily disapproved
tyrosine	summarily disapproved
uva-ursi	summarily disapproved
uva-ursi, potassium extract	summarily disapproved
valine	summarily disapproved
vegetable	summarily disapproved
vitamin A acetate	summarily disapproved
vitamin B_2	summarily disapproved
vitamin B_6	summarily disapproved
vitamin C	summarily disapproved
vitamin D_2	summarily disapproved
vitamin E	summarily disapproved
wheat germ	summarily disapproved
xanthan gum	safe, but not proved effective
yeast	summarily disapproved

*Assessed by the FDA.

Safety and Effectiveness: Combination Products Sold Over-the-Counter as Reducing Aids

Safe and Effective

phenylpropanolamine hydrochloride (PPA) + caffeine or caffeine citrate

**Safety and Effectiveness: Combination Products Sold Over-the-Counter
as Reducing Aids** *(continued)*

Conditionally Safe and Effective

alginic acid + sodium bicarbonate

alginic acid + sodium bicarbonate + carboxymethylcellulose sodium

Not Safe or Effective

contains weight-loss active ingredient at more or less than approved dosage(s)

contains weight-loss active ingredient + vitamins or minerals

contains any active ingredient disapproved as unsafe or ineffective

---

Reducing Aids: Product Ratings

Single-Ingredient Products

Product and Distributor	Dosage of Active Ingredients	Rating[1]	Comment
benzocaine			
Slim Line Gum (O'Connor)	**chewing gum:** 6 mg	**A**	
phenylpropanolamine hydrochloride (PPA)			
Coffee-Break (O'Connor)	**cubes:** 37.5 mg	**A**	
Coffee, Tea & a New Me (Thompson)	**cubes:** 25 mg	**A**	
Control (Thompson)	**drops:** 25 mg per 4 drops	**A**	
Delcopro (Delco)	**tablets:** 25 mg	**A**	
Diadax (O'Connor)		**A**	
Dietac (Menley & James)		**A**	
Diadax (O'Connor)	**capsules, timed-release:** 50 mg	**A**	
Obestat (Lemmon)	**capsules, timed-release:** 75 mg	**A**	
Pro-Dax 21 (O'Connor)		**A**	

Reducing Aids: Product Ratings *(continued)*

Combination Products

Product and Distributor	Dosage of Active Ingredients	Rating[1]	Comment
Anorexin One-Span (SDA Pharm.)	**capsules, timed-release:** 50 mg phenylpropanolamine hydrochloride + 200 mg caffeine	**A**	
Dietac (Menley & James)		**A**	
Appress (North American)	**tablets:** 25 mg phenylpropanolamine hydrochloride + 100 mg caffeine	**A**	
Dexatrim Extra-Strength (Thompson)	**capsules, timed-release:** 75 mg phenylpropanolamine hydrochloride + 200 mg caffeine	**A**	
Extra Strength Grapefruit Diet Plan with Diadax (O'Connor)	**capsules, timed-release** and **tablets, chewable:** 75 mg phenylpropanolamine hydrochloride	**A**	contains 100 mg grapefruit extract
Fluidex Plus (O'Connor)	**tablets:** 25 mg phenylpropanolamine hydrochloride + 65 mg powdered buchu + 65 mg powdered extract couch grass + 32.5 mg powdered extract corn silk + 32.5 mg powdered extract hydrangea	**C**	disapproved combination; many ingredients not safe and/or not effective

1. Author's interpretation of Panel criteria. Based on contents, not claims.

Ringworm Cures

See JOCK ITCH, ATHLETE'S FOOT, AND RINGWORM CURES

Salt Supplements and Substitutes: Preliminary Report

People who sweat a lot—either because they are working (or playing) very hard or are exposed to heat—often take salt tablets to counteract the loss of body salt.

These salt supplements and salt substitutes were to have been evaluated by the Advisory Review Panel on OTC Miscellaneous Internal Drugs, but the group was disbanded before the review could be completed. The FDA or a supplemental Panel may complete this task. Meanwhile, persons on sodium-restricted diets should ask their doctors whether—and how much—of the salt substitutes they can use. Many older persons—particularly those who have kidney or heart ailments—must shun table salt (sodium chloride) and they may be advised to use potassium chloride or potassium iodide instead.

Your family doctor or a sports-medicine specialist may be able to enlighten you on the value of taking salt pills when you are hot and sweating. *Drinking a lot of water* and other fluids may be at least as important as replacing the salt.

Sedatives, Daytime

The class of drugs promoted for use during the day to relieve "simple nervous tension," "nervous irritability," and "simple nervousness due

SALT SUPPLEMENTS AND SUBSTITUTES is based on an FDA study report on the OTC Drug Review.

SEDATIVES, DAYTIME is based on the report of the FDA's Advisory Review Panel on OTC Sedative, Tranquilizer, and Sleep-Aid Drug Products, the FDA's Tentative Final Order and Final Order on Daytime Sedatives, and related documents.

to common everyday overwork and fatigue" has been *eliminated* from the over-the-counter marketplace in the United States.

Reviewers could not find any clearcut medical need for these drugs. Their active ingredients are unlikely to produce calmative, relaxing, or tranquilizing effects—which under certain (medically determined) circumstances might be desirable. Instead, these ingredients make the user drowsy, a condition that could be potentially dangerous.

The FDA banned these products from interstate commerce. This action has not meant, however, that these sedatives have vanished from druggists' shelves. The reason is that the active ingredients in sedatives formerly sold for daytime use are essentially identical to those found in sedatives sold for nighttime use (*see* SLEEP AIDS). The FDA says that some manufacturers simply relabeled their products and now recommend them for use only at night—as sleep aids.

The one published study on the subject compared the 2-week effect of 4 different preparations on moderately anxious patients. One preparation was a nonprescription daytime sedative containing 2 antihistamines + scopolamine. One was a prescription tranquilizer, chlordiazepoxide. One was aspirin. The last was a dummy drug, or placebo. The tranquilizer yielded significantly greater relief of anxiety than the other 3 medications. The nonprescription daytime sedative was no more effective than the dummy drug. So it was concluded that people who require a drug during the day to combat anxiety, nervousness, or tension should consult a physician—who can prescribe a tranquilizer if he or she thinks it is needed.

CLAIMS

"Based on the available evidence," the FDA says, "no ingredient can be generally recognized as safe and effective for use as an OTC daytime sedative. If the labeling on any product represents or suggests it to be used as an OTC daytime sedative . . . that product . . . is not in compliance with [the Federal Food, Drug, and Cosmetic Act and] . . . is subject to regulatory action."

Because products formerly sold as daytime sedatives remain on the market as sleep aids and because of split jurisdiction by the FDA and the Federal Trade Commission, some questionable advertising claims may continue to appear. These could include phrases such as:

"gently soothe away the tension"
"help you relax"
"[when] you're under occasional stress"

Thus, consumers may have to continue to evaluate claims of this nature for themselves.

ACTIVE INGREDIENTS—UNSAFE AND INEFFECTIVE

The active ingredients used in daytime sedatives are unsafe as well as ineffective. The 3 principal groups of active ingredients have been antihistamines, bromide compounds, and scopolamine compounds.

The principal antihistamine used for years was methapyrilene—which was withdrawn from the market in 1979 as a cancer risk. The safety and the effectiveness of pyrilamine maleate, the antihistamine that replaced it in daytime sedatives, have not been confirmed.

The bromides are disapproved as unsafe and ineffective because they fail to produce daytime sedation in a single dose and if taken for a long enough time to reach effective levels they could cause toxic reactions.

Scopolamines are similarly ineffective at doses that were suggested and unsafe at doses that might cause drowsiness.

Other Disapproved Ingredients

Several other components of daytime sedatives are no more effective than the active ingredients. The pain relievers acetaminophen, aspirin, and salicylamide are ineffective and the vitamins niacinamide and thiamine hydrochloride—which were formulated into some of these products—are not only ineffective for sedation but also their inclusion makes no sense for that purpose.

Safety and Effectiveness: Ingredients in Sedatives Sold Over-the-Counter for Daytime Use

Ingredient	Panel and FDA's* Assessment
antihistamines	
methapyrilene fumarate	not safe
methapyrilene hydrochloride	not safe
pyrilamine maleate	not safe or effective
bromides	
ammonium bromide	not safe or effective
potassium bromide	not safe or effective
sodium bromide	not safe or effective
scopolamine compounds	
scopolamine aminoxide	
hydrobromide	not safe or effective
scopolamine hydrobromide	not safe or effective
miscellaneous compounds	
acetaminophen	not effective

**Safety and Effectiveness: Ingredients in Sedatives
Sold Over-the-Counter for Daytime Use** *(continued)*

Ingredient	Panel and FDA's* Assessment
aspirin	not effective
niacinamide	not effective
salicylamide	not effective
thiamine hydrochloride	not effective

*Judgments reaffirmed or modified by the FDA, or originated by it.

Daytime Sedatives: Product Ratings

All daytime sedatives have been removed from the market in the U.S.

Sleep Aids

Many people have difficulty from time to time falling asleep or staying asleep. Therefore, both the FDA and the Panel see a valid need for
safe and effective nonprescription medication to induce and sustain
sleep.

CLAIMS

Accurate
    For adults only, the FDA says, the only claims that can legitimately be made
for a safe and effective over-the-counter sleep aid are:
    "helps [you] fall asleep"
    for "relief of occasional sleeplessness"
    "helps to reduce difficulty in falling asleep"

    SLEEP AIDS is based on the report of the FDA's Advisory Review Panel on OTC
Sedative, Tranquilizer, and Sleep-Aid Drug Products; the FDA's Tentative Final Orders
for OTC Nighttime Sleep-Aid and Stimulant Products; the Final Order on OTC Daytime
Sedatives; and official addenda in the OTC Drug Review.

Unproved

"reduces time required to fall asleep or number of awakenings"
"prolongs sleep"

False or Misleading

references to: "natural sleep" or "normal sleep," "sound sleep," or "refreshing sleep"
"non-habit forming"
"relaxes"

BENEFITS AND RISKS

The principal active ingredients in sleep aids have been drugs of the class called *antihistamines*. They make many people drowsy. How they achieve this is not clear. It is known that antihistamines depress the activity of the central nervous system; this may in part explain how they act.

A nonprescription drug that induces drowsiness and sleep can be useful and convenient. Unfortunately, however, the Panel's assessment is that most active ingredients that have been used in sleep aids are unsafe, ineffective, or both and that many of the claims made for these products are false and misleading. The FDA, by and large, agreed and proposed severe restrictions in the ingredients and in the claims that could be made for such preparations. However, the FDA has recently granted approval to 3 antihistamines as sleep-aid active ingredients. They are doxylamine succinate, diphenhydramine hydrochloride and diphenhydramine monocitrate.

The most widely used—and apparently safest and most effective—sleep-aid active ingredient, the antihistamine methapyrilene, had been marketed by prescription and over-the-counter for more than a quarter of a century. In 1973, 543 million tablets and capsules containing methapyrilene were sold in the United States alone. In 1979 the United States National Cancer Institute confirmed that methapyrilene was "a potent cause of liver cancer in rats, and, as such, of potential human hazard." After the cancer risk was confirmed, drug makers, at the FDA's behest, recalled some 600 products containing methapyrilene. More than 300 were nighttime sleep aids or daytime sedatives that contained essentially the same amounts of essentially the same ingredients. Included in this group were:

Compoz (Jeffrey Martin)
Nytol (Block)

Sominex (J. B. Williams)
Sleep-Eze (Whitehall)
Quiet World (Whitehall)
Excedrin P.M. (Bristol-Meyers)
Cope (Glenbrook)
Nervine (Miles)

The manufacturers of these products either reformulated them with other antihistamines and returned them to the marketplace or dropped them. No such product containing methapyrilene is sold in the United States today.

There is one antihistamine that is conditionally approved, pyrilamine maleate. As its name suggests, it is a close chemical relative of the banned methapyrilene. "There are no conclusive studies regarding the carcinogenicity [cancer-causing nature] of pyrilamine," the FDA declared. "However, consumers should note that scientists have raised questions about the possible carcinogenicity of pyrilamine." Accelerated studies have been undertaken to probe pyrilamine's safety, which, however, has yet to be proved.

WHEN TO CONSIDER SLEEP AIDS

Brain-wave recordings made while subjects are asleep in a laboratory have become the principal means that scientists use to study normal sleep and sleep disturbances. The recordings show the exact moment that a subject falls asleep and then the minute-by-minute progression through what have come to be well-recognized sleep stages. Most people go through essentially the same sequences, although there is considerable variation in sleep patterns from person to person.

A person's normal sleep patterns tend to be similar night after night. An occcasional sleep disturbance is valid reason for buying and using an over-the-counter sleep aid, the Panel says. The medication can be expected to help one fall asleep, or remain sleeping, if the problem is untimely awakenings at night or early in the morning. But it should not be used longer than 2 weeks. Persons with severe or continuing insomnia should consult a doctor, who can offer more potent remedies.

The effectiveness of over-the-counter sleep aids can be determined in part by users' subjective reports or by trained observers who watch them sleep. But all-night sleep recordings made in sleep laboratories are the preferable, most objective method for assessing the action of these drugs. Such action should not seriously interfere with the behavioral and brain-wave patterns of normal sleep, the Panel warns. Neither should the drug's effects persist into the following day to interfere with normal daytime tasks.

Sleep aids specifically depress brain activity. So the FDA warns that they may act additively and prove to be particularly hazardous for persons drinking alcoholic beverages, which have a similar, depressant effect.

Antihistamines used in sleep aids also have the effect of reducing fluid secretions throughout the body. This can be particularly dangerous to persons with asthma or glaucoma and to men with enlarged prostate glands. Such individuals therefore should avoid taking sleep aids except under the advice and supervision of a physician. These preparations are also inappropriate for children under 12 years, whom they may stimulate rather than sedate.

ANTIHISTAMINES

Antihistamines, as their name implies, block the action of the body protein histamine, which triggers runny nose, watery eyes, and a variety of other allergic symptoms. These drugs were introduced in the 1940s and are widely used for allergic relief.

It soon was discovered that sedation is one of the antihistamines' principal side effects. This may produce an inability to concentrate, dizziness, incoordination, and drowsiness, all the way to deep sleep.

This sedative effect was soon recognized as a hazard: antihistamine users are routinely warned not to drive, operate heavy machinery, or do other jobs that require mental alertness while taking these drugs. On the other hand, pharmacologists soon recognized that this soporific side effect might also be used to advantage. Antihistamines began to be formulated into sleep-aid products, which quickly became quite popular. An estimated 10 million Americans use antihistamine-based sleep aids and related daytime sedatives, for which, in 1981, they were estimated to spend $30 million per year.

Different chemical groups of antihistamines have different sedative effects, the most pronounced in a group of potent antihistamines called *ethanolamines*. This group includes diphenhydramine hydrochloride, and doxylamine succinate—2 antihistamines recently approved by the FDA as safe and effective.

A second group of antihistamines, the ethylenediamines, are highly effective histamine antagonists. But the Panel says they "do not have

a strong central-nervous-system action and may not produce a therapeutic somnolence even though a fair number of patients will exhibit
drowsiness." *Ironically, the 2 antihistamines that until recently were
the backbone of the sleep-aid market—methapyrilene and pyrilamine
maleate—belong to this group.*

Despite those side effects listed below, billions of doses of antihistamines are used each year, with relatively few *serious* results and very
few deaths reported to manufacturers and government agencies. On
the other hand, the cancer risk of methapyrilene that has been convincingly demonstrated in animals would be difficult to confirm directly in
humans, given that the incubating period for most human cancers is 20
years or longer.

Common side effects of antihistamines include:

    dizziness
    ringing in the ears
    lassitude
    fatigue
    blurred or double vision
    mood changes (e.g., euphoria, anxiety, disorientation, confusion,
        and even delirium)

Other side effects:

    loss of appetite
    nausea
    vomiting
    both constipation and diarrhea
    dry mouth
    heart palpitations and irregularities in heart rate or rhythm
    frequency or difficulty in urination
    skin rashes
    rare but serious events (e.g., convulsions, coma, even death)

Formulating antihistamines into safe and effective sleep aids can be
a challenge. "The problem," says the FDA, "is to ensure that the dosage
recommendation is adequate for the intended sedative effect desired,
yet not so large that toxic effects result. The [FDA] Commissioner is
concerned that in currently available antihistamine over-the-counter
products promoted for sleep, dosage may have been reduced by the
manufacturer to borderline or ineffective levels to avoid toxicity." The
FDA goes so far as to recommend that *higher* doses be studied for
possible introduction to the nonprescription market.

ACTIVE INGREDIENTS IN SLEEP AIDS

The active ingredients in sleep aids can be divided into 4 major groups. All drugs in 2 of them—bromides and scopolamine compounds —are categorically rejected by the Panel and the FDA as unsafe, ineffective, or both. A third, miscellaneous category includes pain relievers, a vitamin, and a substance called *passion-flower extract*—none of which is effective as an aid to sleep. So, only one group, antihistamines, contains approved and conditionally approved ingredients.

Approved Active Ingredients

No active ingredient evaluated by the Panel was listed as safe and effective for over-the-counter sale and use as a sleep-aid active ingredient. Subsequently, however, the FDA, acting on the basis of new data submitted by manufacturers, approved two types of antihistamines for this purpose.

Diphenhydramine: diphenhydramine hydrochloride and diphenhydramine monocitrate The antihistamine diphenhydramine has a pronounced tendency to induce drowsiness. The Panel granted it conditional approval and it then was approved by the FDA as safe and effective as a nonprescription nighttime sleep aid in 1981.

This decision was reached because of two studies conducted by a manufacturer in which healthy people who occasionally had trouble sleeping alternated the use of diphenhydramine hydrochloride and a dummy medication to fall asleep. Neither the subjects nor the researchers dispensing the drugs knew which tablets contained the active drug and which did not. The diphenhydramine turned out to be "significantly better" than the dummy drug in terms of shortening the time it took users to fall asleep, the depth of sleep they obtained, and their assessment of how well they slept.

A dozen manufacturers' studies that were submitted to the agency "resolved" outstanding issues on diphenhydramine's safety and effectiveness. Its analysis of the studies showed the side effects to be minimal and mild, so the drug is judged safe when used to induce sleep. The FDA approved dosages of 50 mg diphenhydramine hydrochloride and 76 mg diphenhydramine monocitrate, which is rapidly converted to the hydrochloride in the stomach. The monocitrate is weaker than the hydrochloride, so that the two dosages are equivalent.

Doxylamine succinate This antihistamine, like diphenhydramine, has a marked tendency to induce drowsiness. While it has a long record of use as a prescription drug—for a variety of purposes—it had not previously been marketed as an over-the-counter sleep aid. Following the Panel and the FDA's decision that none of the existing nonprescription sleep aids was safe and effective, a manufacturer submitted a New Drug Application and supporting data requesting the FDA's permission to market doxylamine succinate as a nonprescription sleep aid. This application was studied and approved, under the rigorous scientific standards applicable to all new drugs examined in the late 1970s. The drug quickly became the top-selling over-the-counter sleep aid.

The approved dosage is 25 mg. While it has not yet been proved dangerous to pregnant women, neither has it been proved to be safe for them or for their babies. For this reason, the label warns that pregnant or nursing women should not use this sleep aid.

Conditionally Approved Active Ingredient

Pyrilamine maleate   Ironically, this conditionally-approved antihistamine has been evaluated by the American Medical Association, as well as by the FDA, as an antihistamine whose use is associated with a *low* incidence of sedation. Yet when methapyrilene was withdrawn, many manufacturers quickly reformulated their products with pyrilamine as the sole and principal active ingredient. The FDA says that so far there is no evidence that pyrilamine can or does cause cancer.

The Panel and the FDA agree that there is insufficient evidence to show that pyrilamine is either safe or effective when used as a nighttime sleep aid in the manufacturers' suggested dosages of 25 up to a maximum of 50 mg at bedtime. Even at these relatively low doses loss of appetite, nausea, and vomiting are commonly encountered side effects and huge overdoses have been fatal to infants.

The Panel could find only one 25-year-old published report on the ingredient's effect when used by itself. This study showed by brain-wave tracings that air-force personnel taking naps in the daytime fell asleep more quickly when given pyrilamine than when given dummy medication. But when questioned afterward, the airmen were not aware that pyrilamine had helped them fall asleep faster.

Disapproved Active Ingredients

The list of unsafe and/or ineffective sleep-aid active ingredients is a long one. Its principal items are the bromides, the antihistamine methapyrilene, and the scopolamine compounds.

Acetaminophen and aspirin   No evidence was submitted to show that acetaminophen or aspirin, which are pain relievers, are effective aids to sleep.

Bromides The ammonium, potassium, and sodium bromides are similar in their pharmacological action, and so are described together. They are toxic at the dosage levels used in nighttime sleep aids, and may cause birth defects when taken by pregnant women.

Both the medicinal value and the toxicity of the bromides were discovered in the 19th century, when these drugs first were used to treat epilepsy. Their use as aids to sleep dates from 1864. When their poisonous nature became more fully appreciated—some 50 years ago —they were replaced by the barbiturates as the principal prescription sleep inducers. Bromides have since been sold mostly over-the-counter and are rarely recommended by doctors.

One bedtime dose of a bromide never is effective in inducing sleep. This is because a bromide must be taken for several days in order for a high enough level to build up in the body to cause drowsiness. However, the effective dose is very close to the toxic dose and bromide poisoning (bromism) can produce overt psychotic behavior as well as coma, maniacal excitation, hallucinations, and sometimes death.

Methapyrilene hydrochloride and methapyrilene fumarate These compounds have been found to be a potential cause of cancer, and so have been withdrawn from the over-the-counter drug market (*see* page 660).

Passion-flower extract The Panel could find no valid scientific data to support the use of this ingredient in sleep aids. A search of the literature failed to identify any sleep-inducing action on the central nervous system.

Salicylamide No evidence was submitted to show that salicylamide, a pain reliever, effectively serves as an aid to sleep.

Scopolamine compounds: scopolamine, scopolamine hydrobromide, and scopolamine aminoxide hydrobromide The actions and risks of these compounds are relatively the same. Scopolamine—which is derived naturally from leaves of deadly nightshade (belladonna)—depresses the activity of the central nervous system. Thus, in adequate doses, it can cause marked drowsiness. The problem is that at the very low dosage levels in which such compounds have been formulated into nonprescription sleep aids, they probably are not effective. On the other hand, in larger, clinically effective doses, they are quite dangerous.

The side effects of therapeutic doses of scopolamine are unpleasant: dryness of the mouth, blurred vision, intolerance of light, as well as speed-ups, slow-downs, and irregularities in the heartbeat.

Documentation of scopolamine's sleep-inducing effects is wanting. Much of the scientific literature deals with its use against motion sickness and the severe neurologic disease parkinsonism.

The compound scopolamine aminoxide hydrobromide is less toxic, but it is also less effective than other scopolamine preparations. Both the Panel and the FDA say it still is too dangerous for use as a nonprescription drug. The Panel recommends, and the FDA concurs, that scopolamine should be banned as an over-the-counter sleep aid.

Thiamine hydrochloride   No evidence was submitted to show that this vitamin is an effective sleep aid.

COMBINATION PRODUCTS

Only one type of combination is now approved—and that approval is only conditional: One safe and effective sleep aid can be combined with a safe and effective dose of one approved pain reliever—for example, aspirin. To keep combinations of this type on the market, the FDA says manufacturers will have to prove that there are enough people that need both a sleep aid and a pain reliever, and that the combination in fact fills their need.

Some sleep-aid products combine an antihistamine with another sleep-inducing ingredient—for example, scopolamine. Since scopolamine and most other active ingredients have been rejected by the Panel and the FDA as either unsafe, ineffective, or both, these combinations will be disallowed. Other products have combined 2 antihistamines. But the FDA disapproves of combinations of 2 active ingredients of the same class, particularly when they both are antihistamines and may act in concert to depress activity in the brain.

Combining a sleep-aid active ingredient with vitamins or with passion-flower extract is also held not to make sense since neither vitamins nor passion-flower extract have been shown to induce sleep.

Safety and Effectiveness: Active Ingredients in Over-the-Counter Sleep Aids

Active Ingredient	Panel and FDA's* Assessment
antihistamines	
diphenhydramine hydrochloride	safe and effective
diphenhydramine monocitrate	safe and effective
doxylamine succinate	safe and effective
methapyrilene fumarate	not safe

Safety and Effectiveness: Active Ingredients in Over-the-Counter Sleep Aids *(continued)*

Active Ingredient	*Panel and FDA's* Assessment*
methapyrilene hydrochloride	not safe
pyrilamine maleate	not proved safe or effective
bromides	
ammonium bromide	not safe or effective
potassium bromide	not safe or effective
sodium bromide	not safe or effective
scopolamine compounds	
scopolamine aminoxide hydrobromide	not safe or effective
scopolamine hydrobromide	not safe or effective
miscellaneous compounds	
acetaminophen	not effective
aspirin	not effective
passion-flower extract	not effective
salicylamide	not effective
thiamine hydrochloride	not effective

*Judgments reaffirmed or modified by the FDA, or originated by it.

Sleep Aids: Product Ratings

Single-Ingredient Products

Product and Distributor	Dosage of Active Ingredients	Rating[1]	Comment
diphenhydramine hydrochloride			
Nytol with DPH (Block)	**tablets:** 25 mg	A	
Sominex Formula 2 Tablets (J. B. Williams)		A	
Compoz Tablets (Jeffrey Martin)	**tablets:** 50 mg	A	
doxylamine succinate			
Unisom (Pfizer)	**tablets:** 25 mg	A	
pyrilamine maleate			
Nervine (Miles)	**tablets:** 25 mg	B	not proved safe or effective
Nytol (Block)		B	
Sominex (J. B. Williams)		B	

Sleep Aids: Product Ratings *(continued)*

Single-Ingredient Products

Product and Distributor	Dosage of Active Ingredients	Rating[1]	Comment
Relax-U Caps (Columbia Medical)	**capsules:** 25 mg	**B**	
Nytol (Block)	**capsules:** 50 mg	**B**	

Combination Product

Product and Distributor	Dosage of Active Ingredients	Rating[1]	Comment
Quiet World (Whitehall)	**tablets:** 25 mg pyrilamine maleate + 162 mg acetaminophen + 227 mg aspirin	**C**	FDA not convinced of merit of a combination of over-the-counter sleep aid + pain relievers

1. Author's interpretation of Panel/FDA criteria. Based on contents, not claims.

Smelling Salts: Preliminary Report

Fainting—if one believes the classically romantic English novelists—
was once a fashionable method of responding to emotional distress.
Individuals who were subject to fainting spells carried bottles of smelling salts, which, when opened and waved under their nose, appear to
have successfully revived them.

Fainting can signal the presence of a serious underlying illness. It
can also be dangerous in and of itself. People who find themselves
feeling faint, or fainting from time to time, should see a doctor.

These days smelling salts are sold over-the-counter in convenient,
single-use ampules. Their principal active ingredient is ammonia, so
they are called *ammonium inhalants*. A few drops of household ammonia sprinkled on a handkerchief or other cloth that is then passed back

SMELLING SALTS is based on an FDA status report on the OTC Drug Review.

and forth under the nose of a person who has fainted, or who feels faint, may serve the same purpose.

The FDA's Advisory Review Panel on OTC Miscellaneous Internal Drugs was scheduled to assess ammonium inhalants, but it was disbanded before the task could be done. The agency lists the 2 active ingredients in ammonium inhalants as ammonium carbonate and ammonia solution, strong.

Smoking Deterrents

Many people want to stop smoking, and more than 30 million Americans have succeeded in their effort since 1964—when the Surgeon General of the United States Public Health Service first confirmed cigarette smoking's high risk of causing lung cancer. Since then, cigarette smoking has also been documented to be a major contributing factor in heart and artery disease and a variety of breathing disorders.

Most Americans know these facts. Many who have not yet stopped smoking and would like to, ask whether the readily available over-the-counter drugs that are promoted as smoking deterrents actually work. The Panel's answer: maybe, for brief periods of time, and only if you *really* want to stop and are willing to mobilize the self-discipline that may be needed to free yourself from the habit. In fact, it is will power, or at least a desire to stop smoking, that is needed for success. To make this clear, the Panel mandates that each smoking-deterrent product label carry this notice:

This product's effectiveness is directly related to the user's motivation to stop smoking cigarettes.

CLAIMS

Accurate
"a temporary aid to those who want to stop smoking cigarettes"
"helps stop the cigarette urge temporarily"
"a temporary aid to breaking the cigarette habit"

SMOKING DETERRENTS is based on the report "Smoking Deterrent Drug Products for OTC Human Use" by the FDA's Advisory Review Panel on OTC Miscellaneous Internal Drug Products.

False or Misleading
"a temporary aid to cut down on smoking"
"an aid to those who want to reduce the smoking habit"
"curbs the tobacco urge"
"helps to stop smoking without requiring willpower"

THE ALLURE OF SMOKING

In 1623, Sir Francis Bacon noted that "the use of tobacco is growing greatly; it conquers men with a certain secret pleasure so that those who have once become accustomed thereto can hardly be restrained therefrom." The FDA's expert advisers, writing 357 years later, found no reason to dispute Bacon's account.

Rolling up corn silk, coffee grounds, or dried lettuce leaves in cigarette paper and smoking it—as some persons have done—simply will not deliver pleasure comparable to tobacco's. This leads the Panel to conclude that tobacco contains some element that causes druglike behavorial changes—one of which, of course, is difficulty in stopping. The dependency-producing element almost certainly is the nicotine, a substance that strongly stimulates the central nervous system.

PRODUCTS

How, then, to stop, once one comes to accept that the habit is detrimental to health? Many professionally guided and self-help methods have been developed in the last 2 decades. But long-term success rates are low—many people slip back into the habit.

For the smoker seeking the way to go, the Surgeon General's recent findings, published in 1979, may offer a useful clue. He estimates that of the 30 million persons who have successfully stopped smoking since 1964, over 95 percent have done so *without counseling or using a structured program*. In other words, the do-it-yourself method has proved to be the most successful.

How much nonprescription or prescription drugs can contribute to this effort remains unclear. Reviewers were unable to approve any of the over-the-counter smoking deterrents they examined. But a few have showed promise in clinical tests, so they might provide a margin of success for the smoker who has seriously set himself or herself to the hard—but certainly not impossible—task of stopping.

All over-the-counter smoking deterrents claim one of two possible mechanisms. Either they change the taste of tobacco smoke so that smoking is no longer pleasurable or they substitute a nicotinelike drug in an oral form—as candy or gum, for example. This latter method creates an alternative habit pleasurable enough to help the smoker forsake cigarettes.

These drugs may also be promoted to help a person "cut down" on smoking. The Panel takes a strongly disapproving stand on this goal. Reviewers feel this is a waste of time and money because such efforts are doomed to failure. The only meaningful role for a smoking deterrent is to help a smoker *stop*.

The hardest time will be the first few weeks, so this is when the aids will be of most value. It's because of this time element that evaluators assessed the effectiveness of these drugs in terms of how they work during the 3 weeks after people throw away their last pack of cigarettes.

INGREDIENTS IN SMOKING DETERRENTS

Of the many active ingredients in smoking deterrents, some are spices and aromatics that are combined in candylike preparations. And in this unit some combination products are discussed below as if they were individual ingredients.

Approved Active Ingredients

None

Conditionally Approved Active Ingredients

Lobeline preparations: lobeline sulfate, natural lobeline alkaloids, and Lobelia inflata herb   These are plant products and extracts whose active substance, lobeline, is similar to—though weaker than— nicotine. *How* they help is not altogether clear from the Panel's description, but it appears that lobeline may provide a temporary and alternative oral gratification while one is trying to lessen the craving for inhaling nicotine.

Large doses of lobeline can cause belching, heartburn, stomach ache, and other symptoms. But in the small 2 mg recommended doses, few such symptoms result and, going by the handful of studies available, the Panel declares lobeline safe. The drug is often combined with tribasic calcium phosphate or magnesium carbonate, both antacids, which are purported to increase blood levels of the drug. They are safe, but their value remains to be proved.

In one double-blind, scientifically controlled study, over 80 percent of smokers who used lobeline had stopped smoking after 5 or 6 days compared with fewer than 10 percent who stopped smoking among the group taking dummy medication. But of 10 other controlled studies assessed, only 2 confirmed these results; the other 8 did not. So the reviewers believe further testing is in order. Conclusion: lobeline preparations are safe but not proved effective.

Silver acetate A silver compound, this drug has no known adverse effects—except that it can discolor the skin, turning it bluish. The Panel therefore calls it safe.

Silver acetate is usually formulated into a chewing gum, to prolong its presence in the mouth. It reputedly affects the mucous membranes of the mouth so that cigarette smoke has a nasty, metallic sweet taste, which smokers find discouragingly unpleasant. This aversive effect may last up to 4 hours.

Three double-blind placebo-controlled studies were submitted as evidence that silver acetate gum is effective; none of them was considered to be objective enough. In the first, 11 of 30 smokers who used the medicated gum said they had stopped smoking by the end of 2 weeks, a significantly greater percentage than was recorded among members of a control group who chewed a dummy, nonmedicated gum. But the investigators relied on mail-in answer forms and telephone interviews to obtain these results, and evaluators say self-reports of this kind are highly suspect. So the Panel concluded that while silver acetate is safe, it has not been proved effective.

Disapproved Active Ingredients

For lack of data about safety and effectiveness, a number of ingredients were summarily dismissed (*see* SAFETY AND EFFECTIVENESS chart at the end of this unit). Other disapproved compounds are discussed below.

Quinine ascorbate This compound was submitted to the Panel as part of a product that also contains vitamins and a dry alcoholic extract of hawthorne. Panel members decided that the quinine ascorbate was the intended active ingredient. They could not, however, find quinine ascorbate—which is quinine with vitamin C—listed as a drug in any reference volume. But, since small amounts of both vitamin C (ascorbate) and quinine are generally recognized as safe, the Panel was willing to give an affirmative nod to quinine ascorbate's safety.

The manufacturer of this product failed to provide any clinical studies showing that quinine ascorbate is an effective smoking deterrent. Most of what was sent along was dismissed by the Panel as "testimonials" that fail to meet current standards of scientific investigation. Another firm that submitted a product containing quinine ascorbate included a scientific study—but it was poorly constructed. The Panel therefore concluded that while safe, quinine ascorbate is not generally recognized as an effective smoking deterrent—and has not been marketed as such in the United States.

The combination of licorice-root extract + ground coriander + ground Jamaica ginger + ground cloves + lemon oil (terpeneless) + orange oil   This combination product consists of common spices and essential oils that are used as food; reviewers regard the substances as safe. Sucking one of these medicinal tablets is claimed to overwhelm and satisfy the senses of smell and taste, so that one no longer desires a cigarette and will put it aside unlit. One uncontrolled study was submitted to show that this product works, but its design was too poor to permit the Panel to take it seriously. Furthermore, participants also received supportive person-to-person therapy—which the purchaser and user would not necessarily have. So, pending better studies, evaluators conclude that this aromatic combination product is safe but has not been proved effective.

The combination of methyl salicylate + eucalpytus oil + menthol + thymol   Because of its pleasant aroma, methyl salicylate is attractive to children. This is risky in principle, since the chemical is also highly toxic. But in the tiny amounts present in these products, the Panel believes it poses no risk—so it calls this combination product safe. However, no scientific evidence was submitted to show that the mixture really works to deter smoking. Conclusion: safe but not proved effective.

Safety and Effectiveness: Active Ingredients in Over-the-Counter Smoking Deterrents

Active Ingredient	Panel's Assessment
alcohol	summarily disapproved
aloin	summarily disapproved
aluminum chloride	summarily disapproved
aluminum hydroxide	summarily disapproved
ammonium chloride	summarily disapproved
belladonna leaves (extract of)	summarily disapproved
benzocaine	summarily disapproved
calcium phosphate tribasic (adjuvant)	safe, but not proved effective
capsicum	summarily disapproved

Safety and Effectiveness: Active Ingredients in Over-the-Counter Smoking Deterrents *(continued)*

Active Ingredient	Panel's Assessment
cascara sagrada (extract of)	summarily disapproved
chlorophyllins	summarily disapproved
cimcifuga	summarily disapproved
cloves (ground; *see* licorice-root extract . . .)	
co-carboxylase	summarily disapproved
coriander (ground; *see* licorice-root extract . . .)	
cornstarch	summarily disapproved
eucalyptus oil (*see* methyl salicylate . . .)	
gentian (solid extract of)	summarily disapproved
ginger (ground Jamaican; *see* licorice-root extract . . .)	
gum arabic (powdered)	summarily disapproved
hawthorne (dry alcoholic extract of)	summarily disapproved
lactose	summarily disapproved
lemon oil (terpeneless; *see* licorice-root extract . . .)	
licorice-root extract + ground coriander + ground Jamaica ginger + ground cloves + lemon oil (terpeneless) + orange oil*	safe, but not proved effective
lobeline preparations: lobeline sulfate, natural lobeline alkaloids, and *Lobelia inflata* herb	safe, but not proved effective
magnesium carbonate (adjuvant)	safe, but not proved effective
magnesium stearate	summarily disapproved
menthol (*see* methyl salicylate . . .)	
methapyrilene hydrochloride	summarily disapproved
methyl salicylate + eucalyptus oil + menthol + thymol*	safe, but not proved effective
nicotinic acid	summarily disapproved
nux vomica (extract of)	summarily disapproved
orange oil (*see* licorice-root extract . . .)	
potassium gentian root	summarily disapproved
potassium nux vomica	summarily disapproved
propylene glycol	summarily disapproved
pyridoxine hydrochloride	summarily disapproved
quinine ascorbate	safe, but not effective
silver acetate	safe, but not proved effective
silver nitrate	not safe or effective
sodium ascorbate	summarily disapproved

Safety and Effectiveness: Active Ingredients in Over-the-Counter Smoking Deterrents *(continued)*

Active Ingredient	*Panel's Assessment*
sodium chloride	summarily disapproved
sugar	summarily disapproved
talc	summarily disapproved
thiamine mononitrate	summarily disapproved
thymol (*see* methyl salicylate . . .)	

*As noted in the text, combination products are assessed in this unit as if they were single-ingredient entities.

Smoking Deterrents: Product Ratings

Product and Distributor	*Dosage of Active Ingredients*	*Rating[1]*	*Comment*
Bantron (Campana)	**tablets:** 2 mg lobeline	B	not proved effective
Healthbreak (Lemar)	**gum:** silver acetate + ammonium chloride	B	not proved effective
Nicocortyl Tablets (Anti-Tobacco Information Center)	**tablets:** licorice + ginger + coriander + cloves + orange oil + spices + lemon oil	C	not effective
Tabmint Chewing Gum (Edgefield)	**gum:** 6 mg silver acetate	B	not proved effective

1. Author's interpretation of Panel criteria. Based on contents, not claims.

Soaps, Antimicrobial

Millions of people routinely wash and bathe using expensive bar soaps that contain potent chemical ingredients that kill microbes (germs) or inhibit their growth on the skin. These soaps are promoted and used to

SOAPS, ANTIMICROBIAL is based on the report of the FDA's Advisory Review Panel on OTC Antimicrobial Drug Products Used for Repeated Daily Use (Antimicrobial I Panel), the initial Tentative Final Order on OTC Topical Antimicrobial Products, and related documents.

prevent body odor, particularly underarm odor; for general cleanliness; and to a lesser extent to forestall skin infections.

An antimicrobial is an agent which kills or inhibits the growth and reproduction of microorganisms. An antimicrobial bar soap contains one or more of these ingredients.

DO THEY WORK?

Antimicrobial bar soaps do kill germs and so are able to help control underarm and other body odors. However, despite the huge sales of these soaps, there is little data on the number of microorganisms they kill. Soap and drug industry experts and research scientists were unable to provide evidence that directly shows the percentage of underarm bacteria that need to be killed to reduce body odor, or the concentration of antimicrobial agents in soaps that are required to produce this effect.

The best the experts could do was to estimate—on the basis of tests —that about a 70 percent reduction in bacteria is required to control armpit and other body odors. While it remains to be proved, some antimicrobial soaps may in fact reduce underarm bacterial counts by 70 percent, or even up to 90 percent. But a second major question—one of safety—has arisen, and remains unanswered today: Is it wise or healthy to use such potent germ killers on a day-to-day basis for many years of one's life?

One concern, which was strongly expressed by the Panel in its report, is that some of these chemicals are absorbed into the body through the skin, even when the skin is not broken. They may accumulate in the liver and other organs—with dangerous consequences.

The other principal worry is that most antimicrobial substances very effectively kill microorganisms in the class called *gram-positive bacteria* that normally inhabit the skin. But they are far less effective against the class called *gram-negative bacteria* (see page 47). The Panel's hypothesis, which it says is supported by several scientific studies, is that these soaps may kill relatively harmless gram-positive bacteria only to make room for and encourage the growth of gram-negative flora that can cause serious infection. A microbiologist at the National Institute of Health says, however, that there's no evidence that this compensatory overgrowth of other organisms occurs on the skin. The Panel urged the FDA to classify and regulate all antimicrobial soaps and other products that contain these ingredients as *drugs*—not as cosmetics—so that the more stringent drug safety and effectiveness standards can be applied to them.

It initially was concluded that none of the antimicrobial agents used in these bar soaps is safe and effective. Only conditional approval was granted to a half-dozen antimicrobials, including the substances cloflucarban, triclocarban, and triclosan. These ingredients have been, and continue to be, widely used in antimicrobial bar soaps.

A New Look

These adverse judgments provoked a flood of protest and of new scientific research and data—much of it from major soap manufacturers, including Procter & Gamble and Colgate-Palmolive, and from drug companies such as Upjohn and Ciba-Geigy, which make antimicrobial substances. The manufacturers claimed their new data confirm the safety and effectiveness of triclocarban and other antimicrobial ingredients.

The FDA agreed in 1979 that much significant new data needed to be assessed. It therefore took the unusual step of reopening the administrative record. In effect the agency rolled back the review process on these and other antimicrobial products to an earlier stage so that new evidence could be submitted and evaluated. Final decisions on the safety and effectiveness of antimicrobial soaps cannot be expected until a later date. The doubts originally raised by the Panel, and for the most part seconded by the FDA, remain unresolved.

SAFETY OF HEXACHLOROPHENE AND OTHER ANTIMICROBIALS

The development of potent antimicrobial chemicals for medical use before and during World War II soon led to the introduction of these substances into consumer products. One of the most effective and widely used antimicrobials was hexachlorophene or HCP. By 1972—the year that the review process and the Antimicrobial Panel was established—hexachlorophene was being formulated into 1500 over-the-counter cleansers, and other products. But that same year it became clear that hexachlorophene was a toxic substance. Significant amounts of the agent were found to be absorbed through the skin into the blood. In one study concentrations ranging from 0.02 to 0.14 micrograms of hexachlorophene per milliliter (mcg/ml) of blood were found. The level rose to 0.38 mcg/ml in one volunteer who bathed in the substance.

Hexachlorophene was shown to cause systemic toxicity. The greatest danger was to newborn babies. The substance had become widely used for bathing newborn babies to prevent infections and some infants were washed with it 2 or more times daily. But hexachlorophene was found to dig Swiss-cheese-like holes in the brain tissue after it was absorbed through the skin and then carried there by the bloodstream. In France, in the summer of 1972, 36 babies died after they were powdered with a baby powder that was accidentally contaminated at the manufacturers with up to 6.3 percent hexachlorophene. Some 168 other babies who were poisoned, but did not die, are still being studied (1982) to determine whether they suffered permanent brain damage from their exposure to hexachlorophene.

Babies, it has been found, have difficulty eliminating hexachlorophene from their bodies. Older persons probably are better able to excrete it, and so are less at risk. Nevertheless, the margin between the safe and effective hexachlorophene dose on the one hand and the dangerously poisonous dose on the other clearly is far too narrow. So, as its first substantive act in the over-the-counter drug-review process, the FDA removed hexachlorophene from over-the-counter sales in the United States in September 1972.

The dismaying history of hexachlorophene no doubt prompted the Antimicrobial I Panel to look very critically at other antimicrobial substances formulated into products designed for prolonged daily use—particularly bar soaps. The Panel proposed new testing guidelines to assess the safety of ingredients, and formulated a set of assumptions—strongly contested by the soap industry—about how much of these chemicals would be absorbed into the body in a bath or shower.

The Panel calculated that 7 grams (roughly ¼ of an ounce) of soap is used by an adult in bathing. A bar soap containing a 3 percent concentration of an antimicrobial would thus expose the user to 210 mg of the agent per bath. If it is assumed that all of the antimicrobial sticks to the skin, and that 3 percent of it is quickly absorbed through the skin to wind up in the bloodstream, a 150-pound man or woman would then be carrying about 1.26 mcg of the agent per 1 ml of blood. In the case of hexachlorophene, this is a potentially toxic dose.

EFFECTIVENESS

In Reducing Odor

The unresolved questions of antimicrobials' safety are matched by the paucity of convincing scientific data on their effectiveness. While the Panel and the FDA concur that these chemicals do reduce bacterial flora on the skin, this effect has never been directly correlated with reduction in body odor. The FDA now will require that claims relating to deodorant effectiveness be based on demonstrated ability to reduce microbes or inhibit the growth of those microbes responsible for odor production.

In Preventing Infection

Besides cleanliness and control of body odor, the other benefit claimed for antimicrobial ingredients in bar soaps is the prevention of skin infections. Several tests have been conducted, including ones at West Point and Annapolis. At West Point, cadets who showered with an antimicrobial bar soap containing tribromsalan, triclocarban, and cloflucarban had 44 percent fewer boils, but had more fingernail infections (paronychia) than men who used ordinary bar soap. Moreover, a soap containing triclocarban and hexachlorophene did not lower the incidence of boils in naval cadets at Annapolis. A Panel consultant called these results equivocal and it was decided they were insufficient to support the conclusion that these soaps were effective in preventing infection. Too, if the products do indeed *increase* the potential for gram-negative or gram-positive streptococcal infection, any "deodorant benefit would probably be considerably outweighed by the potential hazard . . . when alternative methods of odor control are available."

CLAIMS

Accurate
"antimicrobial soap" or "antibacterial soap" (Elsewhere on the label manufacturers can say "reduces odor" or "deodorant soap.")

False or Misleading
Because no antimicrobial ingredient can truly ensure germ-free skin—and such a goal may not be desired anyway—the FDA says that the claim "ensures bacterially clean skin" should *not* be made.

WARNING   Do not use on infants under 6 months of age.

COMBINATION PRODUCTS

Two chemically similar antimicrobial ingredients, triclocarban and cloflucarban, continue to be combined in some antimicrobial bar soaps. The FDA gives only *conditional* approval to this combination, pending proof that the 2 individual ingredients are safe and effective and do not become more toxic when mixed in a soap. The combination of triclosan and tribromsalan is *disapproved* because tribromsalan is not safe.

ANTIMICROBIAL AGENTS

Approved Active Ingredients

None

Conditionally Approved Active Ingredients

Chloroxylenol (PCMX)   Very little data on this substance—which also is designated parachlormetaxylenol, or PCMX—were submitted for evaluation. Even the additional material sent later to the FDA leaves questions of safety and effectiveness unresolved. Chloroxylenol, like hexachlorophene, is a phenol derivative. Thus it should be very active against bacteria. But the evidence, in fact, is conflicting and inadequate. One report, published half a century ago, indicates that the substance is not very effective against bacteria on the skin. A more recent—but inconclusive—study shows that choroxylenol reduces microbial flora by 70 percent after 10 days' use. More studies are definitely needed.

Cloflucarban   There are no *known* hazards associated with use of this antimicrobial, which is often combined with triclocarban in antimicrobial bar soaps. But data to confirm its safety are wanting, and it is conditionally approved only in concentrations up to 1.5 percent.

Cloflucarban, when ingested, is only about one-fiftieth as toxic as hexachlorophene. It also may be absorbed less readily through the skin, but data on blood levels following one or more baths and information about absorption in the body are still lacking. Finally, certain substances chemically related to cloflucarban may cause skin problems discussed below under DIBROMSALAN.

Phenol (under 1.5 percent aqueous/alcoholic)   It is phenol—better known as carbolic acid—that lent the medicinal odor to some of the soap products that for many years were used to control body odor. While phenol is an effective germ killer, it is also highly toxic to the skin. Once absorbed through the skin, phenol can damage internal organs (*see* PHENOL). Since safer antiseptics are available, the Panel says that phenol—as sodium phenolate or secondary amyltricresols—is now far less commonly used.

The Panel evaluates phenol in bar soaps as only conditionally safe and effective at concentrations under 1.5 percent in water or alcoholic solutions, and definitely unsafe at levels over 1.5 percent in those liquids. When phenol is formulated with camphor, which retards absorption and availability, it is permissible in concentrations of up to 5 percent. Phenol also is allowed in very low concentrations—of up to 0.5 percent—as an inactive ingredient, to give the product a medicinal smell.

WARNING FOR PHENOL   Phenol in any form should never be used on diapers or on babies' skin, since an infant may be unable to excrete it. Phenol also should not be used under bandages or other coverings.

Triclocarban   Triclocarban's effectiveness in killing microbial organisms has been demonstrated. But a clear correlation between reduced microbial counts and reduced body odor has not been demonstrated, so the FDA declines to certify triclocarban as effective.

"The available evidence does not indicate that the use of triclocarban in bar soaps presents any known hazard to the general public," the FDA declared in 1978. "Based on blood-level data, [it] does not appear to be as toxic as hexachlorophene [which has been banned from OTC products]."

Studies conducted according to the Panel's guidelines show that a person who showers once or twice daily with a triclocarban soap will absorb roughly 500 to 1000 times *less* than the minimal toxic dose—a wide safety margin. However, because the enzyme pathways responsible for getting rid of triclocarban from the body develop only slowly after birth, this substance should not be used on babies under 6 months of age.

The possibililty that triclocarban causes cancer has not been disproved. So the FDA grants only conditional approval in terms of safety, and it limits the amount of triclocarban—alone, or in conjunction with cloflucarban—to 1.5 percent of the bar soap in which it is formulated.

Triclosan   Although this is an effective antimicrobial, it has not been demonstrated that it kills the bacteria that cause body odor. So triclosan's effectiveness for this purpose in soaps remains to be proved.

About 12 percent of the triclosan deposited on the skin during a shower is absorbed into the skin—the highest amount for any antimicrobial now used in bar soaps. Most people excrete this chemical very rapidly. But some individuals are what the FDA calls "slow metabolizers" of triclosan. Their safety is of concern because, if triclosan is retained, high doses can damage the liver.

There is another cause for concern: Triclosan is used in a variety of consumer products. It is formulated into cosmetics, infant clothing, and diaper rinses but the wisdom of such wide availability has been questioned. However, because the hazards of using triclosan have not been clearly established, it is one of the substances being reevaluated. The FDA has lingering doubts about triclosan's effectiveness, apparently because it is not effective against *Pseudomonas*, which is one of the most dangerous gram-negative bacteria.

Disapproved Active Ingredients

Several antimicrobial agents have been ruled unsafe when formulated into antimicrobial bar soaps for consumers' daily use. The issue, in all cases, is that of safety. Some of these chemicals, identified below, already have been ruled off the market by the FDA.

Dibromsalan (DBS) This is a chemical in the group called *halogenated salicylanilides* that once was widely used in antimicrobial bar soaps marketed in the United States. It can sensitize the skin so that rashes and other skin disorders appear when the skin is later exposed to light (photosensitization). The FDA has banned dibromsalan from antimicrobial products sold in the United States.

Fluorosalan Little data was presented to support the safety and effectiveness of this substance. The Panel says fluorosalan could be a photosensitizer in humans, and its use could result in a serious skin condition known as *persistent light reaction*. So it is deemed to be unsafe and is no longer marketed in the United States.

Hexachlorophene (HCP) The FDA banned hexachlorophene as an over-the-counter product some years ago, as the Panel recommended (*see* SAFETY OF HEXACHLOROPHENE AND OTHER ANTIMICROBIALS, above).

Phenol (over 1.5 percent aqueous/alcoholic) The Panel found phenol (carbolic acid) unsafe in concentrations greater than 1.5 percent. While studies referred principally to formulations other than soap, phenol can be formulated as bar soap and evaluators wanted to rule out its use in these high concentrations to avoid risk of serious hazards such as severe skin burns, gangrene, and other forms of tissue damage (*see* PHENOL).

Tetrachlorosalicylanilide (TCSA) This halogenated salicylanilide, which has been widely used in antimicrobial soaps and other products, is a potent photosensitizer capable of causing serious skin disorders. The FDA ruled the substance, which is chemically similar to tribromsalan, off the over-the-counter drug market.

Tribromsalan (TBS) Manufacturers' data suggested that tribromsalan's only established value was in counteracting body odor—for which safer agents are available. Even in concentrations as low as $\frac{1}{10,000}$ of 1 percent, tribromsalan can elicit an allergic reaction. It can cause rashes and other skin eruptions upon contact with the skin, and can also sensitize the skin so it will erupt when exposed to the sun or other light. The Panel's concern about this incidence of disabling photo-dermatitis prompted the FDA to ban tribromsalan from the over-the-counter drug market in the United States.

Safety and Effectiveness: Active Ingredients in Antimicrobial Bar Soaps

Active Ingredient	Panel and FDA's† Assessment
chloroxylenol (PCMX)	not proved safe or effective
cloflucarban	not proved safe or effective
dibromsalan (DBS)*	not safe
fluorosalan*	not safe
hexachlorophene (HCP)*	not safe
phenol (under 1.5% or less in aqueous/alcoholic)	not proved effective
phenol (under 1.5% in camphorated oil)	not proved effective
phenol (over 1.5% aqueous/alcoholic)	not safe
tetrachlorosalicylanilide (TCSA)*	not safe
tribromsalan (TBS)*	not safe
triclocarban	not proved safe or effective
triclosan	not proved safe or effective

*No longer marketed over-the-counter in the United States.
†Judgments reaffirmed or modified by FDA, or originated by it.

Antimicrobial Bar Soaps: Product Ratings

Product and Distributor	Dosage of Active Ingredients	Rating[1]	Comment
Coast Deodorant Soap (Procter & Gamble)	**bar soap:** triclocarban	B	not proved safe or effective
Dial Gold (Armour Dial)	**bar soap:** triclocarban	B	not proved safe or effective
Irish Spring (Colgate)	**bar soap:** triclocarban + triclosan	B	neither ingredient proved safe or effective
Lifebuoy Coral (Lever Bros.)	**bar soap:** triclosan	B	not proved safe or effective

Antimicrobial Bar Soaps: Product Ratings *(continued)*

Product and Distributor	Dosage of Active Ingredients	Rating[1]	Comment
afeguard (Procter & Gamble)	**bar soap:** triclocarban	B	not proved safe or effective
est (Procter & Gamble)	**bar soap:** triclocarban	B	not proved safe or effective

Author's interpretation of Panel/FDA criteria. Based on contents, not claims.

Sore-Throat and Mouth Medicines

A sore throat—according to the National Center for Health Statistics—is the most common complaint that brings patients to doctors' offices. It is a frequent symptom of the common cold and also accompanies many other diseases, some serious, some not. Sore mouth, which may produce pain, discomfort, or sensations of burning or scratching, can result from an even wider variety of causes, including denture injuries, burns from hot soup, scrapes from chewing on hard objects—as well as infections and other conditions.

All the drugs described in this unit are intended for topical use—that is, they are applied directly to throat and mouth mucous membranes. (For information about drugs taken internally that may relieve sore throat, *see* PAIN, FEVER, AND ANTI-INFLAMMATORY DRUGS TAKEN INTERNALLY.) The Panel warns that many of the drugs, particularly antimicrobials, are of dubious worth at best. Some are frankly dangerous and many are unnecessary or inappropriate for treating self-diagnosed throat and mouth soreness. Prolonged or severe soreness in the throat or mouth may signal the onset of serious illness that should be looked after by a doctor, not self-treated.

CLAIMS

False or Misleading
"helps kill mouth germs"
"healing aid for minor oral inflammation"

SORE-THROAT AND MOUTH MEDICINES is based on the report of the FDA's Advisory Review Panel on OTC Oral Cavity Drug Products.

"promotes flow of saliva"
"antimicrobial cleansing agent"
"quiets rasping cough due to colds which may be causing discomfort"
"healing aid"
"relieves dryness"
"soothing to smoker's throat"
"acts fast" (time can't be demonstrated)
"fast healing aid"
"kills germs in minutes"
"long-lasting relief"
"quick comfort to irritated throats"
"for temporary relief of pain associated with canker sores" (medical diagnosis should be made)
"temporary relief of pain of stomatitis"
"relieves pain due to tonsillitis"

WARNING   Severe or persistent sore throat accompanied by high fever, headaches, nausea, and vomiting may be serious. Consult a physician promptly. Do not use these drugs for more than 2 days or administer to children under 3 years of age unless directed by a physician.

ORAL-CAVITY MUCOUS MEMBRANES

The oral cavity, as the term is used in this unit, means the soft tissues of the mouth and throat—starting just behind the lips and moving downward past the Adam's apple. The teeth and gums, major anatomic structures in the mouth, are discussed in other units concerned with dental problems.

The insides of the mouth and the throat are lined with mucous membranes. These tissues, unlike skin, must be bathed constantly by saliva and other secretions to remain healthy. They differ from ordinary skin in another important respect: they readily absorb many drugs and other chemicals that are then transported into the lymph and the blood. These body fluids in turn carry the drugs and other compounds throughout the body. This capacity for absorption means that a drug like the anesthetic dibucaine—which can cause convulsions and cardiac arrest if it reaches the central nervous system and heart—cannot safely be used in the mouth. Yet the same drug is safe for self-treatment of small areas of skin, because ordinary skin acts as a barrier to absorption. To spare consumers unnecessary risk the Panel has ranked such anesthetic drugs unsafe for use in the throat and mouth.

SORE THROAT

Most sore throats are a symptom of some underlying infection or other illness. They are particularly common in sufferers of colds and other upper-respiratory infections that produce thick secretions which adhere to and irritate the throat's mucous membranes. The streptococcal bacteria that cause scarlet fever and rheumatic fever (most often in children) may first make themselves felt as a sore and reddened "strep throat." Other serious illnesses—like Vincent's disease (an ulcerating infection that kills gum tissue), oral gonorrhea, measles, and some cancers—also produce sore-throat symptoms. Fish bones, glass, or other sharp objects taken in with food can injure the throat so that pain and infection may follow.

The discomfort of mild sore throat can be successfully treated with over-the-counter drugs. Reviewers warn, however, that these drugs provide only *temporary* relief of symptoms. They do not correct the underlying conditions.

SORE MOUTH

Unlike sore throat, few sore-mouth problems lend themselves either to self-diagnosis or self-treatment. Yet labels on many nonprescription oral health-care products make treatment claims that the Panel would ban. Immediately below the reader will find descriptions of mouth infections and information about whether the Panel thinks they can be self-diagnosed and treated with nonprescription preparations.

Mouth Infections

Aphthous stomatitis (Bechet's syndrome)   A recurring form of ulcerative sore mouth, this condition may occur because of an immunologic disease. Medical or dental diagnosis is required, and so is professional treatment.

Candidiasis   This is a common fungal infection of the mouth. It is characterized by white bumps and reddish, inflamed patches on the mucous membrane. This infection can be diagnosed only by a physician or dentist, through laboratory tests.

Gonococcal sores of the mouth   A diagnosis of venereal disease can be made only by a doctor, and only a doctor can provide appropriate treatment.

Herpangina   A common disease in young children, herpangina is especially prevalent in late summer. Tiny ulcers appear at the back of the mouth and in the throat. They soon rupture, causing a burning sensation or pain. Herpangina must be treated by a dentist or doctor.

Primary herpetic stomatitis   This is a viral illness that causes extremely painful blisters on the cheek, tongue, palate, and floor of the mouth. The gums may be swollen, bright red, and may bleed easily. A dentist or doctor must diagnose and treat this ailment.

Secondary herpetic infections   These recurrent herpes attacks are caused by the same virus as primary herpetic stomatitis (*see* immediately above). The sores usually erupt on the roof of the mouth or on the lips—where they cause a burning sensation or pain. The Panel fails to say whether it thinks consumers can self-diagnose and self-treat this condition.

Syphilis   Sore mouth and throat can occur in the early, delayed, or late stages of this venereal disease. If the infection results from oral sex, the primary ulcer (chancre) may appear in the mouth. Wherever the disease starts, the second stage—about 6 weeks after onset—is often characterized by sore throat, possibly by sore mouth, and by grayish mucous patches. This disease cannot be self-diagnosed or self-treated with over-the-counter products.

Tuberculosis lesions   A chronic ulcer or sore on the tongue or inside the cheek may be caused by this serious lung disorder, or a form of it that originates within the mouth. Self-diagnosis and treatment are simply not possible. Medical supervision is the answer.

Vincent's disease (acute necrotizing ulcerative gingivitis [ANUG])   This infection produces between-teeth sores that secrete a grayish, puslike substance. The gums bleed easily. A doctor's or dentist's diagnosis and antibiotic therapy are usually needed to relieve the symptoms and to clear up the infection.

COUGH

Some over-the-counter products used to treat sore throat and sore mouth contain drugs intended to loosen thick mucus and relieve throat irritation and coughing. Most coughs can be more effectively treated with cough suppressors, antitussives, or expectorants that are taken internally (*see* COUGH SUPPRESSORS AND EXPECTORANTS in COLD, COUGH AND ALLERGY DRUGS). But there may also be some value in treating the throat directly with topical drugs (*see* DEBRIS REMOVERS, DECONGESTANTS, and EXPECTORANTS, below).

EFFECTIVE WAYS TO USE THESE MEDICATIONS

Over-the-counter drugs that are applied directly to the mucous membranes for relief of sore throat, sore mouth, and coughs are classified as *oral health-care products*. They are intended for brief use, over a few days, to relieve specific symptoms of injury or disease. The Panel reserves the phrase *oral hygiene products* to describe mouthwashes, rinses and sprays that are recommended for routine daily use (*see* MOUTHWASH FOR ORAL HYGIENE).

Oral health-care products are made in a variety of ways for application to the mouth or throat. Some are formulated to be swished around the mouth, then spit out. Spray bottles are a particularly effective way to get medication to the back of the mouth and the throat.

A gargling solution—or, simply, gargle—is used to rinse or bathe the upper part of the throat. The best way to gargle is to take some of the fluid into the mouth, tilt the head back, and then force air from the lungs up through the liquid to splash it around before spitting it out. A useful trick is to try "singing" through the rinse.

The Panel, however, does not think gargling is an effective way of medicating the throat. Tests with dyes and X-rays show that gargled liquids often do not reach the back of the throat, where the soreness is likely to occur, and may bathe even the front of the throat only briefly. Evaluators believe that sprays are more effective.

The trouble with mouthwashes, rinses, and sprays is that saliva quickly washes them away. For treating small, discrete areas in the mouth, it may be more effective to swab the medication onto the sore spot with a clean cotton applicator. For wider soreness, the most effective method may be to use candylike lozenges (troches), which dissolve slowly so that they may bathe the irritated areas with the medicine for 5 or 10 minutes or more. The Panel adds, however, that no well-controlled studies have been performed to really prove the advantage of this method.

TYPES OF ACTIVE INGREDIENTS

Seven different kinds of drugs are formulated into products meant to be swished around, sprayed on, or dissolved inside the mouth.

- *Anesthetics/Analgesics* temporarily relieve pain or discomfort.
- *Antimicrobials* kill or inhibit infectious microorganisms.
- *Astringents* bind and remove irritating protein-type substances.

- *Debris removers* or *debriding agents* loosen and remove mucus and debris.
- *Decongestants* are meant to shrink mucous membranes and relieve congestion.
- *Demulcents* ("soothers") coat and protect sore spots.
- *Expectorants* are intended to soften and liquefy thick mucus.

The individual drugs for sore throat and mouth are described below under these general headings, and Panel findings are summarized in the SAFETY AND EFFECTIVENESS chart at the end of this unit. Any active ingredient that has not been specifically judged by the Panel is automatically listed as disapproved when used to relieve sore-throat and sore-mouth symptoms.

COMBINATION PRODUCTS

Reviewers expressed caution about combination products, even though they are extremely popular with over-the-counter oral-health-care product makers—as well, apparently, as with consumers. The Panel would, however, approve combinations that include 2 active ingredients of the same drug class—for example, 2 anesthetics—if they provided a real gain in treatment. The combination would have to be *proved* to be more effective, safer, better accepted by consumers, or have some other clear advantage over the individual active ingredients that are formulated separately.

Evaluators were able to find safe and effective active ingredients in only 4 of the 7 groups of drugs used to relieve sore throat and sore mouth. Only 2 types of presently marketed combination products can be designated as safe and effective:

1 approved anesthetic/analgesic + 1 demulcent (soother)
1 approved anesthetic/analgesic + 1 approved astringent

In combinations that include 2 safe and effective drugs from different categories, effective doses of both should be present. The Panel's specific decisions are summarized in the SAFETY AND EFFECTIVENESS: COMBINATION PRODUCTS chart at the end of this unit.

ANESTHETICS/ANALGESICS

Pain relief is the most clear-cut benefit that can be obtained from over-the-counter oral-health-care products. Many commonly used ingredients are safe and effective for this purpose. Some are powerful enough to inhibit all sensory impulses from the mucous mumbranes— including not only pain, but also feelings of coldness, warmth, touch, and pressure. Less potent ones relieve or dampen pain, but spare the other senses. The former effect is technically called *anesthesia* (numbness); the latter, *analgesia* (pain relief). But in the common parlance accepted by the Panel, "anesthesia" has come to cover both these types of sensory relief.

CLAIMS FOR ANESTHETICS/ANALGESICS

Accurate
for "the temporary relief of occasional minor irritation, pain, sore mouth, and sore throat"

False or Misleading
"first aid for throat irritation" and "soothing to smoker's throat"

"quick comfort," "fast-acting local anesthetic action," and "fast temporary relief"

"soothes tired throats"

"for temporary relief of sore throat associated with colds and excessive smoking"

relief of "tonsillitis and pharyngitis," "canker sores," "aphthous ulcers" (to be diagnosed by a doctor)

Types
The anesthetics/analgesics in medications for sore throat and sore mouth fall into 4 pharmacological groups:

Nitrogenous anesthetics Most of these drugs are recognizable because their names end in the suffix *-caine*, as in lidocaine, or in *-ine*. They are the most potent but also the most potentially dangerous pain relievers formulated into nonprescription oral-health-care products. They act by temporarily short-circuiting sensory nerve receptors in the mucosa so that "pain messages" cannot be transmitted toward the brain.

When absorbed into the system, stronger nitrogenous anesthetics affect the central nervous system. They can cause convulsions, coma, and death. They slow the heartbeat, and may cause it to stop altogether. These serious side effects, fortunately, have been rare.

Alcohol-type anesthetics These are older drugs, some of which have been used over the ages in folk medicine. They tend to be less potent than the nitrogenous anesthetics. But they are also safer, because they do not carry the risk of central-nervous-system side effects.

Antihistamines   By blocking the activity of histamine and other irritating body substances, antihistamines relieve pain, itching, and inflammation. The Panel does not believe that the substances act directly on the mucous membranes of the mouth and throat. Rather, they appear to be absorbed into the bloodstream from mouth-throat mucosa, as well as from lower parts of the gastrointestinal tract. So the drugs appear to act systemically (*see* ANTIHISTAMINES in COLD, COUGH, AND ALLERGY DRUGS).

Salicylates   This group includes aspirin and related drugs. They do not block nerve impulses, as the nitrogenous and alcoholic anesthetics do. They act on pain centers in the brain, and, the Panel asserts— despite controversy—they also act directly to relieve inflammation and pain when applied to mucosal tissue in the throat and mouth.

WARNING   These anesthetic drugs should not be used for more than 2 days, or given to children under 3 years of age, except as directed by a physician. When the anesthetic ingredient is included in a gargle, mouthwash, or mouth rinse that is intended to be spit out, the Panel adds this warning:

"Avoid swallowing this product as much as possible."

Approved Active Ingredients

The Panel decided that the following active ingredients are safe and effective in relieving irritation and soreness in the mouth and throat. Two are nitrogenous anesthetics, one is a salicylate and the others are alcohols.

Aspirin in chewing gum   Aspirin is the most widely used medicinal ingredient, and a mountain of data indicates that it is safe and effective when swallowed. In the doses in which aspirin is usually formulated into chewing-gum products, it is also safe—unless the inside of the mouth or throat is highly inflamed, cut, or torn. In that case the aspirin may induce bleeding. The Panel also warns that persons with underlying bleeding problems should not use topical aspirin products.

There is no convincing scientific evidence that aspirin is at all effective when applied directly to mouth-throat mucosal surfaces. It does not block nerve transmission of pain, as nitrogenous anesthetics do. Whatever pain-relieving benefit the drug may offer when used locally is said to result from its absorption through the mucosal lining of the gastrointestinal tract and into the bloodstream—from which it is carried to the brain and other internal organs.

The Panel majority's assessment is that aspirin has a local analgesic effect in the oral cavity and is useful in relieving mild to moderate pain, in part due to its effect on the pained and inflamed mucosal tissue surfaces. Chewing-gum aspirin is thus safe and effective in approved dosages. For adults, the approved dosage is 2 pieces of gum (which contain 420 mg of aspirin) when needed; or 16 pieces of gum in 24 hours (up to 3360 mg). For children 6 to 12, the recommended dosage is 1 or 2 pieces of gum (210 to 420 mg) when needed, not to exceed 8 pieces per day. For children 3 to 6, the recommended dosage is 1 piece, 210 mg, when needed, not to exceed 3 pieces, 630 mg, per day. For children under 3 there is no recommended dosage except as directed by a dentist or doctor.

The Panel adds this warning:

"Provide good fluid-intake when aspirin or aspirin-containing preparations are used."

Benzocaine   A widely used *-caine* type of anesthetic, benzocaine is extremely safe because it is quite insoluble in water. When applied to the skin or mucous membranes of the mouth or throat, very little of the drug is absorbed into the body. So there is almost no risk of injury to the nervous system, heart, or other vital organs.

Wide and varied studies as well as case reports attest to both safety and effectiveness. When benzocaine is applied to the mucous membranes of the mouth and throat, in a lozenge or spray, it produces pain relief in 30 to 60 seconds. Given the normal dilution and washout by saliva, each application should block pain for 5 to 10 minutes; continuous application, in lozenges, will produce continuing relief.

Benzocaine acts only on the sensory receptors of the mucous membranes. It does not penetrate into these membranes, and so will not relieve deep-seated inflammatory pain or dental pain originating deep in the teeth or gums.

The approved dosage for adults and children over age 3 is 5 to 20 percent benzocaine in a gel or spray for use not more than 4 times daily, or 0.05 to 0.1 percent concentration in lozenges taken not oftener than every 2 hours for up to 2 days. Each lozenge should contain 2 to 15 mg benzocaine.

Benzyl alcohol   This alcoholic anesthetic does not carry the risk of central-nervous-system and cardiac complications that are a problem with some nitrogenous anesthetics, and evaluators judged it safe largely on the basis of long use and the rareness of side effects.

While benzyl alcohol is less potent than benzocaine, it is nevertheless effective in relieving irritation and soreness in the mouth and throat. It takes 2 minutes to produce pain relief, which then may last for 5 to 10 minutes. By itself, benzyl alcohol is irritating to the mucous membranes, and must be diluted.

For adults and children over age 3, the safe and effective dose is 0.05 to 10 percent benzyl alcohol as a rinse, mouthwash, drops, or sprays, used no more than 3 or 4 times daily for up to 2 days. Lozenges may be taken up to once every 2 hours. Each lozenge should contain 100 to 500 mg of benzyl alcohol.

Dyclonine hydrochloride Of the nitrogenous anesthetics, this is the most effective that can be safely used in the mouth and throat. It has been modified chemically from a *-caine* to an *-ine* compound—a step that eliminates the risk of convulsions and other central-nervous-system side effects that is present with many of the *-caine* drugs (although not benzocaine) when they are absorbed through the mucous membranes into the body.

A variety of animal and human tests indicates that dyclonine hydrochloride is safe for use in the mouth, reviewers say. Studies are available that show, too, that it is quite an effective anesthetic when used on mucosal surfaces. According to one investigation, 2 to 3 minutes after application a 1 percent concentration of this drug produces numbness that lasts almost half an hour. Used as a rinse or gargle, it may provide an hour's relief. When it is sucked from a lozenge, relief may last several hours or longer.

The Panel says the safe and effective dosage for adults and children over age 3 is a 0.05 to 0.1 percent solution of dyclonine hydrochloride in a rinse, mouthwash, gargle or spray, used not more than 3 or 4 times daily. The approved dosage in lozenges is 0.05 to 0.1 percent up to once every 2 hours for up to 2 days. Each lozenge should contain 1 to 3 mg dyclonine hydrochloride.

Hexylresorcinol This is a sharp-tasting, aromatic alcohol that has been used as an anesthetic (as well as for other medicinal purposes) for more than 40 years. It is chemically related to phenol, but is less irritating to skin and mucous membranes than either phenol or resorcinol. Animal tests, and long marketing experience with few reports of allergic reactions or other complications, led evaluators to rank hexylresorcinol as safe.

The data on hexylresorcinol's effectiveness is less impressive. It appears to be less potent than benzocaine and shorter-acting than dyclonine hydrochloride (*see* above). Nevertheless, the Panel finds that hexylresorcinol is effective (as well as safe) for adults and children over age 3, when used every 3 or 4 hours for up to 2 days. Dosages should be 0.05 to 0.1 percent in rinses, gargles, sprays, and mouthwashes, and 2 to 4 mg per lozenge. The lozenges may be taken as often as once every 2 hours.

Menthol   A pepperminty alcohol, today menthol is more likely to be manufactured synthetically than extracted from mint plants. Its wide use in candies and other foods (as well as in medicine) persuades evaluators that menthol is safe. The Panel warns, however, that menthol products should not be given to children under 2 because they have been known to choke some infants and toddlers.

No well-controlled studies are available to document menthol's effectiveness in quelling irritation and soreness in the throat and mouth. But reviewers believe its wide use, its acceptance by doctors and consumers, and the paucity of adverse effects reported permit classification as an effective ingredient. In liquid preparations, this relief usually lasts no longer than 5 to 10 minutes; lozenges may extend this time.

The safe and effective dosage of menthol for adults and children over 3 is 0.04 to 2 percent concentrations of menthol in rinses, mouthwash, gargles or sprays, to be used not more than 3 or 4 times daily for up to 2 days. For lozenges, the dosage is one lozenge with 2 to 20 mg menthol, taken up to once every 2 hours if necessary.

Phenol   An alcohol, this coal-tar derivative has been used in medicine for more than a century, and its safety has been carefully studied. Although the drug can be quite toxic in higher doses, evaluators regard it as safe in the low doses approved for oral-cavity use.

Phenol penetrates the sensory nerve endings in the mucosal surfaces of the mouth and throat, temporarily blocking transmission of impulses for pain and other sensations. This blockage begins in 1 to 2 minutes and may go on for 5 to 10 minutes—or longer if the phenol is being continuously released from a lozenge. As the drug is washed away by saliva, the numbness recedes and the pain may return.

The Panel approves as safe and effective for persons over age 3 water-base (aqueous) solutions of from 0.5 to 1.5 percent phenol not more than 3 or 4 times daily for up to 2 days. It warns that aqueous solutions stronger than 2 percent can be dangerously irritating to the mucous membranes. (Stronger mixtures of phenol in glycerin are claimed to be safe because the glycerin releases phenol only slowly; but the Panel questions the safety of these mixtures.) The safe and effective dose of phenol in lozenges is 10 to 50 mg per lozenge, to be taken as often as once every 2 hours if necessary.

Phenolate sodium (sodium phenolate) The active material in this ingredient is phenol (*see* immediately above) and its safety and effectiveness are largely the same. In liquid preparations, sodium phenolate is active for 5 to 10 minutes; in lozenges it may act longer.

The approved dosage for persons over age 3 is phenolate sodium that is equivalent to 0.5 to 1.5 percent phenol in rinses, mouthwash, gargles, or sprays, used up to 3 or 4 times daily for up 2 days. Lozenges containing phenolate sodium equivalent to 10 to 50 mg of phenol are safe and effective when taken as often as once every 2 hours for 2 days.

Salicyl alcohol Except in over-the-counter preparations, this alcohol is no longer widely used and there are few scientific studies that indicate it is safe and effective. Going by what is known, however, the Panel says that the drug "appears" to have no adverse effects on the mucous membranes in concentrations under 6 percent. It is also assessed as an effective—albeit short-acting—anesthetic. Relief comes within 2 to 3 minutes and lasts 5 to 10 minutes when liquid dosage forms are used; lozenges may afford longer relief.

The safe and effective dosage of salicyl alcohol is 1 to 6 percent concentrations in aqueous solutions in the form of mouth rinses, mouthwash, gargles or sprays, to be used up to 2 days. It is safe and effective self-medication to use a lozenge containing 50 to 100 mg of salicyl alcohol every 2 hours for 2 days.

Conditionally Approved Active Ingredients

The Panel granted only conditional approval to 3 pain-relieving drugs that are applied topically to sore throats and mouths. All are safe. The unanswered question is: Are they effective?

Eucalyptol This spicy-smelling, cool-tasting eucalyptus-leaf oil, also known as *cineol*, *cineolcayeptol* or *cajuptol*, has been widely used in over-the-counter drug products in small amounts, with no signs that such doses are hazardous. The Panel says that eucalyptol is safe, but it says that the substance has no analgesic qualities, so that its effectiveness for pain relief remains to be proved.

Methyl salicylate This substance has a pleasing wintergreen taste and fragrance that young children find attractive, yet it may be deadly if they swallow it. Because of this hazard, only tiny amounts of methyl salicylate are formulated into over-the-counter products—and the Panel says that these preparations are safe. Effectiveness is another matter. The Panel finds there are too little data to conclusively show that methyl salicylate is effective in relieving sore throat and mouth pain. Verdict: safe but not proved effective.

Thymol   The Panel believes that this aromatic substance, which smells like thyme, is safe. While the Panel says that thymol *might* have a pain-relieving property, it maintains that scientific studies need be done to establish whether this is true. So the verdict for now is that thymol is safe, but has not been proved effective as an anesthetic for sore throat or sore mouth.

Disapproved Active Ingredients

On the basis of available evidence the Panel recommends that the following active ingredients that have been formulated into oral-health-care products be banned. Safety is the principal issue.

Antipyrine   This is a century-old anesthetic that is no longer widely used in the United States because of suspect safety. Antipyrine produces severe skin reactions. Also, careful studies that might establish safe dosages have not been done. In addition, the drug has the added handicap of not being effective in relieving sore throat and sore mouth. So the Panel says antipyrine is both unsafe and ineffective.

Camphor   Despite its long use, several of the Panels are deeply concerned about this substance's toxicity (*see* CAMPHOR). This Panel concurs; it maintains that camphor is too dangerous to be used to treat sore throat and mouth—even though the drug has been shown to be a pain reliever when applied to the skin. Lacking data showing that camphor is similarly effective on the mucous membranes of the throat and mouth, evaluators judged the ingredient both unsafe and ineffective.

Cresol   A phenol derivative, cresol is not safe as an anesthetic active ingredient for use in the mouth and throat. The Panel allows that cresol does have anesthetic properties when applied topically in dilute solutions, but it does not recommend it for such use. Verdict: not safe and not effective.

Dibucaine   This is a very potent—but also very risky -*caine*-type anesthetic. The chemical is readily absorbed through the mucous membranes of the mouth and throat, and evaluators are concerned that this could lead to serious toxic consequences—including convulsions and other central-nervous-system symptoms, or slowed heart rate. This risk is regrettable, since the Panel says there is no doubt that dibucaine is an effective anesthetic when used in the mouth. Verdict: not safe, and disapproved on that account.

Dibucaine hydrochloride   This compound's use in the mouth is about as risky as that of dibucaine (*see* immediately above). So while dibucaine hydrochloride is an effective anesthetic, the Panel says it is unsafe and unsuitable for use in over-the-counter remedies for sore throat and mouth.

Lidocaine   A much-used nitrogenous anesthetic, lidocaine is considered safe when used on small injured areas of skin. But it is readily absorbed through the mucous membranes of the throat and mouth. This could cause fatal central-nervous-system or cardiac complications. Well-controlled studies have clearly demonstrated lidocaine's effectiveness in quelling throat and mouth pain. The Panel proposes that it be available for this purpose only as a prescription drug. It is ruled unsafe for use in over-the-counter products.

Lidocaine hydrochloride   The risks of using this anesthetic are similar to the risks of lidocaine (*see* immediately above). Although lidocaine hydrochloride is an effective anesthetic on mucous membranes, the Panel disapproved it as not safe.

Pyrilamine maleate   This antihistamine has been carefully studied and widely used since its introduction into medical practice more than 3 decades ago. In recommended doses, side effects have been rare. So the Panel judges pyrilamine maleate to be safe. But it says that while some antihistamines have been demonstrated to have anesthetic properties when they are applied to mouth and throat mucous membranes, this one has not. So the drug is assessed as safe but ineffective.

Tetracaine   The Panel says that tetracaine is a very effective nitrogenous anesthetic. But the drug is readily absorbed through the mucous membranes of the mouth and throat, and can cause sudden, serious side effects—including fainting and cardiac arrest. Because such reactions may occur suddenly and with no warning, and can result in death, the Panel concluded that tetracaine is unsafe.

Tetracaine hydrochloride   This compound has the same liability as does tetracaine (*see* immediately above). So while it certainly is effective when used as an anesthetic for the mouth and throat, the Panel disapproved it as not safe for self-use in over-the-counter preparations.

ANTIMICROBIALS

An antimicrobial kills or inhibits the growth and spread of bacteria and other microorganisms. These drugs are also known as *antiseptics* or *germ killers*. Antimicrobials are present in many oral-health-care products sold to relieve sore throat and mouth. Panel evaluators say, however, that there is little evidence that these substances really work—and that they may interfere with the healing process of both clean and infected wounds.

Each of the antimicrobial agents available in over-the-counter products is effective against only a relatively few disease-producing organisms. Most are wholly ineffective against viruses, which are a principal cause of sore throats associated with colds. Health-product consumers have no way to decide which organisms are causing their complaint— since medical tests are required for this purpose—and they cannot make an informed choice about which antimicrobial to use. So self-treating sore throat or mouth conditions with antimicrobials is just as inappropriate as self-diagnosis, according to the experts.

Swishing an antimicrobial around in one's mouth—even if it happens to be one that acts against the offending "germ"—is likely to be fruitless. The drug probably cannot penetrate into the deeper layers of the mucous membranes, where holed-up microorganisms are causing inflammation and pain. No sooner is the antimicrobial gone from the mouth than the microorganisms reproduce their numbers anew.

Too, most antimicrobials kill *useful* microorganisms as well as harmful ones. Their continuous use may encourage the growth of resistant breeds that may be more difficult to control—and thus be more dangerous—than the ones that originally were there. These drugs also may counteract the action of the body's natural protective mechanisms.

For these various reasons, antimicrobials should never be used for preventive purposes—particularly not on a routine, daily basis as some manufacturers advise (*see* MOUTHWASH FOR ORAL HYGIENE). And, since none of the antimicrobial active ingredients in these products has been demonstrated to be safe and effective for relieving sore throat or sore mouth, the Panel suggests that none be used for that purpose. Instead of antimicrobials, evaluators suggest that small wounds or sores in the mouth or sore throats be treated by gently swishing clean, cool water over the inflamed area, then spitting out the water. (A cotton swab can be used to remove foreign matter from a wound.) Or one might use a gentle water spray.

CLAIMS FOR ANTIMICROBIALS

Accurate

for "the temporary relief of minor sore mouth and sore throat by decreasing the germs in the mouth" (*if* any were safe and effective, which none is)

False or Misleading
   provides "relief of pain and discomfort due to minor sore throat," "healing aid"
   "fast temporary relief," "kills germs by the millions on contact"
   for "temporary relief of minor sore throat due to common cold" (diagnosis can be made only by a doctor)
   "an aid to professional care" (a doctor should provide the care)
   "prevents infection" or "helps provide breath protection" (proof of preventive action is lacking)
   "inhibits odor-forming bacteria," "for oral hygiene," and "management of mouth odors, bad breath" (these are cosmetic, not drug, actions)

WARNING Avoid swallowing, as much as possible.

Approved Active Ingredients

   None

Conditionally Appproved Active Ingredients

   Benzalkonium chloride This chemical is a quaternary ammonium compound (quat). It is a white to yellowish powder or gel, which is soluble in both water and alcohol. It has been shown to be safe in a variety of studies, although few of these investigations involved use on mucous membranes of the throat and mouth. No acceptable evidence is available concerning the safety of long-term, day-to-day use. Nor is it known if the chemical may cause cancer, birth defects, or genetic damage when used in this way. The Panel nevertheless rates benzalkonium safe when used—very briefly—in an attempt to kill organisms that can cause sore throat and sore mouth.
   However, benzalkonium chloride controls only a limited range of these microorganisms. It is of dubious value when applied to the surface of an infected area—as is the intended use for some mouthwashes and rinses. So, while this agent is designated safe, reviewers say its effectiveness in relieving sore throat and sore mouth remains to be proved.
   Benzethonium chloride This compound is similar to benzalkonium chloride, (*see* immediately above). It is absorbed into the bloodstream when it is applied to the mucous membranes of the mouth and throat. Since the results, if any, of this absorption remain to be determined, the Panel ranks this agent's safety as unproved—although, generally speaking, benzethonium chloride is not highly toxic.
   The drug has been shown to be highly effective against bacteria and other microorganisms in many infectious settings. But its value in

killing microorganisms when applied directly to the mouth or throat has yet to be proved. It may, in fact, increase rather than decrease inflammation. Also, no data are available to justify its long-term use on a daily basis. In sum: both the safety and effectiveness of benzethonium chloride are yet to be proved.

Benzoic acid   Benzoic acid is widely used medicinally and as a food preservative. It is also known as phenylcarboxylic acid, phenylformic acid, and flowers of benzamine. A number of studies have shown that benzoic acid is relatively nontoxic to humans, and the present Panel agrees the drug is safe. The experts do note, however, that it may be mildly irritating to the mucous membranes of the throat and mouth.

Benzoic acid kills microorganisms under many laboratory and real-life conditions. But, by and large, it does not work against organisms that are responsible for sore throat and sore mouth. Results cited by manufacturers in support of the ingredient were found to be both outdated and unconvincing. So the Panel's verdict is that benzoic acid is safe, but its effectiveness needs to be shown.

Carbamide peroxide in anhydrous glycerin (urea peroxide) The anhydrous (water-free) glycerin is a vehicle that keeps carbamide peroxide dry. When carbamide peroxide is exposed to saliva and enzymes in the mouth, it breaks down to hydrogen peroxide. This, in turn, breaks down into bubbling, foaming oxygen and water. The oxygen released this way is alleged to kill bacteria.

Reviewers noted, however, that most organisms are relatively resistant to the action of peroxides, and they doubted that the bacteria and viruses which cause sore throats and sore mouths are much affected by these preparations.

Little evidence from scientific studies is available on this mixture's safety when it is used in the mouth and throat. But since the breakdown products—urea, oxygen, and water—all occur naturally in the body, the Panel accepts carbamide peroxide as safe. Conclusion: safe but not proved effective.

Cetalkonium chloride   This is another quaternary ammonium compound that disrupts the cell surfaces of many bacteria and funguses. So it is employed to control both kinds of microorganisms. In the dilute form in which this compond is used in mouthwashes and other oral-health-care products, it is odorless and practically tasteless. It may be mildly irritating, the Panel says—but not to a harmful degree. But cetalkonium chloride's effectiveness against the microorganisms that cause sore throat and sore mouth is questionable. Because the tests were poorly constructed, the Panel rejected results submitted by manufacturers who hoped to show that the substance rapidly kills bacteria in human saliva. So while cetalkonium chloride is safe, it remains to be proved effective.

Cetylpyridinium chloride   Yet another quaternary ammonium compound, this drug was introduced into clinical use in 1942. Since that time, it has been shown to kill or inhibit some species of bacteria and fungus, and some other microorganisms as well. However, many important questions have never been resolved: long-term and cumulative effects, metabolism, and information on excretion. Furthermore, the compound works against only a limited number of bacteria, and its lethal effect on these organisms can be blocked by natural or introduced chemicals present in the mouth. Finally, even if the drug does reduce bacterial counts, it remains in doubt whether curative effects are achieved. So the Panel ruled that both the safety and the effectiveness of cetylpyridinium chloride for mouth-throat use need to be proved.

Chlorophyll   Since chlorophyll is a major part of food, experts ruled it reasonable to assume that the substance is safe in the amounts present in oral-health-care products. Some forms of chlorophyll marginally inhibit bacterial growth, but there is no evidence that this is really useful in the context of throat-mouth use. (Even as far as cosmetic use goes, chlorophyll has been shown to relieve bad breath in dogs—but not in people.) Verdict: safe but not proved effective in combating the bacteria and viruses that cause sore throat and mouth.

Dequalinium chloride   This quaternary ammonium compound is believed to be relatively nontoxic. But few toxicologic-test results were submitted to the Panel. So it could not certify that use of the compound in mouthwashes and other oral-health-care products is safe. Dequalinium chloride kills both bacteria and funguses. But it is not effective against very many species of bacteria. Even this limited activity may be further sabotaged since the drug is easily neutralized by natural body secretions, debris in the mouth, and other materials that may be introduced into the mouth by the preparation itself. Both the safety and the effectiveness of dequalinium chloride remain to be proved.

Domiphen bromide   A compound that has been widely tested in animals and in humans, domiphen bromide appears to cause few if any toxic reactions in the dosages recommended for throat-mouth products. But studies that might rule out the risk that it can cause cancer, birth defects, or genetic damages appear not to have been done. Evaluators therefore regard safety as unproved.

According to manufacturers' data, this chemical will kill the bacteria present in dental plaque. But the experts say this does not establish its ability to kill bacteria that are on or embedded in nearby mucous membranes of the mouth and throat. Like other quaternary ammonium compounds, domiphen bromide is inactivated by tissue debris and body fluids. To really work, it may require far longer exposure to infected surfaces than is realistically possible—given that saliva rapidly dilutes drugs applied to the mouth. Also, currently marketed mouthwashes contain 1:20,000 dilutions of domiphen bromide, which may be too weak to kill significant numbers of bacteria under any circumstances. For these reasons, the Panel says domiphen bromide's safety and effectiveness have yet to be demonstrated.

Ethyl alcohol   Although use of this alcohol is safe in the concentrations—up to 35 percent—that are used in over-the-counter oral health products, these relatively low concentrations have not been shown to be effective against bacteria. Higher concentrations, which *are* effective, cause burning and intense discomfort—so they are too irritating to be used to treat sores and inflammation in the mouth or throat. The Panel concludes: ethyl alcohol is safe but of unproved effectiveness in relieving sore throat and mouth.

Eucalyptol   An oil obtained by boiling fresh eucalyptus leaves, eucalyptol has a pungent smell and a spicy, cooling taste. It is widely used in folk and nonprescription medicines, and long marketing experience indicates that small amounts of it are probably not harmful. The Panel could find little information about which bacteria eucalyptol may kill—or how, and how rapidly it might do so. While one manufacturer submitted data showing that a mixture of eucalyptol and several other agents will kill more microbes than the same mixture without the eucalyptol, reviewers say this does not prove that eucalyptol is an effective antimicrobial agent when used by itself. Verdict: eucalyptol is safe but its effectiveness as an antimicrobial agent must be demonstrated.

Gentian violet   This greenish-purple dye will kill some bacteria, funguses, and other microorganisms. Currently, it is less widely used than it once was because more effective drugs have been developed and because doubts have been raised about its safety (*see* GENTIAN VIOLET, page 852). Gentian violet has the added disadvantage that it stains false teeth and other dental appliances, as well as mucous membranes. The Panel decided that 1 percent gentian violet is safe when swabbed directly onto sore and infected areas in the mouth and throat 2 or 3 times daily for a few days at a time. But there is little or no evidence from controlled scientific studies to show that it acts effectively as an antimicrobial, compared with other agents that are available on prescription, or that it really relieves sore throat and mouth. So the Panel rates gentian violet safe but of still-unproved effectiveness.

Hydrogen peroxide   Basing their decision on another Panel's ranking, this Panel accepts this bitter-tasting substance as being safe for brief, occasional use in the mouth at concentrations up to 3 percent (*see* HYDROGEN PEROXIDE, page 357). It warns, however, that continuing use of hydrogen peroxide can damage the calcium in teeth.

High concentrations of hydrogen peroxide will kill bacteria. But these concentrations may also be dangerous, and evaluators say it is difficult to imagine the circumstances under which the compound will kill bacteria without injuring mucous membranes of the throat and mouth. Lower concentrations have been shown to be bactericidal, too —but only if they remain in contact with the microorganisms for relatively long periods (say, one hour). Because of natural salivary dilution, it seems unlikely that a safe dose of the drug will remain in the mouth —in effective amounts—for this length of time. So, the Panel accepts hydrogen peroxide as safe but is skeptical about its antimicrobial effect in treating sore throat and mouth.

Iodine   This element has been used medicinally since 1819, and is an extremely potent antimicrobial agent that works against bacteria, viruses, and funguses. The major difficulty with iodine is its toxicity. It is deadly if swallowed in large amounts. Even lesser amounts, if used repeatedly, can lead to a chronic poisoning called *iodism*. (The principal symptom is pain or a sense of heaviness in the sinuses around the nose.) Iodine also stings, irritates, and inflames the skin—and its effects on mucous membranes in the mouth and throat are even more severe. So the Panel would limit the allowable concentration to 1 to 2 percent in gargles, rinses, sprays, or swabs, and says that good evidence must be obtained to confirm that even these low doses are safe.

Despite iodine's potent germicidal effect, the Panel says studies have yet to be done to obtain proof that it works effectively as an oral-cavity drug to relieve sore throat and mouth. Thus iodine is "on probation" both in terms of safety and effectiveness.

Menthol   A fragrant alcohol obtained from oil of peppermint and other mint oils, menthol is a common ingredient in candy and other foods as well as medicines. Few serious adverse effects have been reported, so the Panel assessed it as safe.

Menthol is germicidal—but little or no data are available on *which* germs it kills, or how rapidly. One manufacturer submitted test results which showed that a mix of aromatic substances—including thymol, menthol, camphor, and methyl salicylate—had more antimicrobial power than the same mixture without the menthol. The Panel dismisses this finding, saying the test does not establish the antimicrobial value of menthol used as a single ingredient. At this time, therefore, menthol is categorized as safe but in need of proof about effectiveness.

Methyl salicylate   This aspirinlike compound has the fragrance and taste of wintergreen and teaberry. Its taste appeal has been a problem: a number of accidental poisonings occurred when children ate methyl salicylate products. Newer safety packaging requirements have greatly reduced this risk—so the Panel calls it safe. But no controlled scientific study is available to demonstrate that methyl salicylate has useful antimicrobial action when used in over-the-counter drugs applied to the mucous membranes of the throat and mouth. The Panel's verdict: the effectiveness of this pleasant-smelling compound still needs to be established.

Oxyquinoline   sulfate   (8-hydroxyquinoline)   Also known as oxine, quinphenol-8-hydroxyquinoline, and bioquin, this drug is widely used in industry because of its ability to bind to metals. Medicinally, the action is believed to involve picking up and binding copper from body tissues. The copper bound to the oxyquinoline sulfate in this way readily enters bacterial cells. Once inside these cells, the copper is released and it kills the bacteria.

Oxyquinoline and related compounds have seen wide use as antimicrobials. But they pose 2 problems. On the one hand, they are toxic —although oxyquinoline sulfate may be less poisonous than some others. The second problem is the lack of scientific data that clearly establish the chemicals' safety. The Panel says it received no results from well-controlled scientific studies to show oxyquinoline sulfate's value as a broad-spectrum antimicrobial agent. Its value in relieving sore throat and mouth is similarly unclear. The judgment: both the safety and the effectiveness of this compound remain to be demonstrated.

Phenol   This compound has been widely used in over-the-counter medications to relieve pain and control microorganisms. The present Panel finds phenol in very low concentrations safe as well as effective as an anesthetic for relief from the pain of sore throat and sore mouth. So safety is not the issue here.

But phenol's effectiveness as an antimicrobial *is* in question. While the drug (also known as *carbolic acid*) is the antiseptic that was used over a century ago to prove that antiseptic practices reduce postsurgery infections, phenol has by and large been replaced in this use by more effective antiseptics. And as for its effects against microorganisms causing sore throat or mouth, phenol's supporters gave no specific evidence to the Panel. So the verdict is: safe (in very low concentrations) but not proved effective.

Phenolate sodium   Similar to phenol (*see* immediately above), this compound has comparable actions. Approved as a pain reliever, sodium phenolate also possesses "germ-killing" properties. But reviewers say they received insufficient evidence to show that the chemical effectively kills the specific microorganisms responsible for sore throat and sore mouth. In sum: safe but not proved effective for over-the-counter oral-health-care products.

Povidone-iodine   Because iodine is extremely irritating to the skin and mucous membranes, manufacturers have combined it with other substances, like povidone, in order to reduce the amount of free iodine that reaches the body surface at any one time. The povidone is practically nontoxic, the Panel says, and experimental and marketing data indicate that 1 or 2 applications of povidone-iodine to the throat or mouth are also safe. But the compound's safety on a regular-use, long-term basis has not been established. Too, the rate at which povidone-iodine is absorbed into the bloodstream from the mouth and throat is not known.

Effectiveness also remains in question—even though a number of studies on its use on the skin and in the mouth have been published. In particular, it is not clear how much of the iodine's germicidal effect is lost when its activity is inhibited by the presence of povidone. It is not clear, either, whether povidone-iodine slows or actually enhances wound healing. Conclusion: neither the safety nor the effectiveness of povidone-iodine has been confirmed.

Secondary amyltricresols   These are phenollike compounds that are a hundred or more times more potent than phenol itself against some bacteria. They have been used in medicine for half a century.

Animal studies show that secondary amyltricresols are slightly irritating to mucous membranes. Evaluators were given only one study concerning the use of these substances for human mouth wounds. No clear signs of toxicity were noted, but the report contained no information about rate of absorption from the mucous membranes, mucosal irritation, or the breakdown and excretion of the drug from the body. The Panel says it knows too little to declare secondary amyltricresols safe for use in the mouth and throat. Further, no data were submitted demonstrating that secondary amyltricresols are effective in combating bacteria responsible for mouth or throat soreness. Conclusion: both safety and effectiveness need to be shown.

Sodium caprylate   This is a fatty acid that has been demonstrated to work against fungal infections of the mouth and of the skin (including athlete's foot and jock itch). Although there is little scientific evidence of its safety when used as an oral drug, the Panel notes that fatty acids are in many foods and they appear to cause no harm. So it says that one can assume that the substance is safe for throat-mouth use.

Effectiveness is another matter. While the dental literature contains several reports of dramatic cures of thrush—a disease that raises painful white bumps in the mucous membranes of the throat and mouth—there are no properly conducted studies to show that sodium caprylate kills the microorganisms responsible for sore throat and mouth. The judgment: safe but not proved effective.

Thymol   Standard toxicology tests and long use indicate that serious side effects are very rare when thymol, a pleasant-smelling alcohol, is taken in the doses commonly available in over-the-counter preparations. So the Panel puts it into the "safe" category—noting, however, that thymol can irritate mucous membranes. Thymol has been shown to kill both bacteria and funguses. But its potency is reduced when it interacts with the natural organic material that is always present in the mouth and throat. Little contemporary data demonstrate thymol's effectiveness in relieving sore throat and mouth. The Panel rejected one study that seemed to demonstrate greater antimicrobial potency of a thymol-containing mixture compared with the same mixture minus the thymol. In short: thymol is safe, but effectiveness needs to be shown.

Thymol iodide   A combination of thymol and iodine—also known as dithymol diiodide—thymol iodide is a red-yellow or red-brown powder. It is often dissolved in peanut oil for application inside the mouth. The Panel expressed the same doubts about thymol iodide's safety when applied topically in the mouth as it did about iodine's (*see* IODINE, page 704). Evaluators said they received no reliable test results demonstrating that thymol iodide effectively limits or destroys microorganisms responsible for sore throat and mouth. Conclusion: both safety and effectiveness remain unproved.

Tolu balsam   This sap extract has a pleasant, vanillalike aroma and has been used medically for many years. But its therapeutic properties have rarely been assessed according to acceptable scientific standards. While it is not considered to be dangerous, it also is not thought to be really effective in killing or inhibiting the growth of microorganisms that cause sore throat and sore mouth. Verdict: safe but not proved effective.

Disapproved Active Ingredients

Boric acid   This drug is derived from the nonmetallic element boron—a potent nerve poison. Skin can block boric acid's absorption but mucous membrane cannot. The early signs of boron poisoning—or boric-acid poisoning—are nausea, vomiting, diarrhea, and stomach pain.

Furthermore, boric acid is only weakly effective, at best, in killing microorganisms in the mouth and throat. The Panel therefore classifies boric acid—and the related compounds sodium borate and borax—as both unsafe and ineffective.

Borogylcerin glycerite   As its name suggests, this is a compound of boric acid and glycerin. No convincing scientific evidence is available on its worth in the case of sore throat and sore mouth, and it also shares the toxic risk of boric acid (*see* immediately above). The Panel's verdict: not safe and not effective.

Camphor   Serious safety questions have been raised about this aromatic substance (*see* CAMPHOR). Since it is easily absorbed through the mucous membranes of the mouth and throat, the present Panel rates it unsafe. Nor was any valid scientific study submitted to demonstrate that camphor works as an antimicrobial when used in the mouth and throat. So it is judged to be both unsafe and ineffective.

Cresol   This is a phenol derivative that may be more irritating to body surfaces than phenol itself is. Cresol is readily and rapidly absorbed into the body through mucous membranes and produces local damage to tissues even in dilute solutions. For these reasons, it is declared unsafe. It is more active against some bacteria than is phenol, but the Panel did not rule on cresol's effectiveness. It disapproved cresol wholly on grounds of safety.

Ferric chloride   An iron salt that is reddish or brownish in color, ferric chloride is irritating to the mucosal lining of the gastrointestinal tract. It is fairly toxic, and large doses accidentally swallowed could cause death. So the Panel rules it unsafe. Also, since evaluators were provided no data indicating that ferric chloride effectively combats microorganisms that cause sore throat and mouth, the Panel declared ferric chloride ineffective as well as unsafe.

Meralein sodium   This substance, commonly called *merodicein*, is a mercury derivative that may vary in color from green to dark red. It can poison the kidneys, and one expert cited by the Panel rates it as being highly toxic. Meralein sodium slows bacterial growth and reproduction. But it requires many hours to kill the bacteria, which means that swabbing it once onto sore spots in the mouth and throat is not likely to be of much therapeutic value, because saliva quickly dilutes and washes away drugs applied in this way. Verdict: unsafe and not effective.

Nitromersol   Although, like meralein sodium (*see* immediately above), this drug is derived from mercury, its different chemical nature makes it more active against bacteria and less irritating and less toxic. This difference does not, however, persuade the Panel that nitromersol is safe for self-use in nonprescription oral-health-care products. To the contrary, reviewers categorized it as unsafe because of the damage that even small amounts of mercury can do to the fine, inner structures of the kidney after it has been absorbed through the mucous membranes. In addition to these risks, there is no evidence to convince the Panel that nitromersol effectively kills or inhibits microorganisms specifically responsible for sore throat and mouth. Verdict: unsafe and ineffective.

Potassium chlorate   According to the experts, chlorate poisoning was common when the drug enjoyed widespread medicinal use after its introduction as a seemingly innocuous substance. Potassium chlorate specifically damages the gastrointestinal tract, kidneys, and red blood cells. On top of that, chlorates show no germ-killing activity when studied in the test tube, and reviewers were puzzled as to how such drugs ever came to be used as antimicrobials. The Panel judges potassium chlorate as both unsafe and ineffective.

Sodium dichromate and sodium bichromate   Both sodium dichromate and sodium bichromate are derivatives of the element chromium. Both are exceedingly dangerous because they are corrosive to skin and mucous membranes. They can cause violent stomach pain, circulatory collapse, dizziness, headaches, muscle cramps, coma, and even death. The Panel's verdict is that chromium derivatives should have *no* use as therapeutic agents because of this tremendous danger of toxic reactions. In short: unsafe.

Tincture of myrrh   The ancients used this gum resin as medicine and as a component of embalming mixtures. Myrrh is irritating to the skin and mucous membranes. In recent years it has been dropped from major drug reference books and the Panel could find no sound scientific data to show that the substance kills microorganisms that cause sore throat and sore mouth. The Panel disapproved myrrh on counts of safety and effectiveness.

ASTRINGENTS

An *astringent* is a chemical that will bind to or hold proteins that are present in saliva and other body fluids and then pull them out of these solutions. When swished around the mouth, astringent preparations briefly form a thin layer on mucosal cell surfaces. They draw together proteins on these cells' surfaces—causing a puckery, astringent sensation—and protect this area from painful and irritating substances.

Used in recommended doses, astringents act only on the surface of the outer layer of these mucosal cells. They do not penetrate into the cells' interiors or into deeper layers of tissue, so they carry little or no risk of poisoning one's system. (More highly concentrated astringent solutions—which are *not* recommended for use without prescription—may, however, reach and damage cell interiors and internal organs.)

Drawing inspiration from the simple, short-acting benefits that astringents provide, manufacturers have come up with what the Panel suggests are outlandish claims for over-the-counter sore-throat and sore-mouth remedies that contain these substances. Some of the more general claims for these products that the Panel disapproves of are listed in the introductory portion of this unit. Others, which refer more specifically to astringent active ingredients, are outlined below.

CLAIMS FOR ASTRINGENTS

Accurate
"aids in the temporary relief of occasional discomfort due to minor irritations of the mouth and throat"

False or Misleading
"works directly on throat membranes"
"formula in use over ninety years"
"relief of uncomfortable conditions of the mouth and throat"
"relief of pain from aphthous ulcers [canker sores]"
"helps the mouth feel clean"
"provides protective coating to mouth sores"

Approved Active Ingredients

Alum   As its name implies, alum is a preparation of the metallic element aluminum. Three different aluminum compounds are sold as alum. The most common is *potassium aluminum sulfate*. Other forms include sodium aluminum sulfate and ammonium aluminum sulfate. These three preparations have essentially the same therapeutic properties.

Alum is widely used in foods, being a part of baking powder. Extremely large doses may irritate the stomach lining or produce diarrhea, but side effects are rare or nonexistent when recommended dose levels are maintained. So the Panel says alum is safe.

Although the Panel cites no specific studies that demonstrate alum's effectiveness as an oral astringent, it calls dilute solutions workable aids in relieving sore throat or mouth because the drug provides a protective layer over irritated areas. The evaluators say that these drugs do not cure—they provide relief only.

The safe and effective dosage for adults and children over 3 is 0.2 to 0.5 percent alum in water-base rinses, gargles, sprays, or swabs, applied to the affected site up to 4 times daily. The excess drug should be spit out, and such preparations should not be used longer than 2 days.

Zinc chloride   This water-soluble zinc compound is sometimes called *butter of zinc*. Like other forms of zinc, it is quite harmless when swallowed; zinc is an essential nutritional ingredient and is present in many foods. For these reasons, evaluators judged zinc chloride safe— in the recommended medicinal dosages—for use to relieve sore throat and mouth. As is the case with alum (*see* immediately above), no scientific studies are cited, but the substance is said to effectively provide temporary relief (not "cure") of mouth and throat soreness.

The approved astringent dosage of zinc chloride is a 0.1 to 0.25 percent concentration applied up to 4 times daily in rinses, mouthwashes, or on cotton swabs.

Conditionally Approved Active Ingredients

None

Disapproved Active Ingredients

Tincture of myrrh   This aromatic, bitter-tasting plant product can be highly irritating and there is no evidence to support its use as an astringent. The Panel's verdict: unsafe and ineffective.

DEBRIS REMOVERS (DEBRIDING AGENTS)

Colds and other conditions that cause sore throat or irritation and soreness in the mouth usually produce accumulations of mucus, phlegm, and other secretions that stick to and build up on the mucous membranes. These secretions can be irritating and are apt to cause coughing. They may also cause pain.

Effective drugs are available to remove these unpleasant exudates: technically they are called *debriding agents*. They act in several ways. Some release tiny bubbles of oxygen that lift the offending matter off the tissue surface. Other, mineral-containing compounds may act mechanically to wash the gunk away. Gargling with sodium bicarbonate—ordinary baking soda—seems to help in this way. Sodium bicarbonate also increases the alkalinity of mucus and appears to soften and loosen it so that it is easier to swallow, cough up, or blow out through the nose. Salt water is widely used as a debris remover. The salt draws water out of the mucous membranes, which dilutes mucus and acts to cleanse the membrane surfaces. The Panel stresses, however, that the debriding agents act only briefly; they do not cure the underlying condition. The relief provided, however, may last for several hours.

CLAIMS FOR DEBRIS REMOVERS

Accurate
"aids in the removal of phlegm, mucus, or other secretions in the temporary relief of discomfort due to occasional sore throat and sore mouth"

False or Misleading
"quickly removes phlegm and other secretions"
"superior cleansing agent"
"foaming, cleansing rinse for irritated throats"

Approved Active Ingredients

Carbamide peroxide This substance is formulated with anhydrous glycerin or propylene glycol. When it comes into contact with the mouth's mucosal surfaces, saliva, blood, or other body fluids will set off a reaction that transforms the carbamide peroxide into hydrogen peroxide. This in turn breaks down into water, urea, and little bubbles of oxygen (*see* immediately below). Small amounts of glycerin are safe, and other breakdown products—water, urea, and oxygen—are all naturally present in the body. So the Panel says this preparation is safe.

The frothing and foaming of oxygen bubbles released help to dislodge dead and decaying mucosal cells, tissue bits, and pus and other secretions from infected wounds and sores. Without citing evidence from experiments, the Panel maintains that carbamide peroxide acts effectively in this way. The safe and effective dosage is 10 to 15 percent carbamide peroxide in anhydrous glycerin or in a spray, rinse, or gargle, up to 4 times daily for 2 days.

Hydrogen peroxide   The present reviewers agree with another Panel: a 3 percent concentration of this substance is safe for use in the mouth.

Hydrogen peroxide effectively cleanses the mucosal surfaces through its effervescent action. When it contacts tissue, certain enzymes act to convert it into water and oxygen. This reaction is quick, so the oxygen bubbles bounce around and loosen various kinds of debris-type materials. This action may aid in relieving the pain and discomfort of sore throat or mouth.

The Panel recommends that 3 percent hydrogen peroxide preparations be diluted with water before use. One part of the drug should be mixed with one part water. Then the solution can be swished around the mouth, used as a gargle, or be applied to the throat or mouth with a spray or a swab. This safe and effective dose should not be used more often than 3 or 4 times daily, and not for longer than 2 days.

Sodium bicarbonate   This remedy is familiarly known as baking soda. Since it has seen long use in preparing food—as well as in antacids —the Panel regards it as safe. Persons with high blood pressure or kidney disease should not overuse sodium bicarbonate, however, since they probably ought to limit their sodium intake.

Because it is highly alkaline, sodium bicarbonate appears to soften mucus deposits so they can be dislodged by gargling or rinsing. Without citing any specific studies, evaluators declared sodium bicarbonate to be effective (as well as safe) in concentrations of 5 to 10 percent. For gargling, the Panel recommends mixing one teaspoonful of sodium bicarbonate and ½ teaspoonful of salt in a glass of warm water. To get at mucus secretions far back in the mouth and throat, which may not be reached by gargling, the Panel suggests attaching an eyedropper to the tubing of a clean enema bag or other plastic squeeze bag, so that the mixture can be sprayed down the throat.

Conditionally Approved Active Ingredients

None

Disapproved Active Ingredient

Sodium perborate   This ingredient releases boric acid, which is absorbed through the mucous membranes and can be a potent poison because of its boron content (*see* BORIC ACID, page 708). Any effectiveness of sodium perborate as an oral-cavity drug has been attributed to the release of oxygen that occurs when it comes in contact with the soft tissues—and, possibly, to its alkalinity, which might help loosen gooey mucus. But the Panel says too little oxygen is released for the drug to be of much value. Verdict: unsafe and ineffective.

DECONGESTANTS

When one has a red, sore throat due to a cold, air pollution, or some other problem, the tiny blood vessels in the mucous membranes tend to be dilated and engorged with blood. This causes swelling, which in turn narrows the airway to and from the lungs. Decongestants act on the smooth muscle in the mucosal tissues, and particularly in the capillary blood vessels, causing them to tighten up. This reduces the capillary passageways and the amount of blood present in the tissue. The result is a shrinking of tissue and the probable release of thick mucus secretions that become caked on the throat's surface.

Decongestants are often taken orally or inhaled. Thus they act throughout the body. The present Panel referred all such preparations to another group of reviewers, whose findings are summarized in COLD, COUGH, AND ALLERGY DRUGS, under NASAL DECONGESTANTS. However, some oral-health-care products containing decongestants are intended for direct application to the throat and inside of the mouth—as lozenges, liquids, or sprays. So it was decided that these ingredients ought to be evaluated in terms of local effects on the mucous membranes of the throat and mouth.

The Panel could find no sound evidence to show that decongestants are effective when applied topically. So none are approved for this purpose as both safe and effective. On the other hand, it found no data contradicting manufacturers' claims for these ingredients—so it granted them conditional approval. Applying these preparations directly to the throat actually might be safer than swallowing them in pills or other preparations, since they may be potent poisons when taken internally. But this seeming advantage remains to be proved.

CLAIMS FOR DECONGESTANTS

Accurate
"aids in the temporary relief of occasional discomfort due to congestion in the mouth and throat" (if applied to safe and effective decongestants, of which there are none)

False or Misleading
  "superior decongestant"
  "makes breathing easier"
  "reduces inflammation"

Approved Active Ingredients

None

Conditionally Approved Active Ingredients

Phenylephrine hydrochloride The safety and effectiveness of this compound, when taken internally, has been carefully assessed by another Panel. This Panel concurs that it is safe for topical use in the doses customarily found in lozenges and sprays—although preservatives used with it may cause local irritation or allergic reactions.

No well-controlled studies are available to prove that phenylephrine hydrochloride really works when applied topically. So the evaluators concluded that its effectiveness needs to be shown. The safe dosage is set at one teaspoonful (5 ml) of a 0.25 percent solution or 5 mg in a lozenge every 4 hours, up to 4 times daily.

WARNING FOR PHENYLEPHRINE HYDROCHLORIDE (above) AND PHENYLPROPANOLAMINE HYDROCHLORIDE (below) The Panel warns that persons taking monoamine oxidase (MAO) inhibitors should not use this drug. (Monoamine oxidase inhibitors are a class of drugs sometimes prescribed for depression and other psychiatric symptoms, as well as for certain medical conditions.) One should also discontinue using phenylephrine hydrochloride or phenylpropanolamine hydrochloride if dizziness, headache, fast pulse, tremors, or nervousness develop. A doctor should be consulted if these symptoms persist. Do not use these drugs if you have thyroid disease, high blood pressure, diabetes or heart disease—except under a doctor's supervision.

Phenylpropanolamine hydrochloride This is a central-nervous-system stimulant—an amphetaminelike drug—that has been judged to be safe as a nasal decongestant. This Panel concurs that this drug is safe in a dosage of one teaspoonful (5 ml) of a 0.25 percent solution every 3 or 4 hours, or up to 10.5 mg in a lozenge once every 4 hours.

This compound has been widely and carefully studied from a number of perspectives. But how well it works when formulated into lozenges and slow-release capsules has not been demonstrated scientifically.

Disapproved Active Ingredients

None

DEMULCENTS (SOOTHERS)

Thick, syrupy, soothing substances are formulated into oral-health-care products to cover and protect sore tissues in the throat and mouth. They also offer protection from chemicals, fluids, air, and other irritants. Some of these soothers—which are technically called *demulcents*—will bind and hold irritating substances, thus neutralizing them.

Demulcents are largely or wholly inert (chemically inactive); their major benefit rests in their soothing physical properties. They are not absorbed through the mucous membranes, or, if absorbed, are excreted unchanged. So no breakdown products are produced that might prove toxic to internal organs. As a result these drugs cause few, if any, adverse reactions.

CLAIMS FOR DEMULCENTS

Accurate
   "aids in the temporary relief of minor discomfort and protects irritated areas in sore mouth and sore throat"

False or Misleading
   for "relief of sore throat due to smoking"
   "produces a soothing coating that gives quick comfort to irritated throats"
   "soothes tired throats"

Approved Active Ingredients

Elm bark   This traditional remedy, obtained from the dried inner bark of the slippery-elm tree, is harvested in spring. When boiled, it produces a gluey substance with a currylike aroma. Not much information is available on safety. But since the bark breaks down into a variety of harmless sugars and since, too, there have been no reports of adverse effects from using it, the Panel judges the substance safe. When sucked from troches and lozenges, the elm-bark mucilage appears to cover and protect inflamed and irritated mucous membranes in the throat and mouth. This may temporarily help relieve sore throat or sore mouth. Elm bark has no curative or pain-killing properties.

The safe and effective dosage consists of lozenges or troches that contain 10 to 15 percent elm bark in agar or another water-soluble gum base. Adults and children over 3 can suck 1 or 2 of these lozenges every 2 hours for up to 2 days.

Gelatin   Because the substance is widely used in foods as a jelling agent the Panel judges it to be safe for occasional medicinal use.

Gelatin will provide a protective coating over irritated or ulcerated areas in the mouth and throat. It also inhibits one's ability to feel cold, warmth, pressure, or pain, although it has no curative or wound-healing powers. A special dosage form called an absorbable gelatin sponge may be used to medicate the insides of the cheeks and upper throat.

The safe and effective dosage for adults and children over age 3 is 5 to 10 percent gelatin in aqueous (water) solutions. It can be used as a rinse, gargle, spray, or with a swab as often as needed. On a specific sore area, the gelatin may be applied with the tip of the finger; one should use enough to form a solid or semisolid layer over the affected tissue.

Glycerin   This is a clear, colorless, syrupy liquid that is used to protect the skin as well as the mucous membranes. A century's medicinal use with no reported adverse effects persuades the Panel that glycerin is safe as a topical drug. When applied to the mouth in a rinse, wash, spray, or on a swab, it forms a thin protective layer that adheres to the mucous membranes. It insulates sensory nerve endings from hurtful stimuli, but it does not promote healing or "cure."

Glycerin should be diluted with 2 or 3 parts of water before use. It can be applied freely, as often as necessary.

Pectin   The fruit extract that makes fruit jellies jell, pectin has a long record of use in foods and medicines, and no record of known adverse effects. This convinces the Panel that pectin is safe. Forming a protective covering over raw or ulcerated areas in the mouth and throat, it protects the sensation receivers from further stimulation and the tissue from further irritation. Pectin does not, however, enhance healing or actually cure the soreness in the tissue it is covering. The substance is safe and effective, used as often as necessary—in rinse, gargle, spray, lozenge, or gel form. A thick enough preparation should be used to form a solid or semisolid coating over the irritated tissue.

Conditionally Approved Active Ingredients

None

Disapproved Active Ingredients

None

EXPECTORANTS

An expectorant loosens and aids in the expulsion of phlegm and other secretions from the respiratory tract. It may increase the volume of the respiratory-tract secretions, or soften them. Both actions may make it easier to cough up these secretions. Some expectorants promote coughing, which makes it easier to clear material from the throat. Of course, coughing up can be induced without taking a drug. The Panel reports that sour liquids or foods—including, specifically, small pieces of pickle—may stimulate salivary flow and help loosen and remove sticky secretions.

Although expectorants have been used medically for decades, there is little solid evidence that they effectively move phlegm from the lower end of the bronchial tree, which is why some dozen expectorant active ingredients fail to merit classification as both safe and effective (*see* EXPECTORANTS in COLD, COUGH, AND ALLERGY DRUGS). This Panel says there is even less evidence to indicate that expectorants are of value in the mouth and throat.

If used to excess or swallowed, expectorants may irritate the stomach lining. They may also aggravate the discomfort of sore mouth or sore throat by causing one to cough, and they may be directly irritating to inflamed mucous membranes.

CLAIMS FOR EXPECTORANTS

Unproved
"aids in the removal of secretions and in the temporary relief of discomfort due to occasional sore throat and sore mouth"

False or Misleading
"superior expectorant"
"promotes needed expectoration"

Approved Active Ingredients

None

Conditionally Approved Active Ingredients

Ammonium chloride This ammonium compound, which is also known as *muriate of ammonia* and *sal ammoniac*, has been used for medicinal purposes for many years. Although no controlled studies were submitted to document the drug's safety for use on throat-mouth mucous membranes, the lack of reported adverse effects persuaded the Panel that it is safe.

Ammonium chloride is formulated into many expectorant mixtures. What's the rationale? It irritates the stomach lining, causing the respiratory tract to increase fluid secretions into the airway. This loosens tenacious mucus. The drug's high alkalinity may also aid in liquefying the mucus and stimulating the respiratory tract to move it up toward the nose and mouth, where it can be blown out or spit out.

But the Panelists and other pharmacological experts say that the evidence for ammonium chloride's effectiveness is scant and inconclusive. So while ammonium chloride is safe, its effectiveness remains to be proved.

Horehound Used for years, horehound—also known as hoarhound, gypsy wart, harbane and madwort—is a plant extract. No controlled scientific-test results are available to confirm either the safety or effectiveness of horehound. Its venerable history of use convinces the Panel to accredit horehound as safe. But the substance has been dropped from many drug reference guides, and evaluators believe it does not play any significant role in removing secretions from the throat and mouth. So, while safe, horehound's effectiveness needs to be proved—even at this late date.

Tolu balsam The Panel judges this plant product to be safe. Despite its long use in cough mixtures, the Panel says the substance works only feebly as an expectorant, and not a single reference could be found in the scientific literature concerning its use in treating throat and mouth symptoms. Verdict: safe but not proved effective.

Disapproved Active Ingredients

Potassium iodide This compound has been widely used as an expectorant. In effective doses—if there were such—it is not safe, according to the Panel, because of its iodine content. Iodine poisoning (iodism) may produce serious symptoms—including inflammation of the mucous membranes, swelling, sores, and even breathing difficulties —in highly sensitive individuals who take only a few doses. More commonly, nausea and gastric discomfort are adverse effects.

While the Panel found evidence suggesting that potassium iodide increases the secretion of fluids into the respiratory tract—which theoretically could help loosen thick mucus deposits—it noted that this evidence is from uncontrolled studies and is too sparse to be convincing. So it decided that while this agent's effectiveness remains to be determined, its lack of safety is well established.

INACTIVE INGREDIENTS

Inactive ingredients are sometimes formulated into products for reasons of manufacturing process. Those found in sore-throat and sore-mouth medicines are:

acetanilid
anise oil
aromatics
calcium chloride
calcium silicate
cinnamon oil
dextrose
essential oils
honey
isobornyl acetate
methylparaben
peppermint oil

phosphate buffers
plasticized
  hydrocarbon gel
  (polyethylene in
  mineral oil)
potassium chloride
propylene glycol
propylparaben
sage oil
sodium bitartrate
  buffer

sodium
  carboxymethyl-
  cellulose
sodium chloride
sodium saccharin
sorbitol base
spearmint oil
sugar
talcum powder
vegetable stearate
water

Safety and Effectiveness: Active Ingredients in Over-the-Counter Sore Throat and Mouth Medicines

Active Ingredient	Panel's Assessment
Anesthetics/Analgesics	
antipyrine	not safe or effective
aspirin (in chewing gum)	safe and effective
benzocaine	safe and effective
benzyl alcohol	safe and effective
camphor	not safe or effective
cresol	not safe or effective
dibucaine	not safe
dibucaine hydrochloride	not safe
dyclonine hydrochloride	safe and effective
eucalyptol	safe, but not proved effective
hexylresorcinol	safe and effective
lidocaine	not safe

Safety and Effectiveness: Active Ingredients in Over-the-Counter Sore Throat and Mouth Medicines

Active Ingredient	*Panel's Assessment*
Anesthetics/Analgesics	
lidocaine hydrochloride	not safe
menthol	safe and effective
methyl salicylate	safe, but not proved effective
phenol	safe and effective
phenolate sodium (sodium phenolate)	safe and effective
pyrilamine maleate	safe, but not effective
salicyl alcohol	safe and effective
tetracaine	not safe
tetracaine hydrochloride	not safe
thymol	safe, but not proved effective
Antimicrobials	
benzalkonium chloride	safe, but not proved effective
benzethonium chloride	not proved safe or effective
benzoic acid	safe, but not proved effective
boric acid	not safe or effective
boroglycerin glycerite	not safe or effective
camphor	not safe or effective
carbamide peroxide in anhydrous glycerin (urea peroxide)	safe, but not proved effective
cetalkonium chloride	safe, but not proved effective
cetylpyridinium chloride	not proved safe or effective
chlorophyll	safe, but not proved effective
cresol	not safe
dequalinium chloride	not proved safe or effective
domiphen bromide	not proved safe or effective
ethyl alcohol	safe, but not proved effective
eucalyptol	safe, but not proved effective
ferric chloride	not safe or effective
gentian violet	safe, but not proved effective
hydrogen peroxide	safe, but not proved effective
iodine	not proved safe or effective
menthol	safe, but not proved effective
meralein sodium	not safe or effective
methyl salicylate	safe, but not proved effective
nitromersol	not safe or effective
oxyquinoline sulfate (8-hydroxy-quinolone)	not proved safe or effective
phenol	safe, but not proved effective
phenolate sodium	safe, but not proved effective
potassium chlorate	not safe or effective
povidone-iodine	not proved safe or effective
secondary amyltricresols	not proved safe or effective

Safety and Effectiveness: Active Ingredients in Over-the-Counter Sore Throat and Mouth Medicines *(continued)*

Active Ingredient	*Panel's Assessment*
Antimicrobials	
sodium bichromate	not safe
sodium caprylate	safe, but not proved effective
sodium dichromate	not safe
thymol	safe, but not proved effective
thymol iodide	not proved safe or effective
tincture of myrrh	not safe or effective
tolu balsam	safe, but not proved effective
Astringents	
alum	safe and effective
tincture of myrrh	not safe or effective
zinc chloride	safe and effective
Debris Removers (Debriding Agents)	
carbamide peroxide	safe and effective
hydrogen peroxide	safe and effective
sodium bicarbonate	safe and effective
sodium perborate	not safe or effective
Decongestants	
phenylephrine hydrochloride	safe, but not proved effective
phenylpropanolamine hydrochloride	safe, but not proved effective
Demulcents (Soothers)	
elm bark	safe and effective
gelatin	safe and effective
glycerin	safe and effective
pectin	safe and effective
Expectorants	
ammonium chloride	safe, but not proved effective
horehound	safe, but not proved effective
potassium iodide	not safe
tolu balsam	safe, but not proved effective

Safety and Effectiveness: Combination Products Sold Over-the-Counter for Sore Throat and Sore Mouth

Safe and Effective

(Each active ingredient must be present within the dosage range approved by the Panel.)

1 approved anesthetic + 1 approved antimicrobial (of which there is none at present)

**Safety and Effectiveness: Combination Products Sold
Over-the-Counter for Sore Throat and Sore Mouth** *(continued)*

Safe and Effective

1 approved soother + 1 approved antimicrobial (of which there is none at present)
1 approved decongestant (of which there is none at present) + 1 approved
   antimicrobial (of which there is none at present)
1 approved astringent + 1 approved antimicrobial (of which there is none at present)
1 approved anesthetic + 1 approved soother
1 approved anesthetic + 1 approved decongestant (of which there is none at present)
1 approved anesthetic + 1 approved soother + 1 approved antimicrobial (of which
   there is none at present)
1 approved anesthetic + 1 approved astringent
1 approved anesthetic + 1 approved astringent + 1 approved antimicrobial (of which
   there is none at present)
1 approved anesthetic + 1 approved decongestant (of which there is none at present)
   + 1 approved antimicrobial (of which there is none at present)

Conditionally Safe and Effective

any approved ingredient is present in less than the approved dose
1 or more of the ingredients is only conditionally approved
2 or more approved ingredients are included from the same drug class, but the
   combination has not been proved to have a therapeutic advantage (e.g., to be safer,
   more effective, better-accepted by consumers or have some other clear advantage
   over each of the active ingredients, individually, at full therapeutic doses)

Unsafe or Ineffective

contains any disapproved ingredient
contains any ingredient at more than the maximum allowed dose
1 or more approved antimicrobials + 1 or more approved expectorants (since the
   expectorant will dilute or diminish the contact time of the antimicrobial)
1 or more antimicrobials + 1 debris remover (since the debris remover will dilute or
   wash the antimicrobial from the diseased surface)
1 or more approved antimicrobials + 1 approved expectorant + 1 approved debris
   remover (since the combination drug will tend to be washed away from the
   mucous-membrane surface)
1 approved anesthetic + 1 approved debris remover (since the anesthetic will be
   washed away, diluted, or mixed with the debris raised by the debris remover and will
   be inactivated)
1 or more approved anesthetics + 1 or more approved expectorants (since the drug
   will be diluted and removed from the site of action)
1 or more approved anesthetic ingredients + 1 or more approved expectorants + 1
   or more debris removers (since the anesthetic will be diluted or removed from the
   intended site)
1 or more approved astringents + 1 or more approved debris removers (since the
   latter will prevent the former from exerting its effect on protein matter)

Safety and Effectiveness: Combination Products Sold
Over-the-Counter for Sore Throat and Sore Mouth *(continued)*

Unsafe or Ineffective

1 or more approved astringents + 1 or more expectorants (since the expectorants will dilute and wash away the astringent)

1 or more approved decongestants + 1 or more approved expectorants + 1 or more approved debris removers (since these drugs will nullify and wash each other away)

1 or more decongestants + 1 or more expectorants (because the expectorant would dilute or nullify the decongestant)

Sore Throat and Mouth Medicines: Product Ratings

Medicated Gum

Product and Distributor	Dosage of Active Ingredients	Rating[1]	Comment
aspirin			
Aspergum (Plough)	**chewable gum tablets:** 210 mg	**A**	

Mouthwash, Sprays, and Gargles

Product and Distributor	Dosage of Active Ingredients	Rating[1]	Comment
cetylpyridinium chloride			
Cēpacol (Merrell-Dow)	**mouthwash:** 1:2000	**B**	not proved safe or effective
hexylresorcinol			
S. T. 37 (Beecham Products)	**solution:** 0.1%	**A**	
hydrogen peroxide			
hydrogen peroxide 3% (generic)	**solution:** 3%	**A**	
Hydrogen Peroxide 3% (Parke-Davis)	**solution:** 3%	**A**	
PerOxyl Mouth Rinse (Hoyt)	**solution:** 1.5%	**A**	
phenol			
Cēpastat (Merrell-Dow)	**mouthwash/gargle, throat spray:** 1.4% + glycerin	**A**	

Sore Throat and Mouth Medicines: Product Ratings _(continued)_

Mouthwash, Sprays, and Gargles

Product and Distributor	Dosage of Active Ingredients	Rating[1]	Comment
Chloraseptic Liquid (Norwich-Eaton)	**mouthwash/gargle, spray:** 1.4% as phenol and sodium phenolate	A	
povidone-iodine Isodine (Blair Labs.)	**mouthwash and gargle:** approx. 10% free iodine	B	not proved safe or effective
secondary amyltricresols Pentacresol 1:1000 (Upjohn)	**mouthwash:** 100 mg per 100 ml	B	not proved safe or effective

Lozenges and Troches

Product and Distributor	Dosage of Active Ingredients	Rating[1]	Comment
Cēpacol Troches (Merrell-Dow)	**lozenges:** 0.3% benzyl alcohol + 1:1500 cetylpyridinium chloride	B	latter ingredient not proved safe or effective
Cēpastat (Merrell-Dow)	**lozenges:** 1.45% phenol + 0.12% menthol + eucalyptus oil	B	eucalyptus not proved effective
Children's Chloraseptic (Norwich-Eaton)	**lozenges:** 5 mg benzocaine	A	
Trocaine (North American)		A	
Chloraseptic (Norwich-Eaton)	**lozenges:** 32.5 mg phenol	A	
Colrex (Rowell)	**troches:** 10 mg benzocaine + 2.5 mg cetylpyridinium chloride	B	latter ingredient not proved safe or effective
Conex (O'Neal)	**lozenges:** 5 mg benzocaine + 0.5 mg cetylpyridinium chloride	B	latter ingredient not proved safe or effective
Isodettes Super (Norcliff-Thayer)	**lozenges:** 10 mg benzocaine + 4 mg cetalkonium chloride	B	latter ingredient not proved effective
Listerine Antiseptic (Warner-Lambert)	**lozenges:** 2.4 mg hexylresorcinol	A	

Sore Throat and Mouth Medicines: Product Ratings *(continued)*

Lozenges and Troches

Product and Distributor	Dosage of Active Ingredients	Rating[1]	Comment
Sucrets Sore Throat (Beecham Products)		A	
spec-T Anesthetic (Squibb)	**lozenges:** 10 mg benzocaine	A	
Thantis (HW&D)	**lozenges:** 64.8 mg salicyl alcohol + 8 mg meralein sodium	C	latter ingredient not safe or effective

Debris Removers (Debriding Agents)

Product and Distributor	Dosage of Active Ingredients	Rating[1]	Comment
carbamide peroxide in anhydrous glycerin			
Gly-Oxide (Marion)	**drops:** 10%	A	
Proxigel (Reed & Carnrick)	**gel:** 11%	A	
hydrogen peroxide			
hydrogen peroxide 3% (generic)	**solution:** 3%	A	
Hydrogen Peroxide 3% (Parke-Davis)	**solution:** 3%	A	
PerOxyl Mouth Rinse (Hoyt)	**solution:** 1.5%	A	
sodium bicarbonate			
Arm & Hammer Baking Soda (Church & Dwight)	**powder**	A	
sodium bicarbonate (generic)	**powder**	A	
sodium perborate			
Amosan (Cooper)	**powder:** 1.2 g per packet	C	not safe or effective

1. Author's interpretation of Panel criteria. Based on contents, not claims.

Stimulants

Everybody seems to have an idea of what stimulants are. The Panel defines them as drugs that keep one awake and alert, and it decided that occasional use of safe and effective nonprescription stimulant preparations is not harmful to adults. In some cases these mild nonprescription stimulants may usefully counteract the boredom and fatigue of long, tedious work that requires vigilance. The Panel singled out the "highway hypnosis" that long-distance truck and auto drivers sometimes experience as one of these cases. When greater stimulation is required, prescription drugs—including amphetamines and desoxyephedrine—are available through a doctor.

To qualify as safe and effective, the Panel declared, an over-the-counter stimulant should:

- enable the user to perform whatever tasks are necessary even if he or she is drowsy or fatigued
- last long enough for the task to be completed
- provide a very wide margin of safety between a helpful dose and a dangerous one
- not unduly excite the heart
- not make the user restless or irritable
- not interfere with normal sleep
- not interact in an unpleasant or dangerous way with ordinary food or beverages

CLAIMS

Accurate
"helps restore mental alertness or wakefulness when [one is] experiencing fatigue or drowsiness"

STIMULANTS is based on the report of the FDA's Advisory Review Panel on OTC Sedative, Tranquilizer, and Sleep-Aid Drug Products, and the FDA's Tentative Final Order on Stimulants.

NONPRESCRIPTION STIMULANTS

Approved Active Ingredient

Caffeine The only over-the-counter stimulant that meets the Panel's requirements is caffeine. The FDA concurred that caffeine is both safe and effective. The recommended dosage is 100 to 200 mg every 3 or more hours. Caffeine preparations should not be used for longer than a week or two at a time, and they should not be used by children.

Caffeine stimulates both the heart and the central nervous system. This effect is greater when one is tired than when one is rested and alert. The claim that caffeine "enhances performance" when one is not fatigued has not been proved. One scientific review concludes, however, that it can increase precision in a "wide range of behavior . . . from putting the shot to monitoring a clock face."

The Panel noted: "In contrast to the irritating qualities of many coffee extracts, caffeine itself does not seem to cause irritation of the gastrointestinal tract in the usual doses. This is an advantage when the drug is used for its stimulant properties." However, taking large amounts at one time—more than about 240 mg—can cause nervousness, headache, and irritability. Anxiety may develop. Since caffeine is also present in coffee, tea, and cola drinks, supplements of this drug should be used cautiously when one is drinking large amounts of these beverages. The recommended medicinal dose of 100 to 200 mg is comparable to the caffeine in a cup of coffee (roughly 125 mg) or strong tea (roughly 100 to 115 mg) or four 8-ounce glasses of cola drinks (25 to 30 mg per glass).

Caffeine can be habit-forming, but severe problems of addiction appear to be rare. Sudden withdrawal, however, can produce severe headaches. Caffeine dependency was explored in an interesting set of experiments a few years ago. Researchers found that chronic coffee drinkers became sleepy and irritable when given decaffeinated coffee. But they felt alert and contented when given coffee containing caffeine. Regular coffee drinkers did not miss much sleep at night, but noncoffee drinkers who took coffee during the experiment could not sleep. Moreover, they became jittery and suffered stomach aches while the habituated users reported only "contentment." The conclusion seems to be that coffee does not adversely affect regular coffee drinkers but may cause some problems in other people.

There has been concern that coffee drinking—and by implication other uses of caffeine—may cause genetic or developmental defects in unborn babies, or may cause heart ailments in older persons. The FDA believes these fears to be unfounded. The FDA also notes that no fatal caffeine poisonings have ever been reported as the result of oral overdosage; it is calculated that an adult male would have to swallow the equivalent of 100 cups of coffee or more at one time to kill himself with caffeine.

Conditionally Approved Active Ingredients

None

Disapproved Active Ingredients

Three substances besides caffeine have been formulated into over-the-counter stimulant combination products. They are not effective as stimulants by themselves and the Panel and the FDA agree that there is no reason for combining them with caffeine.

Ammonium chloride   The Panel reported that it is unaware of any data that show a role for ammonium chloride as a stimulant, with or without caffeine.

Ginseng   No evidence was found to show that this traditional Oriental root medication—alone or with caffeine—acts as a stimulant. One product label submitted to the Panel claimed that caffeine and ginseng in combination "increase sensual awareness and pleasure." The Panel reported that a review of the available scientific literature failed to provide a reasonable documentation supporting this claim.

Vitamin E   Claims have been made that vitamin E is a stimulant and that, in conjunction with caffeine, it intensifies sexual feelings. The Panel, after an extensive review of research reports, found no reasonable evidence to support this claim. The FDA adds that there is no acceptable pharmacological reason for combining vitamins, and especially the very widely available vitamin E, with caffeine.

**Safety and Effectiveness: Active
Ingredients in Over-the-Counter
Stimulants**

Active Ingredient	Panel and FDA's* Assessment
ammonium chloride	not effective
caffeine	safe and effective
ginseng	not effective
vitamin E	not effective

*Judgments reaffirmed or modified by the FDA, or
originated by it.

Stimulants: Product Ratings

Product and Distributor	Dosage of Active Ingredients	Rating[1]	Comment
caffeine			
caffeine (generic)	**tablets:** 100 mg	A	
NōDōz (Bristol-Myers)		A	
caffeine (generic)	**capsules, timed-release:** 200 mg	A	
Caffedrine (Thompson)		A	
Kirkaffeine (Moore/Kirk)	**tablets:** 250 mg	C	higher than recommended dosage
Vivarin (J. B. Williams)	**tablets:** 200 mg	A	

1. Author's interpretation of Panel/FDA criteria. Based on contents, not claims.

Stomach Acidifiers

In normal individuals, the sight, smell, and taste of food cause the
stomach to expand to accommodate the meal being eaten. These same
factors also stimulate hydrochloric acid secretion into the stomach. A

STOMACH ACIDIFIERS is based on the report "Stomach Acidifier Drug Products"
by the FDA's Advisory Review Panel on OTC Miscellaneous Internal Drug Products.

weak solution of this acid is produced in the stomach lining and then secreted into the stomach itself at the rate of 30 to 40 milliliters (ml) each hour; this is little more than an ounce per hour. As one might imagine, this action is at its height during and soon after a meal.

The acid is believed to assist digestion by converting pepsinogen (a substance produced by glands in the stomach) into pepsin (the digestive juice). The hydrochloric acid and the pepsin apparently then act together to break up connective tissue and cell membranes in foodstuffs and to reduce the size of food particles. Despite these roles that the acid is thought to play, reviewers claim that it is *not* essential to the digestion or absorption of food.

When people produce too little hydrochloric acid, the condition is called *hypochlorhydria*. Some individuals produce none at all, a condition called *achlorhydria*. Several hydrochloric acid supplements are available over-the-counter to treat these situations. But the experts who assessed these drugs say that the drugs actually provide very little hydrochloric acid and are not really necessary because low or nonexistent secretion of the acid is not a disease: it does not cause nutritional or medical problems. This means, too, that diminished secretion of hydrochloric acid cannot be self-diagnosed. For these reasons, all over-the-counter stomach acidifying drugs are listed as ineffective. The Panel further says that all claims made for these preparations are both inappropriate and misleading. If the FDA follows the reviewers' recommendations, it will ban stomach acidifiers from the nonprescription marketplace.

CLAIMS

False or Misleading

for "hydrochloric acid deficiency"

for "replacement therapy in deficiencies of hydrochloric acid"

"stomach acid medication"

for "achlorhydria"

"assists digestion in gastric hypoacidity by gradual release of hydrochloric acid and pepsin"

"digestant"

STOMACH ACIDIFYING PRODUCTS

Approved Active Ingredients

None

Conditionally Approved Active Ingredients

None

Disapproved Active Ingredients

Betaine hydrochloride   Reviewers found no reports of adverse effects from using this chemical, so they concluded that it is safe. But the recommended doses of currently marketed products contain only about ⅓₀ of the amount of hydrochloric acid that is normally secreted into the stomach in an hour's time. This is too little to be of value. Worse, evaluators were not given—nor could they find—any convincing evidence to show that hydrochloric acid supplements from betaine hydrochloride (or any other drug) will really aid digestion. Verdict: safe but not effective—a combination that, to this Panel, warrants disapproval.

The combination of betaine hydrochloride + pepsin   No data were submitted to show that pepsin functions as a stomach acidifier or that it enhances the acidifying effect of betaine hydrochloride. While safe, the preparation was deemed ineffective.

Glutamic acid hydrochloride   No ill effects have been associated with use of this drug at the doses usually taken by people who secrete too little hydrochloric acid. So it is safe. But there are no controlled studies to show that the amount of acid delivered by this drug—or any drug—aids digestion, so it was disapproved.

Hydrochloric acid, diluted   The usual dose of hydrochloric acid is 5 ml, diluted with 125 to 250 ml of water. This fluid—unlike the drugs mentioned above—must be sipped through a glass straw to keep the acid from damaging tooth enamel. Reviewers say that the preparation may have some effect on the acidity of the stomach, but that most of it binds to the food itself and does not add any appreciable amount of free stomach acid. No evidence was presented that dilute hydrochloric acid aids digestion. So although it is considered safe, the preparation was disapproved because it is not effective.

Safety and Effectiveness: Active Ingredients in Over-the-Counter Stomach Acidifiers

Active Ingredient	Panel's Assessment
betaine hydrochloride	safe, but not effective
betaine hydrochloride + pepsin	safe, but not effective
glutamic acid hydrochloride	safe, but not effective
hydrochloric acid, diluted	safe, but not effective

Stomach Acidifiers: Product Ratings

Product and Distributor	Dosage of Active Ingredients	Rating[1]	Comment
:idulin Pulvules (Lilly)	**capsules:** 340 mg glutamic acid hydrochloride	C	not effective
Jutamic Acid HCl (Fibertone)	**tablets:** 325 mg glutamic acid hydrochloride	C	not effective
uripsin (Norgine)	**tablets:** 500 mg glutamic acid hydrochloride + 35 mg pepsin	C	not effective

Author's interpretation of Panel criteria. Based on contents, not claims.

Styptic Pencils and Other Astringents

When a man nicks himself shaving, touching the cut with the moistened end of a styptic pencil produces a stinging sensation—and usually coagulates the blood so that bleeding stops. This is an astringent effect —as are other actions of drugs in this class that slow or stop oozing, discharge, or bleeding from the skin or mucous membranes.

When astringents are defined in this way, the drugs' benefits seem clearcut. But the Panel that grappled with evaluating them concedes that they appear to act in several interrelated ways. They confer benefits that are partly *medicinal* and also perhaps partly *cosmetic*—in the sense that they create clean, puckery, refreshed feelings.

The principal astringent chemicals are the compounds of aluminum, zinc, manganese, iron, and bismuth, and other chemical groups that contain these metals (such as permanganates). The tannins, like tannic acid, are also astringents. Some acids, alcohols, and phenols also separate out proteins, but they also readily penetrate cell surfaces and

STYPTIC PENCILS AND OTHER ASTRINGENTS is based on the unadopted draft report "OTC Astringent Drug Products" by the FDA's Advisory Review Panel on OTC Miscellaneous External Drug Products.

may damage cells and tissues. So according to the Panel's standards they are not technically astringents.

HOW THEY WORK

Although some astringent substances are potent chemicals, they do not enter human body cells. Rather their activity all occurs at the cell surface—where they may block noxious substances from entering the cell—or in the space between cells. At the sites where they act, they coagulate by precipitating proteins—which means that they pull the proteins out of blood, serum, sweat, and other body fluids so that they form clots, crusts, or other solid deposits. If the serum is carrying an irritating body substance (histamine, for example), the astringent appears to trap and remove it. That way it can no longer enter its target cells, where it would provoke inflammation and itching.

Some benefit of the astringents may result from direct action on the protein-type surface molecules of body cells. Astringents are said to draw these molecules—and cells—together, reducing their surface area. This accounts for the puckering sensations they produce. Certain foods—like unripe persimmon or lemon—cause what appear to be comparable sensations when they "pucker the inside of the mouth."

In drawing together and shrinking cells or cell-membrane surfaces, astringents block the passage of blood, serum, and other fluids from one body compartment to another. To go back to the original example of the man who cuts himself while shaving, an astringent styptic pencil not only precipitates the solids out of the blood so that they dry and block further flow, but it also shrinks and tightens cells of the injured capillary vessels, staunching the blood flow.

COMBINATION PRODUCTS

The Panel says it is unaware of any products that combine 2 or more astringent substances, but does know of combinations with other classes of active ingredients. These combinations are safe and effective only if they meet the over-the-counter review standards, which require that both active ingredients contribute to the claimed effect(s) of the combination product and do not counteract or diminish each other's effectiveness or safety. The combination must provide concurrent therapeutic benefit for a significant number of people who require the action of *both* active ingredients.

CLAIMS

Accurate for Styptic Pencils
for "use in stopping bleeding caused by minor surface cuts, particularly those caused during shaving"

Accurate for Aluminum Acetate (modified Burow's solution)
for "use as a wet dressing for relief of inflammatory conditions of the skin such as poison ivy"

WARNING   Astringents should be kept away from the eyes and are meant for external use only.

PRODUCTS CONTAINING A SINGLE INGREDIENT

Approved Active Ingredients

Aluminum acetate (modified Burow's solution)   This aluminum compound is used medicinally in an aqueous solution; it is called modified Burow's solution. When the solution is applied to the skin, as it should be, the Panel says complications are rare or nonexistent. However, drinking aluminum acetate solution can result in poisoning.

As to effectiveness, the medical record on aluminum acetate is more anecdotal than scientific. In the one study cited by the reviewers, a researcher induced poison ivy in 6 persons who were highly sensitive to this plant poison. Two days later, he treated the blisters with compresses containing tap water, salt water, aluminum acetate 2.5 percent, or aluminum acetate 5 percent. The latter, stronger aluminum acetate solution was the only one that significantly reduced the inflammation and itching. Basing its conclusion on that study and on wide clinical experience with this preparation, the Panel says that aluminum acetate is safe and effective for relieving poison ivy and other inflammatory skin conditions. The solution should contain 1 part aluminum acetate to 20 parts water and other ingredients (2.65 mg/ml).

Witch hazel   This fragrant plant extract is also called *hamamelis water*, and is a popular aftershave lotion. So little of the witch hazel is left in the final product that the Panel does not quibble about its safety. As for effectiveness, reviewers at first felt that the 14 percent alcohol that is typically present in witch hazel preparations may be responsible for whatever astringent benefit they possess. However, a witch-hazel manufacturing company presented a study demonstrating that witch hazel in 14% alcohol speeds up the clotting of human plasma while plain 14 percent alcohol does not. This indicates, the company said, that witch hazel is "superior."

The Panel concurred and assessed witch hazel as safe and effective. (The approved dosage is not available in the Panel's draft report, upon which this unit is based.)

Conditionally Approved Active Ingredients

Aluminum sulfate   This ingredient—also known as *cake alum* or simply *alum*—is used to make styptic pencils. It stings when applied to the cut, but this Panel, in contrast to the Antiperspirant Panel, says it does not irritate the skin. In the 75 years styptic pencils have been marketed, reviewers say, there are no reports of side effects from their use. So aluminum sulfate is judged safe for this purpose.

However, despite wide use, no modern-day clinical studies have been conducted on aluminum sulfate as an astringent. So the Panel says that while the drug is safe, it has not been scientifically proved effective for stopping bleeding from shaving nicks or other minor surface cuts.

Tannic acid   A tanning agent, this drug will harden the skin and form a protective coating over mucous membranes, curtailing the oozing of blood and other body fluids.

When used over large areas of damaged skin, tannic acid can be dangerous because it is absorbed into the body and acts as a liver poison. But it has little if any action on unbroken skin, and the Panel believes it is safe when applied to small painful areas such as an ingrown toenail (*see* TANNIC ACID, page 442).

The only studies submitted to the evaluators cover tannic acid's use for treating ingrown toenails. But the panelists believe it may also be useful in treating cold sores and fever blisters, and would like to see it tested for such use. Meanwhile, they grant it only conditional approval: safe but not proved effective as an astringent.

Disapproved Active Ingredients

A variety of compounds are summarily rejected by the Panel because no information was submitted or otherwise made available concerning safety and effectiveness (*see* SAFETY AND EFFECTIVENESS chart that follows).

**Safety and Effectiveness: Active Ingredients
in Over-the-Counter Astringents**

Active Ingredient	Panel's Assessment
acetone	summarily disapproved
alcohol	summarily disapproved
alcohol 14%	summarily disapproved
alum	safe, but not proved effective
aluminum acetate (modified Burow's solution)	safe and effective
aluminum chlorhydroxy complex	summarily disapproved
aluminum sulfate	safe, but not proved effective
ammonium alum	summarily disapproved
aromatics	summarily disapproved
benzalkonium chloride	summarily disapproved
benzethonium chloride	summarily disapproved
benzocaine	summarily disapproved
benzoic acid	summarily disapproved
borax	summarily disapproved
boric acid over 0.6%	summarily disapproved
Burow's solution, modified; (see aluminum acetate)	
calcium acetate	summarily disapproved
camphor (gum camphor)	summarily disapproved
colloidal oatmeal	summarily disapproved
cresol	summarily disapproved
cupric sulfate	summarily disapproved
eugenol	summarily disapproved
ferric subsulfate	summarily disapproved
honey	summarily disapproved
isopropyl alcohol	summarily disapproved
menthol	summarily disapproved
oil of cloves	summarily disapproved
oil of eucalyptus	summarily disapproved
oil of peppermint	summarily disapproved
oil of sage	summarily disapproved
oil of wintergreen	summarily disapproved
oxyquinoline sulfate	summarily disapproved
para-tertiary-butyl-meta-cresol	summarily disapproved
phenol (carbolic acid)	summarily disapproved
polyoxyethylene monolaurate	summarily disapproved
potassium alum	summarily disapproved
potassium ferrocyanide	summarily disapproved
powdered alum	summarily disapproved
silver nitrate	summarily disapproved
sodium diacetate	summarily disapproved
starch	summarily disapproved

Safety and Effectiveness: Active Ingredients in Over-the-Counter Astringents *(continued)*

Active Ingredient	*Panel's Assessment*
talc	summarily disapproved
tannic acid	safe, but not proved effective
tannic acid glycerite	summarily disapproved
thymol	summarily disapproved
witch hazel	safe and effective
zinc chloride	summarily disapproved
zinc oxide	summarily disapproved
zinc phenolsulfonate	summarily disapproved
zinc stearate	summarily disapproved
zinc sulfate	summarily disapproved

Astringents: Product Ratings

Product and Distributor	*Dosage of Active Ingredients*	*Rating[1]*	*Comment*
alum			
Powdered Alum (Medic)	**powder:** ammonium alum, N.F.	C	disapproved because no data on safety or effectiveness
aluminum acetate			
Buro-Sol Powder (Doak)	**powder:** 2.36 g yields 1 pint 1:15 Burow's solution + 4.4% benzethonium chloride	B	benzethonium chloride n proved safe or effectiv
Burow's solution (generic)	**solution:** aluminum acetate solution	A	
aluminum sulfate			
Bluboro Powder (Herbert)	**powder:** aluminum sulfate + calcium acetate	C	latter ingredient not safe and/or not effective
Flowery Large Styptic Pencil (Flowery)	**stick:** aluminum sulfate	B	not proved effective
tannic acid			
Amertan (Lilly)	**jelly:** 5% tannic acid + thimerosal 1:5000	C	tannic acid not proved effective; thimerosal no safe or effective
tannic acid (generic)	**powder**	B	not proved effective

Astringents: Product Ratings *(continued)*

Product and Distributor	Dosage of Active Ingredients	Rating[1]	Comment
witch hazel			
Tucks (Parke-Davis)	**cream** and **ointment:** 50%	**B**	not proved effective
witch hazel (generic)	**solution**	**B**	not proved effective

. Author's interpretation of Panel criteria. Based on contents, not claims.

Sunscreens

Judged by their active ingredients, most sunscreen products sold in the United States are safe—and remarkably effective. Some can block 99 percent of the ultraviolet (UV) light rays, which cause sunburn, before they strike the skin.

Sunscreens have only one direct role: they prevent sunburn. Sunbathers who use them can spend more hours of more days in the sun —pursuing a tan if they choose to.

CLAIMS

Accurate
"filters out the sun's burning rays to prevent sunburn"
"screens out the sun's harsh and often harmful rays to prevent sunburn"

False or Misleading
"promotes suntanning"
facilitates "rapid," "deeper," "darker," or "longer-lasting tans"

The tan-seeker in a sense must tempt fate. The Panel says that with or without a sunscreen, the fastest way to tan is to expose the skin daily to the sun up to the point where it becomes vividly red, before covering

SUNSCREENS is based on the report "Sunscreen Drug Products for OTC Human Use," prepared by the FDA's Advisory Review Panel on OTC Topical Analgesic, Antirheumatic, Otic, Burn, and Sunburn Prevention and Treatment Drug Products.

up or going indoors. It takes twice as long to get a painful, blistering burn as it does to achieve the initial nonpainful reddening. For example, after an hour of sunning, if your skin is bright red but not sore, then you can anticipate that after just one more hour of exposure you will be badly burned. Using a sunscreen slows this process and so widens a sunbather's margin of error.

Unlike most over-the-counter drugs, using too little of a sunscreen is more dangerous than using too much. Apply the product liberally to cover the skin and reapply after swimming or other activities that may wash it away, or after sweating.

SKIN PROTECTION FACTOR (SPF)

Many manufacturers—following the Panel's recommendation—now provide a guide number on product labels to help consumers pick an appropriately graded product to fulfill his or her immediate need for protection. To use this guide number, one first must determine one's Skin Protection Factor or SPF. This is an estimate, based on past sunbathing and sunburning experience, of how sensitive one's skin is to the sun. It in turn indicates how strong a sunscreen one will need. SPFs range from a low of SPF 2, which means one has a dark and insensitive skin that needs little or no sunscreen protection, to SPF 15, for a supersensitive skin that must be heavily shielded almost all of the time to prevent painful, blistering sunburn. The average white-skinned American is SPF 4.

SPFs have been correlated by the Panel with the descriptive words *minimal*, *moderate*, *extra*, *maximal*, and *ultra*. A product that provides *minimal* protection will permit tanning but will also allow burning. A *maximal* product will protect against sunburn but also will prevent tanning, even in very sun-sensitive persons.

Skin Types and Recommended Sunscreen Products

Skin Sensitivity on First 30- to 45-Minute Exposure (e.g., after winter)	Skin Protection Factor (SPF)	Recommended Sun Product
Highly sensitive—always burns very easily, never tans	SPF 15 or above	ultra
Sensitive—always burns easily, never tans	SPF 8 to under 15	maximal
Sensitive—always burns easily, tans minimally	SPF 6 to under 8	extra

Skin Types and Recommended Sunscreen Products *(continued)*

Skin Sensitivity on First 30- to 45-Minute Exposure (e.g., after winter)	Skin Protection Factor (SPF)	Recommended Sun Product
Normal—burns moderately, tans gradually to light brown	SPF 4 to under 6	moderate
Normal—burns minimally, always tans well to moderate brown	SPF 2 to under 4	minimal
Insensitive—rarely burns, tans profusely to dark brown	SPF 2	minimal
Very insensitive—never burns, skin is deeply pigmented	Under SPF 2	(none needed)

Using the Skin Type and Recommended Sunscreen Products chart below, you can devise a handy chart for yourself and each family member.

Family Member	Skin Sensitivity	Skin Protection Factor (SPF)	Product Category
Self	_____	_____	_____
Spouse	_____	_____	_____
Child _____	_____	_____	_____
Child _____	_____	_____	_____
Child _____	_____	_____	_____

SPFs do more than tell you which product to buy. They indicate how long it is safe to stay out in the sun with use of the recommended sunscreen and they also show which product to use if one needs or wants to stay out *longer*.

Using no sunscreen, average light-skinned persons—SPF 4—will get red, but not painfully burned, after about 40 minutes of sun on his or her first beach outing of the season. So the Panel says that by using a *moderate* sunscreen, labeled SPF 4, these people can extend their safe exposure time by a factor of 4—that is, to 160 minutes, or 2 hours and 40 minutes.

$4 \times 40 = 160$

If, however, they use a *maximal* product, SPF 8, they can extend their safe time to 320 minutes, or more than 5 hours.

$8 \times 40 = 320$

Thus a person will be protected throughout the dangerous midday period (from 10:00 a.m. to 2:00 p.m.), when the sun is high in the sky. A fisherman with an SPF 4 who plans a day in an open boat on the ocean, where there is little shade, thus should select a maximal or ultra protective product—SPF 8 or above—if he hopes to eat his fish dinner in comfort.

Using like calculations, a fair-skinned person who usually burns after 20 minutes by the pool can extend his or her protected period to 2 hours by using an extra protective sunscreen with SPF 6.

$6 \times 20 = 120$

If, however, he uses a darker-skinned friend's sunscreen, SPF 4, to avoid burning, he must cover up with clothing after only 1 hour and 20 minutes

$4 \times 20 = 80$

or risk a burn.

A suntanned skin, like an inherently dark one, provides protection against burning. So as the season advances and one's skin darkens, it is safe to stay longer in the sun each day. Alternatively, one can switch to a less-protective sunscreen—one with a lower SPF—which in turn will enhance tanning. Most white people, nevertheless, will require repeated daily exposure to the sun for about 2 weeks to darken their skin.

"Tanning," the Panel cautions, "cannot be rushed!" Armed with this knowledge, a person taking a long summer vacation may decide to limit his or her daily sun exposure at the start, in order to slowly build a satisfying tan. But on a 5-day winter jaunt to a sunny climate, people might renounce tanning as unattainable, and instead use a *maximal*- or *ultra*-protective product in order to play safely all day in the tropical sunshine.

SUNLIGHT AND THE SKIN

Sunburns and Suntans

Sunburn and suntan both are caused by UV light rays, which cannot be seen with the naked eye. They are not caused by the sun's visible light rays. UV rays that are between 290 and 320 nanometers (nm)—or about one ten-millionth of an inch in length—are the most dangerous. Burning occurs because this solar radiation is transformed into heat as it strikes the skin. Tanning occurs—much more slowly—because these same UV rays stimulate pigment-producing cells called *melanocytes* to produce the dark pigment (melanin) in the skin. It is melanin that makes black people's skin black. It is melanin that white sunbathers seek to enhance their appearance.

Melanin blocks UV rays from reaching and burning the deep inner layers of the skin. White people who have achieved good tans can, like black people, stay in the sun longer without burning. But the Panel warns that untanned light-complexioned white persons—particularly redheads and blondes of Northern European descent—are about 33 times more susceptible to sunburn than dark-skinned persons from Africa. Thus both vulnerability to sunburn and the ability to tan are to a large extent inherited traits.

The closer one goes to the Equator, by and large, the more intense the sun's UV light. A fair-skinned person who will be vividly red after 40 minutes of June sun in New Jersey (which is 40° N) will reach the same vivid redness after only 25 minutes of sun exposure in the Florida Keys (25° N).

The UV light rays are filtered by the earth's atmosphere. So the higher upward one goes, the more intense they become—a fact that persons skiing in high mountains should keep in mind. Ice, snow, water, and desert sands that reflect a lot of UV light also decrease the safe interval before sunburn.

Harmful Effects

The most immediate effect of overexposure to sunlight is sunburn, which can be an excruciatingly painful—even dangerous—condition. One's skin is reddest some 6 to 20 hours after sunning.

Skin cancer   Exposure to sunlight is a major causative factor in the 400,000 incidences of skin cancer diagnosed in the United States each year. In one recent year, there were an estimated 1409 deaths due to sun-induced cancers (excluding melanomas). These cancers may take several decades to develop. White people have a higher risk of skin cancer than blacks, and men a higher rate than women—perhaps because they have traditionally spent more time working out-of-doors. Farmers, sailors, and construction workers are at greatest risk. The incidence of skin cancer doubles for every 3 or 4 degrees one travels toward the Equator.

The Panel found it ironic that sunscreens for the most part are promoted to—and used by—women engaged in recreational pursuits. Yet it is men working outdoors who need them most. But the experts had few suggestions on how to persuade outdoorsmen to use these products.

Premature Aging of the Skin   The sun exposure that produces tanning also thins, dries, and wrinkles the skin. This condition is called *premature aging of the skin*, although at the cellular level these skin changes are different from normal aging. The UV sunlight appears to stimulate the growth of elastic fibers in the skin. These fibers eventually disintegrate into an amorphous mass—which deprives the skin of its elasticity and gives it an aged appearance.

A majority of the Panel members, in a close vote, proposed that all sunscreen products carry a statement that says in effect: "Overexposure to the sun may lead to premature aging of the skin and skin cancer. The liberal and regular use over the years of this product may help reduce the chance of these harmful effects." A minority of the Panel—3 of its 7 members—disagreed. "Sunlight can cause premature aging and cancer," they said, "but because [the] data are not yet conclusive that skin cancers are preventable by these over-the-counter products . . . a claim of . . . preventing cancer is unwarranted at this time."

SUN-BLOCKING AGENTS AND SUNBURN PREVENTIVES

If sunburn is bad news, the good news is that a remarkably large number of drugs will effectively protect the skin from the sun.

Opaque sunblock agents—often used to cover the nose, ears, toes, or other vulnerable small areas of the body—reflect or scatter all light that strikes them from both the visible and UV spectra.

Two other types of sunscreen admit some UV light. A *sunscreen-sunburn* preventive agent contains an active ingredient that absorbs 95 percent or more of UV light in the dangerous 290 to 320 nm range. A *sunscreen-suntanning* agent absorbs between 85 percent and 95 percent of these rays—and hence lets more UV light get through to the skin. Clearly the protective agent permits faster tanning—and burning —than a preventive product.

The safety and effectiveness of a sunscreen depends in part on the concentration, or dosage, of active ingredients that it contains. The Panel's decisions on the safe and effective dosage for each approved active ingredient is presented in the Safety and Effectiveness chart at the end of the unit.

The evaluators say the majority of sunscreen products contain only 1 or 2 sunscreen active ingredients. More may be contained if each is present in a safe and effective concentration and contributes to the product's effectiveness without interacting with or compromising any other ingredient's effectiveness or safety. A combination of a safe and effective sunscreen with a safe and effective component of another drug category—for example, a skin protectant or insect repellent—is also safe and effective if it meets these requirements.

Dosage

Many people suffer serious sunburns each summer. Yet most sunscreen products sold in the United States contain effective protective ingredients. So it must be concluded that many people use too little of these products, or none at all.

The remedy, the Panel says, is to apply these products generously—before sunning and again after swimming or doing sweat-inducing exercises. The preparations must be spread over and *cover* body surfaces in order to protect them.

Because sunscreens are quite safe, the Panel proposed no upper limits to the amounts adults and older children can use. Youngsters' skin is more sensitive to the sun than adults'. So products that provide only minimal protection—SPF less than 4—should not be used on children under 2 years of age, except with medical supervision. Products that offer more protection—SPF 4 and above—may be used for babies 6 months to 2 years old. Except with the advice and supervision of a doctor, sunscreens should not be used on younger babies; rather, they should be kept out of the sun. Their tender skin and eyes can be badly injured by the sun.

The way a sun product is formulated can strongly influence its effectiveness and durability, including the preparation's resistance to sweating and washing off during swimming. A person who becomes sunburned while using a particular product should consider switching to another product that is prepared in a different way (lotion, cream, ointment, or solution) or one that has a higher, more protective SPF.

Ingredient Names in Over-the-Counter Sunscreen Products

Standard Names	Alternate Names and Abbreviations
The combination of allantoin + aminobenzoic acid	allantoin-*p*-aminobenzoic acid ALPABA
aminobenzoic acid	*p*-aminobenzoic acid PABA
cinoxate	2-ethoxyethyl-*p*-methoxycinnamate
diethanolamine *p*-methoxycinnamate	*p*-methoxycinnamic acid diethanolamine salt

Ingredient Names in Over-the-Counter Sunscreen Products *(continued)*

Standard Names	Alternate Names and Abbreviations
dioxybenzone	2,2′-dihydroxy-4-methoxybenzophenone
ethyl 4-[bis(hydroxypropyl)] aminobenzoate	2-mole propoxylate of aminoethylbenzoate ethylhydroxypropyl PABA
2-ethylhexyl 2-cyano-3,3-diphenylacrylate	2-ethylhexyl-alpha-cyano-beta-phenylcinnamate
ethylhexyl *p*-methoxycinnamate	2-methoxycinnamic acid 2-ethylhexyl ester
2-ethylhexyl salicylate	octyl salicylate
glyceryl aminobenzoate	glyceryl *p*-aminobenzoate
homosalate	3,3,5-trimethylcyclohexyl salicylate homomenthyl salicylate
the combination of lawsone + dihydroxyacetone	
lawsone	2-hydroxyl,4-naphthoquinone
dihydroxyacetone	1,3-dihydroxy-2-propanone DHA
oxybenzone	2-hydroxy-4-methoxybenzophenone benzophenone-3
padimate A	amyl *p*-dimethylaminobenzoate isoamyl *p-N,N* dimethylaminobenzoate pentyl 4-(dimethylamino) benzoate
padimate O	2-ethylhexyl *p*-dimethylaminobenzoate 2-ethylhexyl 4-(dimethylamino) benzoate octyl dimethyl PABA 2-ethylhexyl PABA
red petrolatum	red veterinary petrolatum
sulisobenzone	2-hydroxy-4-methoxybenzophenone-5-sulfonic acid

Approved Active Ingredients

Aminobenzoic acid (PABA)   While this substance, commonly known as PABA, was not widely used in commercial sunscreen preparations until the last decade, careful and exhaustive tests have recently shown that aminobenzoic acid is very effective—and also very safe—as a sunscreen. It has become the standard against which other sunscreens now are compared. One study revealed aminobenzoic acid to be more effective than 100 other sunscreen formulations; another found it superior to 24 commercially available sunscreen products.

This ingredient provides day-long protection if the user does not swim or sweat heavily. Accounts vary on its retention after swimming, and the Panel recommends that it be reapplied when one emerges from the water.

Aminobenzoic acid appears to be more effective when applied 2 hours *before* sunning. This gives it time to diffuse into the outer layer of the skin, where it is retained.

Considerable data show that aminobenzoic acid is safe and that incidence of adverse reaction is rare. As to effectiveness, it can protect the skin against sunburn in cases of extremely strong UV irradiation such as found on glaciers or on the ocean.

Cinoxate   A 1 percent preparation of this substance totally absorbs UV light rays in the dangerous 290 to 320 nm range. Several studies have shown that most users get good to excellent tans when they use cinoxate. Its effectiveness depends in part on the vehicle in which it is formulated; one study showed that a lotion provided much better protection against exposure to fluorescent sunlamps than did a slightly weaker liquid solution.

Extensive tests in animals and in humans have failed to turn up serious toxic or allergic reactions. One manufacturer reported no complaints from the sale of 400,000 units of a 2 percent cinoxate sunscreen lotion and only 9 complaints—of which 8 were minor—for the sale of 2 million units of a 1.7 percent cinoxate solution. The Panel's verdict: safe and effective.

Diethanolamine p-methoxycinnamate   This tannish substance, also known as p-methoxycinnamic acid diethanolamine salt, is highly water-soluble. So it may wash off when one swims or perspires. Studies in animals show that it is not irritating to the eyes or skin, and does not trigger allergic sensitization. These studies, plus wide use without reports of adverse effects, persuade the Panel that it is safe. Several tests on human subjects indicate that this sunscreen provides significant protection against the burning UV rays of the sun; it is most effective against rays that are 290 nm in length. The Panel judges it safe and effective at dosages of 8 to 10 percent for adults and children over 6 months of age.

Digalloyl trioleate   A derivative of tannic acid, this substance has been used as a sunscreen for 40 years. No scientifically controlled experiments were submitted to demonstrate its effectiveness. But a number of less rigorous studies have shown that it blocks sunburn, even in people with extremely sun-sensitive skins. Digalloyl has been an "approved" sunscreen agent under United States Army specifications.

Safety tests have uncovered no major risks. One company that sold 2 million units of a digalloyl trioleate sunscreen product over 20 years reported only 6 consumer complaints—only one of which may have been serious. The Panel evaluates digalloyl trioleate as safe and effective.

Dioxybenzone   Dioxybenzone has been widely marketed in a combination product with padimate A (*see* page 751), over which it has a wider spectrum of UV wavelength coverage. Several double-blind studies—conducted in real-life situations in which participants sat, played, or went swimming in the sun—indicate that this combination is an effective sunscreen, comparable to combinations of padimate A and aminobenzoic acid. A wide variety of safety tests failed to identify any significant risk with its use, so the Panel concludes that dioxybenzone is both safe and effective.

Ethyl 4-[bis(hydroxypropyl)] aminobenzoate   This formulation of aminobenzoic acid in a waxy ointment remains on the skin and will block UV light effectively after immersion and vigorous activity in the water. So it may be preferable to other aminobenzoic acid preparations for sunbathers who go in and out of the water frequently or sweat profusely. Animal and human tests, doctors' clinical experience with the substance in sun-sensitive patients, and manufacturers' marketing experiences all indicate that it effectively blocks UV light rays. Yet it causes little irritation or other untoward effects, even when used in liberal amounts and for several days at a time. The Panel calls the compound safe and effective.

2-Ethylhexyl 2-cyano-3,3-diphenylacrylate   A water-soluble sunscreen ingredient, this compound is formulated into a variety of oil, alcohol, and cream-base products. Tests in animals show that it is not an allergic sensitizer and one manufacturer said he had received no complaints about sensitivity or intolerance to it after he marketed 15,000 product units. Studies show that it is very effective in absorbing UV light and in protecting the skin, albeit less effectively than aminobenzoic acid. The Panel's judgment: safe and effective.

Ethylhexyl p-methoxycinnamate   This is an almost odorless, pale-yellow liquid with a slightly oily feeling. Diluted in alcohol, a 2 percent solution absorbs 84 percent of UV light rays; a 5 percent solution absorbs 98.8 percent of these rays before they reach the skin.

Extensive tests show that it is nonirritating and does not cause allergic sensitization, and the Panel could find no reports of adverse effects in the medical literature. In comparative tests, products containing ethylhexyl p-methoxycinnamate "performed well" against aminobenzoic acid, so the Panel evaluated this substance as safe and effective as a sunscreen active ingredient.

2-Ethylhexyl salicylate   A clear, pale, odorless liquid, 2-ethyl-hexyl salicylate meets the technical requirements (light absorption) for an effective sunscreen. It is widely used; one company sells 55,000 pounds of it in sunscreens each year.

While 2-ethylhexyl salicylate was introduced in 1938, when safety testing requirements were less rigid than they are now, there have been no reports of adverse effects in the medical literature. Continuing consumer demand confirms the theoretical and experimental data which show that it effectively absorbs UV light rays, so the Panel pronounced it safe and effective.

Glyceryl aminobenzoate   The virtue of this substance is that, un-like the related aminobenzoic acid, it is not soluble in water. Tests show that in some product formulations—albeit not in all of them—it remains present and protective even after an ocean swim. It commonly is combined with a chemically related substance, p-dimethylaminobenzoate, but one study submitted to the Panel indicates that 3 percent glyceryl aminobenzoate by itself is as protective as 3 percent of each of these 2 aminobenzoates together.

Tests in animals and in humans, as well as sunbathers' reports, suggest that some people will experience very mild itching in the eyes and minor skin irritation from glyceryl aminobenzoate preparations. But no serious or long-lasting problems have been reported. The Panel says that this is a safe and effective sunscreen active ingredient—one that could be particularly useful for swimmers.

Homosalate   This oily, faintly yellow liquid blocks out less UV light than aminobenzoic acid. Therefore it may be more appropriate for persons who are actively seeking a suntan than for people with extremely sensitive skin who are trying to avoid sunburn at all cost. Sweating and washing with water decrease homosalate's protective value so that it then needs to be reapplied.

The way that homosalate products are formulated will influence their effectiveness. In one test, a cream that contained 4 percent homosalate provided greater protection than a lotion that contained an 8 percent concentration.

In safety tests, homosalate has been shown to be nonirritating and nonsensitizing. One manufacturer reported that, over a decade of marketing experience, homosalate-containing products prompted about one letter of complaint for every quarter-million units sold. No serious ill effects were reported, so homosalate is judged by the Panel to be safe as well as effective.

The combination of lawsone + dihydroxyacetone (DHA)   These chemicals are dyes. Lawsone is the principal dye component of henna, the red hair-dye. When the 2 substances are used in sequence—the DHA first, then the lawsone—they bind to the skin and effectively protect it from the sun's UV rays. People whose skin is so sensitive that they can tolerate very little sunlight at all use this combination. It allows some—though not all of them—to go outside, travel, and even swim and play out-of-doors in daylight without danger. This combination is effective even for people who are not adequately protected by aminobenzoic acid.

The exact way this double-dye method works to block UV light is not known. The 2 ingredients are effective sunscreens *only* when used together. They do not cause allergic sensitization and serious complications are quite rare; accordingly the Panel finds the combination of lawsone with DHA to be safe and effective.

It is claimed that this combination also acts to tan the skin even *without* exposure to sunlight. The DHA does, in fact, interact with the horny substance keratin in the outer layer of skin, and dyes the skin reddish brown. *No sun exposure is needed.* Repeated DHA applications progressively darken the skin. This "coloration" persists for some time, the Panel said. But it may be uneven because thicker skin—on the palms of the hands, for example—contains more keratin than thinner skin and so becomes darker. Coloring the skin with DHA is a cosmetic and not a medical activity, the Panel decided, and so is outside its purview.

DHA also may have a delayed effect on sun exposure. A person who has "pre-tanned" with it on one day will burn less readily the next day. However, this protection is no greater than might be obtained with a single safe and effective sunscreen active ingredient by itself and the cost may be an artificial and uneven DHA "dye job" rather than a sun-induced natural tan. Nevertheless, DHA does darken the skin more quickly than sunlight—without risk of sunburn.

Methyl anthranilate Although its name does not immediately suggest it, this compound is an aminobenzoate. It is much less effective in blocking UV light rays than aminobenzoic acid, the standard against which other sunscreens are judged. But it has the advantage that it is less likely to irritate or sensitize the skin than some other aminobenzoates, so the Panel assessed it as safe and effective.

Oxybenzone This compound is virtually insoluble in water. It is often combined with a second active ingredient. The evidence relating to its effectiveness is sparse, and less convincing than the evidence for some other sunscreen active ingredients. But its safety has been better studied and on the basis of available evidence, the Panel judged oxyben-zone to be both safe and effective.

Padimate A   While chemically related to aminobenzoic acid, padimate A is insoluble in water; thus it is more resistant to the effects of swimming and sweating. One researcher finds it comparable to aminobenzoic acid in effectiveness. (The 2 compounds are combined in some sunscreen products.) In a test, a 1 percent preparation of padi-mate A blocked 90 percent of dangerous UV rays; a 2 percent prepara-tion was a total sunblock. On the negative side, padimate A has been shown to irritate the skin of some individuals. However, these reactions have not proved serious, so the Panel considers the ingredient safe and effective.

Padimate O   Like padimate A (*see* immediately above), padimate O is a chemical relative of aminobenzoic acid. But it is not soluble in water. It is, in fact, more water-resistant than most sunscreen agents that have been tested. For example, more than half the padimate O remained on test subjects' arms after they swirled them around in tap water for half an hour. The Panel cites one researcher who says that a combination of padimate A, padimate O, and oxybenzone should pro-vide at least a half-day's protection against sunburn, even after swim-ming. Like padimate A, padimate O will irritate the skin of some users. But since these reactions tend to be mild, the Panel says padimate O is safe and effective.

2-Phenylbenzimidazole-5-sulfonic acid   This fine, white, crystal-line powder has been used for a long time as a sunscreen, usually in combination with other active ingredients. Controlled tests show that these combination products tend to provide effective protection against sunburn. The compound's safety has been established in many tests in animals and humans. One manufacturer told the Panel that in a recent 10-year period 50 tons were marketed around the world, with no ad-verse effects reported. So the ingredient was judged both safe and effective.

Red petrolatum   As the name suggests, this is a petroleum prod-uct—one of the residues that remain after gasoline and home heating oil are removed from crude oil. The red color, an intrinsic pigment, is what blocks the UV sun rays. Long-term successful use confirms that it is effective. During World War II the United States Army Air Corps chose red petrolatum as the most effective protective substance for men marooned on life rafts or in the desert after plane crashes, because of its effectiveness and because a little bit covers a lot of skin. Surpris-ingly, while red petrolatum contains some paraffin wax and other petroleum byproducts, it spreads to a smooth, almost invisible film on the skin and leaves no visible greasy film as other forms of petrolatum may do.

Red petrolatum is considered to be inert and so safe that it is used as the vehicle for a number of drug and cosmetic products. The manufacturer reports fewer than one complaint per 100,000 product units sold. As a sunscreen active ingredient, red petrolatum is safe and effective, according to the Panel.

Sulisobenzone   This is a chemical derivative of oxybenzone that has been shown in tests to be safe and effective as a sunscreen active ingredient. But it appears to be less protective than the aminobenzoates and it is highly soluble in water. So it provides virtually no continuing protection after swimming, although the Panel evaluates it as safe and effective.

Titanium dioxide   Most sunscreen active ingredients block UV light by absorbing it. This one—a brilliant white powder—reflects and scatters the UV light, much as whitewash will; it is an opaque sun block. Titanium dioxide is used in face powders and beauty creams, as well as in sunscreen ointments, lotions, and protective powders. One skin specialist says it is "perhaps the most suitable and widely-used" light-scattering ingredient employed to protect people from the sun.

Titanium dioxide is chemically inert, and wide use confirms that it is safe. Some 3.5 million units of a sunscreen containing titanium dioxide were sold between 1949 and 1972, and the manufacturer says no complaints were received that were attributable to the substance. The Panel's view: titanium dioxide is safe and effective.

Triethanolamine salicylate (trolamine)   This substance has been studied less rigorously than some other active ingredients in sunscreens, but the tests that have been done indicate that it's effective. The available data show that while it may irritate the skin of some users, these reactions tend to be rare and mild. So the preparation was assessed as both safe and effective.

Conditionally Approved Active Ingredients

The combination of allantoin + aminobenzoic acid   A manufacturer claims he has combined these 2 substances in a single molecular complex. The Panel was not convinced that such is the case; neither was it convinced that there is any additional protective benefit to be gained from such a combination. The available data indicate that the combination is safe; they simply do not establish that allantoin—a tannic acid derivative—enhances the already great protective power of aminobenzoic acid. Pending such proof, the Panel rates this combination as conditionally approved.

5-(3,3-Dimethyl-2-norbornyliden)-3-penten-2-one   The Panel received no studies documenting the effectiveness of this agent as a sunscreen active ingredient—even though it had been marketed for this purpose since 1973, and seemed safe.

Dipropylene glycol salicylate   While animal tests indicate that this substance is not highly toxic, no data were submitted to the Panel on its safety or its effectiveness as a sunscreen. So it is given only conditional approval.

Disapproved Active Ingredients

The Panel finds that 3 sunscreen active ingredients are neither safe nor effective. While none of them is used in sun products marketed in the United States, travelers abroad should be aware of the disapprovals.

2-Ethylhexyl 4-phenylbenzophenone-2'-carboxylic acid   No experimental or marketing data on the safety of this compound, when used by humans, was submitted. Neither were there studies concerning its effectiveness. So the Panel concluded that it is not safe and not effective, and recommends that it not be marketed in the United States until adequate studies are submitted to the FDA.

3-(4-Methylbenzylidene)-camphor   The safety of this compound has been studied in mice, rats, and rabbits, but not in humans. There is no data to show that it is effective as a sunscreen. So the Panel judged it as neither safe nor effective.

Sodium 3,4-dimethylphenyl-glyoxylate   There are no data on the safety and effectiveness of this substance when used as a sunscreen agent. The Panel says: not safe and not effective.

Inactive Ingredients

There is more to most sunscreen products than their active ingredients. The sun-blocking chemical is usually dissolved or suspended in a vehicle—an ointment, lotion, cream, or solution—so that the sunscreen can be applied to the skin. Perfumes, skin-softening compounds, and other inactive components also may be added.

Some of these inactive ingredients have complex chemical names —just as the active ingredients do. So it can be difficult to decide which is which by reading the label. To help the consumer differentiate, these inactive components are:

alcohol
allantoin
beeswax
benzyl alcohol
BHA
BHT
2-bromo-2-
   nitropropane-l,
   3-diol
camphor
carbomer 934
carboset
cellulose gum
cetyl alcohol
cetyl palmitate
cetyl stearyl glycol
citric acid
clove oil
cocoa butter
color
dimethicone
dimethyl polysiloxane
ethyl alcohol
FD&C yellow No. 5

FD&C red No. 4
fragrances
glycerin
glyceryl stearate
isopropyl myristate
isopropyl palmitate
lanolin
lanolin alcohol
lanolin derivatives
lanolin oil
menthol
methylparaben
microcrystalline
   titanium-coated
   mica platelets
microcrystalline wax
mineral oil
oleth-3-phosphate
parabens
paraffin
PEG 2 stearate
petrolatum
polyoxyl-40-stearate
polysorbate 60

propellant 46
propellant 12/114
propylparaben
propylene glycol
propylene glycol
   stearate
quaternium 15
SD alcohol 40
sesame oil
silica
sodium carbomer
sorbitan oleate
sorbitan stearate
stabilized aloe vera gel
stearyl alcohol
synthetic spermaceti
triethanolamine
triethanolamine
   stearate
water
wax
zinc oxide

Safety and Effectiveness: Active Ingredients in Over-the-Counter Sunscreens

Ingredient	Panel's Assessment	Concentration (%)
allantoin + aminobenzoic acid	safe, but not proved effective	
aminobenzoic acid (PABA)	safe and effective	5–15
beta carotene (taken internally)	not safe or effective*	
canthaxanthin (taken internally)	not safe or effective*	
cinoxate	safe and effective	1–3
diethanolamine		
p-methoxycinnamate	safe and effective	8–10
digalloyl trioleate	safe and effective	2–5
5-(3,3-dimethyl-2-norbornyliden)-		
3-penten-2-one	not proved effective	
dioxybenzone	safe and effective	3
dipropylene glycol salicylate	not proved safe or effective	
ethyl 4-[bis(hydroxypropyl)]		
aminobenzoate	safe and effective	1–5

Safety and Effectiveness: Active Ingredients in Over-the-Counter Sunscreens
(continued)

Ingredient	Panel's Assessment	Concentration (%)
2-ethylhexyl 2-cyano-3, 3-diphenylacrylate	safe and effective	7–10
ethylhexyl p-cinnamate	safe and effective	2–7.5
ethylhexyl p-methoxycinnamate	safe and effective	2–7.5
ethylhexyl salicylate	safe and effective	3–5
2-ethylhexyl 4-phenylbenzophenone-2′-carboxylic acid	not safe or effective	
2-ethylhexyl salicylate	safe and effective	3–5
glyceryl aminobenzoate	safe and effective	2–3
homosalate	safe and effective	4–15
lawsone + dihydroxyacetone (DHA)	safe and effective	
lawsone		0.25
dihydroxyacetate		3
methyl anthranilate	safe and effective	3.5–5
3-(4-methylbenzylidene)-camphor	not safe or effective	
oxybenzone	safe and effective	2–6
PABA (*see* aminobenzoic acid)		
padimate A	safe and effective	1–5
padimate O	safe and effective	1.4–8
2-phenylbenzimidazole-5-sulfonic acid	safe and effective	1–4
red petrolatum	safe and effective	30–100
sodium 3,4-dimethylphenyl-glyoxylate	not safe or effective	
sulisobenzone	safe and effective	5–10
titanium dioxide	safe and effective	2–25
triethanolamine salicylate (trolamine)	safe and effective	5–12

*FDA assessment.

Sunscreens: Product Ratings
(Listed in Diminishing Order of Protectiveness)

Product and Distributor	Dosage of Active Ingredients	SPF	Rating[1]	Comment
Super Shade Sunblocking (Coppertone)	lotion: 7% padimate O + 3% oxybenzone	15	A	
Sundown Sunblock Ultra Protection (Johnson & Johnson)	lotion: 7% padimate O + 5% octylsalicylate + 4% oxybenzone	15	A	
PreSun 15 (Westwood)	lotion: 5% PABA + 5% padimate O + 3% oxybenzone	15	A	
PreSun Lip Protector (Westwood)	lipstick: 8% padimate O	15	A	
Block-Aid (Elder)	cream: 6% ethyl dihydroxypropyl PABA + 5% oxybenzone	14	C	too much of first ingredient
Pabanol (Elder)	lotion: 5% PABA	14	A	
RVPaba (Elder)	lipstick: 5% PABA + red petrolatum	10	A	
Improved Uval (Dorsey)	lotion: 6% oxybenzone + 5% ethyl-p-methoxycinnamate	10	A	
A-Fil (Cooper)	cream: 5% menthyl anthranilate + 5% titanium dioxide	8–15	A	

Product	Formulation	SPF	Grade[1]	Note
Sundown Maximal Protection (Johnson & Johnson)	lotion: 7% padimate O + 5% octylsalicylate + 2% oxybenzone	8	A	
Shade Plus (Coppertone)	lotion: 7% padimate O + 3% oxybenzone	8	A	
PreSun 8 (Westwood)	lotion: 5% PABA	8	A	
PreSun 8 Creamy (Westwood)	lotion: 5% PABA	8	A	
PreSun 8 (Westwood)	gel: 5% PABA	8	A	
Sus-tan (Elder)	lotion: 2.4% ethyl dihydroxypropyl PABA	8	C	
Maxafil (Cooper)	cream: 4% cinoxate + 5% menthyl anthranilate	6–8	C	too much cinoxate
Sundown Extra Protection (Johnson & Johnson)	lotion: 5.3% padimate O + 1.75% oxybenzone	6	C	too little oxybenzone
pabaGel (Owen)	gel: 5% PABA	6	A	
sunDare Creamy (Cooper)	lotion: 2% cinoxate	4–6	A	
sunDare Clear (Cooper)	lotion: 1.75% cinoxate	4–6	A	
Sundown Moderate Protection (Johnson & Johnson)	lotion: 3.8% padimate	4	A	
PreSun 4 (Westwood)	lotion: 4% padimate O	4	A	

1. Author's interpretation of Panel criteria. Based on contents, not claims.

Sweet Spirits of Nitre: Special Warning

Sweet spirits of nitre has been sold and swallowed for a variety of symptoms, appears to relieve none of them, and, what is worse, is hazardous. Therefore, its sale over-the-counter has now been banned in the United States at the recommendation of the Panel that assessed this compound.

The active ingredient in sweet spirits of nitre is 3.5 to 4.5 percent ethyl nitrite in alcohol. The preparation is also known as *spirits of nitre*, *nitrous ether*, and *ethyl nitrite spirit*. *Medicine bottles labeled with any of these names should be discarded*.

Manufacturers of this preparation appear not to have heeded the FDA's repeated requests that all nonprescription drugs be submitted for evaluation. A University of Chicago pediatrician wrote the FDA to report that a 4-month-old infant had died after being given about a teaspoonful of the substance in an effort to control "fussiness." At least one other lethal poisoning case, in a 3-year-old child, is known to have occurred—and there may have been others. In both reported cases, death was due to methemoglobinemia, a serious blood disorder. In addition, 16 nonfatal poisonings from the use of sweet spirits of nitre were reported in one recent 4-year period. Evaluators believe this is a gross underestimation of the number of poisonings that actually occurred.

The attraction of sweet spirits of nitre as a medicinal remedy is that it causes dramatic body changes—even when taken in doses that are far *less* than were given to the 2 fatally poisoned children. For example, it causes sweating—so it was used in attempts to reduce fever. The effect is real, but one researcher reported as long ago as 1893 that the drop in temperature is negligible unless one consumes quantities apt to be toxic. The drug also was given as a diuretic, to promote urination—which the Panel says it does not do. It was also given to relieve gut spasms in infants with colic. Some nitrites and nitrates have this capacity, but there is no current evidence showing that sweet spirits of nitre

SWEET SPIRITS OF NITRE is based on the report "Sweet Spirits of Nitre" by the FDA's Advisory Review Panel on OTC Miscellaneous Internal Drug Products and on the FDA Final Rule on this substance.

is effective (let alone safe) for this purpose. When the drug is mixed with the acid in the stomach, it forms a gas, nitrous oxide, which is relieved only by copious belching, or by flatulence (passing gas).

Because of definite concern about lack of safety as well as the absence of scientific data concerning effectiveness, the Panel recommended banning such products. Concurring, the FDA issued a ban that became effective on June 27, 1980.

Safety and Effectiveness: Sweet Spirits of Nitre

Active Ingredient	Panel and FDA's† Assessment
ethyl nitrite*	not safe or effective
sweet spirits of nitre*	not safe or effective

*Such a preparation may be labeled with either term as well as nitrous ether or ethyl nitrite spirits. Any medicine so labeled should be disposed of (see text).
†Judgments reaffirmed or modified by the FDA, or originated by it.

Sweet Spirits of Nitre: Product Ratings

Products containing sweet spirits of nitre have been banned from interstate commerce in the U.S., so none should be offered for sale. Those remaining in medicine cabinets should be discarded. They may be labeled as:

Ethyl Nitrite
Nitre Spirit
Spirit of Nitre
Spirit of Nitrous Ether
Sweet Spirits of Nitre

Teething Easers

When a several-months-old baby suddenly becomes fussier than usual, it is a good bet that he or she is cutting a tooth. Teething babies need to "work" their gums by chewing on crib edges, teething rings, bottle nipples, or parents' fingers—or their own. They also may need occasional relief from the pain, which can be provided by cooling the gums with a bit of crushed ice or giving the infant a baby bottle containing a few ounces of cool water. A numbing—or anesthetic—teething medication also may help.

The approved claim for safe and effective teething easers is

For the temporary relief of sore gums due to teething in infants and children 4 months of age or older.

ANESTHETICS FOR PAIN OF TEETHING

Approved Active Ingredients

Only a single, widely used anesthetic, benzocaine, is approved for use—without consulting a doctor—to relieve teething distress in infants from 4 months to 2 years of age. Phenol should be used only if one is advised to do so by a doctor.

Benzocaine   This drug acts within seconds when applied to the gums and it provides pain relief that may last 5 to 10 minutes or longer. Benzocaine is widely used as an anesthetic and is considered very safe (*see* BENZOCAINE, page 361) and also effective for the relief of teething distress. However, it should not be used on infants younger than 4 months without first checking with the baby's doctor.

The safe and effective dosage is 5 to 20 percent benzocaine, applied with a swab or small piece of cotton, up to 4 times daily.

Phenol (0.25% to 1.5%)   This alcohol is regarded as safe and effective when applied in small amounts to the gums. It blocks nerve conduction of pain impulses. But because even small doses of phenol may

TEETHING EASERS is based on the report "Drug Products for the Relief of Oral Discomfort for OTC Human Use" by the FDA's Advisory Review Panel on OTC Dentifrice and Dental-Care Drug Products.

be more hazardous than benzocaine, the Panel specifically limits the approved dosage to 300 mg per day of 0.25 to 1.5 percent phenol in an appropriate base, and stipulates that it should only be used as directed by a doctor.

Conditionally Approved Active Ingredients

None

Disapproved Active Ingredients

None

Safety and Effectiveness: Active Ingredients in Over-the-Counter Teething Easers

Active Ingredient	Panel's Assessment
benzocaine	safe and effective
phenol (0.25 to 1.5%)	safe and effective

Teething Easers: Product Ratings

Product and Distributor	Dosage of Active Ingredients	Rating[1]	Comment
abee Teething (Pfeiffer)	**lotion:** 2.5% benzocaine + 0.02% cetalkonium chloride + 20% alcohol + urea + witch hazel + menthol + camphor	C	inadequate concentration of benzocaine; none of other ingredients appear to have been submitted to or assessed by Panel as teething aids
aby Orajel (Commerce Drug)	**gel:** 7.5% benzocaine	A	
rajel Extra Strength (Commerce Drug)	**gel:** 20% benzocaine	A	

. Author's interpretation of Panel criteria. Based on contents, not claims.

Thyroid Protectors for Nuclear Emergencies

Leaks of radioactive gases and liquids from atomic power plants and other nuclear facilities can occur suddenly and without warning—as was demonstrated by the Three Mile Island mishap several years ago. This accident carried dangerous materials into the surrounding environment.

A self-treatment drug, potassium iodide, which once was a standard ingredient in over-the-counter cough remedies, can provide significant protection from radiation damage. *But it must be taken within the first hours of exposure in order to work effectively.*

VULNERABILITY OF THE THYROID GLAND

In nuclear accidents some of the released material is almost certain to be radioactive iodines, particularly the nuclide called iodine-131. After these iodines—which may be gases, liquids, or solid particles—are inhaled from the air or taken in with milk or other foods, they are picked up by the blood. The bloodstream carries them to the thyroid gland, which normally helps regulate food intake and digestive metabolism. This gland quickly takes up and holds radioactive iodine. (It normally takes up and holds other nonradioactive iodines, which it needs, in tiny amounts, to function.)

Thyroid uptake of radioactive iodine is particularly dangerous because this gland is highly sensitive to radiation damage. Radiation can cause thyroid cancer, although the cancer may not become evident for a decade or more after exposure. It also can cause noncancerous growths, called *thyroid nodules*, and can inhibit thyroid function. Children are more vulnerable to this injury than adults.

THYROID PROTECTORS FOR NUCLEAR EMERGENCIES is based on the FDA Summary of Basis for Approval for New Drug Applications 18-307 and 18-308, and on final recommendations for the use of potassium iodide as a thyroid-blocking agent in a radiation emergency, prepared by the FDA's Bureau of Radiological Health and Bureau of Drugs.

PROTECTIVE PREPARATIONS

Despite its great vulnerability, the thyroid can function in preventing damage from radiation fallout. To protect itself from iodine overload, the gland will stop taking up iodine once it has as much as it needs.

So thyroid specialists and the FDA proposed a way of taking advantage of this mechanism. The method is to supply the thyroid with enough *non*radioactive iodine to make it stop taking the element up before the radioactive iodine arrives and is absorbed by one's body. To be effective, the blocking dose must be taken very quickly.

A protective dose taken before or at the time that radioactive fallout or other leaked material reaches one's body will provide 90 to 100 percent protection. A substantial benefit—a block of 50 percent— is attainable during the first 3 to 4 hours after exposure, the FDA says. Longer delay will further diminish benefits.

The need to act quickly means that persons who live close to nuclear facilities probably should have potassium iodide close at hand in the home.

The FDA recommends that decisions on who should take potassium iodide—and when—be made by public health officials. But given the confusion and the delay in issuing public health warnings that have marked recent nuclear mishaps, persons who hear credible radio or TV reports about current or impending exposure may wish to make decisions on their own.

A number of other iodine compounds as well as some other drugs will block thyroid uptake of radioactive iodine. In an emergency, if you do not have potassium iodide on hand, phone your doctor or pharmacist for advice, and listen to health advisory warnings on the radio or TV.

CLAIMS

Accurate
for "thyroid blocking in a radiation emergency only"

WARNING   Potassium iodide should not be used by people allergic to iodine. In case of overdose or allergic reaction, contact a physician or the public health authority.

THYROID-BLOCKING AGENTS

While a variety of iodines may provide protection against radioactive iodine, only one is well studied and approved.

Approved Active Ingredient

Potassium iodide This iodine compound is present in small amounts in ordinary food and in iodized table salt. It has been widely used medicinally as a salt substitute, and is available by prescription as an expectorant for persons with bronchial asthma. It used to be commonly formulated into nonprescription cough medicines, but is far less often used this way since the Cold, Cough and Allergy Panel ruled the ingredient unsafe because of risks of *iodism* (iodine poisoning).

The doses used to treat bronchial asthma and other respiratory diseases are from 300 to 1200 mg daily for adults. This is far higher than the dosage recommended for the use in the brief period following a nuclear emergency. The National Council on Radiation Protection estimates that even with the higher doses only one in every 1 to 10 million users will suffer an adverse reaction; the complication rate can be assumed to be lower with lower doses. So the FDA says potassium iodide is safe as well as effective in recommended dosages. For persons who are allergic to iodine, the risk probably outweighs the potential benefit!

The approved dosage for adults, including pregnant women, and for children over one year of age is 130 mg once daily. The approved dosage for babies up to a year old is 65 mg once daily. Treatment should continue for 10 days unless public health officials say it should be stopped.

Two potassium iodide preparations, a tablet and a liquid, were approved for nonprescription sale soon after the Three Mile Island accident.

Conditionally Approved Active Ingredients

None

Disapproved Active Ingredients

None

Safety and Effectiveness: Active Ingredients in Over-the-Counter Thyroid-Protecting Agents

Recommended Daily Dosage

Active Ingredient	Infants Under Age 1	Adults and Children Over Age 1	FDA's Assessment
potassium iodide	65 mg	130 mg	safe and effective

Thyroid Protectors: Product Ratings

Product and Distributor	Dosage of Active Ingredient	Rating[1]	Comment
potassium iodide			
Thyro-Block (Wallace Labs.)	**tablets:** 130 mg	A	distributed by health agencies, not sold over-the-counter
Iosat (Anbex)	**tablets:** 130 mg	A	mail order
Potassium Iodide Oral Solution (Roxane)	**liquid:** 130 mg per 6 drops	A	

Author's interpretation of FDA criteria. Based on contents, not claims

Toothache Relievers

Quick relief is what everybody wants when a tooth suddenly starts aching. A number of drugs are sold for this purpose. Their instructions say to apply the drug to the cavity or crack in the tooth, or temporarily use it to plug the hole until a dentist can be seen.

Most of these drugs are unsafe, ineffective, or both, according to Panel reviewers. The one ingredient, eugenol, that *does* win approval is so irritating to dental pulp—soft nerve tissue at the core of the tooth —that the experts would limit its use to teeth that are irreparably damaged. It can destroy still viable ones that otherwise could be saved.

TOOTHACHE RELIEVERS is based on the report "Drug Products for the Relief of Oral Discomfort for OTC Human Use," by the FDA's Advisory Panel on OTC Dentifrice and Dental-Care Drug Products.

So it seems from the evaluators' findings that anyone who hopes for the repair and saving of an aching tooth ought to avoid over-the-counter drugs that are applied to the teeth. Instead a toothache sufferer should make an emergency dental appointment and in the meantime use ice cubes, aspirin, or prescription pain killers to relieve pain.

The only tooth that the experts believe is a candidate for treatment with topical nonprescription toothache relievers is the one that is so badly damaged that the dentist is going to have to extract it. How does one decide? If the pain is intermittent—coming and going—the tooth is probably still alive and salvageable. If the pain is throbbing and relentless, the tooth is likely to be irreversibly damaged—so no further harm can be done by using a pain reliever that may further irritate the pulp.

One way of treating tooth pain is by counterirritation. By setting up what is presumably a more tolerable irritation or pain in the nearby gum, one is supposed to forget the pain in the tooth. Reviewers have reservations about using counterirritants in treating toothaches as well as about the drug—essence of red pepper—that is used for this purpose (*see* below).

The Panel also assessed over-the-counter drugs sold to relieve a more chronic problem: *dental hypersensitivity*—in which mild stimuli cause recurrent tooth pain because the protective outer enamel has been chipped or the tooth root has eroded. The evaluators registered strong doubts about the effectiveness of tooth desensitizers marketed over-the-counter for these complaints (*see* below).

CLAIMS FOR TOOTHACHE RELIEVERS

Accurate

for "the temporary relief of throbbing, persistent toothache due to a cavity until a dentist can be seen"

False or Misleading

for "temporary relief of cavity toothache"
"eases pain due to cavities fast"
"quickly forms temporary filling"
"fast relief from toothache due to cavities"

WARNING   Do not use for intermittent pain. Toothaches and open cavities indicate serious problems, which need prompt attention by a dentist. A dentist must be seen as soon as possible, whether the pain is relieved or not.

The Panel adds an additional warning about toothache relievers that are marketed in small, porous bags (poultices) designed to be held in the mouth so that the drug will be released slowly onto the sore tooth and surrounding gum. To avoid danger of choking, do not leave a poultice in the mouth during periods of sleep.

TYPES OF TOOTHACHE RELIEVERS

Some toothache remedies are intended to act as "temporary fillings" which allegedly protect the tooth pulp by shielding it against saliva, food particles, and other things that can provoke pain. The serious problem with this approach is that the dental pulp easily becomes inflamed. When this happens, it swells and may secrete fluids and gases that need to be drained. Without proper drainage, pressure within the tooth can be created and cause further, perhaps uncorrectable, damage. Putting beeswax, sandarac, or other semisolid temporary fillings into the tooth prevents necessary drainage and decompression. The Panel says such temporary fillings are unsafe and are also unlikely to be effective in relieving pain.

Many toothache relievers are alcohols, which dry out the calcified hard material (the dentin) that forms the bulk of the tooth. Some of these drugs are also irritants. The drugs have a medicinal taste and smell, and, as irritants, cause a new, and perhaps helpful, sensation of pain. "These properties distract the patient and may provide some psychological feeling of benefit," the Panel says, "but the major problems of deep cavities, pulp inflammation, and infection remain untreated."

COMBINATION PRODUCTS

The Panel listed no safe and effective combinations, and granted conditional approval only to 3.

A combination of 2 approved or conditionally approved toothache relievers that act by different mechanisms

1 approved or conditionally approved toothache reliever + 1 gingival (gum) anesthetic

1 approved or conditionally approved gingival anesthetic + 1 approved or conditionally approved counterirritant

All other combinations that include toothache-relief drugs are disapproved.

TOOTHACHE PAIN RELIEVERS

Approved Active Ingredients

Eugenol preparations: 85 to 87 percent eugenol in clove oil or a bland, fixed oil These pungent, spicy-tasting preparations are obtained from cloves—although now eugenol can also be extracted from other sources. Clove oil contains 85 to 87 percent eugenol; the Panel stipulates that only full-strength—85 to 87 percent—preparations contain enough eugenol to effective.

Eugenol's pain-deadening property has been known for 300 years. For many years the drug has been used by dentists as a local anesthetic. Eugenol was previously available only as a prescription drug. The reviewers decided—with some misgivings—that it should be made available without prescription. A major argument in favor of this step was the evaluators' lack of confidence in the safety and effectiveness of existing nonprescription toothache drugs. A major argument against it was that eugenol acts as an extreme irritant to nerve tissue of the tooth pulp. *Because of this tooth-destroying trait, the Panel warns strongly that eugenol preparations should be used only on teeth that already are irreparably damaged.*

The decision to approve eugenol was made despite a lack of well-controlled contemporary studies on its use as a self-treatment drug. Approval was based largely on the clinical experience of Panel members and the views of consultants.

Eugenol preparations should be used as follows: the tooth should first be rinsed with water to flush out any food particles or other debris. Then a *tiny* bit of cotton should be moistened with 1 or 2 drops of an 85 to 87 percent eugenol preparation and placed into the tooth cavity or fracture for 1 minute, then removed. This treatment can be repeated up to 4 times daily. Great care should be taken to keep eugenol off the gums because it is irritating. Children under 12 should be supervised when they use this treatment, and eugenol should not be used for children under 2 except under medical or dental supervision. In sum: safe and effective when used as directed.

Conditionally Approved Active Ingredients

Benzocaine Generally speaking, this is a safe anesthetic, and also a highly effective one. But there are little data about its value when applied directly to dental nerve tissue in the cavity of a tooth. Verdict: safe but not proved effective.

Benzyl alcohol   This drug irritates tissues, so that its safety—even in the low concentrations of 1 to 3 percent in which it is formulated into toothache remedies—remains to be proved. No scientific evidence is available to show that it effectively relieves toothache when applied directly to the decayed or broken tooth. In sum, benzyl alcohol is not proved safe or effective for this purpose.

Butacaine sulfate   An anesthetic, this substance is safe and effective when applied to the gums, as is benzocaine. But there is insufficient documentation to show that it is either safe or effective when put directly onto sensitive nerve tissue inside a diseased or injured tooth. Conclusion: not proved safe or effective.

Creosote   This is a distillate of wood tar. Because it paralyzes sensitive nerves—and so acts anesthetically—it has been reported to provide temporary relief from toothache. But it is an irritant, and a safe dosage has never been established. Creosote is usually formulated into toothache remedies as dilute solutions, and evidence is lacking to show it is effective in these dilutions. So the Panel says: not proved safe or effective.

Cresol   This is a phenollike alcohol that is fairly irritating to tissues, so the Panel cannot vouch for its safety. The Panel searched widely for a scientific study demonstrating cresol's effectiveness as a dental anesthetic, but it could find none. So cresol is listed as not proved safe or effective as a toothache remedy.

Eugenol preparations: 1 to 84 percent eugenol   Since higher concentrations of this aromatic substance are scored by the Panel as safe, it follows that these are, too. But there is no evidence that the lower concentrations of eugenol will actually relieve toothache. Conclusion: safe but not proved effective.

Phenol   This anesthetic is safe and effective for use on the gums. But it has never been established through acceptable scientific studies that it is either safe or effective when instilled into a rotten or broken tooth.

Thymol preparations: thymol and thymol iodide   These medicinal extracts of thyme are aromatic, like clove oil and eugenol. In dentistry they are used after a cavity is drilled clean, to form a protective layer between the dentin and the inlay (filling) that will be packed in. They are also used as deodorant ingredients in antiseptic mouthwash and gargles. So, despite little scientific data that establish safety, reviewers judged the drugs safe. But the Panel could not find sufficient evidence to demonstrate thymol's effectiveness as a toothache remedy. So these preparations are listed as not proved effective.

Disapproved Active Ingredients

Capsicum   This red-pepper extract is highly irritating to the tooth pulp, gums, and other tissues. The Panel says the substance will injure viable tooth pulp, and is unsafe. Also, no studies could be found to show that currently marketed capsicum toothache drops or gum effectively relieve pain. Verdict: neither safe nor effective.

Menthol   This pepperminty substance is extremely irritating to living tissues, so it is not safe for the temporary relief of toothaches. Evidence shows that it is also ineffective. Verdict: menthol is unsafe and ineffective.

Methyl salicylate   This minty alcohol is extremely irritating to soft tissues and should not be put into a tooth cavity. In addition, there is no evidence whatsoever that the drug acts as a pain killer. In sum: methyl salicylate is unsafe and ineffective.

COUNTERIRRITANTS

Given the general ineffectiveness of over-the-counter toothache relievers, it is little wonder that some people desperately try to defeat the pain by deliberately irritating the gums that surround a sore tooth. The rationale is that one's attention is shifted from the toothache—or perhaps the tolerable irritation from the counterirritant blocks the intolerable tooth pain. Another theory is that the counterirritant draws additional blood into the area, hastening the removal of poisonous products from the injured tooth. None of these theories has been proved, according to the Panel, and only one counterirritant (capsicum) rates even conditional approval.

CLAIMS FOR COUNTERIRRITANTS

Accurate

for "temporary relief of toothache until a dentist can be seen" (if there were a safe and effective counterirritant—which there isn't)

Approved Active Ingredients

None

Conditionally Approved Active Ingredient

Capsicum   This red-pepper extract is sold in poultices that may also contain a pain-relieving ingredient. It also comes in the form of drops and gums. The capsicum dose is very weak—about 2 parts per 10,000 in the base in which the drug is formulated. So the Panel judges it safe. Several small studies have been done to try to establish whether capsicum relieves toothache pain; the Panel judges the results to be inconclusive. Conclusion: safe, but effectiveness still needs to be proved.

Disapproved Active Ingredients

None

TOOTH DESENSITIZERS

Pain can arise and persist in a tooth without a cavity being present and without the pulp being exposed. Some teeth, in some people, simply seem to be more sensitive—indeed, painfully hypersensitive—to quite minor stimuli such as heat, cold, and pressure that other individuals would not notice. A hypersensitive tooth may feel as painful as one with a cavity. This means the consumer cannot self-diagnose hypersensitivity; the dentist must do so—by ruling out cavities and all other causes of pain. Once the diagnosis has been made, reviewers believe, nonprescription medication should be available to treat dentin hypersensitivity.

The dentin—calcified matter that makes up the bulk of the tooth between the crown enamel and the root cementum—appears to be capable of conveying sensations inward toward the sensitive pulp that lies at the tooth's center. Whether the dentin is laced with microscopic nerve fibers or conveys sensations in some other way remains unclear. What *is* certain, the Panel says, is that even tiny nicks, scratches, or malformations in the enamel or cementum can expose the dentin, making it vulnerable to these unpleasant sensations.

The way that these drugs act is not really clear. Some may alter the tiny nerve endings in the dentin, so they are less sensitive. Some may temporarily cover and block these sensitive endings. Others are claimed to form a new, hard outer layer of tooth that recovers the exposed dentin.

Because the causes of dentin hypersensitivity and the actions of drugs to relieve it are still somewhat of a mystery, the Panel decided that it could not fully approve any active ingredients or any claim made for them. Its draft report does not contain even a conditionally approved indication for use—although one was possibly approved at the Panel's last meeting and will appear in its published report.

CLAIM FOR DESENSITIZERS

Accurate
"to aid in the reduction of painful sensitivity of the teeth to cold, heat, acids, sweets, or contact." (However, no over-the-counter tooth desensitizers have as yet been fully approved for this purpose.)

WARNING Sensitive teeth may indicate a serious problem which needs prompt care by a dentist. See your dentist as soon as possible whether or not relief is obtained from these medications. Continue use beyond 2 weeks only under supervision of a dentist.

Approved Active Ingredients

None

Conditionally Approved Active Ingredients

Citric acid + sodium citrate in poloxamer 407 (Pluronic F-127 gel) The individual ingredients in this preparation, which is marketed abroad as a tooth desensitizer, are widely used in foods and drugs. So the Panel accepts them, together, as safe. But the reviewers received only scant and inadequate data to show that the combination quells discomfort inside sensitive teeth. Verdict: effectiveness remains to be proved.

Fluoride preparations: sodium fluoride, sodium monofluorophosphate, and stannous fluoride These are the fluoride preparations used in cavity preventive dentifrices; in the concentrations used in these products they are safe (*see* TOOTHPASTES, RINSES, AND GELS FOR CAVITY PREVENTION).

Fluorides act by hardening the enamel and perhaps by helping to re-enamel worn areas. It makes sense, then, that they would cover up exposed dentin—reducing sensitivity to heat, cold, pressure, and other stimuli. Several controlled studies suggest that fluorides do, in fact, provide this benefit. But the current reviewers felt these studies were poorly constructed and they proposed additional testing to establish the claim that these drugs reduce hypersensitivity. For the moment, the Panel rates them as safe but not proved effective.

Formaldehyde solution   This is a weak preparation—usually about 1.4 percent formaldehyde by weight in water—of the pungent gas that is also a principal ingredient in embalming fluid. It can be formulated as a toothpaste for treating hypersensitive teeth, and the Panel judged it safe after one manufacturer reported only 27 complaints of mouth reactions or gum injuries following the sale of 3,681,000 tubes of his product.

Formaldehyde's actual effectiveness in soothing hypersensitive teeth is less clearcut. Some controlled scientific studies indicate that a small percentage of users experience reduced sensitivity compared with subjects who used a dummy medication. But reviewers found defects in the design of the experiments, and commented on the lack of statistical significance. In short, while safe, formaldehyde's effectiveness as a tooth desensitizer remains to be proved.

Potassium nitrate   Since large amounts of nitrates are consumed daily as food—principally from lettuce, beets, celery, radishes, and spinach—reviewers decided that the relatively small amounts that might be ingested from a medicated toothpaste are safe. Dentists have used potassium nitrate—often in higher, 8.5 to 10 percent concentrations—as an office treatment for dental hypersensitivity. But there is scant evidence to demonstrate the effectiveness of the weaker, 5 percent potassium nitrate toothpaste that the Panel recommended for the over-the-counter market. This preparation is "promising" as a home remedy, and it is safe. But evaluators stipulate that its effectiveness as a self-treatment remains to be proved.

Strontium chloride   This mineral compound has been shown to be extremely nontoxic. Published reports over 12 years on a 10 percent strontium chloride hexahydrate toothpaste show no adverse effects. So reviewers concluded that strontium chloride is safe.

The studies that are purported to demonstrate this mineral's effectiveness in relieving tooth hypersensitivity are far less convincing. In the best of these studies—which was double-blind, meaning that neither the patients nor the dentist knew who was using the medicated toothpaste and who was using a dummy preparation—both the test group and the controls showed measurable reductions in hypersensitivity at 4, 8, and 12 weeks. Compared with the control subjects, users of the strontium chloride toothpaste did not have a more statistically significant improvement.

In another, similar study, the investigator obtained similarly inconclusive results after subjects had used medicated and dummy toothpastes for 3 months. Only after 6 months was there a statistically significant advantage—in reduced sensitivity—among those who used the strontium chloride preparation. The lack of early and consistently significant improvement led the Panel to doubt the drug's effectiveness. Conclusion: safe but not proved effective.

Disapproved Active Ingredients

The combination of edetate disodium + sodium fluoride (0.44 percent) + strontium chloride The sodium fluoride level in this preparation is 0.44 percent—which is double the level that the Panel has approved as safe for daily use against cavities (*see* SODIUM FLUORIDE, page 782). Along with the added risk of doubling the fluoride concentration, edetate disodium is unsafe because it could soften the teeth. Furthermore, no evidence showed that the latter drug alone or in this combination of compounds is effective. In sum: not safe and not effective.

Safety and Effectiveness: Over-the-Counter Toothache Pain Relievers, Counterirritants, and Desensitizers

Active Ingredient	Panel's Assessment
Toothache Pain Relievers	
benzocaine	safe, but not proved effective
benzyl alcohol	not proved safe or effective
butacaine sulfate	not proved safe or effective
capsicum	not safe or effective
creosote	not proved safe or effective
cresol	not proved safe or effective
eugenol preparations with 85 to 87% eugenol	safe and effective
eugenol preparations with 1 to 84% eugenol	safe, but not proved effective
menthol	not safe or effective
methyl salicylate	not safe or effective
phenol	not proved safe or effective
thymol preparations: thymol and thymol iodide	safe, but not proved effective
Counterirritants	
capsicum	safe, but not proved effective
Desensitizers	
citric acid + sodium citrate in poloxamer 407 (Pluronic F-127) gel	safe, but not proved effective

Safety and Effectiveness: Over-the-Counter Toothache Pain Relievers, Counterirritants, and Desensitizers (continued)

Active Ingredient	Panel's Assessment
Desensitizers	
edetate disodium + sodium fluoride + strontium chloride	not safe or effective
fluoride preparations: sodium fluoride, sodium monofluorophosphate (0.44%), and stannous fluoride	safe, but not proved effective
formaldehyde solution	safe, but not proved effective
potassium nitrate	safe, but not proved effective
strontium chloride	safe, but not proved effective

Toothache Relievers and Tooth Desensitizers: Product Ratings

Toothache Relievers

Product and Distributor	Dosage of Active Ingredients	Rating[1]	Comment
Anbesol (Whitehall)	**liquid:** 6.3% benzocaine + 0.5% phenol	B	benzocaine not proved effective; phenol not proved safe or effective
Butyn (Abbott)	**ointment:** 4% butacaine + 1% benzyl alcohol	B	neither ingredient proved safe or effective for toothache relief
Num-zit jel (Purepac)	**gel:** benzocaine + menthol	C	menthol not safe or effective
Orajel (Commerce)	**gel:** 10% benzocaine	B	Panel says benzocaine not proved effective for relieving toothache
Orajel-D (Commerce)	**gel:** 7.5% benzocaine + 0.2% clove oil + 1% benzyl alcohol	C	disapproved combination: too many ingredients
Toothache Drops (DeWitt)	**drops:** 5.01% benzocaine + 9.98% clove oil + 4.83% beechwood creosote	C	disapproved combination: too many ingredients

Tooth Desensitizers

Product and Distributor	Dosage of Active Ingredients	Rating[1]	Comment
Aim (Lever)	**toothpaste:** sodium monofluorophosphate	B	not proved effective

Toothache Relievers and Tooth Desensitizers: Product Ratings *(continued)*

Tooth Desensitizers

Product and Distributor	Dosage of Active Ingredients	Rating[1]	Comment
Aqua-fresh (Beecham)	**toothpaste:** sodium monofluorophosphate	B	not proved effective
Colgate (Colgate)	**toothpaste** and **gel:** sodium monofluorophosphate	B	not proved effective
Crest with Fluoristat (Procter & Gamble)	**toothpaste** and **gel:** sodium fluoride	B	not proved effective
Denquel (Richardson-Vicks)	**toothpaste:** 5% potassium nitrate	B	not proved effective
Gleem (Procter & Gamble)	**toothpaste:** sodium fluoride	B	not proved effective
Sensodyne (Block)	**toothpaste:** 10% strontium chloride hexahydrate	B	not proved effective

1. Author's interpretation of Panel criteria. Based on contents, not claims.

Toothpastes, Rinses, and Gels for Cavity Prevention

Treating the teeth with tiny amounts of sodium fluoride—or other fluorine compounds—will significantly decrease the number of cavities that develop. The easiest, cheapest, and most effective form of fluoride supplementation is fluoridation of each community's drinking water. The FDA's reviewing Panel says fluorides in dental products can further reduce the number of dental cavities that do develop in people who live in places where water is fluoridated. And these over-the-counter preparations may be particularly valuable for the majority of Americans who live in towns and cities without fluoridation.

TOOTHPASTES, RINSES, AND GELS FOR CAVITY PREVENTION is based on the report "Anticaries Drug Products for OTC Human Use" by the FDA's Review Panel on OTC Dentifrice and Dental-Care Drug Products.

The technical name for cavities is *caries*. The toothpastes, powders, rinses, and gels sold to prevent cavities are called *anticaries drug products*. They are categorized as drugs—and regulated by the government as such—because they prevent dental disease.

CLAIMS

Accurate
"aids in the prevention of dental caries [decay or cavities]"

False or Misleading
"for a healthier mouth with less decay"
"raising your natural resistance to tooth decay"
"reduces mouth acidity"

WHY TEETH DECAY

Acid is what erodes tooth enamel, causing cavities. This acid is produced by bacteria that are a part of the sticky, gel-like mass called *dental plaque* (or *bacterial plaque*) that builds up on the surfaces of teeth. It sticks stubbornly, gradually hardens, and cannot be adequately brushed away; professional cleaning by a dentist may be the only way to remove it.

Cavities start early. It's estimated that by age 2, half of all American children have at least one cavity. Serious early dental decay has been attributed to propping bottles of milk or juice in babies' mouths so they can suck themselves to sleep. At age 6, more than three-quarters of children have cavities, and by the time they leave school, only 2 percent of young Americans remain free of dental decay. The average 20-year-old American has 14 teeth that are decayed, have fillings, or are already missing.

The conventional wisdom in dentistry is that plaque—and, by extension, cavities—is caused by table sugar (sucrose) and other carbohydrates that nourish the acid-producing bacteria. So it is thought that eating less sugar and maintaining a more balanced diet can help control acid and cavities. But the Panel ruefully concedes that sugar consumption continues to be high despite widespread efforts to educate the public about its effects on dental health. Chewing gum is high on the list of offending substances as are cereals, desserts, soft drinks, and sweet, gooey foods that linger in the mouth and stick to the teeth. But children love them. Given their craving for sweets—which some recent studies suggest may be wholly natural and normal—less restrictive methods seem needed to prevent tooth decay.

FLUORIDES

How They Help

When infants and young children swallow fluoride, it is incorporated into the developing teeth, as hard, insoluble crystals. This substance, fluorapatite, replaces some of the natural outer-tooth enamel and to a lesser extent it is incorporated into the deeper layers of the teeth. Later, after these teeth erupt, the fluoride-enriched enamel resists being dissolved by acid.

Fluoride may do more than simply harden developing teeth, according to recent studies. Fluoride in the saliva, or in overlying dental plaque, may aid in the remineralization of the enamel by encouraging the deposition of calcium and phosphate. So older children and adults may also benefit from continuing use of fluoride products.

The metal tin also protects against acid; the word *stannous* on a dentifrice label means that the product contains tin.

Sources

Americans' principal source of fluoride is drinking water. This is so even if the water is not artificially fluoridated, because most if not all ground, river, and lake waters contain some natural fluoride. Where levels contain about 1 part per million (1 ppm), the prevalence of dental decay is about 60 percent lower than it is in low fluoride areas. This higher level of fluoridation poses no risk to people who drink the water.

Of 105 million people who live in United States communities where the water contains 0.7 ppm or more fluoride particles, 11 million are drinking naturally fluoridated water while 94 million use water that contains fluoride supplements. This supplementation is usually added in the amounts needed to bring the level up to 1 ppm. These statistics, which were cited by the Panel, come from a federal survey of fluoridation that was conducted in 1975 and published in 1977. No dramatic changes in fluoridation practices have occurred since that time.

Alternative sources of fluoride include professional applications by a dentist or dental hygienist; periodic mouth rinsings with fluoride— such as is provided in some schools; and home treatment with fluoride toothpastes, gels, or rinses. It appears likely that 3 rinses and a gel that previously were available only to dentists soon will be sold over-the-counter as the result of the reviewers' decision that they are safe and effective for self-care.

Effectiveness

Which methods are most effective? A study conducted in Sweden a number of years ago ranked 6 different approaches. The first is the most effective, the last method is the least effective.

1. Sodium fluoride rinse once daily
2. Sodium fluoride rinse every 2 weeks
3. Regular use of a stannous fluoride dentifrice
4. Sodium fluoride applied periodically by a dentist
5. Regular use of a sodium bicarbonate fluoride dentifrice
6. Stannous fluoride applied periodically by a dentist

Encouragingly, this study indicates that self-care can be more effective than professionally administered fluoride treatments. It certainly is cheaper. The present Panel says that subsequent studies have largely verified these Swedish findings.

Dosage Forms

Fluoride is commonly formulated into dentrifrices, mouth rinses, and gels.

Dentifrices A dentrifrice is a toothpaste, powder, or other substance that is used with a toothbrush. The first fluoride toothpaste—one containing stannous fluoride—was introduced in the United States in 1955. The main technical obstacle that had to be overcome was to find an abrasive (a cleansing and polishing substance) that did not make the fluoride inactive. The first such abrasive, calcium pyrophosphate, was described in the dental literature in 1954; there have been others since then.

The American Dental Association (ADA) has classified several fluoride toothpastes as "accepted," and allows manufacturers to use its Seal of Acceptance on their products along with an endorsement which says a product "has been shown to be an effective decay-preventive dentifrice that can be of significant value when used in a conscientiously applied program of oral hygiene and regular professional care." Daily use of these toothpastes may reduce the number of cavities that develop by as much as 20 to 30 percent.

Rinses   Fluoridated rinses are newer and less widely investigated than dentifrices. Nevertheless, more than 20 extensive studies noted by the Panel indicate that use of these products can reduce cavities by 20 to 50 percent—that is, perhaps *more* than dentifrices. Some rinses have ADA endorsement.

Gels   The few studies on fluoride gels that had been published when the evaluators wrote their report provided what the Panel called "reasonable documentation" of their effectiveness. Reviewers stipulate, however, that these gels should be used *in addition to* a dentifrice rather than as a substitute for it. Gel formulations are not intended to be used as toothpastes.

Very confusingly, however, some major United States manufacturers, specifically Procter & Gamble (which makes Crest) and Colgate have started to market fluoride toothpastes that also are labeled as "gels." Since these products contain fluoride in the form of sodium monofluorophosphate, and since the only fluoridated dental gel approved by the FDA contains stannous fluoride, it appears that these products are technically toothpastes and *not* fluoride gels.

Risk Factors

At concentrations far above those attained in dental-health programs, fluoride can be quite toxic. As noted, the best cavity-preventing dose in drinking water is 1 ppm. When drinking water contains 2 to 10 ppm of fluoride, it may discolor children's teeth. At far higher concentrations—of 20 to 80 ppm in drinking water—fluoride may severely affect the bones. They become too dense, too fragile, and joints may no longer work properly.

Many dental researchers have studied the question of whether fluoridated water or fluoride dental products will lead to toxic changes. The Panel believes, on the basis of available evidence, that they will not. One investigator found, for example, that in an average brushing no more than 0.25 mg of fluoride would be swallowed—and probably a lot less. Reviewers think that this is considerably below any toxic range.

To forestall the remote possibility that a child would eat the contents of a tube of fluoride toothpaste or drink a bottle of rinse, the Panel recommends that dentifrice packages contain no more than 260 mg total fluoride and dental rinse packages no more than 120 mg. The risk of fluoride-caused tooth discoloration is greatest in childhood years, when adult teeth still are developing under the gums. Therefore experts recommend that fluoride rinses and gels be labeled for use only by adults and children over 6, and that fluoride dentifrices be labeled for use by adults and children only when over the age of 2. Advice is added that children 2 to 6 use these products under parental supervision.

COMBINATION PRODUCTS

It would seem to make sense to combine an antibacterial agent with a cavity-preventive fluoride agent. But no such combination has been shown to be safe and effective, thus none is approved.

Almost all testing of anticaries preparations has been done on products with a single active ingredient. So, pending wholly new studies to establish the safety and effectiveness of combination products, the Panel disapproves of all dental preparations that contain 2 anticaries agents or 1 plus any other active ingredient.

ANTICARIES PREPARATIONS

Approved Active Ingredients

All approved cavity-preventing ingredients are fluorides. For 2 of them—sodium fluoride and stannous fluoride—there are 2 or more approved dosage forms.

Dosages of Approved Ingredients

	Approved Dosage	
Active Ingredient	*In Dentifrice*	*In Rinse*
acidulated phosphate fluoride		0.02%
sodium fluoride	0.22%	0.05%
sodium monofluorophosphate	0.76%	
stannous fluoride*	0.4%	0.1%

*In gel, 0.4% is the approved dosage.

Acidulated phosphate fluoride (rinse)   In the amount of fluoride it delivers and in its safety, this preparation is comparable to the better-studied sodium fluoride rinses (*see* below). Several studies that have been conducted with acidulated phosphate fluoride rinses show no harmful local or systemic effects. This rinse appears to be more effective for people who live in areas without fluoridated drinking water than it is for residents of communities that do have it. People who rinse with acidulated phosphate fluoride preparations may anticipate about a 25 to 30 percent reduction in cavities as reward for their effort.

The Panel joins the FDA's dental advisers and the ADA in endorsing the safety and effectiveness of this rinse. The approved daily dosage for adults and children 6 and over is one 1-minute swishing through the teeth with a rinse containing 2 teaspoonsful of 0.02 percent acidulated phosphate fluoride. This ingredient may not yet be available over-the-counter.

Sodium fluoride (dentifrice)   This fluoride has been broadly studied and test results led evaluators to conclude that it is safe and effective as a cavity-preventive dentifrice ingredient. In six 16-to-36-month clinical trials 0.22 percent sodium fluoride with a 40 percent high-beta-phase calcium pyrophosphate abrasive system was tested against similar toothpastes without the fluoride. Results showed a statistically significant reduction in dental decay.

These preparations also appear to be safe. A 150-pound man would have to eat the contents of 20 to 40 full tubes of sodium fluoride toothpaste to ingest a lethal dose. Lesser amounts conceivably could cause tooth discoloration in young children who regularly swallowed large amounts of the toothpaste and also consumed large amounts of naturally or artificially fluoridated water. Evaluators noted, however, that in the 15 years since these toothpastes were widely marketed, there was no documented rise in the incidence of such discoloration.

The safe and effective dose for children over 2 and adults is one or more tooth-brushings daily with a 0.22 percent sodium fluoride dentifrice that contains a suitable abrasive system.

Sodium fluoride (rinse)   Daily rinsing with a 0.05 percent solution of sodium fluoride has been shown to reduce the number of cavities that develop in children's teeth by 25 to 50 percent.

One early study showed that one of these rinses irritated the gums. But follow-up studies did not confirm this finding. As with sodium fluoride dentifrices (*see* immediately above), many containers of rinse would have to be consumed to cause lethal poisoning. Reviewers agree with the ADA that a 0.05 percent sodium fluoride rinse—swished through the teeth for a minute, once daily—is a safe and effective way to prevent caries. This ingredient may not yet be available over-the-counter.

Sodium monofluorophosphate (dentifrice)   This compound may be less toxic in a single dose than sodium fluoride (*see* immediately above) simply because the fluoride particles are released from it more slowly. But over the long haul the 2 compounds are comparable in safety.

A number of studies, using toothpastes with a variety of abrasives, show that sodium monofluorophosphate effectively reduces the number of new cavities that will develop over a 2- to 3-year period by 20 to 30 percent. The safe and effective dosage for children over 2 and adults is at least one brushing daily with a 0.76 percent sodium monofluorophosphate dentifrice that contains suitable abrasive ingredients.

Stannous fluoride (dentifrice)   This ingredient contains fluoride and tin, both of which act to harden teeth against acid and decay. The tin does not significantly increase the fluoride's toxic potential, but it may stain dental plaque and debris yellow. However, this is a rare occurrence and the stain can be removed.

Stannous fluoride has been widely tested in dentifrices containing several different abrasive mixes. Most—but not all—studies show that it reduces cavities by statistically significant numbers.

The safe and effective dosage for adults and children over 2 is one or more thorough brushings daily with a 0.4 percent stannous fluoride toothpaste containing a suitable abrasive formulation.

Stannous fluoride (rinse)   This type of formulation is judged safe and effective, although the data on effectiveness are less convincing than is the case with other approved stannous fluoride and sodium fluoride formulations. Of the 4 long-term studies evaluated, 2 showed highly positive results; one failed to show consistently positive responses; and the last indicated that the rinse did not lower the occurrence of caries. By and large, reviewers suggest, stannous fluoride rinses are valuable for people who do not have fluoridated water, and perhaps less useful for people whose water is fluoridated.

The safety of stannous fluoride rinses does not differ significantly from that of stannous fluoride dentifrices. The occasional yellow staining that occurs in people who do not brush their teeth often enough can be removed by a dentist and will not recur if the teeth are subsequently brushed well.

The rinse must be made up just before use because the active ingredient is chemically unstable when dissolved in water. The approved dosage for adults and children over 6 is one rinse per day of 10 ml (2 teaspoonsful) of a freshly prepared 0.1 percent rinse. It should be swished around between the teeth for one minute and then spit out.

Stannous fluoride (gel)   Evaluators found suitable documentation for the effectiveness of this preparation, in which the stannous fluoride is formulated in anhydrous (water-free) glycerin. In one ingenious study, teeth that were extracted after their owners had used a stannous fluoride gel over a period of time were found to be harder than teeth extracted from people who did not use the gel. Youngsters wearing braces on their teeth were far less likely to suffer calcium loss from the tooth enamel—which can happen with braces—if they regularly used a stannous fluoride gel.

Gel formulations of stannous fluoride do not significantly differ in safety from the dentifrice formulations described above. The evaluators say a 0.4 percent stannous fluoride gel is safe and effective for adults and children over 6 when it is applied once daily to the teeth. But consumers should remember that gel formulations are not intended to be used as toothpastes. This ingredient not yet may be available over-the-counter.

Conditionally Approved Active Ingredients

None

Disapproved Active Ingredients

Phosphate preparations: calcium sucrose phosphate (CaSP), dicalcium phosphate dihydrate (DCPD), disodium hydrogen phosphate, phosphoric acid, sodium dihydrogen phosphate, sodium dihydrogen phosphate monohydrate, sodium phosphate, and sodium phosphate dibasic, anhydrous reagent These substances are used as abrasives, chemical buffers, and fillers in currently marketed dental products. They are safe *for these purposes*. In animal studies they seem to prevent cavities, possibly by acting on—and hardening—tooth enamel. They may substitute harder forms of mineral calcium for the natural mineral calcium that is present in the teeth.

In humans, the effects of phosphates are less conclusive. Unlike fluorides, for example, phosphates have not been shown to enter into and remain in the tooth enamel. So no satisfactory evidence exists that phosphates effectively fight cavities in humans. The Panel's judgment: safe but not effective.

Sodium bicarbonate This is ordinary baking soda. It is widely used as a tooth powder and certainly is safe. But there is no evidence that it prevents the formation of cavities. In short, sodium bicarbonate is safe but not effective for use against caries.

Sodium monofluorophosphate (6 percent rinse) This rinse contains too much fluoride to be safe for nonprescription use. A standard dose applied with a toothbrush could lead users to take in 2 mg of fluoride daily. Used regularly this amount could not only discolor the teeth but might also cause symptoms of fluorine poisoning. So while this liquid preparation may prevent cavities (i.e., be effective), evaluators say it is unsafe to use as an over-the-counter preparation.

INACTIVE INGREDIENTS

Dentifrices, of course, contain tooth-polishing abrasives—as well as other chemicals. Evaluators did not attempt to assess these inactive ingredients other than to note that one of them, sodium lauryl sarcosinate, may irritate the inside of the mouth. The reviewers did recommend that a special Panel be convened for the purpose of evaluating all the many inactive ingredients listed below.

alcohol
alumina
alumina (aluminum
   oxide trihydrate),
   hydrated
aluminum hydroxide
aminoacetic acid
anethole
benzethonium chloride
blue color
buffers
calcium carbonate
   (chalk)
calcium phosphate
calcium
   pyrophosphate
   (calcium
   pyrophosphate,
   high-beta-phase)
calcium silicate
calcium sucrose
   phosphate
carboxymethyl-
   cellulose
carrageenan (sodium
   and potassium
   carrageenans)

carrageenan gum
carvone
cellulose gum
chewing gum
citric acid
coconut
   monoglyceride
   sulfonates
coloring agents
corn syrup
dentifrice soap
dicalcium phosphate
dicalcium phosphate
   anhydrous
dicalcium phosphate
   dihydrate
dicalcium phosphate
   dihydrate-sugar mix
   1:1
disodium hydrogen
   phosphate
flavoring agents
flavorings, natural
glycerine (glycerol)
gum base
hydrated silica
hydrochloric acid

hydrogen fluoride
magnesium aluminum
   silicate
magnesium carbonate
magnesium hydroxide
menthol
methylparaben
milk of magnesia
mineral oil (light food
   grade)
mint flavor
oil of peppermint
papain
phosphoric acid
   (orthophosphoric
   acid)
polyethylene glycol
polymethyl-
   methacrylate (in the
   form of
   microspheres)
polysorbate 80
potassium hydroxide
precipitated calcium
   carbonate
propylene glycol
pumice

red color
saccharine
SD alcohol 38 B
silica
silica gel
silica gel, dehydrated
silica, hydrated
  precipitated
silicon dioxide
silicon dioxide (with
  low aluminum
  content)
soap powder
sodium alkyl sulfate
sodium alkyl
  sulfoacetate
sodium benzoate
sodium bicarbonate
sodium carbonate

sodium
  carboxymethyl-
  cellulose
sodium
  carboxymethyl-
  cellulose gum
sodium citrate
sodium dihydrogen
  phosphate
sodium dihydrogen
  phosphate
  monohydrate
sodium hydroxide
sodium lauryl sulfate
sodium
  metaphosphate
sodium
  metaphosphate,
  insoluble

sodium monoglyceride
  sulfonate
sodium lauryl
  sarcosinate
sodium phosphate
  dibasic, anhydrous
  reagent
sodium saccharin
sorbitol
spearmint flavor
spice
stannous
  pyrophosphate
sugar
titanium dioxide
water, distilled
wintergreen

Safety and Effectiveness: Active Ingredients in Over-the-Counter Cavity Preventives

Active Ingredient	Panel's Assessment
acidulated phosphate fluoride	safe and effective
calcium sucrose phosphate (CaSP)	safe, but not effective
dicalcium phosphate dihydrate (DCPD)	safe, but not effective
disodium hydrogen phosphate	safe, but not effective
phosphoric acid	safe, but not effective
sodium bicarbonate	safe, but not effective
sodium dihydrogen phosphate	safe, but not effective
sodium dihydrogen phosphate monohydrate	safe, but not effective
sodium fluoride	safe and effective
sodium monofluorophosphate (dentifrice)	safe and effective
sodium monofluorophosphate (6% rinse)	not safe
sodium phosphate	safe, but not effective
sodium phosphate dibasic, anhydrous reagent	safe, but not effective
stannous fluoride	safe and effective

Cavity Preventives: Product Ratings

Product and Distributor	Dosage of Active Ingredients	Rating[1]
sodium fluoride toothpaste		
Crest with Fluoristat (Procter & Gamble)	**toothpaste** and **gel:** sodium fluoride	**A**
Gleem (Procter & Gamble)	**toothpaste:** sodium fluoride	**A**
sodium monofluorophosphate toothpaste		
Aim (Lever)	**toothpaste:** sodium monofluorophosphate	**A**
Aqua-fresh (Beecham)	**toothpaste:** sodium monofluorophosphate	**A**
Colgate (Colgate)	**toothpaste** and **gel:** sodium monofluorophosphate	**A**
stannous fluoride rinse		
StanCare (Block)	**effervescent tablets:** 0.1%	**A**

1. Author's interpretation of Panel criteria. Based on contents, not claims.

Unguents and Powders for the Skin

For centuries certain substances have been used as dusting powders, lotions, ointments, and creams to temporarily cover, protect, or relieve burned, chafed, chapped, scraped, or otherwise irritated and injured skin. These substances—technically referred to as *skin protectants*—differ from most of the medications described in this book. The latter *act* in some way. For example, they may have a biochemical effect on the body's cells and fluids, or on bacteria or other "germs." Skin protectants tend to be *inert*. They form a physical barrier that protects injured, vulnerable skin from dryness, wetness, irritating chemicals, or from external pressure or frictional contact with clothing, bandages, or even other body surfaces. Some skin protectants grab, hold, dilute, or dissolve irritants. In a sense, some of these substances are inactive active

UNGUENTS AND POWDERS is based on the report on "Skin Protectant Drug Products for OTC Human Use" prepared by the FDA's Advisory Review Panel on OTC Topical Analgesic, Antirheumatic, Otic, Burn and Sunburn Prevention and Treatment Drug Products.

ingredients. Yet, as reviewers noted, they can produce dramatic relief —as when a lubricant and antidrying agent is applied to sunburn; when moisture retainers are used for chapped lips; and when lubricants soften the skin and increase pliability.

CLAIMS

Accurate
"aids in the temporary relief of minor skin irritations"
"soothes minor skin irritation"
"gives comfort" and "temporary protection" (to minor skin irritations)

Accurate for Dryness-Protection Ingredients
for relief of "symptoms of chapping, peeling, or scaling due to minor burns, sunburn, windburn, scrapes, abrasions, or cracked lips"

Accurate for Wetness-Relief Ingredients
for relief of "symptoms of oozing or weeping due to contact dermatitis, poison oak, or poison ivy"

Accurate for Friction-Relief Ingredients
for relief of "symptoms of intertrigo, chafing, galling, rubbing, or friction"
for "the temporary protection and lubrication of minor skin irritations"

False or Misleading
any reference to the "cure" of anything
"aids healing" (this is yet to be proved)

USES FOR SKIN PROTECTANTS

Burns

Many of the ingredients used to treat minor burns are skin protectants. Serious burns, where one or more layers of skin have been destroyed, require medical attention. Only first-degree burns, in which the skin is reddened but initially not broken, and mild second-degree burns, where small areas of the outer layer of skin have been destroyed, should be self-treated.

When a person is seriously burned, medical help should be quickly sought. Covering a wide or deep burn with a first-aid product or skin protectant can complicate later treatment, since it may have to be removed by the doctor or emergency-room nurse—a procedure that can make the pain worse.

Fast action is the key to first aid for minor burns. The burned surface should be immediately immersed in a basin of still, cool, or even cold water, or covered *gently* with cold-water compresses (cloths soaked in cold water and wrung out). Do *not* use running water: the pressure and friction of the water stream may increase the pain. Do *not* use ice cubes or ice water: they are too cold, and can cause further injury and pain.

Cold-water treatment of a mild burn should continue for 20 minutes to half an hour. If the burn pain subsides, little further treatment—other than possible use of a skin protectant—will be needed.

A number of household remedies are also used to treat burned skin. These include application of butter, lard, goose grease, and other oily substances. While this offers some initial relief, such substances are not recommended. They are likely to be unsterile, so they may promote infection. Also, they may contain salt, which can increase the pain. The nonirritating skin protectants described in this unit provide a better choice.

Wound Healing

Three active ingredients that are claimed to promote wound healing were assessed in the review process. Two of them—allantoin and zinc acetate—were found to be safe and effective as skin protectants. The other, live-yeast-cell derivative, was evaluated only as an agent to promote healing.

The Panel is extremely skeptical of these wound-healing claims. Similar doubts have been raised by 2 other Panels that evaluated antibiotics and other antimicrobial agents used to treat skin wounds, and also by the FDA. The FDA maintains that none of the antimicrobial products hastens, promotes, or helps in healing.

The present Panel says no controlled study of over-the-counter wound-healing aids has demonstrated that these agents actually accelerate healing. Therefore, these three ingredients are only *conditionally* approved as healing aids (*see* WOUND HEALERS, below). Manufacturers will have to substantiate the healing claims by scientific studies or drop them from labels. (*See* also FIRST-AID PREPARATIONS FOR SKIN WOUNDS).

STANDARDS FOR APPROVAL FOR SKIN PROTECTANTS

Evaluators appear to have been more tolerant in granting approval to skin-protectant ingredients than they (or other OTC reviewers) were with any other class of ingredients. One reason is that protectants traditionally have been popular because they are soothing and nonirritating. Their safety and effectiveness are attested to by druggists and by doctors' clinical experience.

Because these agents are neutral or inert (and so appear safe), several of them are used as vehicles. This means that manufacturers and druggists use them for mixing other, pharmacologically active ingredients to make products that are applied to the skin or mucous membranes. So the Panel recommended to the FDA that it waive its usual test requirements because of (1) wide use, (2) protectants' inclusion in standard drug compendiums, and (3) established effectiveness in providing a mechanical barrier.

A Possible Hitch?

It can be argued, of course, that occasionally a drug that is universally regarded as safe turns out to be a hazard. One noteworthy example is boric acid, which for a long time was used as a skin protectant in diapering powders for babies, as well as in lotions, ointments, and pastes to prevent irritation and infection, speed healing, and relieve the pain of burns. Only after a half-century of widespread use was boric acid found to be potentially lethal. The danger arises because of the ease with which boron—its principal base, which is now known to be very poisonous—is absorbed through the skin. Moreover, on careful reexamination, boric acid has now been found to have little or no protective value. Accordingly, it was assessed as both unsafe and ineffective for nonprescription use.

Conceivably, other skin-protectant ingredients now considered safe and effective despite the lack of definitive scientific proof will one day be discarded.

COMBINATION PRODUCTS

In the liberal spirit with which it assessed skin-protectant active ingredients, evaluators imposed no limit on the number of these substances that can be formulated into a product—provided that each makes a contribution to the whole. No specific concentrations were set as marking an ingredient both safe and effective.

But ingredients in combination products cannot interact with each other or act in an opposing way to each other. The sense of this reasoning—though not explicitly stated in reports—is that an ingredient like cocoa butter, which is moisture-retaining, should not be combined, say, with calamine lotion, which has the opposite (drying) effect.

SKIN PROTECTANTS

Approved Active Ingredients

Allantoin   This is a compound for which few, if any, adverse reactions have ever been reported in the medical literature. It appears to be nontoxic, nonallergenic, and nonirritating when applied to the skin. It has the ability to protect even very young and tender bottoms against the moisture and irritation of diaper rash. Allantoin is also a skin softener.

In one series of controlled experiments, with an emulsion that contained allantoin, silicones, and the now banned germicidal agent hexachlorophene, only 5 percent of several hundred babies developed diaper rash. In a control group of babies who were not so treated, the incidence of diaper rash was 3 times higher. In another part of this study, the skin of 34 out of 38 infants who already had diaper rash or a similar problem cleared up nicely after treatment with the emulsion. The investigators concluded that the allantoin-containing mixture was effective and relatively free from side effects. Allantoin is considered safe and effective for people of all ages when applied in a concentration of 0.5 to 2 percent, as often as needed.

Aluminum hydroxide gel   This white, powdery aluminum compound—also called *aluminum hydroxide* or *aluminum hydrate*—forms a gel when it is kept in contact with water, so it is widely used internally as a nonprescription antacid. It has been marketed as a skin protectant for almost a century with good consumer acceptance and without reported difficulties. Animal-toxicity tests also attest to its safety.

The effectiveness of aluminum hydroxide gel as a skin protectant is based on 2 properties: as an astringent, it pulls bacteria and other noxious substances out of sweat, urine, and other excreted body fluids; then it tightly binds and holds these substances so that they cannot attach and thus irritate, damage, or penetrate the skin. With such action, the ingredient is particularly useful against the irritating wetness found in prickly heat, ringworm, jock itch, and impetigo, as well as weeping, scaly rashes of poison ivy and similar plant poisons.

Reviewers state that aluminum hydroxide gel can be applied generously whenever necessary, to children over 6 months of age and adults. For infants under 6 months, it should be used only under a doctor's orders. The safe and effective concentration is 0.15 to 5 percent.

Calamine (prepared calamine and calamine lotion)   A pinkish-colored remedy, calamine protects the skin by absorbing moisture and chemical irritants; it soothes, too. Calamine is 98 percent zinc oxide, which is white. But it also contains about 0.5 percent—that is, one-half of 1 percent—of the iron compound ferrous oxide. This chemical's red color imparts the pinkish cast, which is wholly "window dressing" according to the experts. The iron contributes nothing to zinc oxide's absorbent and protectant effect, which, like calamine's safety, is principally attested by consumer acceptance and long, trouble-free clinical use. (*See* ZINC OXIDE, page 795.)

The dosage, for all ages, is a 1 to 25 percent concentration of calamine, applied as often as needed.

Cocoa butter   Cocoa butter is a waxy, chocolate-smelling, and chocolate-tasting substance that has the capacity of melting into a soothing, skin-softening oil when warmed by body heat. So it is convenient, as well as quite agreeable, to use cocoa butter both as a lubricant for massages and as a base for medicinal ointments and suppositories.

The ingredient is a fatty extract from the roasted seeds of the cacao plant. The judgments that it is safe and effective are based on long use and wide acceptance rather than on scientific testing.

When applied to sunburned or otherwise injured skin, cocoa butter prevents evaporation and dryness, and keeps the skin soft and pliable. This reduces friction, irritation, and pain. Evaluators say cocoa butter is safe and effective in 80 to 100 percent concentrations. It can be used liberally and as often as needed—on the youngest and tenderest to the oldest and toughest of skins.

Cornstarch   This is a powdery kitchen-cabinet remedy—a food substance. Its protective power lies in its ability to absorb huge amounts of liquids when it is dusted on the skin. Cornstarch absorbs 25 times more moisture than talc, which is also used for this purpose. Bacteria and their poisonous byproducts, as well as other noxious materials, can be absorbed and held away from the skin by cornstarch—and rendered harmless. Too, cornstarch smoothes and lubricates body surfaces that have been irritated by friction.

Cornstarch feels bland to the skin. This helps explain why no adverse effects have as yet been attributed to dusting it on one's body. For adults, children, and infants, the Panel says that a 10 to 85 percent cornstarch preparation can safely and effectively be applied to irritated skin as often as needed.

Dimethicone (dimethyl polysiloxane) An inert, soothing, syrupy silicone, dimethicone is judged to be remarkably free of side effects and any toxicity. It is chemically similar to simethicone, which is taken internally to relieve symptoms of gas. Dimethicone clings to the skin and repels water. It will effectively seal a wound against air, wind, and other drying or frictional irritants. Because it can block the ammonia usually produced by bacterial decomposition of urine, the ingredient can be used to treat and prevent diaper rash. Dimethicone will also seal and protect chapped skin and lips against further drying and chapping. It should *not* be used on puncture wounds or infected wounds, however, because some air must reach wound surfaces in order for them to heal; without air they fester.

Dimethicone is safe and effective in a 1 to 30 percent concentration on the skins of people of all ages. It can be applied in generous amounts and as often as needed.

Glycerin (glycerine and glycerol) This clear, sweetish, syrupy stuff is highly inert, and for the most part innocuous to the human body. Undiluted, as anhydrous glycerin, it absorbs water, so it could dry out and irritate the skin. But in a 20 to 45 percent concentration in water —the recommended amount—hydrous glycerin will hold water against the skin so that it stays moist and is not irritated by air, wind, or other drying forces. Glycerin may be applied generously, whenever needed, by persons of all ages—except infants under 6 months, for whom one should consult a physician.

Kaolin Also called *China clay*, *white bole*, *argilla*, and *porcelain clay*, kaolin is a powdery, earthy, clay-type material. Technically it is purified and hydrated aluminum silicate. It protects the skin through its avid ability to absorb moisture and toxic substances dissolved in it.

Kaolin has been used as an internal and external medication for hundreds of years. There are no reports of toxic reactions following its application to the skin. The substance absorbs perspiration and other moisture, and acts as a dusting powder to dry weepy skin conditions like eczema and the leaky blisters of poison ivy and poison oak. For people of all ages, kaolin is considered safe and effective in concentrations of 4 to 20 percent. It can be applied liberally, when needed.

Petrolatum preparations: petrolatum and white petrolatum These petroleum derivatives can be used to soften, lubricate, and protect the skin. White petrolatum is chemically more refined than yellow or amber petrolatums, but their pharmaceutical properties are the same.

Petrolatum is the base (vehicle) for a variety of internal and external medications, and is regarded as extremely safe. For small, superficial burns, petrolatum by itself—or on a gauze dressing—will keep air out, prevent evaporation of moisture from the wound, and reduce pain. Petrolatum can also be used to relieve sunburn, chapping, and other forms of dry skin, and as an ammonia-blocking agent to prevent diaper rash. It should *not*, however, be used on puncture wounds, lacerated skin, or wounds that have become infected, since the lack of exposure to air retards healing and may cause the wound to form pus.

For persons of all ages, petrolatum preparations are safe and effective in 30 to 100 percent concentrations, and can be applied as often as needed.

Shark-liver oil   This ingredient can be used to cover, soften, and soothe a dry, burned, or otherwise irritated skin surface. It is not scientific, controlled experiments but rather the long-time experience of users, druggists, and doctors that attests to the substance's safety and worth.

Experts recommend that this remedy not be used for children under 2 except on a doctor's advice. Otherwise, a 3 percent shark-liver oil preparation is safe and effective when applied generously and as often as needed.

Sodium bicarbonate   This white crystalline powder with a salty, somewhat alkaline taste, is another kitchen remedy. It is sometimes called bicarbonate of soda, but is more commonly known as *baking soda*. Sodium bicarbonate fizzes into carbon dioxide gas and water when moistened—leaving behind a paste of sodium carbonate. This soothing residue relieves the itching of bee stings and mosquito bites. It is also helpful in treating *minor* burns. Large acid burns, in particular, should not be treated with sodium bicarbonate because the acid-based chemical reaction can further injure the skin. First aid for large acid burns is cold running water or a cold shower—unlike the still water recommended for less serious situations—before quick referral for medical attention.

Persons with widespread itching due to hives, eczema, or similar skin disorders often find relief by bathing in a tub of tepid water that has been well laced with sodium bicarbonate. This relieves the itch, and softens and soothes the skin.

The safety and effectiveness of sodium bicarbonate as a skin protectant is largely based on clinical self-care use and on consumers' satisfaction with the results. No toxic reactions have ever been reported from its use as a topical drug. Evaluators say that a 1 to 100 percent application of sodium bicarbonate can be used, whenever needed, for persons of any age.

Zinc acetate An astringent crystalline compound, zinc acetate precipitates bacteria and other proteins out of solution. This neutralizes their harmful effects. Because of this astringent property, zinc acetate sometimes is formulated into deodorant products. A long marketing record, with no reported untoward reactions, attests to zinc acetate's safety. Wide use and continuing clinical acceptance point to its effectiveness.

While it is not recommended for children under 2 except under medical supervision, for adults a 0.1 to 2 percent preparation is safe and effective. The substance can be applied to the affected skin without restraint and as often as is required.

Zinc carbonate Zinc carbonate is an inert white powder, insoluble in water. It has been widely used—without reported toxicity—to cover and protect the skin. The substance appears to absorb noxious and irritating substances. Evaluators found no specific studies documenting zinc carbonate's effectiveness, but they believe it works because of its wide acceptance and because other zinc compounds—like zinc oxide (*see* immediately below)—are recognized as effective for their astringent properties and their ability to soothe and protect irritated skin. The recommended dose for persons of all ages is 0.2 to 2 percent as needed.

Zinc oxide This fine, white powdery substance—sometimes known as *flowers of zinc* or *zinc white*—is the basic active ingredient in calamine preparations. Zinc oxide is used to cover the skin to protect it from dryness and other harmful environmental stimuli. It also absorbs toxic substances and serves, too, as a lubricant. Zinc oxide is extremely safe—even when taken internally—and there have been no published reports of complications following its use on the skin. Its effectiveness is established by wide use and acceptance by consumers and doctors; it is the sole or principal ingredient in a wide variety of over-the-counter preparations.

Because of its cooling, slightly astringent, antiseptic, antibacterial, and protective actions, zinc oxide is considered particularly effective in treating diaper rash and prickly heat. It is also useful against eczema, impetigo, and many other itchy conditions. The safe and effective dosage for persons of all ages, including infants, is 1 to 25 percent applied liberally to the affected area whenever needed.

Conditionally Approved Active Ingredients

The Panel did not list any ingredient as conditionally safe or conditionally effective as a skin protectant. But 2 approved skin-protectant ingredients—allantoin and zinc acetate, both described above—are also claimed by manufacturers to accelerate wound healing. So is a third ingredient: live-yeast-cell derivative. These 3 substances were judged as conditionally approved as *wound-healing aids* (*see* page 797).

Disapproved Active Ingredients

Bismuth subnitrate This chemical is also known as *basic bismuth nitrate*, *bismuth oxynitrate*, *bismuthyl nitrate*, *white bismuth*, and *Spanish white*. It is a white, odorless, tasteless powder that has been used as an antiseptic, astringent, and skin protectant. Despite its long use and acceptance, bismuth subnitrate has been found to be lethally toxic when taken internally. Also, because there are no persuasive data to show that it is effective as a skin protectant, evaluators decided that the ingredient is unsafe and ineffective for this purpose.

Boric acid When boric acid—also known as *boracic acid* or *orthoboric acid*—is applied to damaged skin in an ointment, its main constituent, boron, is absorbed into the body. Boron from even a relatively small amount of such an ointment can damage the central nervous system; larger amounts can be fatal. Deaths also have been reported in infants powdered before diapering with a borated talc powder—which indicates that boron can be absorbed through unbroken skin as well as through wounds.

Despite boric acid's wide use and great medicinal popularity in decades past, evaluators judged the ingredient to be unsafe as a topical drug and also ineffective.

Sulfur Another time-honored remedy for skin disorders, sulfur has been thrown into disrepute by recent research findings. Reviewers concluded that precipitated sulfur, sublimed sulfur, washed sulfur, and colloidal sulfur are dangerous and likely to be counterproductive in terms of wound healing.

Sulfur has long been known to have 2 different effects on skin: it causes peeling and damage but stimulates skin growth. Using sulfur on a wound will initially exacerbate the problem, rather than relieve it, and could destroy surface epithelium that is freshly healing. So, sulfur is assessed as unsafe and ineffective as a skin protectant.

Tannic acid This tanning agent, traditionally used to cure leather, has been used as an astringent to "pull" foreign protein matter out of burns and other small wounds and to provide a protective covering. Tannic acid has also been used to relieve pain—which in fact it may do.

But bacteria also may flourish under this tannin "crust," inducing infection. What is worse, topical burn preparations made with tannic acid may damage the liver and other organs. A number of reports have appeared in the medical literature concerning deaths following the use of tannic acid sprays, jellies, and solutions in treating burns. Despite previous wide use, therefore, evaluators believe there are now few legitimate medical uses for tannic acid and they judge it unsafe and ineffective in over-the-counter skin-protectant products.

WOUND HEALERS

Approved Active Ingredients

None

Conditionally Approved Active Ingredients

Allantoin   During World War I, battle surgeons noted that wounds that became infested with maggots healed with unexpected speed. This was attributed to the presence of allantoin in the maggots' excretions, and allantoin began to be widely employed to encourage the healing of stubborn wounds. Many studies have since been conducted to assess this phenomenon, but reviewers believe that none offers conclusive evidence that the substance has a wound-healing property, or that such a property is described in scientifically acceptable detail. Neither do these studies show that allantoin contributes to wound healing by speeding the removal of dead tissue (as had been suggested).

Live-yeast-cell derivative   This substance is an alcoholic extract of baker's yeast—the foodstuff that makes bread dough rise. It also is called *skin respiratory factor*, because its purported effect—when applied to wounded skin—is to increase oxygen uptake. This, in turn, claims the manufacturer of live-yeast-cell derivative products, stimulates the growth of new connective tissue and skin.

Some animal tests submitted for review suggest—somewhat equivocally—that live-yeast-cell derivative does possess this property. But only a single, small experiment on humans (involving 18 patients) was presented and evaluators found the study inadequate. Here, too, only conditional approval could be granted.

Zinc acetate   Concentrations of zinc naturally appear along the margins of healing wounds. This has led to tests in which zinc, given orally, has been shown to speed wound healing. But reviewers say that there are no data as yet to show that applying zinc directly to a wound will speed healing. More investigation is needed if zinc acetate is to "graduate" from conditional approval.

Disapproved Active Ingredients

None

ADDITIONAL SKIN REMEDIES: PRELIMINARY REPORT

A dozen active ingredients—many of them used to treat dry and itchy skin—were not assessed by the Panel, but were referred instead to the OTC Review Panel on Miscellaneous External Drug Products. This expert group planned a report on skin remedies, but its federal charter ran out and was not renewed because of budgetary constraints. So the report could not be completed; it will have to be finished by a new panel or by the FDA.

The Miscellaneous External Drug Panel did prepare a rough draft of its write-ups on these ingredients, some of which are widely used in soaps, skin creams, and lotions. These ingredients, their intended purposes (as listed by the FDA in a status report on the over-the-counter drug review), and the Panel's preliminary judgments are noted in the chart that follows:

Active Ingredients in Over-the-Counter Skin Remedy Products: Preliminary Assessments

Ingredient	Purpose	Panel's Tentative Assessment*
aloe vera	wound healer	not proved effective
castor oil	skin softener	not proved safe or effective
cetyl alcohol	chafing and chapping	not effective
chlorphyllins	wound healer	not proved effective
colloidal oatmeal	itch reliever	safe and effective
cottonseed oil	lubricant	not effective
ichthammol	anti-irritant	not proved effective
lanolin	skin softener	safe and effective
methanol	skin preparation	not safe
oxyquinoline	skin preparation	not safe
panthenol	anti-irritant	not proved effective
urea (2 to 10%)	itch reliever	safe and effective

*The Advisory Review Panel on OTC Miscellaneous External Drugs.

Safety and Effectiveness: Active Ingredients in Over-the-Counter Skin Protectants

Active Ingredient	Panel's Assessment	Approved Concentration (%)	For Ages
allantoin*	safe and effective	0.5–2	all
aluminum hydroxide gel	safe and effective	0.15–5	over 6 months†
bismuth subnitrate	not safe or effective		
boric acid	not safe or effective		
calamine (prepared calamine, calamine lotion)	safe and effective	1–25	all
cocoa butter	safe and effective	80–100	all
cornstarch	safe and effective	10–85	all
dimethicone (dimethyl polysiloxane)	safe and effective	1–30	all
glycerin (glycerine and glycerol)	safe and effective	20–45	over 6 months†
kaolin	safe and effective	4–20	all
petrolatum preparations: petrolatum and white petrolatum	safe and effective	30–100	all
shark-liver oil	safe and effective	3	over 2 years†
sodium bicarbonate	safe and effective	1–100	all
sulfur	not safe or effective		
tannic acid	not safe or effective		
zinc acetate*	safe and effective	0.1–2	over 2 years†
zinc carbonate	safe and effective	0.2–2	all
zinc oxide	safe and effective	1–25	all

*These ingredients—along with *live-yeast-cell derivative*—were also evaluated as wound-healing aids, for which they were granted only conditional approval, with the assessment: safe, but not proved effective.

†Approved for younger children when under medical supervision.

Unguents and Powders for the Skin: Product Ratings

Single-Ingredient Products

Product and Distributor	Dosage of Active Ingredients	Rating[1]	Comment
boric acid			
boric acid (generic)	**ointment:** 10%	**C**	not safe
Borofax (Burroughs-Wellcome)	**ointment:** 5%	**C**	not safe
calamine			
calamine lotion (generic)	**lotion:** 8% calamine + 8% zinc oxide	**A**	
cocoa butter			
cocoa butter (generic)	**lotion, cream, oil, soap**	**A**	
cornstarch			
cornstarch (generic)	**powder**	**A**	
glycerin			
glycerin (generic)	**liquid**	**A**	
Glycerin (Purepac)	**liquid**	**A**	
petrolatum preparations			
Vaseline (Chesebrough-Pond's)	**ointment:** white petrolatum, USP	**A**	
sodium bicarbonate			
Arm & Hammer Baking Soda (Church & Dwight)	**powder:** bicarbonate of soda, USP	**A**	
sodium bicarbonate (generic)		**A**	
tannic acid			
Amertan (Lilly)	**jelly:** 5% + thimerosal 1:5000	**C**	not safe or effective
zinc oxide			
Zincofax (Burroughs-Wellcome)	**cream:** 15%	**A**	
zinc oxide (generic)	**ointment:** 20%	**A**	
Zinc Oxide (CMC)		**A**	
Zinc Oxide (Lilly)		**A**	
zinc oxide (generic)	**paste:** 25% + 25% starch	**A**	

‹in protectants are often formulated into combination products containing benzocaine or other itch
ıd pain remedies. *See* pages 470–471.

Author's Interpretation of Panel criteria. Based on contents, not claims.

Vitamins and Minerals

The billion-dollar-a-year vitamin business came under federal purview
as early as 1906. Yet for technical, legal, and other reasons, the safety
and efficacy of such products have not been assessed in a thoroughgoing
way heretofore. The Panel report summarized here is the first FDA-
sponsored systematic review of nonprescription vitamin and mineral
products.

WHO NEEDS SUPPLEMENTS?

Vitamins are organic substances—that is, they are derived from
living matter in the form of plants, animals, or microbial sources. They
may be soluble in water or fats. Minerals and their salts are nonliving
chemicals. They are noncombustible, and so can be recovered from the
ash that is left when certain natural materials are burned at high temperatures.

The human body requires small amounts of vitamins and several
minerals to sustain health and life. Because the body cannot produce
these nutrients by itself, they must be obtained from external sources
—principally from the food we eat. A person may become deficient in
one or more of the essential nutrients for a variety of reasons such as
illness, pregnancy, or the use of special diets (including weight-loss
regimens). About a dozen of these deficiencies—for example, those
reflecting a lack of vitamins A, D, C, several of the B vitamins, calcium,

VITAMINS AND MINERALS is based on the report of the FDA Advisory Review
Panel on OTC Vitamin, Mineral and Hemantic Drug Products and the FDA's final order
withdrawing this document from its rule-making process.

and iron—can be safely and effectively prevented with over-the-counter supplements, once the need for such supplementation has been diagnosed by a doctor. Other deficits, however, require medical management with prescription vitamin products.

Panel findings indicate that over-the-counter vitamins are promoted, purchased, and swallowed out of all proportion to their real value. They are sometimes promoted for conditions they do not relieve and they may be combined with ingredients of dubious nutritional value (such as oyster shell, ox-bile extract, and green-pepper powder).

Many people, the Panel says, take vitamins to relieve self-diagnosed deficiency symptoms that in fact cannot be self-diagnosed because they are quite nonspecific and could be caused by a variety of underlying diseases. Fatigue and stress are good examples.

The common—and promotionally reinforced—belief that everybody needs vitamin supplements is *untrue*. Most children and adults who eat a normally balanced diet do not need them. In the Panel's view, supplements for the most part are required only by groups of people who have special nutritional and metabolic needs. Examples include:

- People on restricted diets whose intake of vitamins and minerals from natural sources may be limited.
- Heavy drinkers whose digestive and metabolic processes may be impaired or who simply do not eat regularly.
- Pregnant and nursing women who may have a heightened requirement for iron.
- People with intestinal disease who have difficulties absorbing vitamins and minerals from food.
- People taking prescription drugs that block nutrient absorption or interfere with their use in the body.
- People with severely limited financial resources who cannot buy the foods necessary for a balanced diet.

In one of its key decisions, the Panel therefore recommends that over-the-counter vitamin and mineral products be used only when the need for them has been established by a doctor. The Panel believes that once a doctor has established a need and has suggested a vitamin or mineral regimen to relieve the deficiency, health consumers can treat themselves by using approved over-the-counter products without further medical supervision. (This use of vitamins and minerals is, of course, different from prescription programs.)

CLAIMS

Accurate Labeling
"when the need for such therapy has been determined by a physician"

False or Misleading
references to "stress" as a condition for use
references to a product's being "natural," "geriatric," or "super-potent"

HOW MUCH IS NEEDED?

The question of how much of each nutrient a normal person needs is answered—on the basis of current scientific knowledge—by the Food and Nutrition Board of the National Academy of Sciences/National Research Council (NAS/NRC). This body periodically updates and reissues a chart of recommended Daily Dietary Allowances, commonly abbreviated as RDAs. Consult the RECOMMENDED DAILY DIETARY ALLOWANCES chart on pages 804–805.

The NAS/NRC claims the RDAs are "designed for the maintenance of good nutrition of practically all healthy people in the U.S.," and adds that "the allowances are intended to provide for individual variations among most normal persons . . . under usual environmental stress."

SOURCES OF VITAMINS AND MINERALS

Internal Contributors

Strictly defined, vitamins are essential organic nutrients that must be obtained from sources *outside* the body. Some vitamins, however, are made internally (even though additional amounts may still be required from external sources). Vitamin D, for example, is manufactured by a fatty biochemical in the skin when the skin is stimulated by sunlight. Some vitamin A and niacin are also made internally.

Some vitamins—particularly vitamin K and biotin—are not made by the body itself but by bacteria that reside in the intestines. Vitamin B_{12} is synthesized by bacteria in the colon. But these bacteria are probably too far down in the gut for people to absorb and use—thus each person must rely on external sources for this vitamin.

Recommended Daily Dietary Allowances (RDAs)

Water-Soluble Vitamins

	Age (years)	Vitamin C or Ascorbic Acid (mg)	Folacin (mcg)	Niacin (mg)	Riboflavin (mg)	Thiamine (mg)	Vitamin B$_6$ (mg)	Vitamin B$_{12}$ (mcg)
Infants	0.0–0.5	35	30	6	0.4	0.3	0.3	0.5
	0.5–1.0	35	45	8	0.6	0.5	0.6	1.5
Children	1–3	45	100	9	0.8	0.7	0.9	2
	4–6	45	200	11	1.0	0.9	1.3	2.5
	7–10	45	300	16	1.4	1.2	1.6	3
Males	11–14	50	400	18	1.6	1.4	1.8	3
	15–18	60	400	18	1.7	1.4	2.0	3
	19–22	60	400	19	1.7	1.5	2.2	3
	23–50	60	400	18	1.6	1.4	2.2	3
	51+	60	400	16	1.4	1.2	2.2	3
Females	11–14	50	400	15	1.3	1.1	1.8	3
	15–18	60	400	14	1.3	1.1	2.0	3
	19–22	60	400	14	1.3	1.1	2.0	3
	23–50	60	400	13	1.2	1.0	2.0	3
	51+	60	400	13	1.2	1.0	2.0	3
Pregnant		+20	+400	+2	+0.3	+0.4	+0.6	+1
Nursing		+40	+100	+5	+0.5	+0.5	+0.5	+1

Adapted from: Recommended Dietary Allowances, 9th ed., 1980 (National Academy Press), with the permission of the National Academy of Sciences, Washington, D.C.

Diet

Most of the vitamins and minerals people need are available in the food they eat if they eat a balanced diet. Ordinary foods provide remarkably large amounts of the recommended daily allowances (RDAs). The product-rating publication *Consumer Reports* has calculated, for example, that one McDonald's 7½ ounce Big Mac sandwich contains the following percentages of the RDAs for an adult woman:

vitamin A	5 percent
thiamine	52 percent
riboflavin	33 percent
vitamin B$_6$	13 percent
vitamin B$_{12}$	63 percent
niacin	55 percent
calcium	23 percent
phosphorus	44 percent
iron	23 percent

Recommended Daily Dietary Allowances (RDAs) *(continued)*

Fat-Soluble Vitamins			Minerals					
Vitamin A Activity (IU)	Vitamin D (IU)	Vitamin E Activity (IU)	Calcium (mg)	Phosphorus (mg)	Iodine (mcg)	Iron (mg)	Magnesium (mg)	Zinc (mg)
1,400	400	4.5	360	240	40	10	50	3
2,000	400	6	540	360	50	15	70	5
2,000	400	7.5	800	800	70	15	150	10
2,500	400	9	800	800	90	10	200	10
3,300	400	10.5	800	800	120	10	250	10
5,000	400	12	1,200	1,200	150	18	350	15
5,000	400	15	1,200	1,200	150	18	400	15
5,000	300	15	800	800	150	10	350	15
5,000	200	15	800	800	150	10	350	15
5,000	200	15	800	800	150	10	350	15
4,000	400	12	1,200	1,200	150	18	300	15
4,000	400	12	1,200	1,200	150	18	300	15
4,000	300	12	800	800	150	18	300	15
4,000	200	12	800	800	150	18	300	15
4,000	200	12	800	800	150	10	300	15
+1,000	+200	+3	+400	+400	+25	+30–60*	+150	+5
+2,000	+200	+4.5	+400	+400	+50	+30–60*	+150	+10

*Supplemental iron is recommended.

Over-the-Counter Vitamins and Minerals

Products for a particular deficiency state that meet the Panel's labeling standards can be used safely and effectively once the need has been established by a doctor, the Panel says. Its viewpoint is that a vitamin or mineral active ingredient becomes a nonprescription drug when it is used to prevent the development of a vitamin or mineral deficiency, or to treat a deficiency state once it has arisen.

A vitamin or mineral can be considered effective for over-the-counter use only if there is a specific disorder or condition that it can remedy or prevent. There must be a dose or dosage range that can be expected to produce this result when the vitamins are taken according to directions on the label. The vitamin or mineral must be present in a chemical form that will permit it to be absorbed from the gut and used by the body: that is to say, it must be bioavailable.

Several factors determine the safety of an over-the-counter vitamin or mineral product. One is the intrinsic safety of the ingredient or combination of ingredients. Since all vitamins and minerals considered (except choline) are essential human nutrients, the Panel believes all are intrinsically safe at recommended dosages. Safety also depends on whether the nutrient is safe for self-treatment. Manufacturers should put no more—or less—than the recommended daily dosage in a dosage unit. But it is up to the consumer not to exceed the dosages recommended in Panel and FDA guidelines as outlined below. Safety depends, too, on the quantity sold and ingested in each pill, capsule, or other dosage unit.

These dosage recommendations should not be confused with the RDAs for healthy individuals. The Panel's recommendations are for specific over-the-counter vitamins and mineral supplements that certain groups in the population require, *medically*, to prevent or correct deficiency states. For example, the RDA for vitamin C is 45 mg per day for adults. The Panel's recommended preventive dosage is 50 to 100 mg per day and for treatment it is 300 to 500 mg per day. The higher medicinal dosages (compared to the RDAs) are calculated to replenish tissue stores, compensate for the fact that not all of a nutrient that is ingested will be absorbed into the body, and provide a safe margin for error.

Prescription Vitamins and Minerals

In serious or severe deficiency states, the supplemental requirement must be identified by a doctor. He or she then must supervise the supplement's use for as long as needed. Pernicious anemia, a severe form of vitamin B_{12} deficiency, and pellagra, a niacin deficiency, are two such conditions that require prescription vitamins, which are generally administered by injection.

Vitamins and Minerals as Nutritional Supplements

Most over-the-counter vitamin products today are sold as *nutritional supplements*, not as drugs. This means that their labels can make no medicinal claims: they cannot say that the product will prevent or cure any symptom or disease. Because no medicinal claims are made, these products are regulated under the *food* section of the U.S. Food, Drug and Cosmetic Act, rather than under the part of that law that concerns drugs. The FDA defines them as foods "purported or represented to supplement a diet by increasing the total dietary intake of one or more essential vitamins or minerals."

The regulations for foods are far less strict than those for drugs. So manufacturers can sell and promote vitamins and minerals as nutritional supplements in larger dosages, and in combinations that the Panel believed would be unsafe or unwise.

The FDA's ability to protect consumers from manufacturers' blandishments for unnecessary and outrageously potent vitamin products was badly weakened by an amendment to the Food, Drug and Cosmetics Act called the "Proxmire Amendment," introduced several years ago by U.S. Senator William Proxmire (Dem.-Wisc.). As interpreted by the FDA, this amendment "essentially mandated that any regulation of the potency of vitamin and mineral products, whether sold as drugs or as dietary supplements, must be based on considerations of human toxicity rather than human need." In other words, the FDA cannot block the sale of over-the-counter products that are ineffective or unwise, unless they contain so much of a vitamin or mineral that they demonstrably endanger users' health.

Since the Panel was empowered to evaluate only drugs, dietary vitamins sold as dietary supplements are not considered here. The Panel says, however, that its conclusions on the safety, effectiveness, and appropriate labeling of vitamins and minerals as drugs may be relevant to their use as dietary supplements as well.

Status of Panel's Report

The Panel's report, upon which this unit is based, created much furor when it was published. Vitamin manufacturers and vitamin users united to condemn it. The FDA received thousands of protest letters.

Some objected to the Panel's conservative message that many more vitamins are taken than are needed. Others believed, incorrectly, that the Panel's proposals, if adopted by the FDA, would restrict the over-the-counter marketing of vitamins as nutritional supplements, as well as their marketing as drugs.

The result of this controversy—sadly—was that the FDA responded to pressures from consumers, manufacturers and Congress by withdrawing the Panel's recommendations from its rule-making procedures. This means that the present Panel's recommendations—unlike those of all other OTC Review Panels—is not being translated into regulations to ensure the safety and effectiveness of over-the-counter vitamin and mineral drug products.

The upshot, at least for a while, is that consumers are less well-protected by the FDA in their use of over-the-counter vitamin and mineral drug products than they are in the use of other classes of over-the-counter drugs. Consumers will have to be more self-reliant.

The Panel's report, summarized here, can be a key guide to making decisions about vitamins and minerals. For while the report has been withdrawn from the FDA's rule-making process, the agency continues to endorse its scientific accuracy and worth. It says "the information in the report will provide valuable guidance to both the agency and industry in the area of vitamins and minerals."

It can serve consumers in this role, as well.

DOSAGE

Maximum-Minimum

Vitamins, like all ingested substances—including water—have an upper limit beyond which they are no longer safe. Supplements should not be taken in doses greater than are needed to achieve the specific desired effect: relief of a deficiency. Taking more increases the risk of side effects. The Panel explicitly rejects the popular notion that if 1,000 units of a vitamin are useful and effective then 2,000 must be better. *This is not so.*

The therapeutic effects of vitamins and minerals are dose-related, so that more drug produces greater benefit *only* up to the point at which the drug saturates the body tissues in which it is stored and used, thus preventing or relieving the deficiency state. Beyond these saturating doses, which in general are the upper limits of the Panel's recommended dosages, some vitamins and minerals simply are excreted—and so are wasted. Others may be stored in such a way that they injure the tissue in which they reside (as in the case of vitamin A), produce undesirable metabolic effects (for example, vitamin D), or mask the presence of a serious underlying disease. High doses of folic acid, for example, will confound the diagnosis of pernicious anemia and vitamin B_{12} deficiency; excessive doses of vitamin C can interfere with commonly used urinary sugar tests for diabetes.

Vitamin and mineral overdoses can produce immediate or delayed toxic effects. Delayed reactions are particularly dangerous: some individuals who continue to overdose themselves with vitamin A experience few, if any, warning signs before they have severely damaged their livers. Vitamin C, which is widely taken in huge amounts, may increase the user's risk of kidney stones.

Because of these dangers, the Panel has identified a *maximum dose* for treatment. It is the level at which all scientifically recognized therapeutic effects can be achieved with minimal risk of side effects. This is the highest daily dose recommended for each individual vitamin when taken for treatment purposes, and the highest amount that should be in a pill or other dosage unit. The lower, or *minimum dose* for treatment is based, when possible, on clinical scientific studies in which the vitamin or mineral was used successfully to treat a deficiency state.

All recommended doses assume a one-a-day dosage schedule as a matter of convenience. Also for convenience, and because advertising campaigns constantly reinforce consumers' tendency to select one-a-day capsules, pills, or other units, the evaluators sought to select dosage levels that can be obtained in this way. For preventive use, the Panel recommends that each pill or other unit contain at least the minimum preventive dose, but no more than the maximum preventive dose. The same rule applies to products intended for therapy, except that for those vitamins and minerals that are not individually approved for treatment purposes, the *preventive* dosages should prevail in combination products.

Prevention-Treatment

While the dosages required to treat a deficiency are larger than those required to prevent it from occurring, the labels on many vitamin products blur or simply fail to say for which purpose the product has been formulated. The Panel believes that either "prevention" or "treatment" should be explicitly stated.

Some vitamins are safe for preventive use but not for treatment. For example, strict vegetarians are vulnerable to vitamin B_{12} deficiency. They can safely and effectively forestall this problem with a daily preventive supplement. But the vitamin B_{12} deficiency state—once it occurs—is a serious medical problem. It responds far better to injections of vitamin B_{12} supplements that are prescription drugs, and requires close medical management. So the Panel disapproves self-treatment of vitamin B_{12} deficiency with over-the-counter preparations and makes no dosage recommendation for this purpose. With other essential nutrients—like the mineral potassium—the margin between an effective dose and a toxic dose is so small that self-dosing simply cannot be recommended without the supervision that accompanies prescription use of the drug.

Biologic Activity

A particular vitamin may be obtainable from several chemical sources that may not always provide equivalent amounts of biologic activity. For example, 100 mg of ascorbic acid provides 100 mg of vitamin C biologic activity. But if sodium ascorbate is the vitamin C source, 112.5 mg are required to provide the same biologic activity. The Panel would like to see these equivalences stated on product labels. Equivalences, when available, are given in this unit where the particular vitamin is discussed.

Megavitamins

Some persons are claimed to need 10, 50, or even 100 times the recommended maximum doses of vitamins in order to achieve maximal health. The Panel doubts this is so, and endorses an NAS/NRC statement that says: "We are aware of no convincing evidence of unique health benefits accruing from consumption of a large excess of any one nutrient."

The claims that megavitamins relieve schizophrenia and other mental disorders have not been confirmed by scientifically valid studies. While some doctors claim excellent results, others have been unable to reproduce these results—which is the test of a therapy's merit.

"The claims made for mega-dose therapy are understandably attractive to individuals seeking symptomatic relief or recovery from conditions with no known cure," the Panel says. "At the present time, however, there is no scientific documentation for the rational use of mega-quantities of vitamins except for those rare individuals with a specific genetic defect."

Lacking such evidence, the Panel disapproves of mega-dosing. As further warning, it adds that acclimating the body to mega-doses will conceivably cause that body to react as if it were deficient in a vitamin or mineral when the mega-dosage is reduced.

NATURAL VITAMINS

There is no evidence to support the claim that vitamins derived from natural products (like dried plants) have any health advantage over manufactured vitamin products. The designation "natural" on the label implies an advantage that in fact is nonexistent.

The Panel disapproved of vitamins and minerals from these sources as inappropriate for use in over-the-counter drug products. The disapproved list includes:

acerola	algin	arginine
alanine	p-aminobenzoic acid	aspartic acid
alfalfa	apricot	beet greens

betaine
bioflavonoids, mixed
black currants
bone meal
bone phosphate,
  edible
brewers' yeast
buckwheat
cabbage
calcium phytate
carrot powder
chaparral
chlorophyll
chlorophyllins
citrus bioflavonoids
cobalamin
  concentrate
cod-liver oil
comfrey root
cystine
dandelion greens
date powder
desiccated liver
dolomite
dulse
duodenal substance
egg albumin
eggshell
egg yolk
fish-liver oil
glutamic acid
glycine
green buckwheat

green-pepper powder
hesperidin
hesperidin complex
histidine
inositol
isoleucine
kelp
lecithin
lemon bioflavonoid
  complex
lemon-grass oil
lettuce
leucine
linoleic acid
linolenic acid
liver fraction
liver fraction, insoluble
liver fractions A and 2
liver preparations
liver substance
liver substance
  concentrate
l-lysine
  monohydrochloride
lysine
magnesium aluminum
  hydroxide
malt extract
methionine
molasses
ox-bile extract
oyster shell
pancreatin

papain
papaya
parsley
peas
pepsin
phenylalanine
proline
protein hydrolysate
prune concentrate
red bone marrow
rice bran
rice oil, cold-pressed
rice polishings
rose-hips powder
rutin
serine
soy flower
spinach powder
sulfur
threonine
tillandsia
torula food yeast
torula yeast
tryptophan
turnip greens
tyrosine
unsaturated fatty
  acids (vitamin F)
valine
watercress
wheat germ
wheat-germ oil
yeast

COMBINATION PRODUCTS

There is a special rationale for multivitamin and vitamin-mineral combination products: deficiency states in pregnant women, dieters, and other vulnerable groups of people rarely affect a single nutrient; they usually involve 2 or more. So these combinations provide a rational means of preventing and treating deficiencies in these high-risk cases —provided that the products contain *all* the vitamins and minerals a target population may require.

Multimineral products are not good medicine, however. Only 3 minerals—iron, calcium, and zinc—are approved for nonprescription use, and deficiencies in these minerals rarely occur together.

To minimize consumer confusion and facilitate the use of combination products, the Panel formulated rules for what these products should contain. They should include only safe and effective ingredients within the recommended dosage ranges, except that pantothenic acid and vitamin E—which both are disapproved as *single*-ingredient products—may be included in combinations.

Combinations for Prevention

Approved

Fat-soluble A or D + *all* singly approved water-soluble vitamins
(C, B_{12}, folacin, niacin, B_6, riboflavin, thiamine). Vitamin E and
pantothenic acid may be added.
Any of the above + 1, 2, or all 3 approved minerals (iron, zinc, calcium).
For pregnant women: all singly approved vitamins + iron in approved
dose range + optional addition of zinc and calcium.
For heavy drinkers: high-dose combinations + zinc

Disapproved   Preparations containing only fat-soluble vitamins
(A, D, E, K)

Combinations for Treatment

Approved

All singly approved water-soluble vitamins (*see* above).
Those vitamins *not* recommended for treatment (B_{12}, folic acid, D) *if*
they are at maximum approved preventive doses. Vitamin E and/or
pantothenic acid may be added.
All B vitamins recommended for treatment (niacin, B_6, riboflavin,
thiamine) + folic acid and B_{12} (at highest preventive doses).
Vitamin C may be added and/or pantothenic acid may be added.

Disapproved   Inclusion of minerals.

OTHER INGREDIENTS

Besides active agents in vitamins and minerals a number of *inactive* ingredients are used in formulating over-the-counter products and are permissible in reasonable amounts. They include:

alcohol	polysorbate	soya lecithin
butyl paraben	polysorbate 20	soy oil, cold-pressed
corn oil	safflower oil	sucrose
formic acid	silicon dioxide (silica	vanilla
gelatin	and silicon)	wild-cherry
lactose	sodium benzoate	concentrate
lecithin	sodium saccharin	
pectin	sorbitol	

Any active ingredient that has not been reviewed by the Panel was automatically classified as not approved—that is, as not safe and/or not effective.

VITAMINS EVALUATED

Approved

Vitamin C (ascorbic acid) Supplements of vitamin C—also called *ascorbic acid*—are safe and effective for the prevention and treatment of vitamin C deficiency diagnosed by a doctor. The preventive dosage for children and adults is 50 to 100 mg per day. The therapeutic dose for children and adults is 300 to 500 mg per day.

Besides ascorbic acid, approved forms of this vitamin are: ascorbyl palmitate, calcium ascorbate, sodium ascorbate, and—for individuals who also need niacin—niacinamide ascorbate.

The reference form of vitamin C is ascorbic acid. The other approved forms are weaker, so that larger doses are required for equivalent results. A milligram of calcium ascorbate, for example, contains only 0.83 as much vitamin C as a milligram of ascorbic acid. So one will need 120 mg of calcium ascorbate to provide the equivalent of 100 mg of ascorbic acid. Similarly, each milligram of sodium ascorbate contains only 0.89 as much vitamin C as a milligram of ascorbic acid. Therefore 110 milligrams of sodium ascorbate will be needed to equal the 100 mg daily preventive dose of ascorbic acid.

The vitamin C deficiency state is called *scorbutic syndrome*, or more popularly, *scurvy*. Early scurvy symptoms include fatigue, spontaneous bleeding from the gums and other tissues, swollen joints, and aching muscles. Later the teeth loosen and may fall out. New wounds heal slowly, old ones tend to reopen. Emotional changes may also occur. Once a scourge of mariners and others who could not obtain fresh citrus fruit, scurvy is extremely rare today. The body contains a large pool of vitamin C—about 1500 mg in the well-nourished adult. Even if the vitamin is wholly withheld, body stores decrease only by about 3 percent per day. Since scurvy does not appear until body stores drop below 300 mg in an adult, this may take 4 or 5 months. Also, early symptoms are confusing because they may reflect many other disorders. Thus, medical tests are required to confirm the diagnosis.

While vitamin C is required by the body to prevent scurvy, it is also used as a helper or cofactor in the formation of connective tissue. It also helps sustain the internal chemical environment in which certain other life processes occur.

Humans, like some animal species, must replenish their vitamin C stores from external sources. But the vitamin is widely available in food. The average diet provides 30 to 250 mg daily of vitamin C. Even the lower amount, 30 mg, is enough to prevent scurvy in otherwise healthy persons. There are 124 mg of vitamin C in 8 ounces of fresh orange juice and 28 mg in a medium-sized tomato. So it is extremely unlikely that essentially healthy, well-fed individuals ever will need vitamin C supplements.

The vitamin C requirement is higher than normal for persons with peptic ulcers, hyperthyroidism, chronic diarrhea, cancer, serious burns, or surgical wounds. Pregnancy and nursing also increase vitamin C needs, as may cigarette smoking, use of oral contraceptives, and heavy ingestion of aspirin and some other drugs. Under none of these conditions, however, does the increased need exceed the amount that can be obtained through a diet that contains citrus fruit or other foods that are rich in vitamin C. There is no evidence to suggest that even people with the problems noted above need or would benefit from vitamin C supplements.

Many people consume large—even huge—amounts of vitamin C for reasons unrelated to the prevention and treatment of scurvy. Taking over 1 gram (1000 mg) daily is potentially hazardous: it may prompt the formation of kidney and bladder stones. This risk may be compounded if one eats foods with high levels of oxalate, a kidney-stone component; these foods include spinach, rhubarb, chocolate, and tea.

Some users take as many as 16 grams (16,000 mg) of vitamin C each day. Yet ingesting even 4 gm (4000 mg) daily can produce upset stomach, nausea, diarrhea, and perhaps more serious complications. Against these risks, there is no evidence that vitamin C—in large or small supplements—will relieve the several other conditions (unrelated to vitamin C deficiency) for which it often is promoted and used. There is no conclusive evidence, for example, that it will prevent or cure the common cold—and it is not approved for this use. Similarly, vitamin C is not effective against schizophrenia or other mental ills, atherosclerosis or blood clots, allergies or bed sores. Similarly, it is not safe and/or not effective as a nonprescription drug to combat blood disorders such as idiopathic methmeglobinemia, megaloblastic anemia, capillary fragility unrelated to vitamin C deficiency, iron deficiency, or the side effects of steroid drugs.

Vitamin B_{12} Vitamin B_{12} is extremely safe. No toxic manifestations have ever been described. Excesses for the most part are excreted in the urine. Vitamin B_{12}, a water-soluble vitamin, is required for the production of DNA, and thus is essential for cell replication. It also plays a number of other important biochemical roles. Animal meat (including liver), and fish, seafood, milk, and eggs are good sources of the vitamin. Vegetarians who add eggs and milk to their diets can ensure adequate B_{12} intake. The use of supplements for women taking oral contraceptives is only conditionally approved.

Vitamin B_{12} deficiency is extremely uncommon—in part because dietary requirements are low. The daily requirements are in the range of 0.3 to 2.5 micrograms (mcg). In a normal healthy adult, the liver can store 1000 to 1500 mcg of this vitamin—a 3- to 5-year supply.

Deficiencies in vitamin B_{12} occur in rare individuals who lack a gastric biochemical that is required for the vitamin's absorption into the body; this is called *pernicious anemia*. Similarly, deficiency can occur when the segment of the small intestine in which absorption occurs is removed or damaged by surgery or disease. Rare bacterial infections and fish-tapeworm infestations of the gut also can lead to vitamin B_{12} deficiencies. All these deficiencies can be treated with B_{12} supplements, but the therapy requires close medical supervision and is much more effective when the vitamin is injected rather than taken orally.

Vitamin B_{12} is approved as safe and effective for use without prescription in the *prevention* of B_{12} deficiency as long as doses are limited to 3 to 10 mcg daily for children over one year of age and adults, and when the need has been established by a doctor. It is disapproved for *treatment* of B_{12} deficiency; this should be managed by a doctor.

Approved oral form: the most commonly used form of vitamin B_{12} is cyanocobalamin. It is the only over-the-counter form approved for self-treatment purposes.

Disapproved oral form: liver extracts, which have been used for B_{12} supplementation, are not approved.

Folic acid Deficiency in folic acid, a B vitamin, leads to anemia

—which can be prevented by supplements. This condition appears to be relatively common and pronounced in pregnant and nursing women, and in heavy drinkers.

When the need for folic acid has been determined by a doctor, the safe and effective dosage is 1 mg daily for pregnant or lactating women and people who consume alcohol in excess. The safe and effective *preventive* dosage of over-the-counter folic acid for other adults and for children is 0.1 mg to 0.4 mg per day—once the need has been determined by a doctor.

In normal volunteers, experimental studies show that the liver stores about 7.5 mg of this vitamin. Less than one one-hundredth of this amount, 0.05 mg, is used each day. But because only a fraction of the folic acid that is ingested becomes available to the body, the approved preventive dose is higher.

Women taking oral contraceptives may be helped to maintain normal folic acid levels by supplements of 1 mg daily, but (as with B_{12}) neither the need for nor the efficacy of this treatment has been established, so such use is only conditionally approved. Self-dosing with over-the-counter supplements is *not* approved for the *treatment* of folic-acid deficiency, which requires medical management.

Folic acid, one form of the vitamin folacin, is also called pteroylmonoglutamic acid (PGA). It is water-soluble. Natural folacin is provided by a variety of foods—especially liver, leafy vegetables, fruits, and yeast. Only the synthetic folic acid is available in supplements.

All folic-acid sources must be broken down inside the body to be of physiological value. They work, in conjunction with Vitamin B_{12}, in the synthesis of DNA and in cell replication. Folic-acid depletion leads to the severe red-blood-cell deficiency state called *megaloblastic anemia*. Clinical signs include sore mouth, diarrhea, irritability, and forgetfulness—all of which are so nonspecific as to make self-diagnosis difficult.

Toxic reactions to folic acid are extremely rare, even when the vitamin is taken in massively large—and unnecessary—doses.

Niacin   Pellagra, which results from a severe deficiency of niacin, is rare. An early investigator described pellagra as being characterized by a "horrible crust" on the skin of the hands and neck; "painful burning of the mouth"; a "perpetual shaking of the body"; and "mania." Once fairly common, this disease has been largely eliminated by the enrichment of commercial flour with niacin supplements. So pellagra now is mostly a problem among some fad dieters, alcoholics, and patients with debilitating illnesses.

However, more modest deficits—manifested by conditions such as loss of appetite, weight loss, and poor milk production in nursing mothers—continue to occur. Also, several recent studies confirmed the popular impression that disadvantaged children suffer some signs of deficient dietary intake of the vitamin. Finally, the cancer drug 6-mercaptopurine and some other drugs have an antiniacin activity that requires patients to take niacin supplements.

Niacin is a B vitamin, which is also sometimes called nicotinic acid. It is water-soluble. Niacin by itself often causes facial flushing, itching, and other side effects when taken as a supplement in standard doses. So the Panel assessed it as unsafe and recommended its removal from the over-the-counter market. An alternative form of niacin, called *niacinamide* or *nicotinamide*, is the preferred and approved form of niacin, along with niacinamide ascorbate (which is approved only for persons who also need vitamin C).

Niacin is naturally obtained directly from food and in the body as a breakdown product of the essential amino acid tryptophan. Both sources are tapped by the ingestion of beef, cow's milk, and eggs, among other foods. Niacin is required for the respiratory activity of all body cells. It also stimulates a number of basic biological processes involving carbohydrates, amino acids, and fats.

Moderate deficiencies can be safely prevented or treated with niacinamide when the need has been determined by a doctor. The preventive dose of niacinamide for adults and for children over age one is 10 to 20 mg per day. The therapeutic dose is 25 to 50 mg per day.

Even very large doses of nicotinamide (niacinamide) can be taken safely; only one case of a toxic reaction appears in the medical literature —in a man who took far more than is needed to maintain health.

Vitamin B₆ (pyridoxine) Several large groups of people have a high incidence of vitamin B_6 deficiency, as measured by assays of vitamin B_6 and related biochemicals in the blood and urine. These groups include:

- *People with poor diets.*
- *Pregnant women.* Pregnancy may cause deficiency because B_6 crosses the placenta and becomes concentrated in the fetus. The RDA for pregnant women is 2.6 mg daily. The Panel believes, however, that this may be too little to restore blood levels to normal.
- *Infants fed heat-sterilized formulas.* Heat may destroy the vitamin.
- *Some women who use oral contraceptives.* As in pregnancy, this low level has not been shown to be dangerous. So, the Panel granted only

conditional approval to the large 20 to 25 mg daily dosage required to normalize blood levels.

- *Alcoholics*. Alcoholics tend to be deficient in vitamin B_6 because they eat poorly, have difficulty absorbing vitamins, and may excrete B_6 abnormally rapidly from their damaged livers.
- *Workers exposed to industrial air pollution*. Preliminary studies from the USSR suggest that such workers may have a greater need for this vitamin.

Vitamin B_6 has been proposed as a treatment for kidney stones. Conclusive evidence is lacking that it will prevent or relieve this condition, which requires medical management. Neither has it been demonstrated that vitamin B_6 will prevent morning sickness during pregnancy —as has been claimed.

Symptoms of B_6 deficiency, which are confusingly close to those for other B vitamin deficits, may (or may not) include inflammation of the tongue and mouth, shakes and seizures, irritability, and mental depression. The similarity of the several B-vitamin deficiency states is the reason why the Panel recommends that nonprescription preventive and B vitamin combinations include all 6 within the vitamin B group.

The B Vitamins

vitamin B_1 (thiamine)
vitamin B_2 (riboflavin)
vitamin B_6 (pyridoxine)
vitamin B_{12}
folic acid
niacin

Vitamin B_6 occurs in nature in a number of chemical forms, but the only commercially available supplemental source is pyridoxine hydrochloride. The vitamin is a cofactor in at least 60 different biologic reactions involved in the digestive breakdown of proteins and amino acids, and, to a lesser extent, with the metabolism of fats and carbohydrates and the synthesis of nucleic acid.

Dietary sources that are rich in B_6 include meat, cereals, lentils, nuts, avocados, bananas, and potatoes. Some of the vitamin is destroyed by cooking.

Large amounts—several hundred milligrams—of vitamin B_6 daily have been taken without observable ill effects. The much smaller doses of up to 25 mg per day recommended for nonprescription use therefore appear quite safe. Even less is actually needed: the RDA for persons on a *low*-protein diet is 1.25 to 1.5 mg per day; for persons on a *high*-protein diet it is 1.75 to 2 mg per day.

The Panel says that supplements to prevent or treat deficiencies are safe and effective when the need for vitamin B_6 has been determined by a doctor. The preventive dose for children and adults is 1.5 to 2.5 mg per day. The therapeutic dose is 7.5 to 25 mg per day.

Vitamin B_2 (riboflavin) Riboflavin deficiencies are rare. They tend to occur in alcoholics and people who eat poorly. Symptoms of vitamin B_2 deficiency include sore mouth and sore throat, pale and cracked lips, swollen tongue, skin disorders, itchy eyes, and cataracts.

The vitamin is available in supplements as riboflavin and as riboflavin-5-phosphate sodium. Both are effective and have a wide margin of safety; no toxic effects have ever been reported. Natural sources of the vitamin include eggs, meat, fish, and liver. The daily requirement for the vitamin is 2 to 2.5 mg daily, with heavy drinkers requiring more. Pregnant women and women on oral contraceptives have been shown to have lower blood levels of riboflavin but this deficit has not been proved to cause problems.

For those whose need for supplements has been determined by a doctor, over-the-counter riboflavin supplements are safe and effective for preventing deficiencies in adults and in children over 1 year of age. Preventive dosage is 1 to 2 mg per day. Safe and effective treatment dosage ranges from 5 to 25 mg per day. Timed-release preparations of riboflavin have been shown to work poorly—and are not approved.

Vitamin B_1 (thiamine) Malnutrition and alcoholism are the principal causes of beriberi—the severe, sometimes lethal form of vitamin B_1 deficiency—but a number of other common conditions, including pregnancy, illness, and old age will produce an asymptomatic deficit state that can be treated and corrected by thiamine supplements.

When the need for thiamine has been established by a doctor, dosages of 1 to 2 mg per day are safe and effective for preventing this deficiency in children and adults. Higher dosages of 5 to 25 mg daily are safe and effective for treatment purposes.

Thiamine is available in over-the-counter vitamins in 2 forms: thiamine hydrochloride and thiamine mononitrate.

The dietary requirement of 1 to 1.5 mg of vitamin B_1 daily for adults—a bit less for children—is principally provided by green vegetables, grains and meat; some comes from commercial vitamin fortification of flour and other food elements.

A rich natural source of thiamine is rice hulls, which is why beriberi was first shown to be a dietary deficiency in Orientals, who polished away the hulls because they liked to serve their rice gleaming white. They suffered nerve disorders, weakness, paralysis, mental degeneration, heart failure, and death as the result. (Some of these problems are seen in severely debilitated alcoholics, who require emergency thiamine replacement to survive.)

The vitamin's principal physiologic role is to help break down sugar for energy. Paradoxically, while poor diets produce thiamine deficiency, it is also true that the more calories one eats, the more thiamine one needs.

Contrary to promotional claims, thiamine is not useful against any condition except those related to thiamine deficiency. False and inaccurate claims have been made that it relieves skin conditions, multiple sclerosis, cancer, impotence, slow-wittedness, and drug toxicity. None of this has been shown to be true. Neither is there any evidence that vitamin B_1 will relieve fatigue or nervous disorders or improve one's thinking ability—unless these conditions were actually caused by thiamine deficiency.

Vitamin A   This vitamin is essential for sustaining the membrane structure and function of all body cells. It prevents night blindness—one of the earliest deficiency signs—as well as drying out of the skin and cornea of the eye and other, more serious problems. But most well-nourished people receive adequate amounts of vitamin A in their diets; deficiencies, which develop only slowly, are rare.

When need for the vitamin has been estalished by a doctor, a daily dose of 1250 IU (international units) to 2500 IU is safe and effective to prevent deficiencies in adults and in children over age one. A daily dose of 5000 to 10,000 IU is effective for treatment. Doses over 10,000 IU might be dangerous and should not be used for self-medication.

The term *vitamin A* actually describes several biochemicals that are found in rich amounts in whole-milk products, eggs, and fish liver, as well as in palm oil and other plant foods. Vitamin A from carotenoids—the orange-red plant pigment found in carrots, tomatoes, and other fruits and vegetables—is absorbed less well than animal sources of vitamin A, and so these sources are not recommended for therapeutic use.

The 3 forms of the vitamin used in nonprescription products are vitamin A (retinol), vitamin A acetate, and vitamin A palmitate. Vitamin A is oil-soluble, but also can be formulated in emulsions and water-soluble forms. For over-the-counter use, it does not matter which form is used. However, claims that cod-liver oil and other natural sources of vitamin A in animals are superior to other forms remain unproved.

In fact, *excessive use* may incur more problems than deficiency! Regular overuse of the vitamin can produce a chronic toxicity characterized by loss of appetite, blurred vision, muscle soreness after exercise, the appearance of reddish pimples on the shoulders and back, and drying out of the skin. Severe liver damage may occur. This chronic syndrome is diagnosed most often in youngsters, and seems to occur when infants are given more than 37,500 IU daily. The condition develops more slowly in adults, who can store large amounts of the vitamin in their livers before it begins to cause damage.

Acute toxic reactions have been reported in adults taking 2 to 5 million IU of vitamin A, and in infants given much smaller doses. The symptoms of this acute poisoning include severe headache centered in the forehead and eyes, dizziness, drowsiness, nausea, and vomiting. These effects occur within 6 to 8 hours. A few hours later the skin reddens and swells. Later it flakes and peels.

The toxic problems of vitamin A supplements are compounded by the fact that the vitamin loses its potency in the bottle. Manufacturers therefore sometimes put up to 40 percent more than the labeled amount into their products; the Panel would like this overage to be reduced to 25 percent.

Many spurious claims have been made for vitamin A. It has not been proven safe or effective as a nonprescription drug for preventing or treating plantar warts, acne, bed sores, respiratory infections, vision problems or eye defects, or dry, scaly, wrinkled, or thickened skin.

Vitamin D The "sunshine vitamin" is synthesized from a cholesterol-like substance in the skin when we are exposed to sunlight. Most people obtain all or almost all the vitamin D they need in this way. Principal sources of the vitamin are fatty fish, egg yolk, liver, and butter. Vitamin D is added by food processors to milk, breakfast cereals, bread, chocolate, and other foods.

Vitamin D helps the body absorb dietary calcium from the gut. It is required, too, for the formation and replacement of bone. So children —with growing bones—need more than adults. The vitamin D deficiency states—which include defective bone growth in children (rickets) and soft bones (osteomalacia) in adults—require careful medical care. So vitamin D deficiencies should not be treated with over-the-counter vitamin D supplements.

Vitamin D deficiency diseases are relatively rare in the United States. They are more likely to occur among people who are malnourished and in dark-skinned persons—who produce less vitamin D of their own in response to sunlight than lighter-skinned persons do. Vegetarians and people who avoid fatty foods are also candidates, as are very premature infants (who, of course, require medical attention). In fact, vitamin D deficiency is so uncommon in relatively well-nourished populations that some experts think that the practice of fortifying foodstuffs with vitamin D may be unwise.

Conclusive evidence is lacking to support claims that vitamin D supplements will prevent or cure osteoporosis in older people, or that it can lower serum cholesterol. Its use is disapproved for these purposes. There is also no evidence that multivitamin preparations containing minerals and vitamin D are better than forms that contain vitamin D without the minerals.

However, *preventive* use of these supplements is safe and effective in dosages of 400 IU for children up to age 18, and 200 IU for adults— provided the need for such supplementation has been established by a doctor.

Two forms of the vitamin are approved for nonprescription use. One is cholecalciferol, which is called vitamin D_3. It is the form made in animal tissues, including human skin. The other is ergocalciferol, a synthetic vitamin derived from plant material. These forms are equally potent. Several other forms of the vitamin are disapproved by the Panel because they are too new, and too little studied for use as over-the-counter drugs. They are listed below.

> 25-hydroxylated vitamin D
> 1,25-hydroxylated vitamin D
> 24,25-hydroxylated vitamin D
> 1-alpha-vitamin D
> 5,6-trans-vitamin D

Excess vitamin D is not excreted in the urine to any great extent. Rather, it continues to build up in dangerous amounts in body tissues. Since vitamin D binds and holds calcium in the body, this may result in disorders associated with excess calcium absorption—including kidney stones, mental deficiencies, heart changes, and the buildup of calcium in the kidneys, heart, and blood vessels. Early symptoms include weakness, fatigue, malaise, dry mouth, aches and pains, and a host of other relatively nonspecific complaints.

Approved Only in Combinations

Vitamin E   This vitamin is widely used—often in enormous doses —for a variety of disease states for which it has not been proved to be helpful. Its principal virtue seems to be its lack of toxicity. Some people have taken thousands and tens of thousands of international units (IU) of vitamin E for extended periods of time, even though the RDA for adults is only 12 to 15 IU daily and that for children is less.

Except in a few premature infants and a few adult victims of severe illnesses that involve medical management, vitamin E deficiency is rare to nonexistent. So vitamin E is disapproved as inappropriate for use by itself. However, it is approved—for preventive use only—in combination products sold for the prevention of multiple vitamin deficiencies of the sort that threaten chronic alcoholics, persons with vitamin malabsorption syndromes, and those who get few nutrients because they eat very badly. Provided such a need has been medically established, the acceptable daily dosage is 30 IU in the form of tocophersolan, alphatocopheryl acetate, alpha-tocopheryl acid succinate, or vitamin E.

Most vitamin E preparations now state the dosage per tablet, capsule or other dosage unit in IUs, as well as in milligrams. Below are the relative potencies of 1 mg of several of the available forms of vitamin E:

1 mg dl-alpha tocopheryl acetate	= 1 IU vitamin E
1 mg dl-alpha tocopherol	= 1.1 IU vitamin E
1 mg d-alpha tocopheryl acetate	= 1.36 IU vitamin E
1 mg d-alpha tocopherol	= 1.49 IU vitamin E
1 mg d-alpha tocopheryl acid succinate	= 1.21 IU vitamin E
1 mg dl-alpha tocopheryl acid succinate	= .89 IU vitamin E

Vitamin E is supplied naturally by soybean products, safflower oil, nuts, cereals, and other foods. It appears to contribute to the function of the muscular, vascular, and nervous systems. But, other than *slight* changes in the survival time of red blood cells, the consequence of vitamin E deficiencies have been hard to document.

Claims have been made that large doses of this vitamin enhance fertility, are of benefit against leg cramps, heart and vascular-system diseases, and several rarer disorders that include the finger-curling condition called Dupuytren's contracture. These claims have not been proved.

Pantothenic acid   This vitamin, ubiquitous in plants and animals, was given a Greek name that means "from everywhere." It is abundant in meat, whole grains, and vegetables.

Pantothenic acid's ubiquity is matched by its biologic importance to humans and other living organisms. It is a precursor of the biochemical coenzyme A, a substance required for a number of biologic transformations including energy release and the metabolism of fat, carbohydrate, and protein.

Deficiency of this vitamin is quite rare and has never been produced experimentally by withholding the vitamin from the diet. A nerve disorder called "burning-feet syndrome" that occurs in malnourished prisoners of war and some rural populations in Asia has been attributed to deficit of the vitamin—but these populations well may suffer from other nutritional lacks that are responsible for such symptoms. Similarly, alcoholics may be deficient in this vitamin—but they, too, are likely to be generally malnourished. Most conditions for which pantothenic acid might prove useful require medical management—so the vitamin has a very limited place in nonprescription medication.

Because the vitamin is so widely available in foods, pantothenic acid deficiency is virtually unknown in the United States. So the Panel disapproves its use as a single-ingredient over-the-counter product. However, if a need for it has been established by a physician, the vitamin may safely be used in amounts of 5 to 20 mg per day in combination products. These combinations contain other essential nutrients for the prevention of multiple vitamin deficiencies that may occur in chronic alcoholics, persons with malabsorption problems, and others who eat very poorly. Approved forms of this water-soluble vitamin, which appears to be relatively nontoxic, include calcium pantothenate and dexypanthenol.

Disapproved Vitamins

Biotin   Biotin is an extremely potent, water-soluble vitamin that is widely distributed in nature in small amounts. The average diet provides 100 to 300 mcg of biotin daily, which appears adequate to meet nutritional needs when added to the still-undetermined amount of this vitamin that is formed naturally in the human gut.

The vitamin is a cofactor in many food and energy transformations. These include the digestion and use of carbohydrates, buildup of fatty acids, and interconversions of amino acids.

Little is known about the toxicity of biotin supplements and no upper limit has been set. But the vitamin appears to be relatively harmless.

Deficiency is marked by a red, scaly skin disease that can be relieved by supplements—but this condition is so rare that only *2 cases* are known to have occurred. Indeed, the only way to induce the deficiency appears to be by eating enormous quantities of raw eggs—and little else—since uncooked egg white contains a chemical that inactivates biotin. Because biotin deficiency is virtually nonexistent, there is no need for supplements—which accounts for the Panel's disapproval of biotin as an over-the-counter drug.

Choline   Strictly speaking, choline is not a vitamin. It is a constituent of several essential fatty substances and serves in the formation of acetylcholine, which is required for the transmission of nerve impulses. The average daily diet contains 150 to 900 mg of choline. Toxic effects have not been reported.

Choline deficits can be induced experimentally in animals, and may have some role in the fatty liver condition that occurs in some children who are starving to death, as well as in alcoholics. But no relationship has ever been demonstrated between dietary choline deficiency in humans and the occurrence or severity of alcoholic fatty liver. Neither is choline beneficial for treating this condition. Since choline deficiency has never been diagnosed, has not been produced experimentally in a human subject, and appears to be virtually nonexistent in the United States, inclusion of choline, choline bitartrate, choline chloride, or choline citrate in over-the-counter vitamin or mineral products was judged to be unwarranted.

Summary of Panel's Recommended Daily Vitamin Doses

Vitamin	Preventive Dose	Therapeutic Dose
vitamin C		
children over 1 and adults	50–100 mg	300–500 mg
vitamin B$_{12}$		
children over 1 and adults	3–10 mcg	not approved
folic acid		
children over 1 and adults	0.1–0.4 mg	not approved
pregnant and lactating women	1 mg	not approved
alcoholics	1 mg	not approved
niacin		
children over 1 and adults	10–20 mg	25–50 mg
vitamin B$_6$		
children over 1 and adults	1.5–2.5 mg	7.5–25 mg
riboflavin		
children over 1 and adults	1–2 mg	5–25 mg

Summary of Panel's Recommended Daily Vitamin Doses *(continued)*

Vitamin	Preventive Dose	Therapeutic Dose
thiamine		
children over 1 and adults	1–2 mg	5–25 mg
pantothenic acid*		
children over 1 and adults	5–20 mg	not approved
vitamin A		
children over 1 and adults	1250–2500 IU	5000–10,000 IU
vitamin D		
children under 18	400 IU	not approved
adults over 18	200 IU	not approved
vitamin E*		
children over 1 and adults	30 IU	not approved

*Approved in combination products *only.*

Vitamins: Comparison of Risk of Deficiency Against Risk of Overdose

OTC Vitamin	Deficiency Risk, U.S. Population	Overdose Risk
Approved		
vitamin C	low	low
vitamin B_{12}	low	nil
folic acid	low (except in pregnancy)	nil
niacin	low	low
vitamin B_6	high	low
riboflavin	low	nil
thiamine	moderate	nil
pantothenic acid	nil	nil
vitamin A	unclear	moderate
vitamin D	low	moderate
vitamin E	nil	nil
Disapproved		
biotin	nil	nil
choline	nil	nil
vitamin K	nil	moderate

Note: Evaluations reflect author's interpretation of Panel report.

Vitamin K   At present, vitamin K (phytonadione) is sold only by prescription. Deficiency states due to low dietary intake rarely if ever occur in the United States. The therapeutic dose for individuals who require it is very close to the toxic dose. So the use of vitamin K needs to be closely supervised by a physician.

MINERALS EVALUATED

Approved

Calcium   Because it is a principal skeletal component and is present in all cells, calcium is one of the most common elements in the human body. The average adult carries 4 pounds of calcium, 99 percent of it in bone. Many people—of all ages and both sexes—may need calcium supplements. When this need has been established by a doctor, over-the-counter calcium supplements are safe and effective for the prevention of deficiency states in these dosages:

Infants up to 6 months: 200 to 400 mg per day
Infants 6 months to 1 year: 300 to 600 mg per day
Children 1 to 10: 400 to 800 mg per day
Children 10 to 12: 600 to 1200 mg per day
Children over 12 and adults to age 51: 400 to 800 mg per day
Adults over 51: 500 to 1000 mg per day
Pregnant and nursing women: 600 to 1200 mg per day

Mineral calcium is available in these 8 approved forms:

calcium carbonate, precipitated   calcium gluconate
calcium caseinate   calcium lactate
calcium citrate   calcium phosphate dibasic
calcium glubionate   calcium sulfate

Calcium supplements within the approved limits are safe. But higher intakes from excessive use of supplements can very quickly lead to the dangerous calcium excess state (hypercalcemia). In some individuals this risk is exacerbated by supplements of vitamin D, which binds to calcium and can enhance its absorption into the body. Hypercalcemia damages the kidneys, heart, blood vessels, and other organs. It can cause painful kidney stones, make the heartbeat dangerously irregular, and impair mental processes. Early signs of this disorder include weakness, fatigue, malaise, dry mouth, vague muscular and skeletal aches and pains, headache, and a metallic taste in the mouth.

In Western countries, the mean daily calcium intake is between 500 and 1200 mg daily; after age 12, males consume more than females.

Many women, in fact, ingest less than the calcium RDA, which is 800 to 1200 mg.

The calcium one takes in through food and the calcium one's body absorbs are not the same thing, because a number of factors influence calcium absorption. Children absorb 75 percent of the calcium they consume, for example, while adults absorb only 30 to 60 percent of their dietary intake. And while vitamin D enhances calcium uptake, ingestion of foods high in phosphate content—including cocoa, soy beans, kale, and spinach—*decrease* intestinal absorption of calcium.

The intestine compensates to some extent for changes in dietary calcium: the less that is consumed, the more that is absorbed. This protective mechanism weakens with age, however, which may be why many older women and some older men suffer from the bone-wasting disease osteoporosis.

Milk and dairy products are a principal source of calcium, particularly for youngsters. Many parents properly insist that young children drink lots of milk, then relax the insistence as the children get older. This may be a mistake, however, for a person's greatest need for calcium—whether in milk and other foods or from supplements—is in the preadolescent years, 10 to 13, when the bones are growing rapidly toward adult proportions.

Pregnant women and nursing mothers also need more calcium because they are providing it for their babies. So do older people, whose bodies absorb and use calcium less effectively than younger people do.

Calcium depletion and the severe deficiency state (hypocalcemia) require medical management. So calcium supplementation is disapproved for treatment of these conditions and is approved only for *preventive* use.

Iron   Iron is an essential component of the heme molecule, in the red pigment (hemoglobin) of red blood cells. It is hemoglobin that transports oxygen to all living body cells. The adult body contains some 4 grams of iron in blood, bone marrow, the liver, and the spleen. While the usual American diet provides 10 to 20 mg daily, many population subgroups appear to be iron deficient. In fact, many of their members may be manifestly anemic.

The need for supplements to prevent iron deficiency thus appears to be greater than for any other essential nutrient supplied in over-the-counter products. The Panel approves supplements as safe and effective—once the need has been medically established—as outlined below:

Infants and children, 6 months to 5 years: 10 to 15 mg per day
Children over 5, men, and nonpregnant women who take a
   combination product: 10 to 20 mg per day
Menstruating and nursing women: 10 to 30 mg per day
Pregnant women: 30 to 60 mg per day

The Panel also conditionally approved the use of preventive doses of 10 to 20 mg per day over-the-counter iron supplements—when recommended by a physician—for adolescent boys (ages 12 to 17) and men and women over age 60. There is evidence, although inconclusive, that many people in these groups need these supplements.

The use of over-the-counter iron supplements is *not* approved for the treatment of iron-deficiency anemia, which is a serious health problem that demands medical attention. The Panel recommends that all iron products carry this warning: *The treatment of any anemic condition should be under the advice and supervision of a physician.*

Iron supplements are sold in a variety of chemical forms, some of which are more readily absorbed than others.

Approved iron sources

ferroglycine sulfate	ferrous gluconate
ferrous lactate	ferrous succinate
ferrous fumarate	ferrous sulfate, dried
ferrous glutamate	

Conditionally approved sources

ferrous citrate	ferric pyrophosphate
ferric ammonium phosphate	ferrous tartrate
ferric phosphate	ferrous carbonate

Disapproved sources

ferric versenate	ferric sulfate
ferric citrate	ferric ammonium citrate
ferrocholinate	

Conditional approval was granted pending proof that the substances are absorbed at least four-fifths as well as the reference form, ferrous sulfate. Poor absorption accounts for the disapprovals.

The reference form—ferrous sulfate—contains 20% iron. Other approved forms contain differing amounts:

- ferroglycinate sulfate contains 16% iron, so that equivalent dose, in milligrams, would be 1.2 times that of ferrous sulfate
- ferrous lactate is 19% iron, so the equivalent dose, in milligrams, would be about the same as that of ferrous sulfate

- ferrous fumarate is 33% iron, so the equivalent dose, in milligrams, is only 0.6 as much as that of ferrous sulfate
- ferrous gluconate is 11.6% iron, so the equivalent dose, in milligrams, is 1.8 times as much as that of ferrous sulfate
- ferrous succinate is 39% iron, so the equivalent dose, in milligrams, is only 0.54, or about half as much as that of ferrous sulfate.

Iron compounds are formulated with a number of other substances, for a variety of reasons. For example, there is some inconclusive evidence that combinations of iron with the laxative dioctyl sodium sulfosuccinate relieve the constipation and other gastrointestinal distress that many people experience when they take iron. Combinations of an approved iron source and dioctyl sodium sulfosuccinate are conditionally approved, pending definitive proof of their efficacy. Other combinations, prepared for a variety of reasons, are disapproved, including iron combined with magnesium trisilicate, cobalt, copper, vitamin B_{12}, intrinsic factor, liver stomach concentrate, and molybdenum.

People taking high doses of iron—in the range of 200 mg—often complain of nausea, abdominal cramps, constipation, and diarrhea. One reason iron is sold in so many different forms is that manufacturers are trying to provide preparations that can be better tolerated. But the Panel says that there is no significant difference in distress in the gastrointestinal tract when doses equivalent in potency of these preparations are taken. Dosages under 100 mg per day are unlikely to cause these side effects.

Zinc   This mineral is required for many body functions, and zinc depletion is reported to occur with a number of serious illnesses. They include retarded growth and sexual development in severe malnutrition, leg ulcers, sickle-cell anemia, and a rare genetic inflammatory disorder of the skin (acrodermatitis enteropathica) that usually occurs in babies. So there is cause for concern in the fact that a number of studies indicate many Americans live on diets marginal-to-deficient in zinc.

The mineral is approved in the form of zinc sulfate as safe and effective for preventive use when the need for it has been established by a doctor. Supplements are not approved for self-treating zinc deficiencies, which are extremely difficult even for doctors to diagnose. The Panel warns specifically that self-medication with zinc should not be attempted for leg ulcers or rheumatoid arthritis and also cautions that zinc depletion associated with sickle-cell disease and other clinical illness requires medical management.

Zinc is an ingredient in more than a dozen of the body's enzymes and coenzymes, and contributes to the synthesis of proteins and nucleic acids. It is required for growth and development, wound-healing, and other important physiologic processes, including the sense of smell.

Protein-rich foods—including meat, eggs, milk products, and shellfish—are also those that tend to be rich in zinc. Unsupplemented vegetarian diets may be deficient in zinc and diets that are high in fiber and in the chemical phytate—which is abundant in grains, nuts, and legumes—appear to specifically reduce the availability of dietary zinc, as do phosphates.

The RDA for zinc is 10 mg in children and 15 mg in adults—except pregnant and nursing women, in whom it is 20 to 30 mg. The danger levels for acute zinc toxicity are several hundred times higher. The question of whether ongoing, lower levels of zinc supplementation may be dangerous has not been fully resolved. Zinc reacts with iron, copper, and other minerals in the body. Thus, too much zinc may cause dangerous imbalances in these substances.

The Panel's approved preventive dosage schedule and the approved forms are:

Children over 1 and adults: 10 to 25 mg per day
Pregnant and nursing women: 25 mg per day

The approved form of zinc is zinc sulfate. Conditionally approved forms include zinc carbonate, zinc chloride, and zinc gluconate. Disapproved forms include zinc hydroxide, zinc oxalate, zinc phytate, and zinc sulfide.

Disapproved

According to the panel, a number of minerals that currently are sold over-the-counter are not safe and/or not effective for self-medication. In the case of some minerals, the deficiency state requires medical diagnosis. For others, both preventive and therapeutic supplementation must be medically supervised because there is a narrow margin between the useful dose and the toxic dose. Too, for some minerals, deficiency states are rare to nonexistent—so there is no need for health consumers to self-treat with over-the-counter products.

Copper Copper, an essential nutrient in trace amounts, is widely available in many foods including nuts, liver, shellfish, kidney, raisins, and dried legumes. The adult body contains 15 to 150 mg of this metal. As a result of the mineral's wide availability, deficiency is extremely rare. (One exception might be in premature infants who have been fed formulas that have little copper.)

The greater danger is excessive intake of copper, which can accumulate in the body and cause a variety of toxic symptoms and can cause death. The early signs of copper intoxication are nonspecific: nausea, vomiting, diarrhea, and headache. These effects may occur even if the intake of copper supplements is relatively low.

For these reasons, the Panel disapproves the use of copper as a nonprescription mineral and recommends that it be removed from over-the-counter products—where it may be present as copper (cupric) gluconate, copper oxide, or copper sulfate.

Fluoride   The body requires trace amounts of fluoride. But this need is met by the drinking of fluoride in fluoridated and non-fluoridated drinking water, and also from the fluoride that is present in a variety of foods. The fluoridation of community water supplies—intended to prevent dental cavities—does not appear to be harmful. But there have been reports of acnelike skin eruptions, hives, itching, and swelling in persons using fluoride-vitamin products and toothpastes enriched with fluoride. Because of these risks, the Panel disapproves of the presence of sodium fluoride or calcium fluoride supplements in over-the-counter vitamin-mineral products and recommends that they be banned.

Iodine   Iodine is required for the synthesis of thyroid hormone. Adults need 100 mcg (micrograms) to 200 mcg daily. But the average American consumes more than 300 mcg each day through tap water, seafood, vegetables, meat, eggs, and dairy products, as well as from iodized salt, salt that has been commercially fortified with this mineral.

Dietary deficiency of iodine can lead to swelling of the thyroid gland, a disease called *goiter*. This disorder was fairly common in the Midwest and Pacific Northwest where the land and its crops are iodine-poor, and seafood was not commonly available. The introduction of iodized salt markedly reduced the incidence of goiter, but recent surveys showed that it continued to occur—usually in women of child-bearing age—in Michigan and Texas. This problem now has been largely ameliorated by public-health measures to promote iodine intake.

The need for ingesting iodine supplements in over-the-counter products thus is small, and the risk may be great since iodine toxicity (iodism) can lead to a number of untoward consequences, including, paradoxically, goiter. For these reasons there is no rationale for including iodine sources like calcium iodate or potassium iodide in over-the-counter drug products used to prevent or treat iodine deficiency. The Panel recommends they be banned.

Magnesium   The body contains about an ounce of magnesium, most of it stored in bone and muscle. It is an important activator for many enzyme systems involved in the utilization of food for energy. It also plays a role in protein synthesis and the maintenance of electrical potentials in the neuromuscular system. Most diets provide 150 to 480 mg of magnesium daily; about 250 to 300 mg per day are required by an average-sized adult man. Cereals, nuts, seafood, peas, beans, corn, and soybeans are rich sources.

The small intestine, through which most of the mineral is absorbed into the body, controls magnesium levels: the amount absorbed decreases as intake rises. The body also has a striking ability to conserve this mineral. When magnesium is absent from the diet, the kidneys retain (rather than excrete) it. Thus less than 12 mg per day is lost in the urine. But when too much is ingested, the kidneys rapidly excrete it.

Because magnesium is widely available in food and efficiently conserved by the body, its deficiency (hypomagnesemia) is essentially nonexistent in the average American. It occurs in a few malnourished alcoholics, and in other persons with problems in absorbing magnesium. These problems require continuing medical care, and, when magnesium supplements are required, they usually must be given by injection because such patients rarely respond adequately to oral magnesium.

For the reasons cited above, there is no reason to put magnesium into over-the-counter drug products. Nor should one self-treat with the mineral. The Panel disapproved—and proposed a ban on—all over-the-counter products that contain magnesium in any of these forms:

magnesium carbonate	magnesium oxide
magnesium chloride	magnesium silicate
magnesium gluconate	magnesium sulfate
magnesium hydroxide	magnesium trisilicate

Manganese   This mineral frequently is put into mineral supplements and preparations of blood-forming substances. But its value as a nonprescription ingredient has yet to be proved.

Manganese is absorbed from the small intestine; carried in the blood; stored in the liver, skin and skeletal muscles; and excreted in the bile. An adult male has about half an ounce of it in his body. Cereal products, leafy fresh vegetables, nuts, and dried fruits are the richest dietary sources.

A principal medical concern about manganese is chronic manganism. This is a disorder of the central nervous system that causes tremors and more severe symptoms. It is most prevalent among manganese miners, but could also afflict people who ingest high levels of the mineral.

Manganese is required by several of the enzymes that regulate the body's food utilization. Manganese may be involved in atherosclerosis and other serious illnesses, but no satisfactory evidence has been proposed to explain how manganese therapy might be helpful. More important—from the average consumer's point of view—no overt and unequivocal case of manganese deficiency has ever been found! Given the absence of any demonstrable need or value for manganese supplements, and considering the very real risks of its use, the panel disapproves manganese as a nonprescription ingredient and proposes that it be removed from the market. It is usually sold in the following forms: manganese chloride, manganese gluconate, and manganese oxide.

Minerals: Comparison of Risk of Deficiency Against Risk of Overdose

OTC Mineral	Deficiency Risk, U.S. Population	Overdose Risk
Approved		
calcium	moderate	moderate
iron	high	high
zinc	moderate	moderate
Disapproved		
copper	low	moderate
fluoride	nil	moderate
iodine	low	moderate
magnesium	low	low
manganese	nil	moderate
phosphorus	nil	moderate
potassium	low	moderate

Note: Evaluations reflect author's interpretation of Panel report.

Phosphorus   This mineral is abundantly present in any diet that includes milk, poultry, fish, and meat. Nonnutritive soft drinks may contain excessive amounts of it in the form of phosphoric acid. Phosphorus and calcium interact in the body, and because of the high phosphorus intake achieved on meat-rich Western diets, the possible consequences of excess phosphorus intake on calcium excretion are of greater public health concern than phosphorus depletion—which appears to be virtually nonexistent. About the only time it is known to occur is in persons who take excessive amounts of certain antacids. Problems of too much phosphorus fortunately are also rare because the kidneys, unless severely diseased, are capable of quickly removing large excess amounts of it. The Panel disapproved of the marketing and use of phosphorus in over-the-counter preparations.

Potassium   Many body organs require small amounts of potassium for normal function. But excessive amounts of this mineral can lead quickly to cardiac arrest and death.

The kidneys largely control potassium balance in the body and usually are able to rapidly get rid of large excesses. Persons with damaged or malfunctioning kidneys cannot so easily rid themselves of excess potasssium and, in fact, large doses of potassium may be hard even for normal kidneys to manage.

There is little if any need for self-dosing with over-the-counter potassium supplements. The mineral is so abundant in animal and vegetable foods that it is difficult to design a diet that provides adequate amounts of calories but does not satisfy the daily potassium requirement. The deficiency state, hypokalemia, rarely if ever occurs simply because one has taken in too little potassium. The usual cause is illness —including diarrhea (the principal cause of hypokalemia in children), severe malnourishment, or perhaps alcoholism. Many alcoholics have low serum potassium levels. So do persons with high blood pressure who routinely take diuretics; this is why doctors often prescribe a supplement for hypertensives on diuretics.

The early symptoms of hypokalemia are common to many illnesses. They include lethargy, irritability, and a decrease in deep tendon reflexes. Laboratory tests are required to establish the diagnosis; thus medical management is clearly required.

Therefore there is no justification for routine self-medication with over-the-counter potassium supplements. The Panel recommended that nonprescription sale of potassium supplements be banned; they are available as potassium chloride, potassium gluconate, and potassium sulfate.

Other Trace Minerals   More than a dozen other mineral elements have been shown to be essential in animals, but not in humans, or are needed by people in such tiny trace amounts that a normally balanced diet is a sufficient source. Some of these minerals can be toxic, including at least one, selenium, that is sold over-the-counter. The Panel says the following substances should not be present in significant amounts in over-the-counter mineral products, since there is no known use for them in this form.

aluminum	chromium	selenium
arsenic	lead	silicon
barium	lithium	strontium
beryllium	molybdenum	tin
cadmium	nickel	vanadium

Safety and Effectiveness: Panel's Assessment of Over-the-Counter Vitamins

Vitamin and Source	Deficiency State	Safe and Effective for Prevention	Safe and Effective for Treatment	Conditions
vitamin C	vitamin C deficiency, scurvy			
ascorbic acid		yes	yes	
ascorbyl palmitate		yes	yes	
calcium ascorbate		yes	yes	
niacinamide ascorbate	niacin deficiency, pellagra	yes	yes	niacin must also be needed
sodium ascorbate		yes	yes	
biotin	biotin deficiency?	no	no	
choline				
choline bitartrate		no	no	
choline chloride		no	no	
choline citrate		no	no	
vitamin B$_{12}$	vitamin B-12 deficiency, megaloblastic anemia			
cyanocobalamin		yes	no	
folic acid	folic-acid deficiency, megaloblastic anemia	yes	no	
niacin	niacin deficiency, pellagra			
niacin (nicotinic acid)		no	no	
niacinamide		yes	no	
niacinamide ascorbate	vitamin C deficiency	yes	no	vitamin C also must be needed
pantothenic acid	pantothenic acid deficiency ?, burning-foot syndrome	yes	no	
calcium pantothenate		yes	no	approved only in combination products (not as single ingredient)

Safety and Effectiveness: Panel's Assessment of Over-the-Counter Vitamins (continued)

Vitamin and Source	Deficiency State	Safe and Effective for Prevention	Safe and Effective for Treatment	Conditions
dexypanthenol		yes	no	approved only in combination products (not as single ingredient)
pantothenic acid		yes	no	approved only in combination products (not as single ingredient)
vitamin B$_6$	vitamin B$_6$ deficiency, dermatitis, nerve disorders, depression, anemia			
pyridoxine hydrochloride		yes	no	
riboflavin	riboflavin deficiency, dermatitis	yes	no	
riboflavin		yes	no	
riboflavin-5-phosphate sodium		yes	no	
thiamine	thiamine deficiency, beriberi			
thiamine hydrochloride		yes	no	
thiamine mononitrate		yes	no	
vitamin A	vitamin A deficiency, night blindness	yes	no	
vitamin A (retinol)		yes	no	
vitamin A acetate		yes	no	
vitamin A palmitate		yes	no	
vitamin D	vitamin D deficiency, rickets, osteomalacia	yes	no	
cholecalciferol (vitamin D$_3$)		yes	no	
ergocalciferol		yes	no	
25-hydroxylated vitamin D		no	no	

1,25-hydroxylated vitamin D		no	no
24,25-hydroxylated vitamin D		no	no
1-alpha-vitamin D		no	no
5,6-trans-vitamin D		no	no
vitamin E tocophersolan	vitamin E deficiency?	yes	no	approved only in combination products (not as single ingredient)
alpha-tocopheryl acetate		yes	no	approved only in combination products (not as single ingredient)
alpha-tocopheryl succinate		yes	no	approved only in combination products (not as single ingredient)
vitamin E		yes	no	approved only in combination products (not as single ingredient)
vitamin K phytonadione	vitamin K deficiency, bleeding	no	no	

Safety and Effectiveness: Panel's Assessment of Over-the-Counter Minerals

Mineral and Source	Deficiency State	Safe and Effective for Prevention	Safe and Effective for Treatment
calcium	calcium deficiency		
calcium caseinate		yes	no
calcium citrate		yes	no
calcium glubionate		yes	no
calcium gluconate		yes	no
calcium lactate		yes	no
calcium phosphate dibasic		yes	no
calcium sulfate		yes	no
precipitated calcium carbonate		yes	no
copper	copper deficiency		
cupric gluconate		no	no
cupric oxide		no	no
cupric sulfate		no	no
fluoride	fluoride deficiency?		
calcium fluoride		no	no
sodium fluoride		no	no
iodine	iodine deficiency, goiter		
calcium iodate		no	no
potassium iodate		no	no
iron	iron deficiency, anemia		
ferric ammonium citrate		no	no
ferric ammonium phosphate		conditionally	no
ferric citrate		conditionally	no
ferric phosphate		conditionally	no
ferric pyrophosphate		conditionally	no
ferric sulfate		no	no
ferric versenate		no	no
ferrocholinate (ferric choline isocitrate)		no	no
ferroglycine sulfate (ferroglycine sulfate complex)		yes	no
ferrous carbonate (ferrous carbonate, stabilized)		conditionally	no
ferrous citrate		conditionally	no

Safety and Effectiveness: Panel's Assessment of Over-the-Counter Minerals
(continued)

Mineral and Source	Deficiency State	Safe and Effective for Prevention	Safe and Effective for Treatment
ferrous fumarate		yes	no
ferrous gluconate		yes	no
ferrous glutamate		yes	no
ferrous lactate		yes	no
ferrous succinate		yes	no
ferrous sulfate (dried)		yes	no
ferrous tartrate		conditionally	no
magnesium	magnesium deficiency		
magnesium carbonate		no	no
magnesium chloride		no	no
magnesium gluconate		no	no
magnesium hydroxide		no	no
magnesium oxide		no	no
magnesium silicate		no	no
magnesium sulfate		no	no
magnesium trisilicate		no	no
manganese	manganese deficiency?		
manganese chloride		no	no
manganese gluconate		no	no
manganous oxide		no	no
phosphorus	phosphorus depletion		
calcium phosphate dibasic		no	no
potassium	hypokalemia		
potassium chloride		no	no
potassium gluconate		no	no
potassium sulfate		no	no
zinc	zinc deficiency		
zinc carbonate		conditionally	no
zinc chloride		conditionally	no
zinc gluconate		conditionally	no
zinc hydroxide		no	no
zinc lactate		conditionally	no
zinc oxalate		no	no
zinc oxide		conditionally	no
zinc phytate		no	no
zinc sulfate		yes	no
zinc sulfide		no	no

Vitamins and Minerals: Product Ratings

An enormous number of single-ingredient and combination vitamin and mineral products currently are marketed. The majority are labeled as nutritional supplements rather than drugs—which means that no claims for the prevention or treatment of illness are made on the label. Many, if not most, labels do, however, list the dosages in milligrams or other units of each vitamin or mineral. Consumers therefore can use the preceding Vitamin-Mineral Safety and Effectiveness Table to identify the vitamins and minerals that they and family members need, and can use that table as a guide for purchasing the appropriate products.

Wart Paints

Warts can be unsightly. Some are quite painful. But the more common kinds of warts—those that arise on the hands, feet, face, and some other body surfaces—are not dangerous. They are not early cancers, they do not develop into cancers, and they never invade deeper layers of tissues.

Many methods have been developed to remove warts, according to the Panel that assessed over-the-counter drug preparations called *wart paints*. Some of these preparations contain the skin-peeling ingredient salicylic acid. This is an aspirinlike drug that was judged not only safe but also effective for wart removal. And while self-treatment with an over-the-counter drug may take weeks as opposed to having a wart removed surgically in minutes, it is likely to be cheaper.

Evaluators did set one important condition to the self-treatment of warts: only the 2 very prevalent and easily identifiable types of warts —common warts and plantar warts—can be self-diagnosed. Therefore, only these 2 types of warts should be self-treated with over-the-counter products.

CLAIMS

Accurate

for "the removal of common warts"
for "the removal of plantar warts on the bottom of the foot"

WART PAINTS is based on the report "Wart-Remover Drug Products" by the FDA's Advisory Review Panel on OTC Miscellaneous External Drug Products.

False or Misleading

"quick" (a week or more may be required)

"painless" (removing a wart with an over-the-counter product may cause pain)

"effective" (many people might erroneously think this means all warts will respond)

WHAT IS A WART?

A wart is a raised area of skin with underlying tissue that often does not go away, or recedes only very slowly. It may be hard or soft. While it can be the color of normal skin, it can also be gray, tan, or some other hue. A single small wart—or even a cluster of them—on some fairly inconspicuous body surface may be of little concern. But some people develop hundreds, and some warts grow into large, bizarre-looking deformities that are the cause of great shame and embarrassment. (This is particularly true of genital warts, which are sexually transmitted and grow on the penis, vagina, rectum, and nearby body surfaces. Genital warts, of course, require medical attention.)

All warts are caused by viruses. They are papova viruses, which infect the nucleus and specifically the DNA (the genetic material) of skin cells. These viruses take over the cells' reproductive mechanisms, causing them to produce warty new cells instead of normal ones.

Warts are contagious: one person catches the virus from someone else. But it is difficult, if not impossible, to say from whom because the incubation period—the time before the virus produces a visible wart —may be as long as a year. The virus can also spread from an existing wart to new sites on the body. This risk was demonstrated several years ago by a dermatologist who conducted a 2-year study of children with warts. He found that two-thirds of the originally diagnosed warts disappeared, without treatment, in that period of time. But, meanwhile, new warts appeared on other body areas in half the children. He blames the reinfection on autoinoculation—which may have occurred when the children scratched or picked at their original warts. Because of this reinfection risk, experts say it is better to treat and try to remove warts rather than wait for them to disappear by themselves.

Warts You Can Diagnose

Common wart This is a small, hard, grayish wart that is easily recognized by the rough, cauliflowerlike texture of its surface. There is a clear margin or demarcation line between the elevated wart and the surrounding normal skin. The technical name for common wart is *Verruca vulgaris*.

Plantar wart   This wart occurs only on the bottom of the feet. It is flat and may be either hard and callused or soft and spongy. A plantar wart (technically called *Verruca plantaris*) can be distinguished from a callus because the normal skin ridges encircle—but do *not* run across —the wart, whereas these footprint ridges continue across the surface of a callus.

Several closely spaced plantar warts may develop into a bumpy, irregularly shaped aggregation called a *mosaic wart*. Individually or in groups, plantar warts can be excruciatingly painful because they are repeatedly compressed by the weight of the body when one stands. They may be so painful that walking becomes impossible.

Warts a Doctor Should Diagnose

All warts that cannot be readily identified from the description of common wart and plantar wart should be shown to a dermatologist or other doctor. If there is the slightest doubt about a wart's identity, it must be surgically excised in a manner that does not destroy the wart tissue. This way it can be examined by a pathologist to rule out the possibility that it is not a wart, but rather skin cancer.

TREATING WARTS

A wart may eventually disappear of its own accord. Many folk remedies and rituals have been used through the centuries to cure warts. One scientifically controlled study even has demonstrated that warts respond to hypnotic suggestion. When placebos (dummy drugs) are used on warts in scientific tests, cure rates of about 25 percent are achieved. This response, too, might be attributed to the power of suggestion or the fact that warts sometimes disappear of their own accord. ("How the mind affects the virus [that causes a wart] is unknown," the report says.)

Medical treatment focuses on destroying the infected cells and the viruses they contain. Surgical methods include removal of the wart by burning, freezing, or cutting out the affected tissue. Drugs that destroy skin tissue also can be used for this purpose and a number of preparations containing such ingredients are sold without prescription.

Because removal of a wart with over-the-counter drug products may take several weeks or longer, the skin-peeling agent or other active ingredient used to accomplish wart removal must be applied to the wart many times. Yet, during this process, nearby skin which may be damaged by the drug must be protected. To do this the active ingredient is formulated into a wart paint, a filmlike substance that can be applied fairly precisely just to the warty tissue. Some of these preparations are called collodions; they contain highly volatile substances like ether or alcohol which evaporate quickly. This action leaves the active drug in a flexible or rigid waterproof film that sticks to the skin. Collodion coverings help hold moisture on the wart, which speeds the action of the wart-removing drugs.

WARNING Wart-remover drug products should not be used on moles, birthmarks, or unusual warts with hair growing from them because precancerous and cancerous growth may be mistaken for warts. Use of these products will aggravate these conditions. If treatment has not succeeded after 12 weeks, discontinue the over-the-counter medication and see a doctor.

COMBINATION PRODUCTS

The Panel does not wholly approve or disapprove of any currently marketed combination, but lists 3 combinations as conditionally approved.

Salicylic acid (5 to 17 percent) + lactic acid (5 to 17 percent) in a collodion base This combination shows good results, yet evaluators doubt that the lactic acid contributes much to the combination and say that evidence must be produced to show that the 2 components together are significantly better than salicylic acid alone before the combination can be fully approved.

Salicylic acid (5 to 17 percent) + glacial acetic acid (11 percent) in a collodion base Available studies do not demonstrate that the acetic acid contributes to the effectiveness of the salicylic acid. Verdict: conditionally approved.

Ascorbic acid (0.16 percent) + calcium pantothenate (0.20 percent) These 2 ingredients, in a starch base, have been sold over-the-counter for a quarter-century; the manufacturer says the product is effective and safe. But reviewers concluded that more data are required on the relative contribution made by each of the 2 ingredients.

WART REMOVERS

Reviewers assessed the active ingredients in 4 wart-removal products submitted for their consideration by pharmaceutical companies. It also evaluated several other ingredients that FDA researchers discovered have been or are being used in such products (*see* SAFETY AND EFFECTIVENESS chart at the end of this unit).

Approved Active Ingredient

Only one ingredient was judged by the Panel to be safe and effective, by itself, in removing common and plantar warts.

Salicylic acid   Billions of doses of salicylic acid are sold each year, principally as aspirin tablets for relieving pain, fever, and inflammatory complaints. Applied to the skin, salicylic acid is useful against warts because it acts as a skin peeler (a keratolytic). The evaluators were not altogether clear in their explanation of how this occurs. They say that the acid destroys the outer layers of the warty skin by drawing in water, which causes the skin to swell, soften, and slough off. The acid is said also to cause an inflammatory reaction that hastens the wart's disappearance—perhaps by stimulating the body's immune defense system to attack the wart.

A concentration of salicylic acid of as low as 1 percent may damage normal skin. Higher concentrations, which act more rapidly against warts, can also cause progressively more serious damage to normal skin around the wart. So for safety's sake, the Panel recommends the use of relatively weak concentrations of the acid over relatively longer periods of time. Only preparations that contain between 5 and 17 percent salicylic acid are approved for use without prescription.

Salicylic acid is a standard medical cure for warts. In one study, 95 patients used a wart paint consisting of 16.7 percent salicylic acid and 16.7 percent lactic acid in a flexible base, nightly, at home, for up to 12 weeks. The cure rate was 67 percent for common warts and 84 percent for plantar warts. These cure rates are comparable with those achieved by freezing and destroying warts with liquid nitrogen—a method many dermatologists consider the treatment of choice.

Persons who are treating a wart with a salicylic acid product should continue the treatment as long as the wart continues to shrink in size —but this treatment should not go on longer than 12 weeks without consulting a doctor. To protect the surrounding skin, evaluators recommend that a donut-shaped ring of white petrolatum be applied to the skin around the wart before the acid-containing wart paint (or other preparation) is applied.

The verdict, in sum, is that salicylic acid is a safe and effective wart remover in concentrations of 5 to 17 percent.

Conditionally Approved Active Ingredients

The Panel granted only conditional approval to 4 active ingredients that are used in nonprescription wart-removing preparations. In each case, the issue was effectiveness, not safety.

Acetic acid, glacial   This is the pungent-smelling acid present in vinegar. Pure acetic acid is diluted for use in treating warts, and concentrations of up to 11 percent are safe—as has been demonstrated in tests on the sensitive skins of shaved albino rabbits.

The acid causes blistering and corrosion so care must be taken to keep it off—or remove it from—normal skin. When applied to a wart with a cotton applicator, an acetic-acid collodion preparation will cause mild-to-severe inflammation, as well as bleeding under the wart. The wart tissue dies and dries up within a week to 10 days. Although acetic acid has been widely used to treat warts, the only scientific data on its effectiveness comes from studies employing wart paints that contain both acetic acid and salicylic acid. So evaluators say acetic acid's value by itself must be proved before it can be called effective.

Ascorbic acid   This substance is vitamin C, which has been shown in many studies to have a low level of toxicity. There is, however, too little data to show that it is effective in removing warts. The only study available for review concerned a combination of vitamin C and calcium pantothenate, so there was no way to differentiate the particular contributions of each of the 2. Verdict: safe but not proved effective.

Calcium pantothenate   A calcium compound of pantothenic acid, this substance is naturally present in low concentrations in virtually all plant and animal tissues. It is essentially nontoxic, so it was judged safe for use in wart paints. But the only evidence of its possible effectiveness comes from studies in which calcium pantothenate was combined with ascorbic acid. Thus, the Panel had no way of deciding if this substance, by itself, contributes to wart removal. In summary: safe but not proved effective.

Lactic acid   This substance is a metabolic breakdown product of glucose and other carbohydrates. It is naturally present in almost all cells of the body. Lactic acid in concentrations of up to 10 percent has been used in treating a variety of skin disorders—causing mild and easily reversible irritations at the worst. So reviewers rate it as safe. But all data on its effectiveness come from studies in which lactic acid was combined with salicylic acid, and evaluators doubt its value to the combination. So the Panel categorizes lactic acid as safe but of unestablished effectiveness in wart therapy.

Disapproved Active Ingredients

Because no supportive data about safety or effectiveness could be found, the following ingredients were summarily disapproved.

benzocaine
camphor
castor oil
iodine (iodine sublimed)
menthol

Safety and Effectiveness: Active Ingredients in Over-the-Counter Wart Removers

Active Ingredient	Panel's Assessment
acetic acid, glacial	safe, but not proved effective
ascorbic acid (vitamin C)	safe, but not proved effective
benzocaine	summarily disapproved
calcium pantothenate	safe, but not proved effective
camphor	summarily disapproved
castor oil	summarily disapproved
iodine (iodine sublimed)	summarily disapproved
lactic acid	safe, but not proved effective
menthol	summarily disapproved
salicylic acid	safe and effective

Wart Paints: Product Ratings

Single-Ingredient Products

Product and Distributor	Dosage of Active Ingredients	Rating[1]	Comment
salicylic acid			
Calicylic Creme (Gordon Labs.)	**cream:** 10%	A	
Mediplast (Beiersdorf)	**plaster:** 40%	C	too much salicylic acid
Off-Ezy (Commerce Drug)	**liquid:** 17%	A	
Wart-Off (Pfipharmecs)	**flexible collodion:** 17%	A	preferred dosage form

Wart Paints: Product Ratings (continued)

Combination Products

Product and Distributor	Dosage of Active Ingredients	Rating[1]	Comment
Compound W Wart Remover (Whitehall)	**flexible collodion:** 14.2% salicylic acid + 9% glacial acetic acid	B	acetic acid not proved effective
Veruka-10 (Syosset)	**flexible collodion:** 10% salicylic acid + 10% lactic acid	B	lactic acid not proved effective

1. Author's interpretation of Panel criteria. Based on contents, not claims.

Worm-Killers for Pinworm Infestation

When a school child awakens to furiously scratch his or her anus during the night and complain of intense itchiness, the cause may well be pinworms. In girls, the itching may extend to the vulva. Adults, too, may be afflicted. In fact, every member of a family with one pinworm victim will need to be treated with a worm-killing drug. But children are the usual sufferers of these infestations.

Pinworms are the most common parasite that afflicts human beings. They are found in all areas of the United States—rural and urban—and in all socioeconomic groups. These worms can be extremely disturbing: children can't sleep, wet the bed, and may get bacterial infections if their persistent scratching breaks the skin. Fortunately these infestations can be successfully treated with prescription drugs. The Panel has recommended that one of these drugs be changed from prescription to nonprescription status. It is extremely effective: a single dose will destroy the worms in most cases.

WORM-KILLERS FOR PINWORM INFESTATION is based on the report "Antihelmintic Drug Products" by the FDA's Advisory Review Panel on OTC Miscellaneous Internal Drug Products, and the FDA Preamble to the report.

CLAIMS

Accurate
for "the treatment of pinworms"

WARNING   If upset stomach, diarrhea, nausea, or vomiting occur with this medication, discontinue use and consult a physician.

PINWORMS

How to Detect Them

A standard procedure to detect pinworms, performed by a technician or a doctor, is to press a short length of Scotch tape against the area just below the anus of the child or adult who is complaining of a suddenly itchy anus. The tape is then inspected under a microscope, which is the only way eggs can be spotted. A second, do-it-yourself detective method involves inspecting the anus and adjacent skin with a flashlight. One looks for movement of a female pinworm as she lays her 11,000 eggs. The pinworm is ¼ to ½ inch in length and can be seen with the naked eye, or, more clearly, with a magnifying glass. If a child is the sufferer it is a good idea to wait an hour or so after the child has gone to sleep to make this inspection.

How They Spread and Symptoms of the Infestation

Pinworms live in the intestinal tract; they have a life span of 4 to 6 weeks. When the time comes to reproduce, the female travels out through the anus to deposit eggs on the nearby skin. This activity causes the itching.

The eggs are extremely light, and can float through the house in the air. They may be picked up from clothes, bedding, or bathroom fixtures and then swallowed. Unfortunately, they are resistant to household disinfectants. Children may reinfect themselves by scratching, which transfers the eggs to their fingernails. The eggs, then, may be dropped onto food, water, or other substances children put into their mouths.

Besides the intense perianal itching, pinworms produce few other symptoms. Nausea and other vague gastrointestinal complaints may occur. Surprisingly, most such infestations cause no symptoms at all, not even the itching. So many people have pinworms without knowing it.

Treatment

Several drugs have been shown to be effective against pinworms. The classic drug, the dye called *gentian violet*, has been available over-the-counter for decades. Although it was approved as safe and effective by the Panel, the FDA has great reservations about its safety. In a preamble to the evaluators' report, that federal agency announced that it soon intends to list gentian violet as disapproved for reasons of safety. So the dye will most likely be removed from the over-the-counter market as a drug for worms. Therefore gentian violet is treated in this unit as a disapproved drug, even though it continues to be available without prescription. Meanwhile, at the Panel's recommendation, the FDA is allowing over-the-counter marketing of a former prescription drug, pyrantel pamoate (*Antiminth*; Pfizer), which is safer and more effective than gentian violet. As of October 1982, however, Pfizer had not decided whether it would market this drug over-the-counter.

All members of the family—except children under 2 or those who weigh less than 25 pounds—should be treated if one family member has an infestation. The decision of whether and how to treat children under 2 should be made by a pediatrician.

Some drugs used to treat pinworms are also effective against other, more serious parasitic infestations—including the large roundworm (*Ascaris lumbricoides*). These worms are more difficult to diagnose and pose a greater health risk, thus these infestations should be treated by a physician. *Pinworms are the only parasites that can be self-diagnosed and then self-treated with nonprescription drugs.*

PINWORM-KILLING PRODUCTS

Approved Active Ingredient

While the Panel initially approved 2 compounds, the FDA disagreed about one of them. Only the following drug meets both of their criteria.

Pyrantel pamoate This is a relatively new drug that was approved for prescription use in 1972, under rigorous FDA licensing standards. There have been no reports of significant toxicity resulting from accidental overdosage. In therapeutic doses, even minor side effects—such as nausea, diarrhea, and cramps—are rare.

The drug acts on the worm by paralyzing muscles it uses to hold on to the intestinal wall; that way it is swept away in the stool. In one large study of 1506 persons, most of them children, a single dose of 5 mg of pyrantel pamoate per pound of body weight eliminated the worms in 97 percent of subjects. Other studies have produced comparably impressive results.

Conclusion: pyrantel pamoate is a safe and effective pinworm-killing drug at the recommended dosage of 5 mg per pound of body weight. A 50-pound child would require a 250 mg dose; a 100-pound child would require 500 mg. As of October 1982, this drug remained a prescription item (*see* TREATMENT, above).

Conditionally Approved Active Ingredients

None

Disapproved Active Ingredients

Of the 2 ingredients described here, one was disapproved by the Panel, the other by the FDA.

Gentian violet   This dye substance, also known as methylrosaniline chloride, kills worms and also turns one's stool purple. The Panel felt that the side effects are not dangerous, despite a high rate of nausea, vomiting, abdominal pain, and diarrhea. But the experts worried that these side effects discourage many people from taking the 20 to 30 doses required over 10 days to complete the recommended course of treatment.

The FDA is concerned about the suggestive—although not conclusive—findings, that gentian violet may cause birth defects and cancer. The agency's particular concern has been that amounts of the dye in foodstuffs eaten over the course of a lifetime could lead to these or other dangerous outcomes. The Panel countered that the benefit of short-term use of gentian violet as an antiworm drug could justify the risk. But the FDA stuck by its contention that using gentian violet as a worm killer may be hazardous.

Because of this danger, as well as the fact that pyrantel pamoate may soon be available without prescription, the FDA declared it would list gentian violet as not safe at some point during the next stage of the drug review.

Piperazine citrate   This prescription drug has been successfully used to treat pinworms for a number of years. Evaluators say it is effective, but it causes neurologic side effects—including confusion, sleepiness, and loss of coordination—in some users and it may provoke epileptic seizures in susceptible individuals. Thus piperazine citrate was assessed as being unsafe.

**Safety and Effectiveness: Active
Ingredients in Pinworm Products**

Active Ingredient	Panel and FDA's Assessment
gentian violet	not safe
piperazine citrate*	not safe
pyrantel pamoate*	safe and effective

*Currently a prescription item.

Worm Killers for Pinworm Infestation: Product Ratings

Product and Distributor	Dosage of Active Ingredients	Rating[1]	Comment
gentian violet			
gentian violet (generic)	**liquid:** 10%	**C**	not safe

1. Author's interpretation of Panel criteria. Based on contents, not claims.

"Yeast" Killers for Feminine Itching

Many women suffer from time to time intense inflammation and itching of the vagina, vulva, and surrounding skin surfaces. According to Antimicrobial Panel II reviewers, one very common cause of this extreme itching is infection by "yeast" organisms of the species called *Candida* —particularly *Candida albicans*. Many women come to recognize yeast infections and can differentiate them from other kinds of vaginitis or vulvovaginitis because yeast also produces a characteristic white, malodorous vaginal discharge.

Contrary to the prevailing belief of many doctors and the FDA, the Panel believes that women should be able to self-diagnose and treat

"YEAST" KILLERS FOR FEMININE ITCHING is based on the unapproved draft report by the FDA's Advisory Review Panel on OTC Contraceptives and Other Vaginal Drug Products, and on the report "Topical Antifungal Drug Products for OTC Human Use," by the FDA's Advisory Review Panel on OTC Antimicrobial Drug Products (the Antimicrobial II Panel).

these conditions themselves, on a first-aid basis, using over-the-counter drugs. Evaluators recommended to the FDA that 3 prescription drugs that have been proved to be safe and effective against *Candida* be switched to nonprescription status. They are haloprogin, miconazole nitrate, and nystatin. The Panel on OTC Contraceptive and Other Vaginal Drug Products has recommended that 2 other prescription drugs that act against yeast—calcium propionate and sodium propionate—be switched, too. Unless the FDA dissents and blocks the change in status, these drugs will automatically become marketable over-the-counter, on a trial basis, when the Panels' reports are published in the *Federal Register*. Thus far the agency has objected to switching nystatin to over-the-counter marketing, so it will remain a prescription drug. The others' status remains unchanged.

Several over-the-counter drugs assessed by the 2 panels have some activity against yeast that is briefly described below.

Dramatic relief from external feminine itching and inflammation —from a variety of causes—can be obtained through the use of over-the-counter hydrocortisone preparations. However, these drugs only relieve symptoms. They do not effectively kill yeast or other microorganisms, so they should be supplemented by an antifungal drug. Hydrocortisone is approved for use in nonprescription products for *external* itching, but not for application into the vagina. It should *never* be used inside the vagina except on doctor's orders.

Some of the drugs that kill yeast will also quell a second, less common source of vaginal itching, inflammation and discharge—the protozoa *Trichomonas vaginalis*, which is commonly called "tric." In one study, several gynecologists reported in the *Journal of the American Medical Association* (vol. 162, pp. 268–71) that among their office patients with vaginitis and vaginal discharge, yeast infections outnumbered tric infections 7 to 1 among nonpregnant women, and 15 to 1 among women who were pregnant.

Some over-the-counter drugs that act against tric are not specifically approved for this purpose by the Contraceptive-Vaginal Panel, except when a doctor supervises the treatment. A heavier dosage may be required than the amount that relieves nonspecific vaginal itching and irritation. So women should seek medical advice before using these drugs to treat a tric infection.

CANDIDIASIS

Yeast infections due to *Candida albicans* and related yeasts are known as candidiasis, moniliasis (from the alternative technical term, *monilia*), or just plain "yeast." The organism thrives on warm, moist areas of the body. It produces itchy, bright-red runny patches with numerous pus-filled pimples along the well-defined outer edge. The entire vulva may become moist, red, and raw; and itching of the vulva may become so intense that the patient must seek emergency medical treatment.

Yeasts also cause eruptions elsewhere on women's bodies, and in the groin and at other body sites on men, too (*see* CANDIDIASIS, page 476).

The antimicrobial II Panel recommends that women use nonprescription yeast-killing drugs as a first-aid measure until they can schedule an appointment with a gynecologist or other physician who can confirm the diagnosis (using readily available tests) and prescribe proper treatment. An NIH specialist adds that seeing a doctor is important because other types of infection, requiring different treatment, may be hard for women to distinguish from yeast. Ideally, the Panel says, effective antiyeast treatment includes a drug applied to the skin and mucous membranes of the vulva, creams or tablets for the vagina, and a drug to be swallowed to clear the yeast out of the gastrointestinal tract—where drugs applied to the surface can't reach.

The Panel proposed that manufacturers be permitted to claim that safe and effective antifungals sold over-the-counter could be used for "treatment of external feminine itching associated with vaginal yeast (candidal) infection." The FDA responded by disapproving this claim, at least until the agency has heard from gynecologists and other experts as to whether they believe candidiasis should be self-treated. The FDA commented as follows. "Self-treating the symptoms of itching around the vagina without knowing or treating the underlying cause . . . could create a serious health hazard. Infections caused by *Candida* must be diagnosed in the laboratory; they cannot be self-diagnosed by consumers."

FEMININE ITCHING MEDICATIONS

Approved Active Ingredients

Three drugs, haloprogin, miconazole nitrate, and nystatin, have been proposed for nonprescription status. They act specifically and effectively to relieve feminine itching due to yeast. Several other topical drugs will also relieve itching caused by yeast or trichomonas infections but they are less effective. The Panel's findings are outlined below.

Calcium propionate See PROPIONATES, below.

Dioctyl sodium sulfosuccinate This drug has been approved by the Contraceptive-Vaginal Panel as a safe and effective vaginal detergent, to remove mucus and other vaginal secretions. The Panel says it is also safe and effective for treating trichomonas infections—when used according to a doctor's recommendations. (For more information, *see* DIOCTYL SODIUM SULFOSUCCINATE and SODIUM LAURYL SULFATE, page 287).

Haloprogin An antifungal, haloprogin was approved as a prescription drug under the stringent requirements for safety and effectiveness enforced by the FDA during the late 1960s and early 1970s. The Antimicrobial II Panel believes that it is both safe and effective for treating feminine itching due to yeast. Evaluators cite laboratory evidence showing that haloprogin will inhibit *C. albicans'* growth in a culture dish, and also cite several dramatic case studies in which large doses of haloprogin produced impressive responses in patients suffering a severe yeast disease called chronic mucocutaneous candidiasis.

The recommended dosage is 1 percent haloprogin in a cream or other base, used twice daily. This drug should not be used on girls under 2 except under medical supervision. If satisfactory results have not occurred within 2 weeks, consult a doctor or pharmacist.

Hydrocortisone and hydrocortisone acetate These anti-inflammatory drugs are now available over-the-counter in concentrations of 0.25 and 0.5 percent. The Antimicrobial II Panel believes 0.5 percent preparations are extremely useful and rapid-acting for relieving the itching and other symptoms of yeast infections. The Panel notes, however, that they usually do not kill the causative organisms—so treatment with an antifungal is also necessary.

WARNING FOR HYDROCORTISONES Do not use inside the vagina.

Miconazole nitrate This antifungal drug was approved as a prescription drug in 1973, under strict guidelines set by the FDA concerning safety and effectiveness of new drugs. The Antimicrobial II Panel believes it has been well tested and would be appropriate for use without prescription. In one Belgian study, 147 out of 165 women treated with miconazole nitrate for vulvovaginitis caused by *C. albicans* were clinically cured and found to be free of *Candida* after the treatment ended; the most successful dosage was 2 percent miconazole cream twice daily for 2 weeks. In 3 later studies, 2 percent miconazole cream yielded cure rates of 76 percent, 91 percent, and 93 percent.

The appropriate dosage for yeast infections, in the Panel's view, is

2 percent miconazole nitrate applied twice daily, in the morning and at night. Girls under 2 should be treated under medical supervision. If satisfactory results are not obtained within a 2-week period, a doctor or pharmacist should be consulted.

Nystatin   *see* DISAPPROVED ACTIVE INGREDIENTS, below.

Potassium sorbate   This drug is approved by the Contraceptive-Vaginal Panel as a safe and effective agent for relieving vaginal irritation. Reviewers note that several studies have shown potassium sorbate to effectively relieve both yeast and tric infections—although the symptoms disappear only gradually, over a week or so. Doctors, however, do not often recommend this drug, an NIH expert says. A 3 percent solution in a vaginal suppository provides more rapid relief than a 1 percent solution. The drug can be applied as a vaginal suppository or in a douche solution.

Propionates: calcium propionate and sodium propionate   Approved as safe and effective anti-irritants by the Contraceptive-Vaginal Panel, these drugs are safe and effective for treating yeast infections when the diagnosis has been established and the treatment is supervised by a physician. These drugs are presently combined in a prescription medicated gel that this Panel has recommended be switched to nonprescription status.

Sodium lauryl sulfate   This chemical is very similar to dioctyl sodium sulfosuccinate (*see* above) and findings and conclusions are the same.

Sodium propionate   See PROPIONATES, above.

Conditionally Approved Active Ingredients

Caprylates: sodium caprylate and zinc caprylate   The Antimicrobial II Panel reports promising but inconclusive experimental results in the use of these drugs against yeast infections. It says they are safe, but their effectiveness remains to be proved.

Edetates: edetate disodium and edetate sodium   These compounds are rated conditionally safe and conditionally effective as anti-irritants by the Contraceptive-Vaginal Panel. They also appear to be effective against tric, and may be recommended for that purpose by a doctor, who should determine the appropriate dosage.

WARNING FOR EDETATES   The edetates should not be used by pregnant women.

Disapproved Active Ingredient

Nystatin   This is an old and useful prescription drug that is very effective against candidiasis. The Panel recommended that it be switched to over-the-counter status, but the FDA rejected this advice —so nystatin will remain a prescription drug.

Safety and Effectiveness: Active Ingredients in Topical Drugs to Relieve Feminine Itching

Active Ingredient	Status December 1982	Assessment	Kills Yeast	Kills Trichomonas
calcium propionate, (see propionates)				
caprylates: sodium caprylate and zinc caprylate	OTC	safe, but not proved effective§	maybe	no
dioctyl sodium sulfosuccinate	OTC	safe and effective‖	no	yes*
edetates: edetate disodium and edetate sodium	OTC	not proved safe or effective‖	no	maybe*
haloprogin	Rxt	safe and effective§	yes	no
hydrocortisone	OTC	safe and effective‡ #	no	no
hydrocortisone acetate	OTC	safe and effective‡ #	no	no
miconazole nitrate	Rxt	safe and effective§	yes	no
potassium sorbate	OTC	safe and effective‖	yes	yes*
propionates: calcium propionate and sodium propionate	Rxt	safe and effective‖	yes	no
sodium caprylate (see caprylates)				
sodium lauryl sulfate	OTC	safe and effective‖	no	yes*
sodium propionate (see propionates)				
zinc caprylate (see caprylates)				

*Condition should be diagnosed and dosage should be set by a doctor.
†Panel evaluators recommend switching to over-the-counter status.
‡Relieves symptoms only.
§Assessment made by the Antimicrobial II Panel.
‖Assessment made by the Contraceptive-Vaginal Panel.
#Assessment made by the Topical Analgesic Panel.

"Yeast" Killers for Feminine Itching: Product Ratings[1]

Product and Distributor	Dosage of Active Ingredients	Rating[2]	Comment
Summer's Eve Medicated (Fleet)	**solution:** 1% potassium sorbate	A	several days' treatment may be needed to ob— relief
	suppositories: 3%	A	
Trichotine-D (Reed & Carnick)	**powder:** sodium chloride + tetrasodium EDTA + sodium lauryl sulfate	B	EDTA sodium not prove— safe or effective

1. None of the highly effective prescription drugs that the Panel recommends be switched to over-the-counter sale ' available to consumers in this way by October 1982. The highly effective hydrocortisone and hydrocortisone ace— products, which may relieve external itching but will not kill the "yeast," are available without prescription, and listed in the Product Ratings Table on page xxx. The 0.5% concentrations of hydrocortisone are recommended, the weaker 0.25% concentrations. See text and warning, page 856.
2. Author's interpretation of Panel criteria. Based on contents, not claims.

General Index

Index to Ratings of Brand Name and Generic Products